# FRCEM PRIMARY

# All-In-One Notes

Compiled Notes of Anatomy, Physiology & Biochemistry, Pharmacology, Microbiology, Pathology, Haematology and Evidence Based Medicine according to the most recent curriculum of the Royal College of Emergency Medicine.

Author:

Moussa Issa

**MBChB MRCEM**

Contributors:

M. Amjad

H. Garda

Z. Ul Abadin

F. Dunne

*Compiled & Edited*

*By Dr Moussa Issa*

*MBChB MRCEM*

*ED Senior Registrar*

# DISCLAIMER

## FRCEM Primary: All-In-One Notes

Authored by **Dr Moussa Issa**

8.27" x 11.69"

ISBN-13: 978-1999957544

BISAC: Medical / Emergency Medicine

Published by: PGB Group Ltd

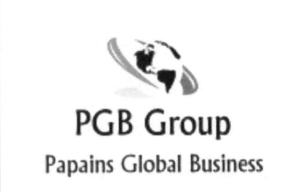

**PGB Group**
Papains Global Business

# PREFACE

The FRCEM Primary 2018 edition is the book you want to have to guide your learning for the FRCEM Primary exams. This new edition comes improved in "full colour" and helps prepare prospective candidates to face the recent changes to the exam format.

Although the previous edition of the book received praise, in the past two years since its publication, readers have given input and suggestions of how this learning tool could be improved. All these suggestions, as well as new exam guidelines and current curriculum were taken into account when compiling this new edition.  Each section of the book has been revised and updated, new chapters added and previously asked exam questions carefully compiled at the end of each chapter to engage the reader and provide a practical approach to emergency conditions.

The new layout and numerous additional colourful images and illustrations will aid the candidate to convert abstract information into easily retrievable mental images using the visualisation and association technique as well as make locating information easier.

Dr Moussa Issa is a member by examination of the Royal College of Emergency Medicine and currently works as a senior ED Registrar. His experience having passed these exams and working daily dealing with emergency conditions has guided him and inspired him to compile this book with such dedication using dozens of reputable resources and the latest guidelines. He is always constantly looking for new ways to update and improve the books to give all prospective candidates the best resource to assist with passing the FRCEM Primary exams.

Meticulous attention to detail was paid to make this new 2018 edition a quality tool that simplifies learning, is in an easy-to-read format with visual aids and contains all the recommended materials for the FRCEM Primary Exams.

**Dr Humayra Garda**
**MBBCh**

# ACKNOWLEDGMENTS

This is an important tool that summarizes, simplifies and presents on an "easy-to-read" format all the recommended materials for the FRCEM Primary Exam.

There is no doubt that such an exercise requires a lot of time and dedication as the author has to extract only what is needed for the FRCEM Primary Exam from more than 10 text books and online publications such as:

- **Life in the Fastlane (ECG)**
- **Physiology at Glance**
- **Lippincott's microbiology**
- **Lance basic and clinical pharmacology**
- **The CDC guidelines and recommendations**
- **WHO: Data, Statistics and Epidemiology**
- **The British National Health System guidelines**
- **The British Committee For standards in Haematology guidelines**
- **The American Heart Association/ACLS Guidelines**
- **The British National Formulary**
- **The SIGN, NICE and Canadian guidelines**

In this 2018 Edition, I have maintained both the high quality and quantity of questions for which the series is known.
I would like to express my sincere thanks towards readers and colleagues who devoted their time to report errors and omissions, to write suggestions, feedbacks leading to the publication of this 2018 Edition.

Nevertheless, I express my gratitude toward my colleagues **Mohammad Amjad, Zain Ul Abadin, Humayra Garda, Faizan Alam and Abdul Sattar** for convincing me to work on a Full colour version of this book, for their kind co-operation and encouragement which help me in completion of this project. Above all I want to thank my best friend and wife **Marlene Issa** and my children **Tatiana, Kevin and Ryan Issa** for their continuous support.

I applaud the following consultants and colleagues for helping me, reviewing the content of this book and for their advice: Humayra Garda, James Visser, Joe Conway, Loay Shalha, Muhammad Amjad, Tatum Ronne, Faizan Alam, , Ahmed Al Rasheed Ahmed, Rehmat Jan, Nassir Mahmood, Abdul Sattar, Fiona Dunne, Ann Campion, Theresa O'Donnell, David Carroll, Aine Williams, DC Swain, Carmel Cox, Maria Kenny, Norma Bergin, Amanda Wickham, Sinead Docherty, Denise Gavin, Margaret Hynes, Katherine Lynch, Ann Walsh, Elaine Neary, Patricia Treacy, Mary Gray, Deirdre Keane, Mary Claire Kelly, Hellen Cullinane, Leigh McMorran, Sinead Crotty, Orla Delahunty, Michael Tierney, Lorraine Kelly, Ciara Grogan, Glenn Allender, Elaine Wall, Martina Brennan, Anita Grace, Triona McKee, Joy Moore, Kerrie Stapleton, Deirdre O'Riordan, Sinead Fox, Ann Cummins , Louise Rafter, Jason Brennan, Marta Brezinska, Bernie Cahill, Anne Hunt and Lorraine Maher.

**Dr Moussa Issa**
**MBChB MRCEM**
**ED Senior Registrar**

# TABLE OF CONTENTS

# PART FOUR: MICROBIOLOGY

## PART A: PRINCIPLES OF MICROBIOLOGY

## PART B: SPECIFIC PATHOGENS

# PART FIVE: PATHOLOGY & HAEMATOLOGY

# PART SIX: EVIDENCE BASED MEDICINE

# Part One: Anatomy

Compiled and Edited by:
Dr Moussa Issa
MBChB MRCEM
Senior ED Registrar

# SECTION 1: UPPER LIMB

## I. PECTORAL REGION

### A. MUSCLES

#### 1. PECTORALIS MAJOR

- **Origin:**
  - Sternal part: sternum and 1<sup>st</sup> six costal cartilages
  - Clavicular part: medial half of the clavicle
- **Insertion**
  - Lateral lip of the bicipital groove of the humerus
- **Action**
  - Flexion, adduction and internal rotation of the shoulder joint
- **Nerve supply:**
  - Lateral pectoral nerve
  - Medial pectoral nerve
  - Clavicular head: C5 and
  - Sternocostal head: C7, C8 and T1

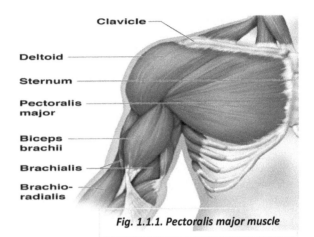

Fig. 1.1.1. Pectoralis major muscle

#### 2. PECTORALIS MINOR

- **Origin:**
  - Anterior ribs 3-5 near the costal cartilages
- **Insertion:**
  - Medial and upper aspect of the coracoid process of the scapula
- **Action**
  - Depresses shoulder
  - When scapula fixed, elevation of ribs 3-5
- **Nerve supply**:
  - Medial pectoral nerve (C8, T1)

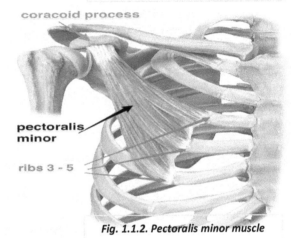

Fig. 1.1.2. Pectoralis minor muscle

#### 3. TRAPEZIUS

- **Surface marking:**
  - External occipital protuberance, nuchal ligament, medial superior nuchal line, spinous processes of vertebrae C7-T12
- **Insertion:**
  - Posterior border of the lateral third of the clavicle, acromion process and spine of scapula.
- **Actions:**
  - Rotation, retraction, elevation and depression of scapula
- **Nerve supply:**
  - Accessory nerve (motor)
  - Cervical spinal C3 and C4 (motor and sensation)

#### 4. LATISSIMUS DORSI

- **Surface marking:**
  - Spinous processes of vertebrae T7-L5
  - Thoracolumbar fascia, iliac crest
  - Inferior 3 or 4 ribs and inferior angle of scapula
- **Insertion:**
  - Floor of intertubercular groove of the humerus
- **Actions:**
  - Adducts, extends and internally rotates the arm
- **Antagonist**:
  - Deltoid and trapezius muscle
- **Nerve:**
  - Thoracodorsal nerve

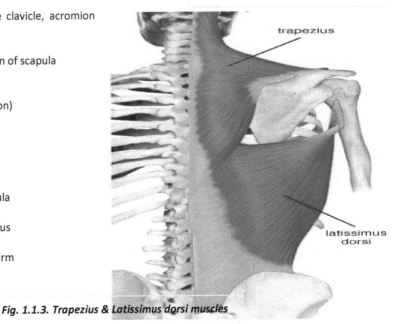

Fig. 1.1.3. Trapezius & Latissimus dorsi muscles

## 5. SERRATUS ANTERIOR

- **Surface marking:**
  - o From the outer surface of upper 8 or 9 ribs
- **Insertion:**
  - o Costal aspect of medial margin of the scapula
- **Actions:**
  - o Protracts and stabilizes scapula
  - o Assists in upward rotation.
- **Antagonist:**
  - o Rhomboid major, Rhomboid minor, Trapezius
- **Nerve supply:**
  - o Long thoracic nerve (from roots of brachial plexus C5, 6,7)

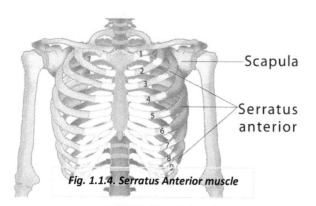

*Fig. 1.1.4. Serratus Anterior muscle*

**FRACTURES OF THE SCAPULA**
- Fractures of the scapula are usually the result of severe trauma, such as occurs in run-over accident victims or in occupants of automobiles involved in crashes. Injuries are usually associated with fractured ribs.
- Most fractures of the scapula require little treatment because the muscles on the anterior and posterior surfaces adequately splint the fragments.

**DROPPED SHOULDER AND WINGED SCAPULA**
- The position of the scapula on the posterior wall of the thorax is maintained by the tone and balance of the muscles attached to it. If one of these muscles is paralyzed, the balance is upset, as in dropped shoulder, which occurs with paralysis of the trapezius, or winged scapula (Fig. 1.1.1), caused by paralysis of the serratus anterior.

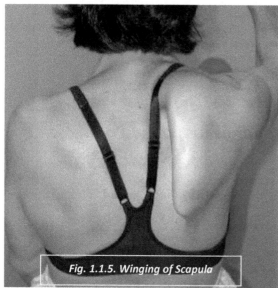

*Fig. 1.1.5. Winging of Scapula*

## B. JOINTS

### 1. STERNOCLAVICULAR

➢ **Joint Capsule**
  - o The **joint capsule** consists of a fibrous outer layer, and inner synovial membrane.
  - o **The fibrous layer** extends from the epiphysis of the sternal end of the clavicle, to the borders of the articular surfaces and the articular disc.
  - o **A synovial membrane** lines the inner surface and produces synovial fluid to reduce friction between the articulating structures.
- **Ligaments:** There are four major ligaments:
  - o **Sternoclavicular ligaments** (anterior and posterior)
  - o **Interclavicular ligament**
  - o **Costoclavicular ligament**

### 2. ACROMIOCLAVICULAR (AC JOINT)
**JOINT CAPSULE:**
- The AC Joint has a thin capsule lined with synovium.
- The capsule is weak and is strengthened by capsular ligaments both inferiorly and superiorly, which in turn are reinforced through attachments from the deltoid and trapezius.
- Without the superior and inferior capsular ligaments, the AC Joint Capsule would not be strong enough to maintain the integrity of the joint.

**LIGAMENTS:**
- **Acromioclavicular ligaments:**
  - o Superior acromioclavicular ligament
  - o Inferior acromioclavicular ligament
- **Coracoacromial ligament**
- **Coracoclavicular Ligaments:**
  - o Conoid ligament
  - o Trapezoid ligament

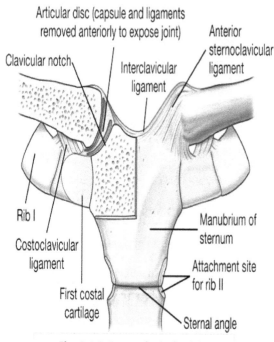

*Fig. 1.1.6. Sternoclavicular joint*

## CLINICAL RELEVANCE

### 1. STABILITY OF THE SHOULDER JOINT

- The shallowness of the glenoid fossa of the scapula and the lack of support provided by weak ligaments make this joint an unstable structure. Its strength almost entirely depends on the tone of the short muscles that bind the upper end of the humerus to the scapula—namely, the subscapularis in front, the supraspinatus above, and the infraspinatus and teres minor behind. The tendons of these muscles are fused to the underlying capsule of the shoulder joint. Together, these tendons form the rotator cuff. The least supported part of the joint lies in the inferior location, where it is unprotected by muscles.

### 2. DISLOCATIONS OF THE SHOULDER JOINT

- The shoulder joint is the most commonly dislocated large joint.

### ANTERIOR INFERIOR DISLOCATION

o Sudden violence applied to the humerus with the joint fully abducted tilts the humeral head downward onto the inferior weak part of the capsule, which tears, and the humeral head comes to lie inferior to the glenoid fossa.

o During this movement, the acromion has acted as a fulcrum.

o The strong flexors and adductors of the shoulder joint now usually pull the humeral head forward and upward into the subcoracoid position.

### POSTERIOR DISLOCATIONS

o Posterior dislocations are rare and are usually caused by direct violence to the front of the joint. On inspection of the patient with shoulder dislocation, the rounded appearance of the shoulder is seen to be lost because the greater tuberosity of the humerus is no longer bulging laterally beneath the deltoid muscle.

o A subglenoid displacement of the head of the humerus into the quadrangular space can cause damage to the axillary nerve, as indicated by paralysis of the deltoid muscle and loss of skin sensation over the lower half of the deltoid.

o Downward displacement of the humerus can also stretch and damage the radial nerve.

### SHOULDER PAIN

o The synovial membrane, capsule, and ligaments of the shoulder joint are innervated by the axillary nerve and the suprascapular nerve. The joint is sensitive to pain, pressure, excessive traction, and distention. The muscles surrounding the joint undergo reflex spasm in response to pain originating in the joint, which in turn serves to immobilize the joint and thus reduce the pain.

o Injury to the shoulder joint is followed by pain, limitation of movement, and muscle atrophy owing to disuse. It is important to appreciate that pain in the shoulder region can be caused by disease elsewhere and that the shoulder joint may be normal; for example, diseases of the spinal cord and vertebral column and the pressure of a cervical rib can cause shoulder pain.

o Irritation of the diaphragmatic pleura or peritoneum can produce referred pain via the phrenic and supraclavicular nerves.

## THE QUADRANGULAR SPACE

- The quadrangular space is a gap in the muscles of the posterior scapular region. It is a pathway for neurovascular structures to move from the axilla to the posterior shoulder and arm.
- Its boundaries are:
  - **Superior** – Subscapularis and teres minor.
  - **Inferior** – Teres major.
  - **Laterally** – Surgical neck of humerus.
  - **Medially** – Long head of triceps brachii.
- The axillary nerve and posterior circumflex humeral artery pass through the quadrangular space.

### MOTOR FUNCTIONS

- The axillary nerve innervates the **teres minor** and the **deltoid** muscles.
- The teres minor is part of the **rotator cuff** muscles of the shoulder. This set of muscles acts to stabilise the glenohumeral joint. Acting individually, the teres minor externally rotates the upper limb. The muscle is innervated the **posterior terminal branch** of the axillary nerve.
- The deltoid is situated at the superior aspect of the shoulder. It performs **abduction** of the upper limb at the glenohumeral joint. The muscle is innervated by the **anterior terminal branch** of the axillary nerve.

### SENSORY FUNCTIONS

- The sensory component of the axillary nerve is delivered via its **posterior terminal branch**.
- After the posterior terminal branch of the axillary nerve has innervated the **teres minor**, it continues as the **upper lateral cutaneous nerve of the arm**. This nerve innervates the skin over the inferior portion of the deltoid (known as the 'regimental badge area').
- In a patient with axillary nerve damage, sensation at the regimental badge area may be impaired or absent. The patient may also report paraesthesia (pins and needles) in the distribution of the axillary nerve.

# II. AXILLA

## A. MUSCLES

### 1. SUBSCAPULARIS
- **Surface marking:** subscapular fossa
- **Insertion:** lesser tubercle of humerus
- **Actions:** internally rotates humerus, stabilizes shoulder.
- **Nerve supply:** upper subscapular nerve, lower subscapular nerve (C5, C6)

### 2. TERES MAJOR
- **Surface marking**: posterior aspect of the inferior angle of the scapula.
- **Insertion:** Medial lip of intertubercular sulcus of the humerus
- **Actions:** adduct humerus, medial rotation humerus, extend humerus from flexed position, protracts scapula and depress shoulder
- **Nerve Supply:** lower subscapular nerve (C5, C6)

## B. AXILLARY NERVE
- Axillary nerve (ventral rami of C5 & C6) arises from the posterior cord of brachial plexus giving muscular branches to teres minor & deltoid.
- It also supplies the shoulder joint and the skin over it.
- The axillary nerve travels through the quadrangular spacewith the posterior circumflex humeral artery and vein.
- **Spinal roots:** C5 and C6.
- **Sensory functions:** carries sensory information from the shoulder joint, as well as the skin covering the inferior region of the deltoid muscle - the "regimental badge" area (which is innervated by the superior lateral cutaneous nerve branch of the axillary nerve).
- **Motor functions:** Innervates the teres minor and deltoid muscles.

### CLINICAL SIGNIFICANCE
- The axillary nerve may be injured in anterior-inferior dislocations of the shoulder joint, compression of the axilla with a crutch or fracture of the surgical neck of the humerus.

An example of injury to the axillary nerve includes axillary nerve palsy. Injury to the nerve results in:
- Paralysis of the teres minor muscle and deltoid muscle, resulting in loss of abduction of arm (from 15-90 degrees), weak flexion, extension, and rotation of shoulder.
- Paralysis of deltoid and teres minor muscles results in flat shoulder deformity.
- Loss of sensation in the skin over a small part of the lateral upper arm (an area known as the regimental badge/patch).

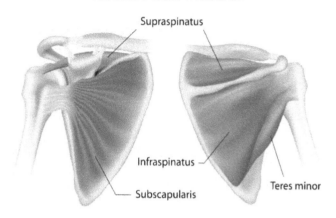

Rotator Cuff Muscles

Anterior view        Posterior view

*Fig. 1.1.7. Rotator cuff muscles*

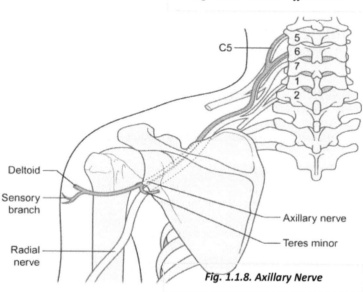

*Fig. 1.1.8. Axillary Nerve*

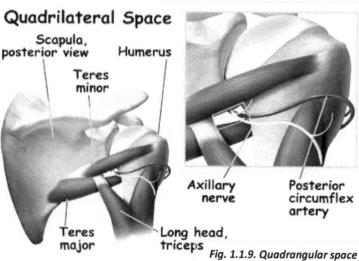

*Fig. 1.1.9. Quadrangular space*

## C. BRACHIAL PLEXUS

### 1. STRUCTURE

**Divided into roots, trunks, divisions, cords and branches.**

### 2. ROOTS

o The five roots are the five anterior rami of the spinal nerves, after they have given off their segmental supply to the muscles of the neck.
o The brachial plexus emerges at five different levels; C5, C6, C7, C8, and T1.

### 3. TRUNKS

Three trunks
o "Superior" or "upper" (C5-C6)
o "Middle" (C7)
o "Inferior" or "lower" (C8, T1)

### 4. DIVISIONS

Each trunk splits in two, to form six divisions
o Anterior divisions of the upper, middle, and lower trunks
o Posterior divisions of the upper, middle, and lower trunks.

### 5. CORDS

Six divisions regroup to become the three cords.
o The posterior cord is formed from the three posterior divisions of the trunks (C5-C8, T1)
o The lateral cord is formed from this anterior divisions of the upper and middle trunks (C5-C7)
o The medial cord is simply a continuation of the anterior division of the lower trunk (C8, T1)

**BRACHIAL PLEXUS: PERIPHERAL NERVES (BRANCHES)**

- **Lateral cord**: Mnemonic **LML**
  o Lateral pectoral nerve
  o Terminal branches:
    ✓ Musculocutaneous nerve
    ✓ Lateral root of the median nerve

- **Posterior cord**: Mnemonic **ULTRA**
  o **U**pper subscapular nerve
  o **L**ower subscapular nerve
  o **T**horacodorsal nerve
  o Terminal branches:
    ✓ **R**adial nerve
    ✓ **A**xillary nerve

- **Medial cord**: Mnemonic **M4U**
  o **M**edial pectoral nerve
  o **M**edial cutaneous nerve of the arm
  o **M**edial cutaneous nerve of the forearm
  o Terminal branches:
    ✓ **M**edial root of the median nerve
    ✓ **U**lnar nerve

- Rugby Teams Drink Cold Beers

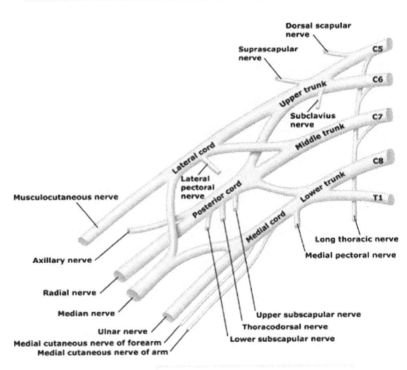

*Fig. 1.1.10. Brachial Plexus*

## CLINICAL RELEVANCE

### INJURY TO THE AXILLARY NERVE

o The axillary nerve is most commonly damaged by trauma to the shoulder or proximal humerus – such as a fracture of the humerus surgical neck.
o **Motor functions**: Paralysis of the deltoid and teres minor muscles. This renders the patient unable to abduct the affected limb.
o **Sensory functions**: The upper lateral cutaneous nerve of arm will be affected, resulting in loss of sensation over the regimental badge area.
o **Characteristic clinical signs**: In long standing cases, the paralysed deltoid muscle rapidly atrophies, and the greater tuberosity can be palpated in that area.

## INJURY TO THE BRACHIAL PLEXUS

- There are two major types of injuries that can affect the brachial plexus.
- An upper brachial plexus injury affects the superior roots, and a lower brachial plexus injury affects the inferior roots.

### 1. UPPER BRACHIAL PLEXUS INJURY (ERB'S PALSY)

- Erb's palsy commonly occurs where there is excessive increase in the angle between the neck and shoulder, this stretches (or can even tear) the nerve roots, causing damage.
- It can occur as a result of a difficult birth or shoulder trauma.
- **Nerves affected:** Nerves derived from solely **C5-C6 roots**; **M**usculocutaneous, **A**xillary, **S**uprascapular and Nerve to **S**ubclavius. **(MASS nerves)**
- **Muscles paralysed:** Supraspinatus, infraspinatus, subclavius, biceps brachii, brachialis, coracobrachialis, deltoid and teres minor.
- **Motor functions:** The following movements are lost or greatly weakened **(FALS)**:
  - ○ **F**lexion at shoulder.
  - ○ **A**bduction at shoulder,
  - ○ **L**ateral rotation of arm,
  - ○ **S**upination of forearm,
- **Sensory functions:** Loss of sensation down lateral side of arm, which covers the sensory innervation of the axillary and musculocutaneous nerves.
- The affected limb hangs limply, **medially rotated** by the unapposed action of pectoralis major.
- The forearm is pronated due to the loss of biceps brachii.
- This is position is known as **'waiter's tip'**, and is characteristic of **Erb's palsy**.

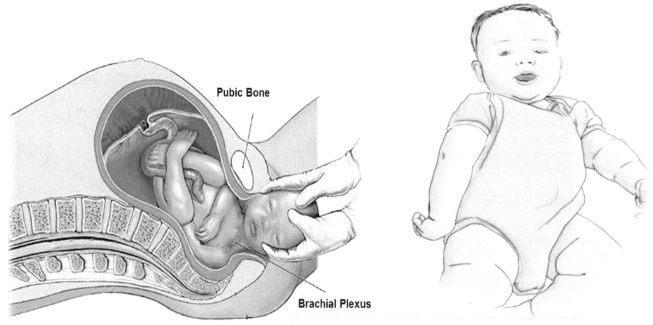

*Fig. 1.1.11. Erb's palsy and Waiter's tip deformity*

### 2. LOWER BRACHIAL PLEXUS INJURY (KLUMPKE'S PALSY)

- A lower brachial plexus injury results from excessive abduction of the arm (e.g. person catching a branch as they fall from a tree).
- It has a much lower incidence than Erb's palsy.
- **Nerves affected:** Nerves derived from the **C8-T1 root: Ulna and Median Nerves.**
- **Muscles paralysed:** All the small muscles of the hand.
  *Note that the flexors muscles in the forearm are supplied by the Ulnar and Median Nerves, but are innervated by different roots.*
- **Sensory functions:** Loss of sensation along medial side of arm.
- The classic presentation of Klumpke's palsy is the **"claw hand" deformity.**
- There is associated **Horner syndrome** if there is involvement of the cervical sympathetic chain.
- There is usually also a disparity in the length of the limbs; the affected limb is usually shorter than the unaffected.

- **Prognosis:** Less than 50% of those affected with Klumpke's palsy will spontaneously recover; the prognosis is worse if there is associated Horner syndrome.
- **Horner syndrome** results from an interruption of the sympathetic nerve supply to the eye and is characterized by the classic triad of **Miosis** (i.e., constricted pupil), **Partial Ptosis**, and Loss of Hemifacial Sweating (i.e., **Anhidrosis**) and **Enophthalmos**.
- **Pancoast syndrome** is characterized by a malignant neoplasm of the superior sulcus of the lung (lung cancer) with destructive lesions of the thoracic inlet and involvement of the brachial plexus and cervical sympathetic nerves (stellate ganglion).

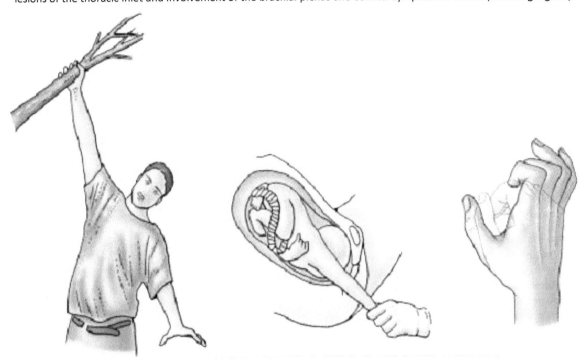

*Fig. 1.1.12. Klumpke's Palsy and Claw hand deformity*

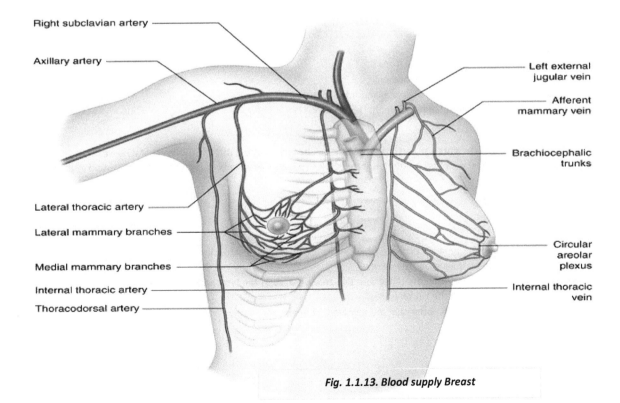

*Fig. 1.1.13. Blood supply Breast*

# III. BREAST

- **OVERVIEW**
  - Located on the anterior thoracic wall. Extends horizontally from the lateral border of the sternum to the **mid-axillary line**.
  - Vertically, it spans between the 2nd and 6th **intercostal cartilages**.
  - Lies superficially to the pectoralis major and serratus anterior muscles.
  - It is composed of mammary glands surrounded by a connective tissue stroma.

- **MAMMARY GLANDS**
  - Modified sweat glands which consist of a series of ducts and secretory lobules (15-20).
  - Each lobule consists of many alveoli drained by a single **lactiferous duct**.
  - Each duct contains a dilated section, (the lactiferous sinus) which is located just behind the **areola**.

- **CONNECTIVE TISSUE STROMA**
  - This is a supporting structure which surrounds the mammary glands. It has a fibrous and a fatty component.

- **PECTORAL FASCIA**
  - The base of the breast lies on the **pectoral fascia**; a flat sheet of connective tissue associated with the pectoralis major muscle.
  - It acts as an attachment point for the suspensory ligaments.
  - There is a layer of loose connective tissue between the breast and pectoral fascia known as the **retromammary space**. This is a potential space, often used in reconstructive plastic surgery.

- ➢ **ARTERIAL SUPPLY**
- The medial aspect of the breast is via the **internal thoracic artery**, a branch of the **subclavian artery**.
- The lateral part of the breast receives blood from four vessels:
  - **Lateral thoracic and thoracoacromial branches:** originate from the axillary artery.
  - **Lateral mammary branches:** originate from the posterior intercostal arteries (derived from the aorta). They supply the lateral aspect of the breast in the 2nd 3rd and 4th intercostal spaces.
  - **Mammary branch**: originates from the anterior intercostal artery.

- ➢ **VENOUS RETURN**
  - Correspond with the arteries, draining into the **axillary** and **internal thoracic veins**.

- ➢ **LYMPHATICS**
  - The lymphatic drainage of the breast is of great clinical importance due to its role in the **metastasis** of breast cancer cells.
  - There are three groups of lymph nodes that receive lymph from breast tissue:
    - ✓ **Axillary nodes (75%),**
    - ✓ **Parasternal nodes (20%)**
    - ✓ **Posterior intercostal nodes (5%).**
- The skin of the breast also receives lymphatic drainage:
  - **Skin**: drains to the axillary, inferior deep cervical and infraclavicular nodes.
  - **Nipple and areola**: drains to the subareolar lymphatic plexus.

- **NERVE SUPPLY**
  - The breast is innervated by the **anterior** and **lateral cutaneous branches** of the 4th to 6th intercostal nerves.
  - These nerves contain both sensory and autonomic nerve fibres (the autonomic fibres regulate smooth muscle and blood vessel tone).

## CLINICAL RELEVANCE:
## BREAST CANCER

- Breast cancer is the most common type of cancer to be diagnosed within the UK. After lung cancer, it has the second highest death rate due to cancer. It is more common in women than men.
- Common presentations associated with breast cancer are due to blockages of the **lymphatic drainage**.
- Metastasis commonly occurs through the lymph nodes.
- It is most likely to be the **axillary lymph nodes** that are involved. They become stony hard and fixed.

# IV. SHOULDER

## A. ROTATOR CUFF MUSCLES
- Include: Teres minor, Infraspinatus, Supraspinatus and Subscapularis.
- Each muscle of the rotator cuff inserts at the scapula, and has a tendon that attaches to the humerus.
- **The rotator cuff is strongest superiorly.**
- Together, the tendons and other tissues form a cuff around the humerus.

### 1. SUPRASPINATUS
- **Actions:** abduction of arm and stabilizes humerus.
- **Artery:** suprascapular artery
- **Nerve supply:** suprascapular nerve

### 2. INFRASPINATUS
- **Actions:** lateral rotation of arm and stabilizes humerus
- **Artery:** suprascapular and circumflex scapular arteries
- **Nerve supply:** suprascapular nerve

### 3. TERES MINOR
- **Actions:** laterally rotates arm, stabilizes humerus
- **Artery:** posterior circumflex humeral artery and the circumflex scapular artery
- **Nerve supply:** Axillary nerve

### 4. DELTOID
- **Actions:** shoulder abduction, flexion and extension
- **Artery:** thoracoacromial artery, ant and post humeral circumflex artery
- **Nerve supply:** axillary nerve

## GLENOHUMERAL JOINT
**LIGAMENTS:**
- Superior, middle and inferior glenohumeral ligaments
- Coracohumeral ligament
- Transverse humeral ligament
- Coraco-acromial ligament

**INNERVATION**
- Suprascapular nerve
- Axillary nerve
- Lateral pectoral nerve

**BLOOD SUPPLY:**
- Anterior and posterior circumflex humeral arteries
- Suprascapular arteries
- Scapular circumflex arteries

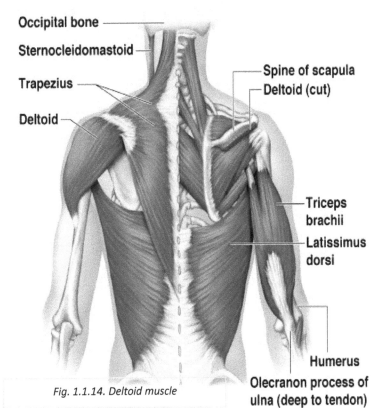

Fig. 1.1.14. Deltoid muscle

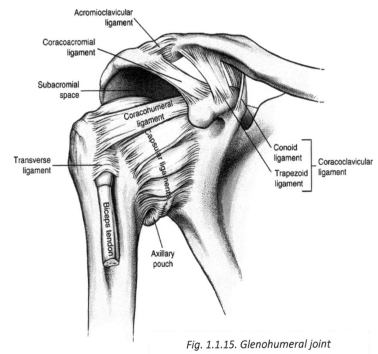

Fig. 1.1.15. Glenohumeral joint

## CLINICAL: ROTATOR CUFF TENDONITIS
- Usually occurs secondary to repetitive use of the shoulder joint. The muscle most commonly affected is the **supraspinatus**.
- Conservative treatment of rotator cuff tendonitis involves rest, analgesia, and physiotherapy. In more severe cases, steroid injections and surgery can be considered.

## B. SHOULDER MOVEMENTS

| ACTION OF THE SHOULDER | PRIMARY MUSCLES |
|---|---|
| Abduction "STD's" | • **S**upraspinatus: first 15°<br>• **D**eltoid: 15° to 90°<br>• **T**rapezius & **S**erratus anterior: > 90° |
| Adduction "PTL" | • **P**ectoralis major,<br>• **T**eres major and<br>• **L**atissimus dorsi |
| Flexion "ABC &P" | • **A**nterior Deltoid,<br>• **B**iceps,<br>• **C**oracobrachialis and<br>• **P**ectoralis major |
| Extension "pTL" | • **P**osterior Deltoid,<br>• **T**eres major and<br>• **L**atissimus dorsi |
| Internal rotation "SPLAT" | • **S**ubscapularis,<br>• **P**ectoralis major,<br>• **L**atissimus dorsi,<br>• **A**nterior Deltoid<br>• **T**eres major |
| External rotation "Itp" | • **I**nfraspinatus,<br>• **t**eres minor and<br>• **p**osterior Deltoid |
| Horizontal abduction "Lp" | • **L**atissimus Dorsi and<br>• **p**osterior Deltoid |
| Horizontal adduction "PA" | • **P**ectoralis major and<br>• **A**nterior Deltoid |

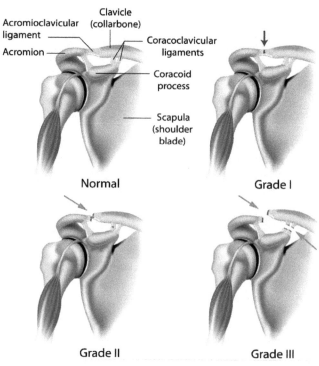

### AC Joint Sprain / AC Joint Separation

Fig. 1.1.16. ACJ injury grades

# V. ARM

# A. THE ANTERIOR ARM

## A.1. MUSCLES

### 1. CORACOBRACHIALIS
- **Actions:** adducts humerus, flexes arm at glenohumeral joint
- **Innervation:** Musculocutaneous nerve (C5,6,7)

### 2. BICEPS
- **Actions:** flexes elbow, flexes and abducts shoulder and supinates radioulnar joint in the forearm.
- **Innervation:** Musculocutaneous nerve (C5,6)

### 3. BRACHIALIS MUSCLES
- **Actions:** flexion at elbow joint
- **Innervation:** Musculocutaneous nerve (C5,6)

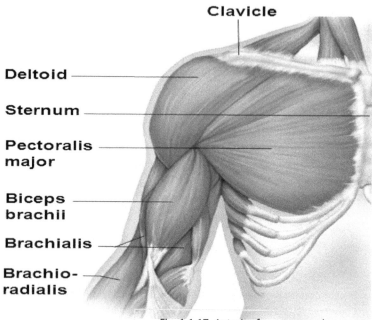

Fig. 1.1.17. Anterior forearm muscles

## A.2. BRACHIAL ARTERY

### A. ORIGIN

- Continuation of the axillary artery at the inferior border of **teres major**. Then lies medial to the humerus where it is accompanied by the **basilic vein** and the **median nerve**. It sits medial to the biceps brachii muscle and anterior to the medial head of triceps.

### B. BRANCHES

- *The profunda brachii* is the first and main branch of the brachial artery.
- Mnemonic: 'PLEASE STAND IN ROW NEAR U'
  - o   **P**rofunda brachii artery
  - o   **S**uperior ulnar collateral artery
  - o   **I**nferior ulnar collateral artery
  - o   **R**adial artery
  - o   **N**utrient branch to humerus
  - o   **U**lnar artery
- Distal to the profunda, the brachial artery gives off nutrient vessels to the humerus as is slowly courses more medially within the upper arm. As it approaches the elbow, it gives off *the superior and inferior ulnar collateral arteries*: Both of the ulnar collateral arteries arise from the medial surface of the brachial artery and course distally towards the medial aspect of the elbow.

### C. TERMINATION

- Bifurcates to form *the radial artery and ulna artery* in the *antecubital fossa* at the level of the radial neck, below the bicipital aponeurosis.

### D. SUPPLY

- The brachial artery supplies blood to the muscles of the upper arm by its branches and to the forearm and hand, by its continuation as the radial and ulnar arteries.

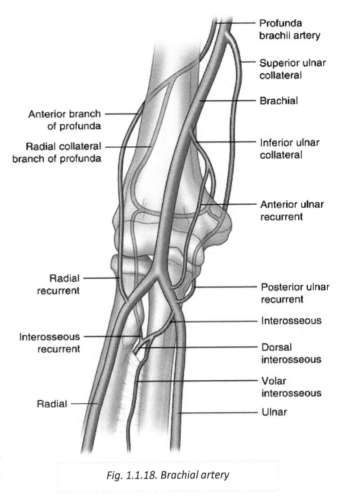

*Fig. 1.1.18. Brachial artery*

## ARTERIAL INJURY

- The arteries of the upper limb can be damaged by penetrating wounds or may require ligation in amputation operations.
- Because of the existence of an adequate collateral circulation around the shoulder, elbow, and wrist joints, ligation of the main arteries of the upper limb is not followed by tissue necrosis or gangrene, provided, of course, that the arteries forming the collateral circulation are not diseased and the patient's general circulation is satisfactory. Nevertheless, it can take days or weeks for the collateral vessels to open sufficiently to provide the distal part of the limb with the same volume of blood as previously supplied by the main artery.

## PALPATION AND COMPRESSION OF ARTERIES

- A clinician must know where the arteries of the upper limb can be palpated or compressed in an emergency.
- **The subclavian artery**, as it crosses the first rib to become the axillary artery, can be palpated in the root of the posterior triangle of the neck. The artery can be compressed here against the first rib to stop a catastrophic hemorrhage.
- **The third part of the axillary artery** can be felt in the axilla as it lies in front of the teres major muscle.
- **The brachial artery** can be palpated in the arm as it lies on the brachialis and is overlapped from the lateral side by the biceps brachii.
- **The radial artery** lies superficially in front of the distal end of the radius, between the tendons of the brachioradialis and flexor carpi radialis; it is here that the clinician takes the radial pulse. If the pulse cannot be felt, try feeling for the radial artery on the other wrist; occasionally, a congenitally abnormal radial artery can be difficult to feel. The radial artery can be less easily felt as it crosses the anatomic snuffbox.
- **The ulnar artery** can be palpated as it crosses anterior to the flexor retinaculum in company with the ulnar nerve. The artery lies lateral to the pisiform bone, separated from it by the ulnar nerve. The artery is commonly damaged here in laceration wounds in front of the wrist.

## ALLEN TEST

- The Allen test is used to determine the patency of the ulnar and radial arteries.
- With the patient's hands resting in the lap, compress the radial arteries against the anterior surface of each radius and ask the patient to tightly clench the fists.

- The clenching of the fists closes off the superficial and deep palmar arterial arches.
- When the patient is asked to open the hands, the skin of the palms is at first white, and then normally the blood quickly flows into the arches through the ulnar arteries, causing the palms to promptly turn pink. This establishes that the ulnar arteries are patent. The patency of the radial arteries can be established by repeating the test but this time compressing the ulnar arteries as they lie lateral to the pisiform bones.

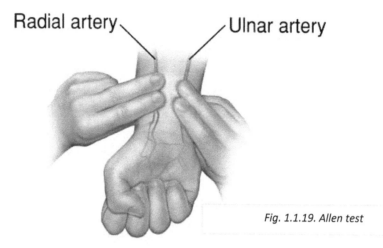

Radial artery          Ulnar artery

Fig. 1.1.19. Allen test

## ARTERIAL INNERVATION AND RAYNAUD'S DISEASE

- The arteries of the upper limb are innervated by sympathetic nerves. The preganglionic fibers originate from cell bodies in the 2nd to 8th thoracic segments of the spinal cord.
- They ascend in the sympathetic trunk and synapse in the middle cervical, inferior cervical, 1st thoracic, or stellate ganglia. The postganglionic fibers join the nerves that form the brachial plexus and are distributed to the arteries within the branches of the plexus.
- For example, the digital arteries of the fingers are supplied by postganglionic sympathetic fibers that run in the digital nerves. Vasospastic diseases involving digital arterioles, such as Raynaud's disease, may require a cervicodorsal preganglionic sympathectomy to prevent necrosis of the fingers.
- The operation is followed by arterial vasodilatation, with consequent increased blood flow to the upper limb

## A.3. MEDIAN NERVE

**Origin: Spinal root C5-T1**
- **Lateral root - Lateral Cord** of the Brachial Plexus
- **Medial root - Medial Cord** of the Brachial Cord

**Course:**
- **Laterally to the axillary artery,** descends in the arm between biceps brachii and triceps brachii muscles, through the forearm with the ulna nerve and vessels before entering the carpal tunnel to the hand.

- **Major Branches: MAP**
    - **M**otor branch in the hand
    - **A**nterior interosseous nerve,
    - **P**almar cutaneous branch,

- **Motor Supply:**
    - Flexor compartment of the forearm, thenar and intrinsic hand muscles.

- **Sensory Supply:**
    - Palmar aspect of the thumb, index, middle and radial half of the ring fingers.

## MEDIAN NERVE vs. ULNAR NERVE

*Median Nerve*
- *Innervates most Flexor Forearm muscles except: Flexor Carpi Ulnaris (FCU) and Flexor Digitorum Profundus (Medial part of FDP), which are both innervated by **Ulnar Nerve.***

*Ulnar Nerve*
- *Innervates most Hand muscles except: Lumbricals 1 &2, Opponens Pollicis, Abductor Pollicis Brevis, Flexor Pollicis Brevis (Superficial head), which are all innervated by **Median Nerve (LOAF).***

## CLINICAL RELEVANCE:
## LESIONS OF THE MEDIAN NERVE

- The median nerve is particularly vulnerable to damage at the elbow and wrist.

➤ **Damaged at the Elbow**
- **Mechanism of injury:**
  - ○ Supracondylar fracture of the humerus.
- **Motor functions:**
  - ○ The Flexors and Pronators in the forearm are paralysed, with the exception of the Flexor Carpi Ulnaris and **medial half** of Flexor Digitorum Profundus.
  - ○ The forearm constantly supinated, and flexion is weak (often accompanied by adduction, because of the pull of the flexor carpi ulnaris).
  - ○ Flexion at the thumb is also prevented, as both the longus and brevis muscles are paralysed.
  - ○ The lateral two lumbrical muscles are paralysed, and the patient will not be able to flex at the MCP joints or extend at IP joints of the index and middle fingers.

- **Sensory functions:**
  - ○ Lack of sensation over the areas that the median nerve innervates.
  - ○ Loss of sensation in lateral 3 ½ digits including their nail beds, and the thenar area.
- **Characteristic signs:**
  - ○ The thenar eminence is wasted, due to atrophy of the thenar muscles. If patient tries to make a fist, only the little and ring fingers can flex completely.
  - ○ This results in a characteristic shape of the hand, known as **Hand of Benediction.**
  - ○ Presence of an **Ape Hand Deformity** when the hand is at rest, due to hyperextension of index finger and thumb, and an adducted thumb.

➤ **Within the Proximal Forearm:**
- Injury to the anterior interosseous branch in the forearm causes **the anterior interosseous syndrome**.
- **Mechanism of injury:**
  - ○ Tight cast, forearm bone fracture.
- **Motor deficit:**
  - ○ Loss of pronation of forearm, loss of flexion of radial half of digits and thumb.
- **Sensory deficit**: None

➤ **Damaged at the Wrist**
- **Mechanism of injury:**
  - ○ Lacerations (Stab wound) just proximal to the flexor retinaculum or Colle's fracture.
- **Motor functions:** LOAF affected
  - ○ Thenar muscles paralysed, as are the lateral two lumbricals.
  - ○ This affects opposition of the thumb and flexion of the index and middle fingers.
- **Sensory functions:**
  - ○ Same as an injury at the elbow.
- **Characteristic signs:**
  - ○ Same as an injury at the elbow.

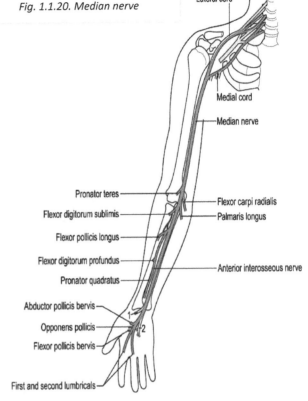

Fig. 1.1.20. Median nerve

Lateral cord
Medial cord
Median nerve
Pronator teres
Flexor digitorum sublimis
Flexor pollicis longus
Flexor digitorum profundus
Pronator quadratus
Abductor pollicis bervis
Opponens pollicis
Flexor pollicis bervis
First and second lumbricals
Flexor carpi radialis
Palmaris longus
Anterior interosseous nerve

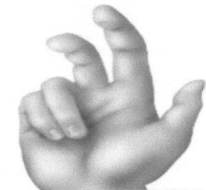

Fig. 1.1.21. Hand of Benediction

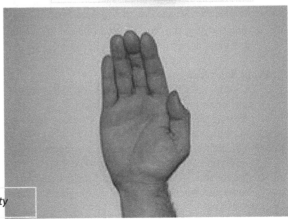

Fig. 1.1.22. Ape hand deformity

## A.4. ULNAR NERVE

- **Origin:**
  - The ulnar nerve is derived from the brachial plexus.
  - It is a continuation of the **Medial Cord.**
  - **Spinal roots**: C8-T1.

- **Course:**
  - After arising from the brachial plexus, the ulnar nerve descends down the medial side of the upper arm.
  - At the elbow, it passes posterior to the medial epicondyle, entering the forearm. At the medial epicondyle, the nerve is easily palpable and vulnerable to injury. In the forearm, the ulnar nerve pierces the two heads of the flexor carpi ulnaris, and travels alongside the ulna.
  - **At the wrist, the ulnar nerve travels superficially to the flexor retinaculum. It enters the hand via the ulnar canal (or Guyon's canal).** In the hand the nerve terminates by giving rise to superficial and deep branches.

- **Sensory functions:**
  - Innervates the anterior and posterior surfaces of the medial 1 ½ fingers, and the associated palm area.

- **Motor functions:**
  - Innervates the muscles of the hand (apart from the thenar muscles and two lateral lumbricals), flexor carpi ulnaris and medial half of flexor digitorum profundus.

- **Three branches arise in the forearm:**
  - **Muscular branch:** innervates some muscles in the anterior compartment of the forearm.
  - **Palmar cutaneous branch:** innervates the skin of the medial half of the palm.
  - **Dorsal cutaneous branch:** innervates the skin of the medial 1 and 1/2 finger, and the associated palm area.

## CLINICAL RELEVANCE:
## LESIONS OF THE ULNAR NERVE

- The ulnar nerve is most susceptible to injury at the elbow and the wrist.
- ➤ **Damaged at the Elbow**
- **Mechanism of injury:**
  - The nerve is most vulnerable to injury at the medial epicondyle, so **fracture of the medial epicondyle** is the most common way of damaging the ulnar nerve.

- **Motor functions:**
  - Flexor carpi ulnaris (FCU) and medial half of flexor digitorum profundus (FDP) paralysed.
  - Flexion of the wrist can still occur, but is accompanied by abduction.
  - The interossei are paralysed, so abduction and adduction of the fingers cannot occur.
  - Movement of the little and ring fingers is greatly reduced, due to *paralysis of the medial two lumbricals*.

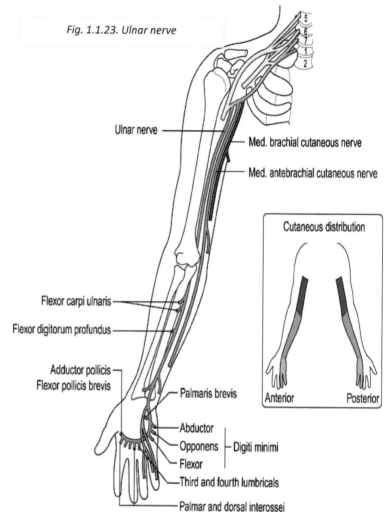

Fig. 1.1.23. Ulnar nerve

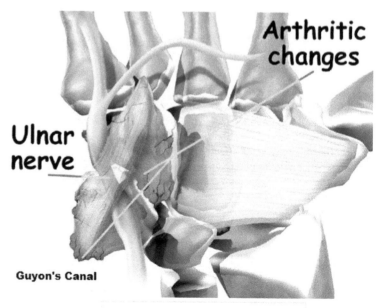

Fig. 1.1.24. Guyon canal

- **Sensory functions:**
  - Loss of sensation in ulnar half of the palm and dorsum of hand, and the medial 1½ digits on both palmar and dorsal aspects of the hand.

- **Characteristic signs:**
  - **Froment's sign** is used to test for a compromised adductor pollicis muscle. Patient cannot grip paper placed between fingers.
  - **Claw hand deformity**
- ➤ **Damaged at the Wrist**
- **Mechanism of injury:**
  - Lacerations to the wrist
- **Motor functions:**
  - **The interossei are paralysed**, so abduction and adduction of the fingers cannot occur.
  - Movement of the little and ring fingers is **greatly reduced**, due to paralysis of the medial two lumbricals.
  - **The two muscles in the forearm are unaffected**
- **Sensory functions:**
  - The palmar branch and superficial branch are usually severed, **but the dorsal branch is unaffected.**
- Sensory loss over palmar side of medial one and a half fingers only. **Characteristic signs:**
  - Patient cannot grip paper placed between fingers.
  - **More pronounced Claw Hand Deformity** at the wrist than the elbow (ulnar paradox).

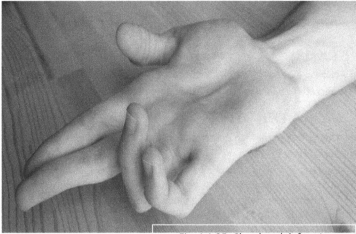

*Fig. 1.1.25. Claw hand deformity*

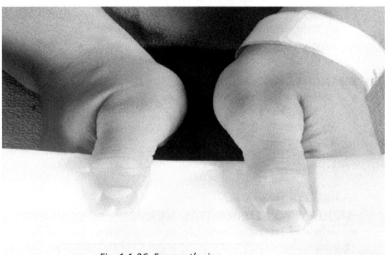

*Fig. 1.1.26. Froment's sign*

## FROMENT'S SIGN

- When the patient grasps a piece of paper between the thumb & index fingertips of both hands and the examiner pulls on the paper, the thumb with ulnar palsy flexes at the interphalangeal (IP) joint, while the uninjured thumb will not flex [or only minimally]. The absence of the AP power removes one of the MP joint flexion/IP joint extension forces, so the flexor pollicis longus (FPL) power becomes more dominate.

## JEANNE'S SIGN

- Similar to Froment's sign, Jeanne's sign is also seen in response to pinch forces. Instead of isolated thumb IP flexion, the IP flexion is accompanied by MP joint hyperextension.

### ULNAR PARADOX

- *The ulnar nerve innervates the medial half of the FDP.*
- *If the ulnar nerve lesion occurs more proximally (closer to the elbow), the FDP may also be denervated.*
- *As a result, flexion of the IP joints is weakened, which reduces the claw-like appearance of the hand. (Instead, the 4th and 5th fingers are simply paralyzed in their fully extended position.)*
- *This is called the "ulnar paradox" because one would normally expect a more debilitating injury to result in a more deformed appearance.*
- ***There is more pronounced Claw Hand Deformity at the wrist than the elbow.***

- **Ulnar claw** consists of:
  - **Hyperextension of the MCP joints** of the little and ring fingers; this is because of the paralysis of the medial two lumbricals, and the now unopposed action of the extensor muscles
  - **Flexion at the interphalangeal joints** (if the lesion has occurred close to the elbow, this might not be evident, as the flexor digitorum profundus will be paralysed)

# B. THE POSTERIOR ARM

## 1. TRICEPS

- **Actions:** extends forearm, long head extends, adducts arm and extends shoulder.
- **Innervation:** Radial nerve and Axillary nerve (long head)

## 2. RADIAL NERVE

- **Origin:** one of the two **Posterior Cords** of the brachial plexus
- **Spinal root:** C5-T1.
- **Course:**
  - Posteromedially with the axillary vessels, behind the humerus, then anteriorly towards the elbow where it divides into Superficial and Deep Branches
- **Terminal branches:**
  - Posterior interosseous (deep).
  - Superficial branch of radial nerve.
- **Motor:**
  - Wrist and finger extension.
- **Sensory:**
  - Dorsal aspect of the thumb, index and middle fingers.

### BRANCHES AND SUPPLY:

- **Mnemonic: Radial nerve innervates** "BEAST"
  - ✓ **B**rachioradialis
  - ✓ **E**xtensors
  - ✓ **A**nconeus
  - ✓ **S**upinator
  - ✓ **T**riceps

## CLINICAL RELEVANCE:

### INJURY TO THE RADIAL NERVE

- Lesions of the radial nerve can be broadly categorised into four groups; depending on where the damage has occurred, and what components of the nerve have been affected.

➢ **IN THE AXILLA**
- **Mechanism of injury:**
  - Dislocation of humerus at the glenohumeral joint or fractures of proximal humerus.
  - Can also happen via excessive pressure on the axilla, e.g. a badly fitting crutch.
- **Motor functions:**
  - Triceps brachii and muscles in posterior compartment are paralysed.
  - Loss of Elbow, wrist and Fingers extensions.
  - Loss of supination
  - Unopposed flexion of wrist occurs, known as **wrist drop**.
- **Sensory functions:**
  - All four cutaneous branches of the radial nerve are affected.
  - There will be a loss of sensation over the lateral and posterior upper arm, posterior forearm, and dorsal surface of the lateral three and a half digits.

➢ **IN THE RADIAL GROOVE**
- **Mechanism of injury:**
  - Fracture of the shaft of the humerus damaging the radial nerve when it is bound in the radial groove.
- **Motor functions:**
  - The triceps brachii may be weakened, but is not paralysed.
  - The deep branch of the radial nerve is affected, so the muscles in the posterior compartment of the forearm are paralysed.

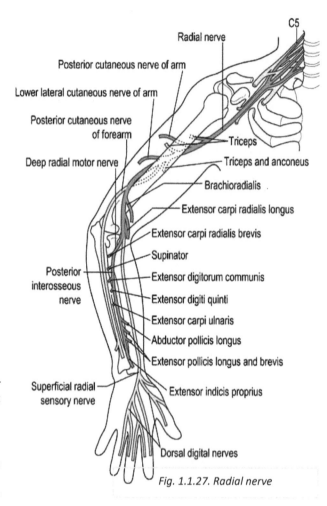

Fig. 1.1.27. Radial nerve

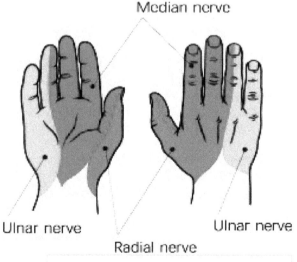

Fig. 1.1.28. Nerves distribution of the hand

- o The patient is unable to extend the wrist and fingers.
- o Unopposed flexion of wrist occurs, known as **wrist drop.**
- **Sensory functions:**
  - o The cutaneous branches to the arm and forearm have already arisen.
  - o The superficial branch of the radial nerve will be damaged, resulting in sensory loss on the dorsal surface of the lateral three and half digits, and their associated palm area.

➤ **AT THE ELBOW AND FOREARM:**
### 1. DEEP BRANCH OF RADIAL NERVE
- **Mechanism of injury:**
  - o Fractures of the radial head, or a posterior dislocation of the radius at the elbow joint.
- **Motor functions:**
  - o Muscles in posterior compartment of the forearm are affected; **except for the supinator and extensor carpi radialis longus.**
  - o The extensor carpi radialis longus is a strong extensor at the wrist, and so **wristdrop does not occur.**
- **Sensory functions:**
  - o None, as it is a motor nerve.

### 2. SUPERFICIAL BRANCH OF THE RADIAL NERVE
- **Mechanism of injury:**
  - o Stabbing or laceration of the forearm.
- **Motor functions:**
  - o None, as it is a sensory nerve.
- **Sensory functions:**
  - o There will be sensory loss affecting the dorsal surface of the lateral three and half digits and their associated palm area.

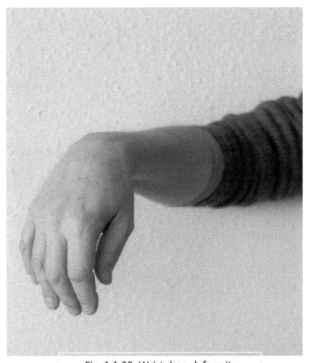

*Fig. 1.1.29. Wrist drop deformity*

## 3. ELBOW JOINT
### A. ARTICULATIONS:
Three articulations **(CRUT)**
- **Radiohumeral:** Capitellum of the humerus with the Radial Head.
- **Ulnohumeral:** Trochlea of the humerus with the trochlear notch (with separate olecranon and coronoid process articular facets) of the Ulna.
- **Radioulnar:** Radial Head with the radial notch of the Ulna (proximal radioulnar joint).

### B. LIGAMENTS
- Medial (ulnar) collateral ligament complex
- Lateral (radial) collateral ligament complex
- Oblique cord
- Quadrate ligament (of Denuce)

### C. BLOOD SUPPLY
- Arterial supply is via anastomotic (medial, lateral and posterior) arcades formed by branches of the radial, ulna and brachial arteries.

### D. NERVE SUPPLY
- Articular branches of the radial, ulna, median and musculocutaneous nerves.

### E. ELBOW MOVEMENTS:
- ✓ **Extension:** **T**riceps brachii and **A**nconeus
- ✓ **Flexion:** **B**rachialis, **B**iceps brachii, **B**rachioradialis

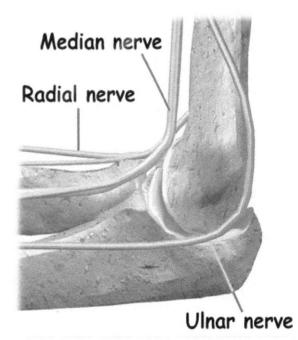

*Fig. 1.1.30. Nerves passing through the Elbow*

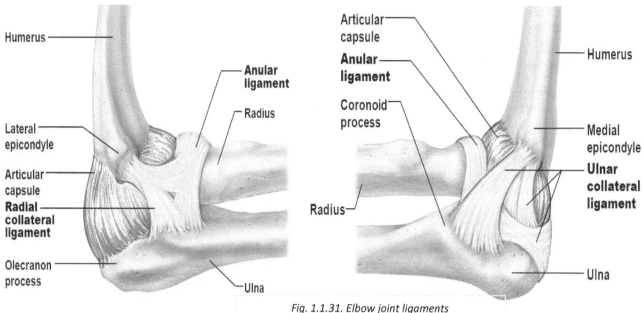

Fig. 1.1.31. Elbow joint ligaments

## 4. THE CUBITAL FOSSA

### 1. BORDERS

- The cubital fossa is triangular in shape, and thus has three borders:
  - **Lateral border**: The medial border of the Brachioradialis Muscle
  - **Medial border**: The lateral border of the Pronator Teres Muscle
  - **Superior border**: An imaginary line between the epicondyles of the humerus.
  - **Floor**: the floor of the cubital fossa is formed
    - **Proximally** by the Brachialis, and
    - **Distally** by the Supinator Muscle.
  - **Roof**: consists of skin and fascia, with is reinforced by the bicipital aponeurosis.
  - Within the roof runs the Median Cubital Vein, which can be accessed for venepuncuture.

### 2. CONTENTS

- The contents of the cubital fossa include vessels, nerves and the biceps tendon *(lateral to medial): RBBM (RaBiBraMe)*
  - **R**adial nerve
  - **B**iceps tendon
  - **B**rachial artery
  - **M**edian nerve

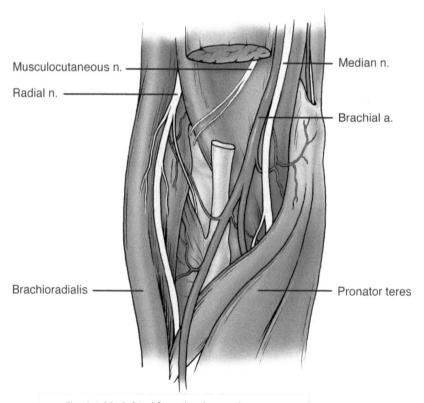

Fig. 1.1.32. Cubital fossa borders and contents

# VI. FOREARM

# A. THE ANTERIOR FOREARM

## A. MUSCLES

Common origin of the Forearm Flexors is the Medial Humeral Epicondyle (Golfers elbow)

### FLEXOR CARPI RADIALIS
- Action: Flexion and abduction at wrist
- Innervation: Median nerve

### FLEXOR CARPI ULNARIS
- Action: flexion and adduction wrist
- Innervation: Muscular branches ulnar nerve

### FLEXOR DIGITORUM SUPERFICIALIS
- Action: flexor of fingers (primarily at PIP joints)
- Innervation: Median nerve

### FLEXOR DIGITORUM PROFUNDUS
- Action: flex hand and both interphalangeal joints
- Innervation: Median nerve (ant. Interosseous) and Muscular branch of Ulnar

### FLEXOR POLLICIS LONGUS
- Action: flexion thumb
- Innervation: anterior interosseous nerve (branch of Median nerve C8, T1)

### PALMARIS LONGUS
- Action: wrist flexor
- Innervation: Median nerve

### PRONATOR TERES
- Action: pronation forearm, flexes elbow
- Innervation: Median nerve

### PRONATOR QUADRATUS
- Action: pronates the forearm
- Innervation: Median nerve (ant. Interosseous)

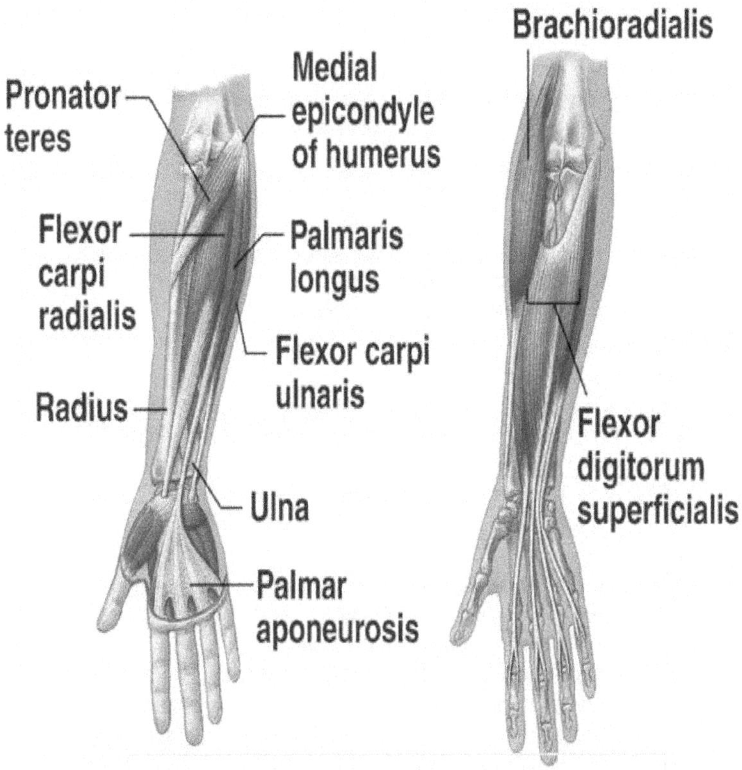

Fig. 1.1.33. Muscles of anterior forearm

## B. VESSELS OF THE COMPARTMENT

## 1. RADIAL ARTERY

**Origin:**
- From the bifurcation of the brachial artery in the cubital fossa. It runs distally on the anterior part of the forearm.
- Then winds laterally around the wrist, passing through the anatomical snuff box and between the heads of the first dorsal interosseous muscle. It passes anteriorly between the heads of the adductor pollicis, and becomes *the deep palmar arch*, which joins with the deep branch of the ulnar artery. It is accompanied by a similarly named vein, the radial vein along its course.

**BRANCHES OF RADIAL ARTERY:**
- **In the forearm:**
  - Radial recurrent artery
  - Palmar carpal branch of radial artery
  - Superficial palmar branch of the radial artery
- **At the wrist:**
  - Dorsal carpal branch of radial artery
  - First dorsal metacarpal artery
- **In the hand:**
  - Princeps pollicis artery
  - Radialis indicis
  - Deep palmar arch

## 2. ULNAR ARTERY

**Origin:**

- The ulnar artery is the main blood vessel, with oxygenated blood, of the medial aspect of the forearm. Arises from the brachial artery and terminates in the superficial palmar arch, which joins with the superficial branch of the radial artery.
- **Branches in Forearm: MARC**
  - **M**uscular branches
  - **A**rterial anastomosis around the wrist joint
  - **R**ecurrent branches
  - **C**ommon Interosseous artery
- *Ulnar artery lies on the lateral side of ulnar nerve and pisiform bone anterior to flexor retinaculum. It gives deep branch and continues into palm as the superficial palmar arch.*

**Superficial palmar arch:**

- It is the direct continuation of ulnar artery and curves laterally behind the palmar aponeurosis, in front of the long flexor tendons. It is completed on the lateral side by the branch of radial artery. The curve of arch lies across the palm at level with the distant border of fully extended thumb.

**Branches in hand:**

- Digital arteries
- Deep branch of ulnar artery: Deep branch lies in front of the flexor retinaculum and passes between the abductor digiti minimi and the flexor digiti minimi.
- It joins the radial artery to complete the deep palmar arch.

## 3. WRIST ANASTOMOSIS

- *Palmar(Anterior) carpal arch*: the anastomosis of two arteries:
  - The palmar carpal branch of radial artery
  - The palmar carpal branch of ulnar artery
  - This anastomosis is joined by a branch from the anterior interosseous artery above, and by recurrent branches from the deep palmar arch below, thus forming a palmar carpal network which supplies the articulations of the wrist and carpus.

- *Posterior carpal arches*
  - The dorsal carpal arch (dorsal carpal network, posterior carpal arch) is an anatomical term for the combination (anastomosis) of:
    - Dorsal carpal branch of the radial artery and
    - Dorsal carpal branch of the ulnar artery near the back of the wrist.
  - It is made up of the dorsal carpal branches of both the ulnar and radial arteries.
  - It also anastomoses with the anterior interosseous artery and the posterior interosseous artery.
  - *The arch gives off three dorsal metacarpal arteries.*

## 4. VEINS

### A. CEPHALIC VEIN:

- **Source:** Dorsal venous network of hand
- **Drain to:** Axillary vein and Median Cubital vein
- Communicates with the Basilic vein via *the Median cubital vein at the elbow.*
- Located in the superficial fascia along the anterolateral surface of the biceps brachii muscle.
- Superiorly the cephalic vein passes between the deltoid and pectoralis major muscles (deltopectoral groove) and through the deltopectoral triangle, where it empties into the axillary vein.

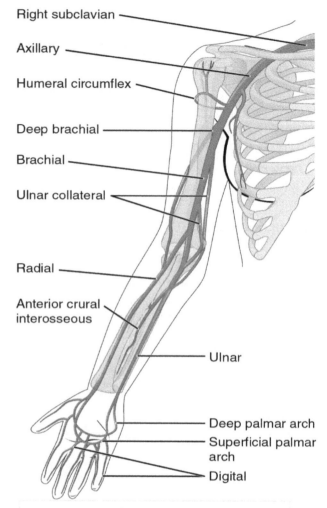

Right subclavian
Axillary
Humeral circumflex
Deep brachial
Brachial
Ulnar collateral
Radial
Anterior crural interosseous
Ulnar
Deep palmar arch
Superficial palmar arch
Digital

*Fig. 1.1.34. Ulnar artery and radial artery*

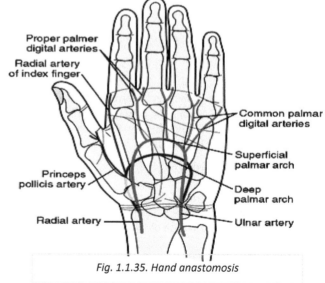

Proper palmer digital arteries
Radial artery of index finger
Common palmar digital arteries
Superficial palmar arch
Princeps pollicis artery
Deep palmar arch
Radial artery
Ulnar artery

*Fig. 1.1.35. Hand anastomosis*

**B. BASILIC VEIN:**
o **Source:** Dorsal venous network of hand
o **Drain to:** Axillary vein

**C. MEDIAN VEIN:**
o **Source:** Cephalic vein
o Drain to:  Basilic vein

## 5.  NERVES OF THE FLEXOR COMPARTMENT
o Lateral and medial cutaneous nerves of forearm
o Median nerve
o Ulnar nerve

## 6. JOINT
o Radioulnar joints

---

**ANATOMY OF BASILIC AND CEPHALIC VEIN CATHETERIZATION**

- **The median basilic or basilic veins** are the veins of choice for central venous catheterization, because from the cubital fossa until the basilic vein reaches the axillary vein, the basilic vein increases in diameter and is in direct line with the axillary vein. The valves in the axillary vein may be troublesome, but abduction of the shoulder joint may permit the catheter to move past the obstruction.

- **The cephalic vein** does not increase in size as it ascends the arm, and it frequently divides into small branches as it lies within the deltopectoral triangle. One or more of these branches may ascend over the clavicle and join the external jugular vein. In its usual method of termination, the cephalic vein joins the axillary vein at a right angle. It may be difficult to maneuver the catheter around this angle.

---

# B. POSTERIOR COMPARTMENT OF THE FOREARM

## A. MUSCLES AND MOVEMENTS
Common origin of the Forearm Extensors is the Lateral Humeral Epicondyle (Tennis elbow)

### 1. BRACHIORADIALIS
- Action: flexion elbow and supination
- Innervation: Radial nerve

### 2. EXTENSOR CARPI RADIALIS LONGUS
- Action: Extensor at wrist joint, abducts hand at the wrist
- Innervation: Radial nerve

### 3. EXTENSOR CARPI RADIALIS BREVIS
- Action: Extensor and abductor of the hand at the wrist
- Innervation: deep branch of Radial nerve

### 4. EXTENSOR DIGITORUM
- Action: Extension of hand, wrist and fingers
- Innervation: Radial nerve

### 5. EXTENSOR CARPI ULNARIS
- Action: extension and adduction wrist
- Innervation: deep branch of Radial nerve C7

### 6. SUPINATOR
- Action: supinates forearm
- Innervation: Deep Radial nerve

### 7. ABDUCTOR POLLICIS LONGUS
- Action: abduction and extension thumb
- Innervation:  posterior interosseous nerve from deep branch of radial nerve C7-8

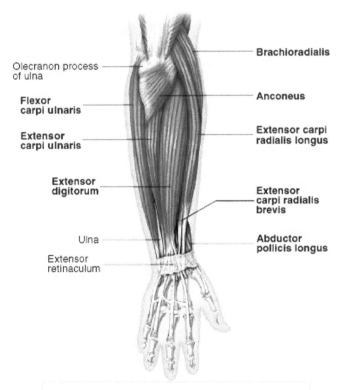

Fig. 1.1.36. Muscles of posterior forearm

### 8. EXTENSORS POLLICIS LONGUS
- Action: extension thumb (MCP and interphalangeal)
- Innervation: posterior interosseous nerve from deep branch of radial nerve

### 9. EXTENSORS POLLICIS BREVIS
- Action: extension thumb at MCP joint
- Innervation:  posterior interosseous nerve from deep branch of radial nerve

### 10. EXTENSOR INDICIS
- Action: extends index finger, wrist
- Innervation: posterior interosseous nerve from deep branch of radial nerve.

## ANATOMICAL SNUFFBOX

- **Borders**
  - **Medial** – Extensor Pollicis Longus **(EPL)**
  - **Lateral** – Extensor Pollicis Brevis and more laterally Abductor Pollicis Longus **(EPB &APL)**
  - **Floor** – Scaphoid, Trapezium Bones; Base of 1ˢᵗ Metacarpal can be palpated distally and the Radial Styloid process can be palpated proximally.

- **Contents**
  - Radial artery
  - Superficial branch of the Radial Nerve
  - Cephalic vein (variable)

## CLINICAL RELEVANCE:

### FRACTURE OF THE SCAPHOID BONE

- It is common in young adults; unless treated effectively, the fragments will not unite, and permanent weakness and pain of the wrist will result, with the subsequent development of osteoarthritis.
- The fracture line usually goes through the narrowest part of the bone, which, because of its location, is bathed in synovial fluid.
- The blood vessels to the scaphoid enter its proximal and distal ends, although the blood supply is occasionally confined to its distal end.
- If the latter occurs, a fracture deprives the proximal fragment of its arterial supply, and this fragment undergoes avascular necrosis.
- Deep tenderness in the anatomic snuffbox after a fall on the outstretched hand in a young adult makes one suspicious of a fractured scaphoid.

### DISLOCATION OF THE LUNATE BONE

- Occasionally occurs in young adults who fall on the outstretched hand in a way that causes hyperextension of the wrist joint.
- Involvement of the median nerve is common.

### FRACTURES OF THE METACARPAL BONES

- Can occur as a result of direct violence, such as the clenched fist striking a hard object.
- The fracture always angulates dorsally.
- The **"boxer's fracture"** commonly produces an oblique fracture of the neck of the fifth and sometimes the fourth metacarpal bones.
- The distal fragment is commonly displaced proximally, thus shortening the finger posteriorly.

### BENNETT'S FRACTURE

- It is a fracture of the base of the metacarpal of the thumb caused when violence is applied along the long axis of the thumb or the thumb is forcefully abducted.
- The fracture is oblique and enters the carpometacarpal joint of the thumb, causing joint instability.

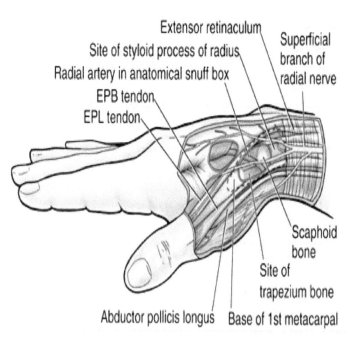

Fig. 1.1.37. Anatomical Snuffbox

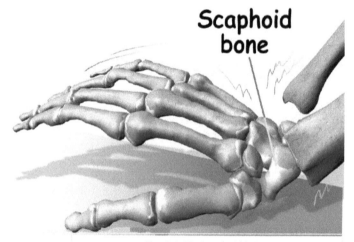

Fig. 1.1.38. Scaphoid injury

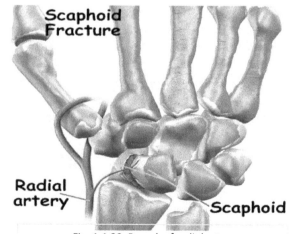

Fig. 1.1.39. Branch of radial artery

# VII. WRIST AND HAND

## 1. MUSCLES WHICH EXERT:

- **Flexion:** Flexor carpi ulnaris, flexor carpi radialis with assistance from the flexor digitorum superficialis.
- **Extension:** Extensor carpi radialis longus and brevis, and extensor carpi ulnaris with assistance from the extensor digitorum.
- **Adduction:** Extensor carpi ulnaris and flexor carpi ulnaris
- **Abduction:** abductor pollicis longus, flexor carpi radialis and Extensor carpi radialis longus and brevis.

## 2. PALMAR APONEUROSIS

Structure (Slips)

- **CENTRAL PORTION:**
    - Occupies the middle of the palm, is triangular in shape, and of great strength and thickness.
    - **Apex:**
        - Is continuous with the lower margin of the transverse carpal ligament, and receives the expanded tendon of the palmaris longus.
    - **Base:**
        - Divides below into four slips, one for each finger.
        - Each slip gives off superficial fibers to the skin of the palm and finger.
        - The deeper part of each slip subdivides into two processes, which are inserted into the fibrous sheaths of the flexor tendons.
        - From the sides of these processes offsets are attached to the transverse metacarpal ligament.

- **LATERAL AND MEDIAL PORTIONS**
    - The lateral and medial portions of the palmar aponeurosis are thin, fibrous layers, which cover, on the radial side, the muscles of the ball of the thumb, and, on the ulnar side, the muscles of the little finger; they are continuous with the central portion and with the fascia on the dorsum of the hand.

- **FUNCTION (MECHANICAL)**
    - Tendinous extension of the palmaris longus
    - strong stabilizing structure for the palmar skin of the hand

## FLEXOR RETINACULUM

- ➤ **Attachments**
    - **Medially:** to the Pisiform and the hamulus of the Hamate bone.
    - **Laterally:** to the tubercle of the Scaphoid, and to the medial part of the volar surface and the ridge of the Trapezium.
    - **Superficially:** with the volar carpal ligament
    - **Deeply:** with the palmar aponeurosis.
        - It is crossed by the ulnar vessels and nerve, and the cutaneous branches of the median and ulnar nerves.
    - **Lateral end:** is the tendon of the Flexor Carpi Radialis.
    - **Volar surface:** the tendons of the Palmaris Longus and Flexor Carpi Ulnaris are partly inserted.
        - **Note: the thenar and hypothenar muscles arise from it.**

- ➤ **Relations**
- **Inferiorly:**
    - contents of the Carpal Tunnel

- **Superiorly**
    - Ulnar artery and nerve (**in Guyon's canal**)
    - Palmar cutaneous branch of the median and ulnar nerves
    - Palmaris longus tendon
    - Superficial palmar branch of the radial artery

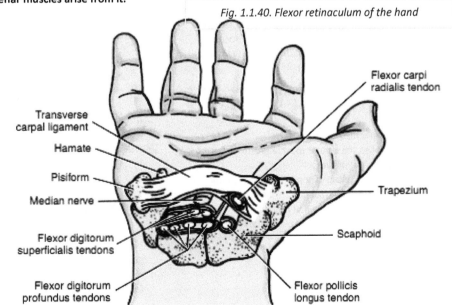

*Fig. 1.1.40. Flexor retinaculum of the hand*

Transverse carpal ligament

Hamate

Pisiform

Median nerve

Flexor digitorum superficialis tendons

Flexor digitorum profundus tendons

Flexor carpi radialis tendon

Trapezium

Scaphoid

Flexor pollicis longus tendon

## CLINICAL RELEVANCE:
## WRIST JOINT INJURIES

- The wrist joint is essentially a synovial joint between the distal end of the radius and the proximal row of carpal bones.
- The head of the ulna is separated from the carpal bones by the strong triangular fibrocartilaginous ligament, which separates the wrist joint from the distal radioulnar joint.
- The joint is stabilized by the strong medial and lateral ligaments.
- Because the styloid process of the radius is longer than that of the ulna, abduction of the wrist joint is less extensive than adduction.
- In flexion–extension movements, the hand can be flexed about 80° but extended to only about 45°.
- The range of flexion is increased by movement at the midcarpal joint.
- A fall on the outstretched hand can strain the anterior ligament of the wrist joint, producing synovial effusion, joint pain, and limitation of movement.
- These symptoms and signs must not be confused with those produced by a fractured scaphoid or dislocation of the lunate bone, which are similar.
- Falls on the Outstretched Hand In falls on the outstretched hand, forces are transmitted from the scaphoid to the distal end of the radius, from the radius across the interosseous membrane to the ulna, and from the ulna to the humerus; thence, through the glenoid fossa of the scapula to the coracoclavicular ligament and the clavicle; and finally, to the sternum. If the forces are excessive, different parts of the upper limb give way under the strain.
- The area affected seems to be related to age. In a young child, for example, there may be a posterior displacement of the distal radial epiphysis; in the teenager the clavicle might fracture; in the young adult the scaphoid is commonly fractured; and in the elderly the distal end of the radius is fractured about 2.5 cm proximal to the wrist joint (Colles' fracture).

## 3. CARPAL TUNNEL

- The carpal tunnel contains a total of **Carpal Bones**, **9 Tendons** surrounded by synovial sheaths, and the **Median Nerve**.
- **Carpal bones: Sam Likes To Push The Toy Car Hard**
  - ✓ **S**: scaphoid, **L**: lunate, **T**: triquetrum, **P**: pisiform
  - ✓ **T**: trapezium, **T**: trapezoid, **C**: capitate, **H**: hamate

- **TENDONS**
  - 1 Flexor Pollicis Longus (**1 FPL**)
  - 4 Flexor Digitorum Profundus (**4 FDP**)
  - 4 Flexor Digitorum Superficialis (**4 FDS**)

- **SYNOVIAL SHEATS**
  - The 8 tendons of the **Flexor Digitorum Profundus** and **Flexor Digitorum Superficialis** are surrounded by a single synovial sheath.
  - The tendon of Flexor Pollicis Longus is surrounded by its own synovial sheath. These sheaths allow free movement of the tendons.
  - Sometimes you may hear that the carpal tunnel contains another tendon, the **Flexor Carpi Radialis** tendon, but this is located within the flexor retinaculum (see above) and not within the carpal tunnel itself.

- **Median Nerve:** Once it passes through the carpal tunnel, the median nerve divides into 2 branches:
  - **The Recurrent branch:**
    - Supplies the thenar muscle group
  - **Palmar digital nerves:**
    - Sensory innervation to the palmar skin and dorsal nail beds of the lateral three and a half digits.
    - Motor innervation to the lateral two lumbricals

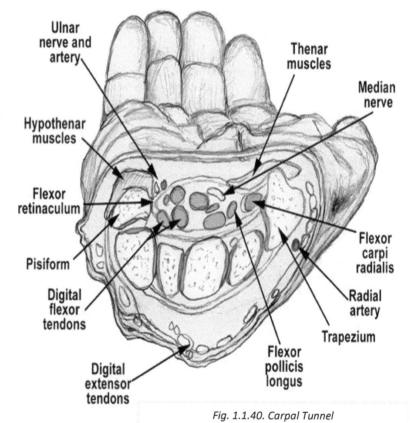

*Fig. 1.1.40. Carpal Tunnel*

# CARPAL TUNNEL SYNDROME

- Compression of the median nerve within the carpal tunnel can cause carpal tunnel syndrome (CTS).
- Its aetiology is most often idiopathic. If left untreated, CTS can cause weakness and atrophy of the thenar muscles.
- The patient's history will comment on numbness, tingling and pain in the distribution of the median nerve.
- The pain will usually radiate to the forearm.
- Symptoms are often associated with waking the patient from their sleep and being worse in the mornings.
- Tests for CTS can be performed during physical examination:
  - **Tinel's Sign:** Tapping the nerve in the carpal tunnel to elicit pain in median nerve distribution.
  - **Phalen's manoeuvre:** Holding the wrist in flexion for 60 seconds to elicit numbness/pain in median nerve distribution.
- Treatment involves the use of a splint, holding the wrist in dorsiflexion overnight to relieve symptoms.
- If this is unsuccessful, corticosteroid injections into the carpal tunnel can be used.
- In severe case, surgical decompression of the carpal tunnel may be required.

## 5. THENAR EMINENCE

- The muscles of the thenar eminence are innervated by the **Median Nerve.**
- 3 muscles: **APB, FPB & OP**
- Abductor Pollicis Brevis is the most proximal muscle of the thenar group.
- Opponens Pollicis lies deep to abductor pollicis brevis.

### 5.1 ABDUCTOR POLLICIS BREVIS
- Action: abduction thumb by acting across the carpometacarpal joint and the MCP joint. It also assists in opposition and extension of the thumb.
- Innervation: Recurrent branch of the median nerve

### 5.2. FLEXOR POLLICIS BREVIS
- Action: flexes the thumb at the 1st MCP joint
- Innervation: Recurrent branch of the Median nerve, deep branch of ulnar nerve (medial head)

### 5.3. OPPONENS POLLICIS
- Action: flexion thumb's Metacarpal at the 1st carpometarpal joint, which aids in opposition of the thumb.
- Innervation: Recurrent branch of median nerve

## 6. HYPOTHENAR EMINENCE: ADM, FDM & ODM
### 6.1. ABDUCTOR DIGITI MINIMI (MOST SUPERFICIAL)
- Action: abducts little finger
- Innervation: Deep branch of Ulnar nerve
### 6.2. FLEXOR DIGITI MINIMI (LATERAL TO THE ADM)
- Action: flexes little finger
- Innervation: Deep branch of ulnar nerve
### 6.3. OPPONENS DIGITI MINIMI (DEEPER MUSCLE)
- Action: draw 5th metacarpal anteriorly and rotates it, bringing little finger (5th digit) into opposition with thumb
- Innervation: Deep branch ulnar nerve C8, T1

## 7. PALMAR ARCHES (OR VOLAR ARCHES)
- **Deep palmar arch:** mainly formed from the terminal part of the radial artery, with the ulnar artery contributing via its deep palmar branch, by an anastomosis.
- *Superficial palmar arch*: predominantly formed by the ulnar artery.

## 8. DIGITAL NERVES:
- Ulnar nerve and Median nerve

## 9. LUMBRICALS AND INTEROSSEI
### 9.1. Lumbricals:
- **Origin:** Flexor Digitorum Profundus **(FDP)**
- **insertion:** extensor expansion
- **Innervation:**
  - 3rd and 4th >> deep branch of **Ulnar Nerve,**
  - 1st and 2nd >> **Median Nerve.**
- **Actions:** Flex MCP joints, extend interphalangeal joints

### 9.2. Interossei:

○ *Dorsal interossei group:*
  - **Action:** Abduct finger
  - **Innervation:** Deep branch of Ulnar nerve
○ *Palmar/Volar interossei group:*
  - **Action:** Adduction, Flexion and Extension Fingers
  - **Innervation:** Deep branch Ulnar nerve.

*Interossei muscles: actions of dorsal vs. palmar in hand "PAd and DAb":*
*The Palmar Adduct and the Dorsal Abduct.*

## 10. THE FLEXOR SHEATHS

- The common synovial sheath for the flexor tendons or the ulnar bursa is a synovial sheath in the carpal tunnel of the human hand.
- It contains tendons of the flexor digitorum superficialis and the flexor digitorum profundus, but not the flexor pollicis longus.

### MALLET FINGER

- Avulsion of the insertion of one of the extensor tendons into the distal phalanges can occur if the distal phalanx is forcibly flexed when the extensor tendon is taut. The last 20° of active extension is lost, resulting in a condition known as **mallet finger**

### BOUTONNIÈRE DEFORMITY

- Avulsion of the central slip of the extensor tendon proximal to its insertion into the base of the middle phalanx results in a characteristic deformity. The deformity results from flexing of the proximal interphalangeal joint and hyperextension of the distal interphalangeal joint. This injury can result from direct end-on trauma to the finger, direct trauma over the back of the proximal interphalangeal joint, or laceration of the dorsum of the finger.

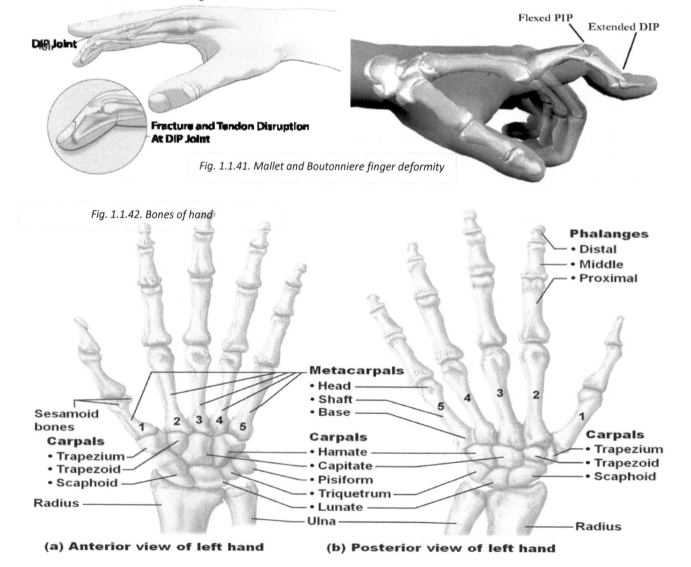

*Fig. 1.1.41. Mallet and Boutonniere finger deformity*

*Fig. 1.1.42. Bones of hand*

(a) Anterior view of left hand

(b) Posterior view of left hand

# 11. DERMATOMES & MYOTOMES

| DERMATOMES | | MYOTOMES | |
|---|---|---|---|
| | Area over the deltoid | **C5** | Shoulder abduction |
| *C6* | Thumb | **C5, C6** | Elbow flexion |
| *C7* | Middle finger | | Elbow extension |
| *C8* | Little finger | **C7** | Wrist extension |
| *T4* | Nipple line | | Finger extension |
| *T8* | Xiphisternum | **C8** | Wrist flexion |
| *T10* | Umbilicus | | Finger flexion |
| *T12* | Symphysis pubis | **T1** | Finger abduction |
| *L4* | Medial aspect calf | **L1, L2** | Hip flexion |
| *L5* | Webspace 1st and 2nd toes | **L5, S1** | Hip extension |
| *S1* | lateral border foot | **L3, L4** | Knee extension |
| *S3* | Ischial tuberosity | **L5, S1** | Knee flexion |
| *S4-S5* | Perianal region | **L4** | Ankle dorsiflexion |
| | | **S1, S2** | Ankle plantarflexion |

| REFLEXES | | | |
|---|---|---|---|
| **S1, S2** | Ankle | Ankle | Great toe extension |
| **L2, L3, L4** | Knee | **S1** | Great toe flexion |
| **C5, C6** | biceps | | |
| **C7,8** | Triceps | | |
| **S3-S4** | Anal wink | | |

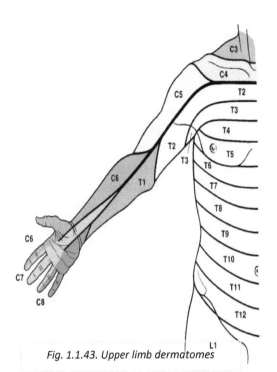

Fig. 1.1.43. Upper limb dermatomes

# 12. REFERRED PAIN

| | STRUCTURES | PAIN TO: |
|---|---|---|
| *1* | Diaphragm | • Ipsilateral shoulder tip |
| *2* | Heart | • T1-5 |
| | | • Left arm and hand |
| *3* | Oesophagus | • T5-6 |
| | Stomach | • T6-9 |
| | | • Chest and substernal area |
| *4* | Pancreas | • T6-10 |
| *5* | Liver and gallbladder | • T7-9 |
| *6* | Small intestine | • T9-10 |
| *7* | Large intestine | • T11-12 |
| *8* | Rectum | • S2-4 |
| | | • Sacrum, lower back and dorsum of leg |
| *9* | Ovaries | • T10-11 |
| | | • Periumbilical area |
| *10* | Uterus | • S1-2 |
| | | • Lower back |
| *11* | Prostate | • T10-11 |
| | | • Periumbilical, penis and scrotum |
| *12* | Kidneys | • T10-L1 |
| | | • Lower back and umbilical area |

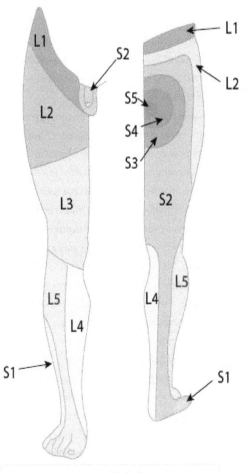

Fig. 1.1.44. Lower limb dermatomes

# PAST ASKED QUESTIONS

### An upper brachial plexus injury

- Is caused by damage to C5 and C6 nerve roots — T
- Mainly affects the small muscles of the hand — F
- Results in loss of supination at the radio-ulnar joint — T
- Is often associated with a Horner's syndrome — F

### Regarding Upper Limbs nerves:

- Axillary nerve function is needed to abduct the shoulder to 90° — T
- The axillary nerve does not have sensory fibres — F
- The Median nerve comes from the Medial and lateral cord of the brachial plexus — T
- Radial nerve compression at the axilla causes weakness of the elbow extension — T
- Radial nerve provides sensation to the thenar eminence — F
- Damage to the Radial nerve from humeral fracture causes loss of pronation — F
- Damage to the radial nerve at the wrist causes wrist drop — F
- Median nerve injury at the elbow causes extensive deformity of the index finger — T
- Carpal tunnel syndrome causes loss of sensation in the palm — F
- Median nerve injury causes loss of thumb opposition — T
- Ulnar nerve injury at the elbow causes worse Clawing than at the wrist — F
- Ulnar nerve injury at the wrist causes loss of sensation from the back of the little finger — F

### An upper brachial plexus injury

- Is caused by damage to C5 and C6 nerve roots — T
- Mainly affects the small muscles of the hand — F
- Results in loss of supination at the radio-ulnar joint — T
- Is often associated with a Horner's syndrome — F

### Regarding Upper Limbs nerves:

- Axillary nerve function is needed to abduct the shoulder to 90° — T
- The axillary nerve does not have sensory fibres — F
- The Median nerve comes from the Medial and lateral cord of the brachial plexus — T
- Radial nerve compression at the axilla causes weakness of the elbow extension — T
- Radial nerve provides sensation to the thenar eminence — F
- Damage to the Radial nerve from humeral fracture causes loss of pronation — F

### Regarding movements at the shoulder joint:

- The muscles of the rotator cuff are supraspinatus, infraspinatus, subscapularis and teres major — F
- Infraspinatus laterally abducts (externally rotates) the shoulder — T
- The scapula acts in abduction of the arm beyond 120 degrees — T
- Axillary nerve damage causes paralysis of deltoid — T
- Difficulty in initiating abduction suggests injury of supraspinatus — T
- Subscapularis externally rotates the arm — F
- The rotator cuff is strongest inferiorly — F
- Damage to the long thoracic nerve may give weakness of shoulder abduction beyond 90° — T
- Many brachial plexus injuries arise from clavicle fracture — F
- Infraspinatus internally rotates the humerus — F
- Axillary nerve damage may give deltoid paralysis — T
- The long head of biceps inserts onto the acromion — F

### Which statements regarding the radial nerve are true?

| | |
|---|---|
| a. It is formed from posterior cord of brachial plexus | T |
| b. It supplies muscles of the posterior upper limb | T |
| c. Radial nerve injury causes weakness of finger extension | T |
| d. It supplies sensation to skin of dorsum of little finger | F |

### Median nerve injury at wrist gives the following functional deficit

| | |
|---|---|
| a. Loss of opposition of the thumb | T |
| b. Paralysis of the third and fourth lumbricals | F |
| c. Wrist flexion is weakened | F |
| d. Median nerve compression in the carpal tunnel gives anaesthesia over the thenar eminence | F |
| e. Loss of thumb adduction (adductor pollicis is innervated by ulnar nerve) | F |

### Regarding the Cubital fossa:

| | |
|---|---|
| • The Brachial artery is medial to the Median nerve | F |
| • The Brachial artery lies medial to the biceps tendon | T |
| • Pronator teres and Brachioradialis form the floor of the ACF | F |
| • The Median Cubital vein connect the Basilic to the Cephalic veins | T |
| • The radial head is subcutaneous | T |
| • The ossification of the trochlea precedes that of the medial epicondyle | F |
| • The trochlea articulates with the radial head | F |
| • The anterior humeral line bisects capitellum at all ages | T |
| • Medial humeral epicondyle is a common site of insertion of extensors | F |

### Regarding the anatomical snuff box

| | |
|---|---|
| a. It is bounded on lateral (radial) side by extensor pollicis brevis and the tendon of abductor pollicis longus | T |
| b. It is bounded on medial (ulnar) side by the tendons of extensor digitorum | F |
| c. Its contents include the radial artery and superficial branch of the radial nerve | T |
| d. Deep to it lies scaphoid and trapezium | T |

### True or False

| | |
|---|---|
| • Innervation of the forearm flexors excluding the FCU is via the Median nerve | T |
| • The common interosseous artery arises from the Ulnar artery | T |
| • The Allen's test is used to assess the patency of the Radial artery | F |
| • Innervation of the ring finger is by the Ulnar and median nerves | F |
| • The volar interossei are responsible for finger adduction | T |
| • The thenar muscles have ulnar innervation | F |
| • The middle finger is in C7 dermatome | T |
| • C5 dermatome is adjacent to T2 dermatome | F |
| • T10: Umbilicus | T |
| • T2: Axilla | T |
| • S1: Big toe | F |
| • C8: Thumb | F |

### Which nerve supplies to the following muscles of the hand are correct?

| | |
|---|---|
| a. Adductor pollicis: Ulnar nerve | T |
| b. 3rd Lumbrical: Ulnar nerve | T |
| c. 2nd Dorsal interosseous: Median nerve | F |
| d. Flexor digiti minimi: Radial | F |

# SECTION 2: LOWER LIMB

## I. ANTERIOR THIGH

### A. SUPERFICIAL ARTERIES

**1. Cutaneous arteries**
- Arise from the femoral artery.

### B. SUPERFICIAL VEINS

- The superficial veins of the lower limb run in the subcutaneous tissue.
- There are two major superficial veins:
  - **The Great Saphenous Vein**
  - **The Small Saphenous Vein.**

### THE GREAT SAPHENOUS VEIN

- The Great Saphenous Vein is formed by the dorsal venous **arch of the foot,** and the dorsal vein of **the great toe.**
- It ascends up the medial side of the leg, passing anteriorly to the medial malleolus at the ankle, and posteriorly to the medial condyle at the knee.
- As the vein moves up the leg, it receives tributaries from other small superficial veins.
- The great saphenous vein then courses anteriorly to lie on the anterior surface of the thigh before entering an opening in the fascia lata called **the saphenous opening.**
- It forms an arch, the saphenous arch, to join the common femoral vein in the region of the femoral triangle at the sapheno-femoral junction.

### THE SMALL SAPHENOUS VEIN

- The Small Saphenous Vein is formed by the dorsal venous **arch of the foot**, and the dorsal vein of **the little toe.**
- It moves up the posterior side of the leg, passing posteriorly to the lateral malleolus, along the lateral border of the calcaneal tendon.
- It moves between the two heads of the gastrocnemius muscle and empties into the popliteal vein in the popliteal fossa.

### C. LYMPH NODES / VESSELS

- **Location:** immediately below the inguinal ligament.
  - There are approximately 10 superficial lymph nodes.
  - They lie deep to Camper's fascia which overlies the femoral vessels at medial aspect of the thigh.
- **Drainage to:** the deep inguinal lymph nodes
- **Source:** They receive as afferents lymphatic vessels from the following:
  - Integument of the penis, scrotum, perineum, buttock, abdominal wall below the level of the umbilicus, back below the level of the iliac crest, vulva, anus (below the pectinate line)
- **Divisions: They are divided into three groups:**
  - **Supramedial or Superomedial**
  - **Superolateral**
  - **Inferior**
- **Location:** Medial to the femoral vein and under the cribriform fascia.
  - There are approximately 3 to 5 deep nodes. Most nodes are located under the inguinal ligament and is called Cloquet's node.
- **Source:**
  - Superficial inguinal lymph nodes
  - Popliteal lymph nodes
- **Drainage:**
  - **Superiorly:** to the external iliac lymph nodes, then to the pelvic lymph nodes and on to the paraaortic lymph nodes.

### D. FEMORAL TRIANGLE

- **Boundaries: Mnemonic SAIL**
  - **Lateral**: medial border of **S**artorious.
  - **Medial**: medial border of **A**dductor longus.
  - **Superior**: **I**nguinal Ligament.
  - **Floor**: Adductor Longus, Iliopsoas, and Pectineus.
  - **Roof**: skin, subcutaneous tissue, a continuation of Scarpa's fascia, Great Saphenous Vein (joins the femoral vein), superficial lymph nodes.
- **Contents: Mnemonic NAVEL (From lateral to medial):**

- o  Femoral **N**erve: Directly behind sheath
- o  Femoral **A**rtery and its branches: within sheath
- o  Femoral **V**ein, and deep lymph nodes: within sheath
- o  Femoral canal (**E**mpty space): between vein and LN
- o  Contains fat and **L**ymph node (Lymph Node of Cloquet)

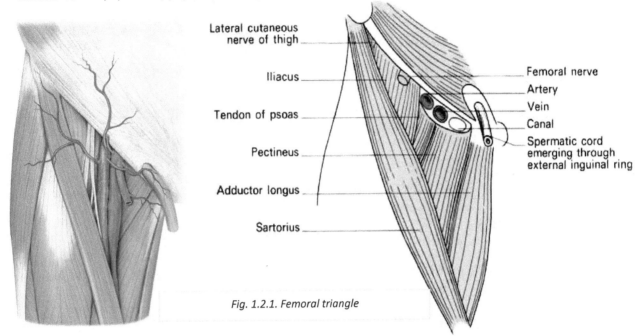

Fig. 1.2.1. Femoral triangle

## E. FEMORAL SHEATH

- o  This oval, funnel-shaped fascial tube **encloses the proximal parts of the femoral vessels**, which lie inferior to the inguinal ligament.
- o  It is a diverticulum or inferior prolongation of the fasciae lining of the abdomen: **Trasversalis fascia anteriorly and iliac fascia posteriorly**.
- o  It is covered by the fascia lata.
- o  Its presence allows the femoral artery and vein to glide in and out, deep to the inguinal ligament, during movements of the hip joint.
- o  *The sheath does not project into the thigh when the thigh is fully flexed, but is drawn further into the femoral triangle when the thigh is extended.*
- o  Subdivided by two vertical septa into three compartments:
  - **Lateral compartment** for femoral artery
  - **Intermediate compartment** for femoral vein
  - **Medial compartment** or space called femoral canal.

## F. FEMORAL CANAL

- **Bordered: LAMP-FILP**
  - o  **L**aterally by the **F**emoral vein.
  - o  **A**nteriorly by the **I**nguinal ligament.
  - o  **M**edially by the **L**acunar ligament.
  - o  **P**osteriorly by the **P**ectineal ligament
- *It contains the lymph node of Cloquet.*
- *The entrance to the femoral canal is the femoral ring, through which bowel can sometimes enter, causing a femoral hernia.*

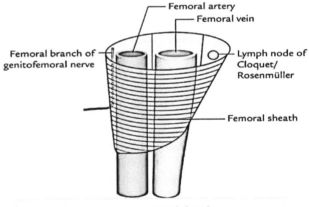

Fig. 1.2.2. Femoral sheath

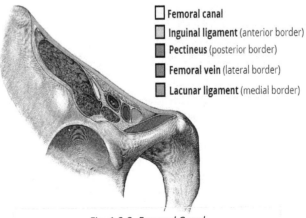

☐ Femoral canal
☐ Inguinal ligament (anterior border)
☐ Pectineus (posterior border)
☐ Femoral vein (lateral border)
☐ Lacunar ligament (medial border)

Fig. 1.2.3. Femoral Canal

## G. MUSCLES AND MOVEMENTS

### A. SARTORIUS
- Action: flexion, abduction and lateral rotation hip, flexion knee
- Innervation: femoral nerve

### B. ILIACUS
- Action: flexes and rotates laterally thigh
- Innervation: femoral nerve

### C. PSOAS MAJOR
- Action: flexion hip joint
- Innervation: lumbar plexus via ant. branches L1-L3

### D. PECTINEUS
- Action: thigh flexion, adduction
- Innervation: femoral nerve, sometimes obturator nerve.

### E. QUADRICEPS FEMORIS
(Rectus femoris, Vasti lateralis, intermedius and medialis)
- Action: knee extension, hip flexion
- Nerve: Femoral

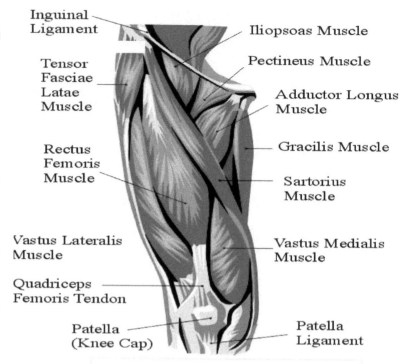

Fig. 1.2.4. Muscles of anterior thigh

## H. FEMORAL ARTERY

- It is a large artery in the thigh and the main arterial supply to the lower limb. It enters the thigh from **behind the inguinal ligament** as the *common femoral artery*, a continuation of the **external iliac artery**. Then lies midway between the anterior superior iliac spine and the symphysis pubis.
- The common femoral artery gives off the *profunda femoris artery* and becomes the *superficial femoral artery* to descend along the anteromedial part of the thigh in the femoral triangle.
- It enters and passes through the adductor (subsartorial) canal, and becomes the *popliteal artery* as it passes through an opening in adductor magnus near the junction of the middle and distal thirds of the thigh.

**BRANCHES:**
- Superficial Epigastric Artery
  - Superficial Iliac Circumflex
  - Superficial External Pudendal
  - Deep External Pudendal
  - Deep Femoral Artery (Profunda Femoris); Its branches:
  Put My Leg Down Please:
  - **P:** Profunda Femoris artery
  - **M:** Medial Circumflex Femoral artery.
  - **L:** Lateral Circumflex Femoral artery.
  - **D:** Descending Branch of The Lateral Circumflex Femoral Artery
  - **P:** Perforating Arteries

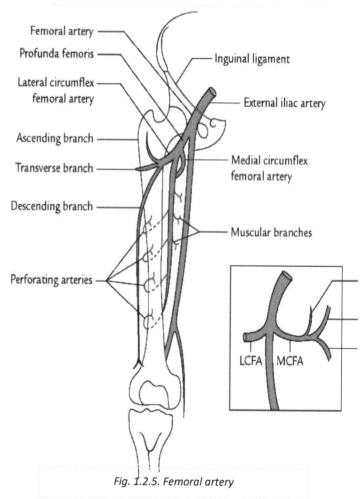

Fig. 1.2.5. Femoral artery

## I. FEMORAL VEIN

- The femoral vein is a blood vessel that accompanies the femoral artery in the femoral sheath. It begins at the **adductor canal** (also known as *Hunter's canal)* and is a continuation of the popliteal vein.
- It ends at the inferior margin of the inguinal ligament, where it becomes the external iliac vein.
- Drainage: Several large veins drain into the femoral vein:
  - **Popliteal vein**
  - **Profunda femoris vein**
  - **Great saphenous vein**

## J. FEMORAL NERVE

- **Derivation:**
  - From the dorsal divisions of the ventral rami of the **L2- L4**.

- **Surface marking:**
  - Descends through the fibers of the psoas major muscle, emerging from the muscle at the lower part of its lateral border, and passes down between it and the iliacus muscle, behind the iliac fascia;
  - It then runs **beneath the inguinal ligament**, into the thigh, and splits into an anterior and a posterior division. Under the inguinal ligament, it is separated from the femoral artery by a portion of the psoas major.

- **Terminal Branches**
  - **Anterior Division Branches**
    - ✓ Medial cutaneous nerve of thigh
    - ✓ Intermediate cutaneous nerve
    - ✓ Motor branch to sartorius
    - ✓ Motor branch to pectineus

  - **Posterior Division Branches**
    - ✓ **Saphenous nerve:** provides sensation to anteromedial aspect of lower leg.
    - ✓ **Motor branches to** Rectus femoris, Vasti medialis, lateralis and intermedius.
    - ✓ **Articular branches to knee:** provides cutaneous innervation to the skin anteriorly over the patella.

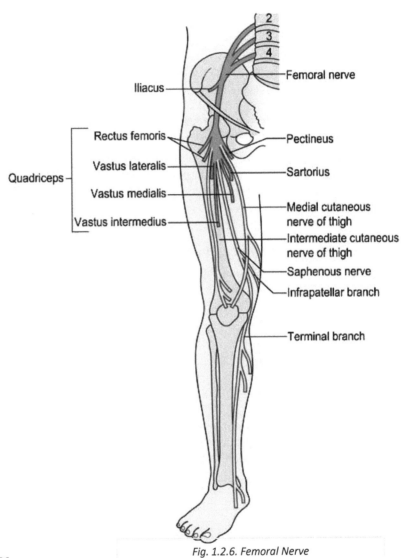

Fig. 1.2.6. Femoral Nerve

## CLINICAL: FEMORAL NERVE INJURY

- **Causes**
  - Direct trauma is most common
  - Iatrogenic (i.e. Percutaneous proximal interlocking screw placement through IM nail)
  - Compression from tumor or hematoma

- **Clinical Signs**
  - **Motor**
    - Quadriceps wasting and Loss of knee extension and some hip flexion (iliacus, pectineus)

  - **Sensory**
    - Loss of sensation over front and medial side of thigh **(anterior and medial cutaneous nerves of the thigh).**
    - Loss of sensation over medial aspect of lower leg and foot **(saphenous nerve).**

# II. MEDIAL THIGH

## A. MUSCLES AND MOVEMENTS

The adductors role: medial femoral rotation

### 1. ADDUCTORS LONGUS
- Action: adduction and flexion hip
- Innervation: anterior branch Obturator nerve

### 2. ADDUCTORS BREVIS
- Action: adduction hip
- Innervation: Obturator nerve

### 3. ADDUCTORS MAGNUS
- Action: adduction hip (both portions), flexion hip (adductor portion), extension hip (harmstring portion)
- Innervation: Posterior branch Obturator nerve (adductor) and tibial nerve (harmstring)

### 4. OBTURATOR EXTERNUS
- Action: adducts thigh, rotate laterally thigh
- Innervation: posterior branch obturator nerve L3-L4

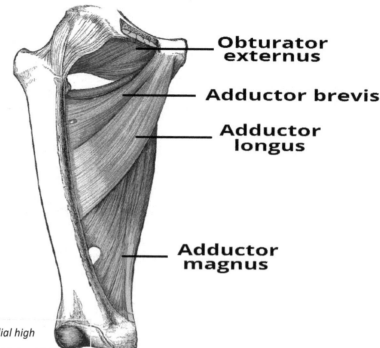

*Fig. 1.2.7. Muscles of Medial high*

## B. ARTERIES AND NERVES

### 1. THE PROFUNDA FEMORIS
- **Source:** Femoral artery.

- **Branches:** My Leg Down Please
  - **M:** medial circumflex femoral artery
  - **L:** lateral circumflex femoral artery
  - **D:** descending branch of the lateral circumflex femoral artery
  - **P:** perforating arteries

### 2. OBTURATOR ARTERY
- **Source:** internal iliac artery
- **Branches:** ant and post branches
- **Supplies:** obturator externus muscle, medial compartment thigh, femur.

### 3. OBTURATOR NERVE
- **From:** lumbar plexus **L2-L4**
- **To:** post branch obturator nerve, Ant branch Obturator
- **Innervates:** medial compartment Thigh

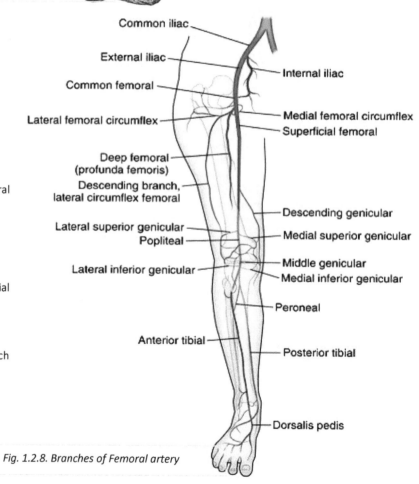

*Fig. 1.2.8. Branches of Femoral artery*

# III. HIP JOINT & GLUTEAL REGION

## A. MUSCLES AND MOVEMENTS

### 1. GLUTEUS MAXIMUS
o  **Action:**
- External rotation and extension hip joint.
- Supports the extended knee through the iliotibial tract.
- Chief antigravity muscle in sitting and abduction of the hip.

o  **Innervation**: inferior gluteal nerve (L5-S2)

### 2. GLUTEUS MEDIUS
o  **Action:** Major abductor of thigh; anterior fibers help to rotate hip medially; posterior fibers help to rotate hip laterally.
o  **Innervation**: superior gluteal nerve (L4-S1)

### 3. GLUTEUS MINIMUS
o  **Action**: Abducts and medially rotates the hip joint.
o  **Innervation**: superior gluteal nerve (L4-S1)

### 4. PIRIFORMIS
o  **Action**: external rotator thigh
o  **Innervation**: inferior gluteal, lateral sacral and superior gluteal

Note:  piriformis, obturator internus and quadratus femoris as synergistic femoral lateral rotators and hip stabilizers.

### 5. TENSOR FASCIAE LATAE
- **Action:**
  o  Thigh: flexion, medial rotation, abduction
  o  Leg: lateral rotation
  o  Torso: stabilization
- **Innervation**: Superior gluteal nerve (L4-S1)
- **Artery:** Primarily lateral circumflex femoral artery, superior gluteal artery.

## B. SCIATIC NERVE
- The Sciatic Nerve originates from lumbosacral plexus **L4-S3**
  o  **Tibial division**
    - Originates from anterior preaxial branches of **L4-S3**
  o  **Peroneal division**
    - Originates from postaxial branches of **L4-S2**

- **COURSE:**
  o  **Exits sciatic notch**
    - Runs anterior or deep to piriformis
    - Runs posterior or superficial to short external rotators (superior and inferior gemellus, obturator internus)

  o  **Posterior leg**
    - It then runs down the posterior leg where it breaks into its three main divisions at the level of the mid-thigh.

  o  **Terminal branches**
    - Common peroneal nerve
    - Tibial nerve

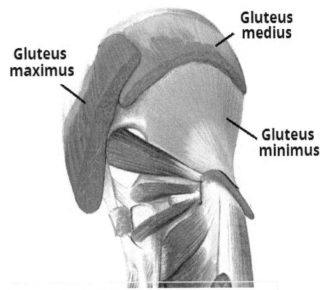

*Fig. 1.2.9. Muscles of Gluteal region*

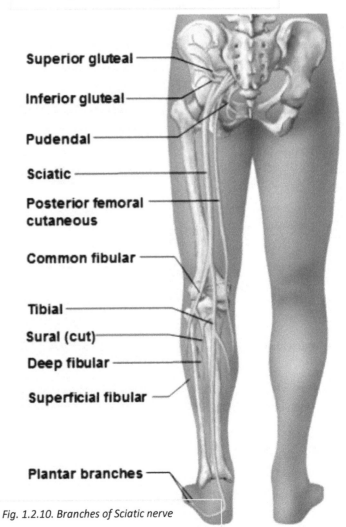

*Fig. 1.2.10. Branches of Sciatic nerve*

## C. HIP JOINT

- The **hip joint** is a synovial joint between the femoral head and the acetabulum of the pelvis.
- **Articulation:** ball and socket joint between the head of the femur and the acetabulum
- **Ligaments:** ischiofemoral, iliofemoral, pubofemoral and transverse acetabular ligaments, and the ligamentum teres
- **Movements:** thigh flexion and extension, adduction and abduction, internal and external rotation
- **Muscles:** There are a number of different muscles that permit flexion/extension, adduction/abduction, and internal/external rotation of the hip joint. (see below)
- **Bursae:** Subtendinous, iliopectineal and greater trochanteric bursae, and bursae between gluteus maximus and vastus lateralis exist near the joint .

### BLOOD SUPPLY

- **Cruciate anastomosis**
  - ✓ Transverse branch of medial circumflex femoral artery
  - ✓ Transverse branch of lateral circumflex femoral artery
  - ✓ Ascending branch of first perforator artery from profunda femoris artery
  - ✓ Descending branch of inferior gluteal artery
  - ✓ Obturator artery
- **Trochanteric anastomosis**
  - ✓ Descending branch of superior gluteal artery
  - ✓ Ascending branch of medial circumflex femoral artery
  - ✓ Ascending branch of lateral circumflex femoral artery
  - ✓ Often joined by inferior gluteal artery

### LYMPHATIC DRAINAGE

- Anterior hip joint drains to deep inguinal nodes
- Posterior and medial hip joint drain to internal iliac nodes

### INNERVATION

- There is nerve supply to the femeroacetabular joint provided by the femoral, obturator and superior gluteal nerves, and the nerve to quadratus femoris .

## D. SUMMARY OF HIP MOVEMENTS

| ACTION | MUSCLES |
|---|---|
| • **Flexion: STRIPA** | ✓ Sartorius<br>✓ Tensor fascia latae<br>✓ Rectus femoris<br>✓ Iliopsoas<br>✓ Pectineus<br>✓ Adductors (A. Magnus only adductor portion) |
| • **Extension: G-BASS** | ✓ Gluteus maximus,<br>✓ Biceps femoris<br>✓ Adductor Magnus (Harmstring portion)<br>✓ Semimembranosus,<br>✓ Semitendinosus |
| • **Abduction: 3G** | ✓ Gluteus medius,<br>✓ Gluteus minimus<br>✓ Deep Gluteals (Piriformis, Gemelli etc.) |
| • **Adduction: APG** | ✓ Adductors (including Obturator externus),<br>✓ Pectineus<br>✓ Gracillis |
| • **Lateral rotation:  BOQS- 3G** | ✓ Biceps femoris,<br>✓ Obturator externus/internus<br>✓ Quadratus femoris<br>✓ Sartorius<br>✓ Gluteus maximus<br>✓ Gluteus medius (posterior fibers only)<br>✓ Deep Gluteals (piriformis, gemelli etc.) |
| • **Medial rotation: 2G 2S** | ✓ Gluteus medius<br>✓ Gluteus minimus,<br>✓ Semitendinosus<br>✓ Semimembranosus |

# IV. POSTERIOR THIGH COMPARTMENT

## A. MUSCLES AND MOVEMENTS

### 1. HAMSTRINGS:

- The tibial and common fibular (peroneal) nerves are both branches of the sciatic nerve

| MUSCLE | ORIGIN | INSERTION | ACTIONS | NERVE |
|---|---|---|---|---|
| Semitendinosus | Ischial tuberosity | Medial surface of tibia | Flexion Knee<br><br>Extension of hip joint | Tibial |
| Semimembranosus | | Medial tibial condyle | | |
| Biceps femoris<br><br>Long head | Ischial tuberosity | Lateral side of the head of the fibula | Flexes Knee<br><br>Laterally rotates knee (when knee is flexed), | Tibial |
| Biceps femoris<br><br>Short head | Linea aspera and<br><br>Lateral supra-condylar line of femur | Lateral side of the head of the fibula (common tendon with the long head) | Extends Hip (long head only) | Common peroneal |

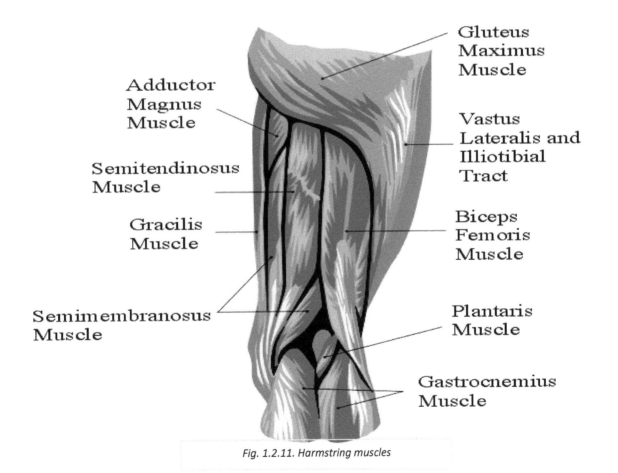

*Fig. 1.2.11. Harmstring muscles*

# V. POPLITEAL FOSSA AND KNEE

## A. BOUNDARIES AND COMPOSITION

- **Borders**
  - ○ **Superiomedial border**: semimembranosus (and semitendinosus)
  - ○ **Superiolateral border**: biceps femoris.
  - ○ **Inferiomedial border:** medial head of the gastrocnemius.
  - ○ **Inferiolateral border:** lateral head of the gastrocnemius and plantaris.

- **Floor:**
  - ○ the posterior surface of the knee joint capsule,
  - ○ By the posterior surface of the femur.

- **Roof:**
  - ○ Popliteal fascia and
  - ○ Skin.

- **Contents** (medial to lateral):
  - ○ Popliteal artery
  - ○ Popliteal vein
  - ○ Tibial nerve
  - ○ Common fibular nerve

*The Tibial and Common Fibular Nerves are the most superficial structures of the popliteal fossa; the deepest structure is the Popliteal Artery.*

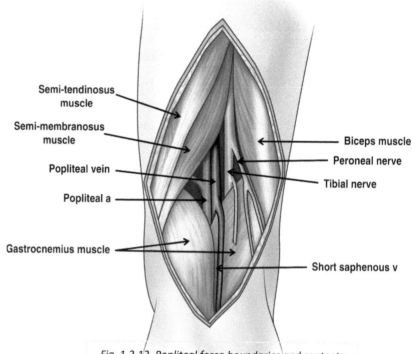

*Fig. 1.2.12. Popliteal fossa boundaries and contents*

## B. MUSCLES AND MOVEMENTS

- ○ **Popliteus:**
  - ▪ **Actions** (on the femur / tibia and its role in lateral meniscus movement):
    - ✓ Medially rotates tibia on the femur if the femur is fixed (sitting down)
    - ✓ Laterally rotates femur on the tibia if tibia is fixed (standing up),
    - ✓ Unlocks the knee to allow flexion (bending),
    - ✓ Helps to prevent the forward dislocation of the femur while crouching.

  - ▪ **Innervation**: Tibial nerve

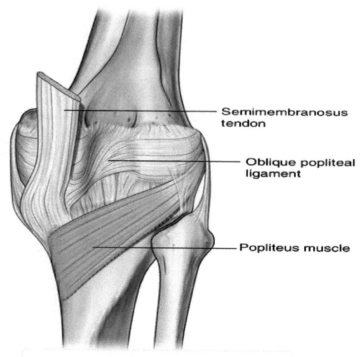

*Fig. 1.2.13. Popliteus muscle*

# VI. KNEE JOINT

## 1. ARTICULATING SURFACES
o   The knee joint consists of two articulations:
- **The Tibiofemoral Joint:** is the weightbearing joint of the knee.
- **The Patellofemoral Joint:** allows the tendon of the quadriceps femoris (the main extensor of the knee) to be inserted directly over the knee, increasing the efficiency of the muscle.

## 2. MENISCI
- The Medial and Lateral Menisci are fibrocartilage structures in the knee that serve two functions:
  o   To deepen the articular surface of the tibia, thus increasing stability of the joint.
  o   To act as shock absorbers.
- *Any damage to the tibial collateral ligament results in tearing of the medial meniscus.*
- The lateral meniscus is smaller and does not have any extra attachments, rendering it fairly mobile.

## 3. BURSAE
- There are five bursae in the knee joint.
  o   **Suprapatella bursa**
  o   **Prepatella bursa**
  o   **Infrapatella bursa (deep and superficial)**
  o   **Semimembranosus bursa**

## 4. LIGAMENTS
- *Patellar ligament:* A continuation of the quadriceps femoris tendon distal to the patella. It attaches to the tibial tuberosity.
- *Collateral ligaments:* They act to stabilise the hinge motion of the knee, preventing any medial or lateral movement
  o   *Tibial (Medial) Collateral Ligament:* Proximally, it attaches to the medial epicondyle of the femur, distally it attaches to the medial surface of the tibia.
  o   *Fibular (Lateral) Collateral Ligament:* attaches proximally to the lateral epicondyle of the femur, distally it attaches to a depression on the lateral surface of the fibular head.

- *Cruciate Ligaments:* these two ligaments connect the femur and the tibia. In doing so, they cross each other, hence the term 'cruciate'.
  o   *Anterior Cruciate Ligament:* attaches at the anterior intercondylar region of the tibia and ascends posteriorly to attach to the femur, in the intercondylar fossa. **It prevents anterior dislocation of the tibia onto the femur.**
  o   *Posterior Cruciate Ligament:* attaches at the posterior intercondylar region of the tibia, and ascends anteriorly to attach to the femur in the intercondylar fossa. **It prevents posterior dislocation of the tibia onto the femur**

## 5. KNEE MOVEMENTS
o   There are 4 main movements that the knee joint permits:
- **Extension:**
  ✓ Quadriceps femoris (inserts into the tibial tuberosity).
- **Flexion: HARMSTRINGS + GPS**
  ✓ Hamstrings,
  ✓ Gracilis,
  ✓ Popliteus
  ✓ Sartorius
  ✓ Also, Gastrocnemius and Plantaris
- **Lateral rotation:**
  ✓ Biceps femoris.

- **Medial rotation:**
  ✓ Semimembranosus and semitendinosus (**+ GPS**)
  ✓ Gracilis,
  ✓ Popliteus
  ✓ Sartorius

*Lateral and medial rotation can only occur when the knee is flexed (if the knee is not flexed, the medial/lateral rotation occurs at the hip joint).*

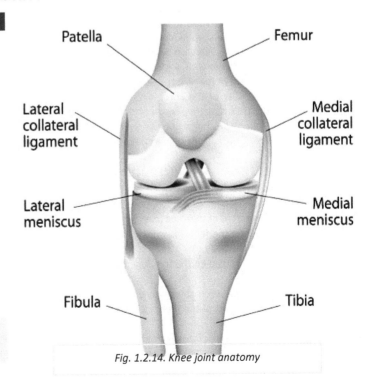

*Fig. 1.2.14. Knee joint anatomy*

## CLINICAL RELEVANCE

### 1. STRENGTH OF THE KNEE JOINT

- The strength of the knee joint depends on the strength of the ligaments that bind the femur to the tibia and on the tone of the muscles acting on the joint.
- The most important muscle group is the quadriceps femoris; provided that this is well developed, it is capable of stabilizing the knee in the presence of torn ligaments.

### 2. KNEE INJURY AND THE SYNOVIAL MEMBRANE

- The synovial membrane of the knee joint is extensive, and if the articular surfaces, menisci, or ligaments of the joint are damaged, the large synovial cavity becomes distended with fluid.
- The wide communication between the suprapatellar bursa and the joint cavity results in this structure becoming distended also.
- The swelling of the knee extends three or four fingerbreadths above the patella and laterally and medially beneath the aponeuroses of insertion of the vastus lateralis and medialis, respectively.

### 3. LIGAMENTOUS INJURY OF THE KNEE JOINT

- Four ligaments—the medial collateral ligament, the lateral collateral ligament, the ACL, and the PCL—are commonly injured in the knee.
- Sprains or tears occur depending on the degree of force applied.
- **MEDIAL COLLATERAL LIGAMENT**
  - Forced abduction of the tibia on the femur can result in partial tearing of the medial collateral ligament, which can occur at its femoral or tibial attachments.
  - It is useful to remember that tears of the menisci result in localized tenderness on the joint line, whereas sprains of the medial collateral ligament result in tenderness over the femoral or tibial attachments of the ligament.
- **LATERAL COLLATERAL LIGAMENT**
  - Forced adduction of the tibia on the femur can result in injury to the lateral collateral ligament (less common than medial ligament injury).
- **CRUCIATE LIGAMENTS**
  - Injury to the cruciate ligaments can occur when excessive force is applied to the knee joint.

- **TEARS OF THE ACL**
  - Are common.
  - It is the most frequently injured ligament in the body, for which surgery is performed.
  - The condition is more common in women and this may be explained by the different alignment of the thigh on the leg in women associated with the wider pelvis.
  - There is also an increased risk in women during the preovulatory phase of the menstrual cycle, possibly due to the influence of the female sex hormones.

- **TEARS OF THE PCL**
  - Are rare. Injury to the cruciate ligaments is always accompanied by damage to other knee structures; the collateral ligaments are commonly torn, or the capsule may be damaged.
  - The joint cavity quickly fills with blood (**hemarthrosis**) so that the joint is swollen.
  - Examination of patients with a ruptured anterior cruciate ligament shows that the tibia can be pulled excessively forward on the femur; with rupture of the posterior cruciate ligament, the tibia can be made to move excessively backward on the femur.
  - Because the stability of the knee joint depends largely on the tone of the quadriceps femoris muscle and the integrity of the collateral ligaments, operative repair of isolated torn cruciate ligaments is not always attempted.
  - The knee is immobilized in slight flexion in a cast, and active physiotherapy on the quadriceps femoris muscle is begun at once. Should, however, the capsule of the joint and the collateral ligaments be torn in addition, early operative repair is essential.

### 4. MENISCAL INJURY OF THE KNEE JOINT

- Injuries of the menisci are common.
- The medial meniscus is damaged much more frequently than the lateral, and this is probably because of its strong attachment to the medial collateral ligament of the knee joint, which restricts its mobility.
- The injury occurs when the femur is rotated on the tibia, or the tibia is rotated on the femur, with the knee joint partially flexed and taking the weight of the body.
- The tibia is usually abducted on the femur, and the medial meniscus is pulled into an abnormal position between the femoral and tibial condyles.
- A sudden movement between the condyles results in the meniscus being subjected to a severe grinding force, and it splits along its length. When the torn part of the meniscus becomes wedged between the articular surfaces, further movement is impossible, and the joint is said to "lock."
- Injury to the lateral meniscus is less common, probably because it is not attached to the lateral collateral ligament of the knee joint and is consequently more mobile. The popliteus muscle sends a few of its fibers into the lateral meniscus, and these can pull the meniscus into a more favourable position during sudden movements of the knee joint

# VII. ANTERIOR LEG COMPARTMENT

**SUMMARY**

- **Common Action:**
  - **Dorsiflex and Invert** the foot at the ankle joint.
  - The Extensor Digitorum Longus and Extensor Hallucis Longus **also extend the toes**.
- **Innervation:**
  - **Deep Peroneal Nerve (L4-L5).**
- **Blood supply:**
  - Anterior Tibial Artery.
- **Muscles: TEEP**
  - **T**ibialis anterior
  - **E**xtensor hallucis longus
  - **E**xtensor digitorum longus
  - **P**eroneus tertius

**STRUCTURES PASSING DEEP TO EXTENSOR RETINACULUM OF FOOT (From medial to lateral side):**

**TEEP + ARTERY + NERVE**

- Tibialis anterior,
- Extensor Hallucis longus,
- Extensor Digitorum longus,
- Peroneus tertius
- Anterior tibial artery,
- Deep peroneal Nerve

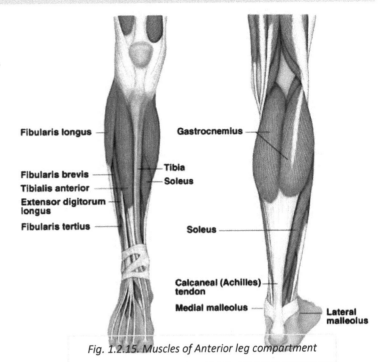

Labels: Fibularis longus, Gastrocnemius, Fibularis brevis, Tibia, Tibialis anterior, Soleus, Extensor digitorum longus, Fibularis tertius, Soleus, Calcaneal (Achilles) tendon, Medial malleolus, Lateral malleolus

*Fig. 1.2.15. Muscles of Anterior leg compartment*

# VIII. DORSUM OF THE FOOT

- The muscles acting on the foot can be divided into two distinct groups:
- **The extrinsic muscles:**
  - Arise from the anterior, posterior and lateral compartments of the leg.
  - They are mainly responsible for actions such as *eversion, inversion, plantarflexion and dorsiflexion of the foot*.
- **The intrinsic muscles:**
  - Located within the foot and are responsible for the more fine motor actions of the foot, for example *movement of individual digits*.

## INTRINSIC MUSLES OF DORSAL ASPECT

- There are only two intrinsic muscles located in this compartment – the Extensor Digitorum Brevis, and the Extensor Hallucis Brevis.
- They are mainly responsible for assisting some of the extrinsic muscles in their actions.
- **Innervation:** Both muscles are innervated by the **Deep Fibular Nerve.**

### 1. EXTENSOR DIGITORUM BREVIS

- **Attachments**: from the calcaneus, the interosseous talocalcaneal ligament and the inferior extensor retinaculum. It attaches to the long extensor tendons of the four medial digits.
- **Actions**: Aids the extensor digitorum longus in extending the medial four toes at the metatarsophalangeal and interphalangeal joints.
- **Innervation**: Deep fibular nerve.

### 2. EXTENSOR HALLUCIS BREVIS

- *The Extensor Hallucis Brevis muscle is medial to Extensor Digitorum Longus and lateral to Extensor Hallucis Longus.*
- **Attachments**: Originates from the calcaneus, the interosseous talocalcaneal ligament and the inferior extensor retinaculum. It attaches to the base of the proximal phalanx of the great toe.
- **Actions**: Aids the extensor hallucis longus in extending the great toe at the metatarsophalangeal joint.
- **Innervation**: Deep fibular nerve.

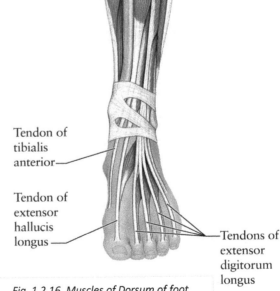

Labels: Tendon of tibialis anterior, Tendon of extensor hallucis longus, Tendons of extensor digitorum longus

*Fig. 1.2.16. Muscles of Dorsum of foot*

# IX. LATERAL LEG COMPARTEMENT

- **Two Muscles:** Fibularis/ Peroneus Longus and Brevis.
- **Innervation:** **Superficial Peroneal Nerve (L4-S1).**
- **Common Action:** **Eversion** and fix the medial margin of the foot during running, and preventing excessive inversion.

## 1. PERONEUS LONGUS

➢ **Attachments:**
  - ○ The fibularis longus originates from the superior and lateral surface of the fibula and the lateral tibial condyle.
  - ○ The fibres converge into a tendon, which descends into the foot, **posterior to the lateral malleolus.**
  - ○ The tendon then crosses under the foot, and attaches to the bones on the medial side, namely the **medial cuneiform** and **base of metatarsal I.**
- **Actions:** Eversion and plantarflexion of the foot. Also, supports the lateral and transverse arches of the foot.
- **Innervation:** Superficial fibular nerve, L4-S1.

## 2. PERONEUS BREVIS

- The fibularis brevis muscle is deeper and shorter than the fibularis longus.
- **Attachments:**
  - ○ It originates from the inferior and lateral surface of the fibular shaft. The muscle belly forms a tendon, which descends with the fibularis longus tendon. It travels into the foot, posterior to the lateral malleolus, passing over the calcaneus and the cuboidal bones.
  - ○ The tendon of the fibularis brevis attaches **to a tubercle on metatarsal V.**
- **Actions:** Eversion of the foot.
- **Innervation:** Superficial fibular nerve, L4-S1.

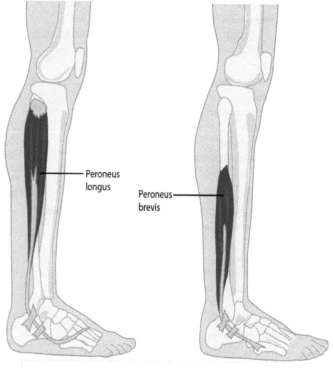

Fig. 1.2.17. Muscles of lateral leg compartment

# X. POSTERIOR LEG COMPARTMENT

- ○ **Action:** **Plantarflex** and **Invert** the Foot.
- ○ **Innervation:** **Tibial Nerve.**
- ○ **Muscles:**
  - ○ **Superficial Group:** **GPS**
    - • **G**astrocnemius
    - • **P**lantaris
    - • **S**oleus
  - ○ **Deep Group:** **TFFP**
    - • **T**ibialis posterior
    - • **F**lexor Hallucis Longus
    - • **F**lexor Digitorum Longus
    - • **P**opliteus

## C. VESSELS & NERVES

### 1. POSTERIOR TIBIAL ARTERY

- **Origin:** continuation of the popliteal artery
- **Main branches:** Fibular artery (peroneal)However, it also branches into:
  - • Circumflex fibular artery
  - • Medial plantar artery
  - • Lateral plantar artery

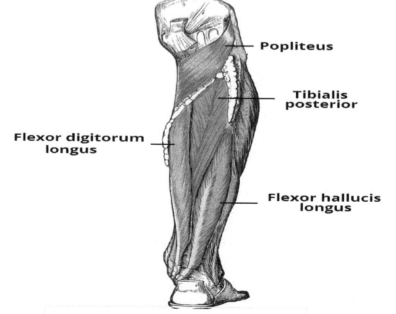

Fig. 1.2.18. Muscles of Posterior leg compartment

# XI. SOLE OF THE FOOT

## PLANTAR ASPECT

- **Common Action:**
  - Act collectively to stabilise the arches of the foot.
  - Individually to control movement of the digits.

- **Innervation:**
  - **Medial Plantar Nerve or**
  - **Lateral Plantar Nerve.**

- **Muscles:**
  - There are 10 intrinsic muscles located in the sole of the foot (3-2-3-2).
  - The muscles of the plantar aspect are described in four layers (superficial to deep).

### A. FIRST LAYER
- **Abductor Hallucis**: Medial plantar Nerve.
- **Flexor Digitorum Brevis**: Medial plantar Nerve.
- **Abductor Digiti Minimi**: Lateral plantar Nerve.

### B. SECOND LAYER
- **Quadratus Plantae**: Lateral plantar Nerve.
- **Lumbricals**: Medial and Lateral Plantar Nerves.

### C. THIRD LAYER
- **Flexor Hallucis Brevis**: Medial plantar Nerve.
- **Adductor Hallucis**: Lateral plantar Nerve.
- **Flexor Digiti Minimi Brevis**: Lateral plantar Nerve.

### D. FOURTH LAYER
- **Plantar Interossei**: Lateral plantar Nerve.
- **Dorsal Interossei**: Lateral plantar Nerve

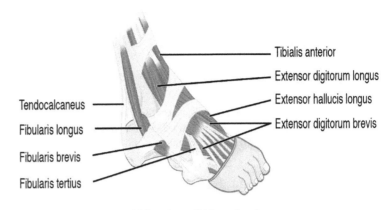

Tibialis anterior
Extensor digitorum longus
Extensor hallucis longus
Extensor digitorum brevis
Tendocalcaneus
Fibularis longus
Fibularis brevis
Fibularis tertius

(a) Dorsal superficial muscles of the right foot (lateral view)

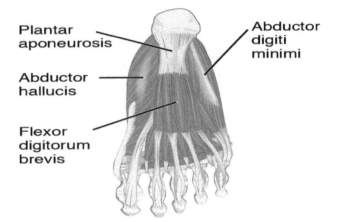

Plantar aponeurosis
Abductor digiti minimi
Abductor hallucis
Flexor digitorum brevis

(b) Superficial muscles of the left sole (plantar view)

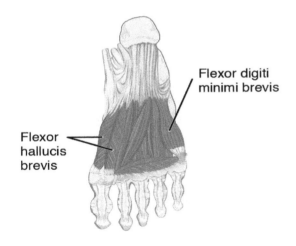

Flexor digiti minimi brevis
Flexor hallucis brevis

(d) Deep muscles of the left sole (plantar view)

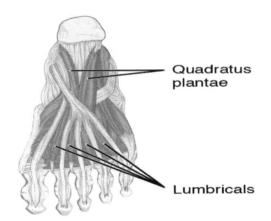

Quadratus plantae
Lumbricals

(c) Intermediate muscles of the left sole (plantar view)

*Fig. 1.2.19. Sole of the foot Muscles*

# XII. ANKLE AND FOOT JOINTS/ JOINT DYNAMICS

## LIGAMENTS

- There are two sets of ligaments, which originate from each malleolus:

### 1. MEDIAL LIGAMENT (OR DELTOID LIGAMENT)

- The ligament is composed of two layers: **The superficial layer** (has variable attachments and crosses two joints) and **the deep layer** (has talar attachments and crosses one joint).
  - ○ **Superficial layer**
    - ▪ Tibiocalcaneal ligament
    - ▪ Tibionavicular ligament
    - ▪ Posterior superficial tibiotalar Ligament (PSTL)
    - ▪ Tibiospring ligament
  - ○ **Deep layer:** this layer is intra-articular and is covered by synovium
    - ▪ Anterior tibiotalar ligament (ATTL)
    - ▪ Posterior deep tibiotalar ligament (PDTL)
- It is much stronger than the lateral ankle ligament
- The primary action of the medial ligament is **to resist over-eversion of the foot**, calcaneus and talus bones.

### 2. LATERAL LIGAMENT

- Originates from the lateral malleolus.
- **It resists over-inversion of the foot**. It is comprised of three distinct and separate ligaments:
  - ○ **Anterior talofibular**: Spans between the lateral malleolus and lateral aspect of the talus.
  - ○ **Posterior talofibular**: Spans between the lateral malleolus and the posterior aspect of the talus.
  - ○ **Calcaneofibular**: Spans between the lateral malleolus and the calcaneus
- Movements at ankle joints are dorsiflexion and plantarflexion.
- Note that inversion and eversion occur at the **subtalar joint**.
- *The ankle joint is very stable at **dorsiflexion**, where the trochlear of the talus is tightly held within the mortise formed by the two malleoli and their attendant ligament complexes.*
  - *The **anterior talofibular ligament** (ATFL) and the **calcaneofibular ligament** (CFL) are sequentially the most commonly injured ligaments when a plantar-flexed foot is forcefully inverted.*
  - *The **posterior talofibular ligament** (PTFL) is rarely injured (stronger), except in association with a complete dislocation of the talus.*
- During plantarflexion, the trochlear of the talus moves anteriorly such that it receives less support from the mortise, and is consequently less stable.
- **Tibialis anterior** attaches proximally to the lateral condyle of the tibia and distally to the medial cuneiform bone and base of the first metatarsal. **It dorsiflexes and inverts the foot.**

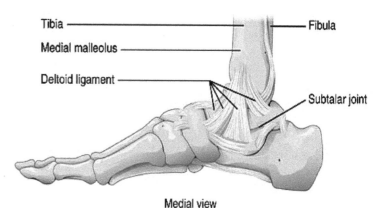

Medial view

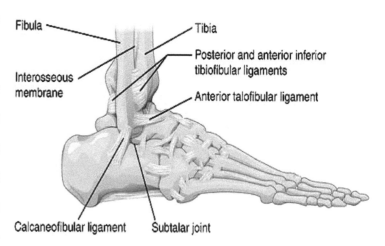

Lateral view

*Fig. 1.2.20. Ankle joint ligaments*

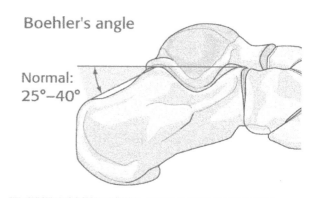

Boehler's angle

Normal: 25°–40°

*Fig. 1.2.21. Bohler's Angle*

## BÖHLER ANGLE (BOHLER ANGLE or BOEHLER ANGLE)
- The angle between two lines tangent to the calcaneus on the lateral radiograph. These lines are drawn tangent to the anterior and posterior aspects of the superior calcaneus. The normal value for this angle is between **20 to 40 degrees**.
- Value less than 20 degrees can be seen in calcaneal fracture.
- However, a normal Böhler angle does not exclude a calcaneal fracture.

## CLINICAL RELEVANCE

### ANKLE JOINT STABILITY
- **The bony architecture of the ankle joint is most stable in dorsiflexion.**
- The most common ankle sprain occurs on the lateral or outside part of the ankle.
- The ankle joint is a hinge joint possessing great stability.
- The deep mortise formed by the lower end of the tibia and the medial and lateral malleoli securely holds the talus in position.

### ACUTE SPRAINS OF THE "LATERAL ANKLE"
- Acute sprains of the lateral ankle are usually caused by excessive inversion of the foot with plantar flexion of the ankle.
- The anterior talofibular ligament and the calcaneofibular ligament are partially torn, giving rise to great pain and local swelling.

### ACUTE SPRAINS OF THE "MEDIAL ANKLE"
- Acute sprains of the medial ankle are similar to but less common than those of the lateral ankle.
- They may occur to the medial or deltoid ligament as a result of excessive eversion.
- The great strength of the medial ligament usually results in the ligament pulling off the tip of the medial malleolus.

### FRACTURE DISLOCATIONS OF THE ANKLE JOINT
- Fracture dislocations of the ankle are common and are caused by forced external rotation and overeversion of the foot. The talus is externally rotated forcibly against the lateral malleolus of the fibula.
- The torsion effect on the lateral malleolus causes it to fracture spirally. If the force continues, the talus moves laterally, and the medial ligament of the ankle joint becomes taut and pulls off the tip of the medial malleolus.
- If the talus is forced to move still farther, its rotary movement results in its violent contact with the posterior inferior margin of the tibia, which shears off. Other less common types of fracture dislocation are caused by forced overeversion (without rotation), in which the talus presses the lateral malleolus laterally and causes it to fracture transversely.
- Overinversion (without rotation), in which the talus presses against the medial malleolus, produces a vertical fracture through the base of the medial malleolus.

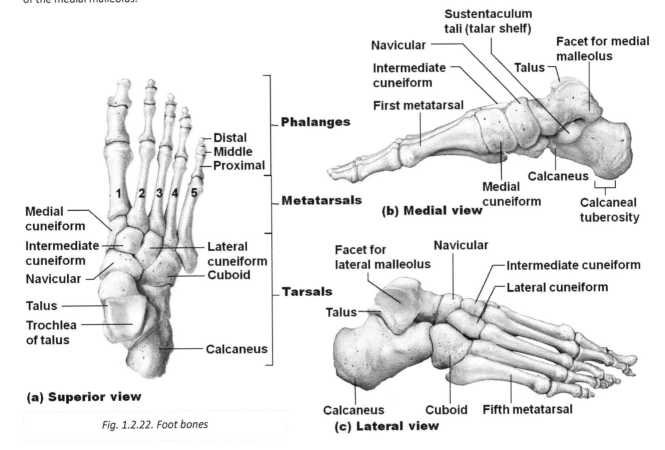

*Fig. 1.2.22. Foot bones*

# XIII. TARSAL JOINTS

- *The forefoot* contains the five toes (phalanges) and the five longer bones (metatarsals).
- *The midfoot* is a pyramid-like collection of bones that form the arches of the feet. These include the three cuneiform bones, the cuboid bone, and the navicular bone.
- *The hindfoot* forms the heel and ankle. The talus bone supports the leg bones (tibia and fibula), forming the ankle. The calcaneus (heel bone) is the largest bone in the foot.

## THE SUBTALAR JOINT

- It is an articulation between two of the tarsal bones in the foot – the talus and calcaneus.
- The joint is classed structurally as a **synovial** joint, and functionally as a **plane synovial** joint.
- This article will look at the anatomy of the subtalar joint – its articulating surfaces, movements and neurovascular supply.

### ARTICULATING SURFACES

- The subtalar joint is formed between two of the tarsal bones:
  - Inferior surface of the body of the talus – the **posterior talar articular surface.**
  - Superior surface of the calcaneus – the **posterior calcaneal articular facet.**
- As is typical for a synovial joint, these surfaces are covered by **articular cartilage**.

### STABILITY

- The subtalar joint is enclosed by a **joint capsule**, which is lined internally by synovial membrane and strengthened externally by a fibrous layer. The capsule is also supported by three ligaments:
  - **Posterior talocalcaneal ligament**
  - **Medial talocalcaneal ligament**
  - **Lateral talocalcaneal ligament**
- An additional ligament – the **interosseous talocalcaneal ligament** – acts to bind the talus and calcaneus together.
- It lies within the **sinus tarsi** (a small cavity between the talus and calcaneus), and is particularly strong; providing the majority of the ligamentous stability to the joint.

### MOVEMENTS

- The subtalar joint is formed on an **oblique axis** and is therefore the chief site within the foot for generation of eversion and inversion movements.
- This movement is produced by the muscles of the lateral compartment of the leg. and tibialis anterior muscle respectively.
- The nature of the articulating surface means that the subtalar joint has no role in plantar or dorsiflexion of the foot.

### NEUROVASCULAR SUPPLY

- The subtalar joint receives supply from two arteries and two nerves.
  - Arterial supply comes from the **posterior tibial** and **fibular** arteries.
  - Innervation to the plantar aspect of the joint is supplied by the **medial or lateral plantar nerve**, whereas the dorsal aspect of the joint is supplied by the **deep fibular** nerve.

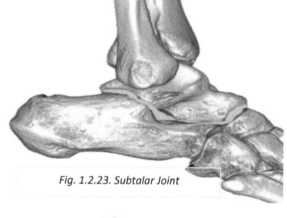

*Fig. 1.2.23. Subtalar Joint*

## CALCANEAL FRACTURE

- The calcaneus is often fractured in a '**crush** 'type injury.
- The most common mechanism of damage is falling onto the heel from a height – the talus is driven into the calcaneus. The bone can break into several pieces, known as a **comminuted** fracture.
- Upon x-ray imaging, the calcaneus will appear shorter and wider.
- A calcaneal fracture can cause chronic problems, even after treatment. The subtalar joint is usually disrupted, causing the joint to become **arthritic.**
- The patient will experience pain upon inversion and eversion – which can make walking on uneven ground particularly painful.

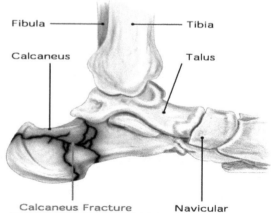

*Fig. 1.2.24. Calcaneal Fracture*

# XIV. LOWER LIMB INNERVATION

## 1. OBTURATOR NERVE (L2-L4)

- **Cause of injury**
  - o Anterior Dislocation of Hip
- **Motor deficit**
  - o Paralysis of adductor muscles
  - o Impaired ability to adduct thigh
- **Sensory deficit**
  - o Sensory Loss on Medial Thigh

## 2. FEMORAL NERVE (L2-L4)

- **Cause of injury**
  - o Pelvic Fracture
- **Motor deficit**
  - o Paralysis of quadriceps femoris
  - o Impaired ability to flex thigh
  - o Impaired ability to extend leg
- **Sensory deficit**
  - o Sensory loss on anterior thigh
  - o Sensory loss on medial leg

## 3. SCIATIC NERVE (L4-S3)

- **Overview**
  - o Forms from the anterior division of the L4-S3 roots (which forms the tibial component) and posterior divisions of the L4-S2 roots (which forms the common peroneal component) of the sacral plexus.
  - o Enters gluteal region via greater sciatic foramen and descends in posterior thigh. Bifurcates into common peroneal nerve and tibial nerve at apex of popliteal fossa.

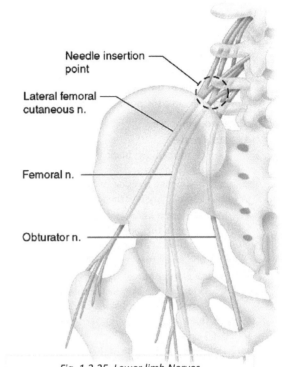
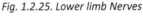

*Fig. 1.2.25. Lower limb Nerves*

## A. COMMON PERONEAL (FIBULAR) NERVE

- **Nerve roots: L4 – S2**
- **Motor:**
  - o **Directly**: Innervates the short head of the biceps femoris (part of the hamstring muscles, which flex at the knee).
  - o **Via Terminal Branches:**
    - **Superficial fibular nerve**: Innervates the muscles of the lateral compartment of the leg (fibularis longus and brevis). These muscles act to evert the foot.
    - **Deep fibular nerve:** Innervates the muscles of the anterior compartment of the leg (tibialis anterior, extensor digitorum longus and extensor hallucius longus).
    - These muscles act to dorsiflex the foot, and extend the digits. It also innervates some intrinsic muscles of the foot.
    - If the common fibular nerve is damaged, the patient may lose the ability to **dorsiflex** and **evert** the foot, and **extend** the digits.
- **Sensory:**
  - o Innervates the skin over the upper lateral and lower posterolateral leg.
  - o Also, supplies (via branches) cutaneous innervation to the skin of the anterolateral leg, and the dorsum of the foot.
  - o There are two cutaneous branches that arise directly from the common fibular nerve as it moves over the lateral head of the gastrocnemius:
    - **Sural communicating nerve**: This nerve combines with a branch of the tibial nerve to form the **Sural Nerve**. The sural nerve innervates the skin over the lower posterolateral leg.
    - **Lateral sural cutaneous neve**: Innervates the skin over the upper lateral leg.

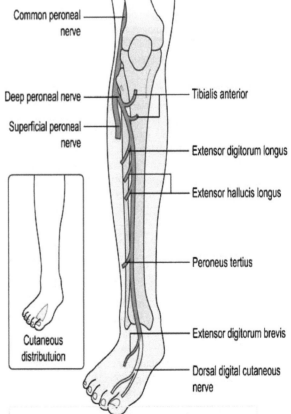

*Fig. 1.2.26. Common peroneal nerve*

- In addition to these nerves, the terminal branches of the common fibular nerve also have a cutaneous function:
  - **Superficial fibular nerve**: Innervates the skin of the anterolateral leg, and dorsum of the foot (except the skin between the first and second toes).
  - **Deep fibular nerve:** Innervates the skin between the first and second toes.

## B. TIBIAL NERVE
- **Nerve roots: L4-S3**
- **Sensory**: Innervates the skin of the posterolateral side of the leg, lateral side of the foot, and the sole of the foot.
- **Motor:** Innervates the posterior compartment of the leg.
  - **Cutaneous branches:**
    - **Sural nerve**
      - Is formed by branches of the tibial and common fibular nerves.
      - It supplies the skin of the posterolateral leg and the lateral margin of the foot.
    - **Medial plantar nerve**
      - Supplies the skin of the medial sole of the foot, and the plantar aspect, nails and sides of the medial three and a half toes.
    - **Lateral plantar nerve**
      - Supplies the skin of the lateral sole, and the plantar aspect, nails and sides of the lateral one and a half toes.
    - **Calcaneal nerves**
      - Supplies the skin of the heel

## 4. SUPERIOR GLUTEAL NERVE (L4-S1)
- **Cause of injury**
  - Posterior dislocation of hip
  - Poliomyelitis damages superior gluteal nerve
- **Motor deficit**
  - Weakened abduction of thigh by gluteus minimus and medius.
  - **Symptoms:**
    - ***Positive Trendelenburg test***
    - Lower limb becomes, in effect, too long and does not clear ground when foot is brought forward in swing phase of walking.
    - Compensation: ***"gluteal gait" or waddling***: person leans away from unsupported side, raising pelvis to allow adequate room for foot to clear ground.
- Sensory deficit: n/a

## 5. INFERIOR GLUTEAL NERVE (L5-S2)
- **Cause of injury**: posterior dislocation of hip damages inferior gluteal nerve
- **Motor deficit:**
  - Paralysis of gluteus maximus muscle
    - Impaired ability to extend hip
    - Impaired ability to laterally rotate hip
  - **Symptoms**
    - Difficulty climbing stairs, difficulty stepping onto a bus.
    - Difficulty jumping, difficulty arising from a chair.
    - Can't push inferiorly (downward).
- **Sensory deficit**: n/a

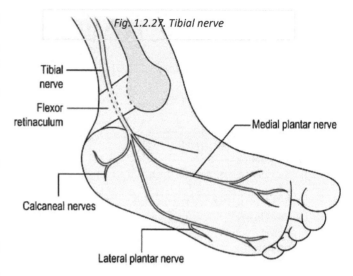

Fig. 1.2.27. Tibial nerve

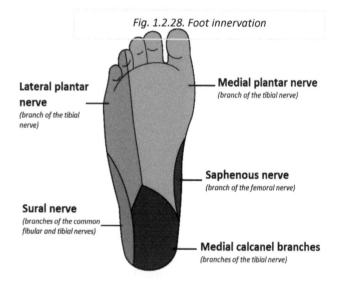

Fig. 1.2.28. Foot innervation

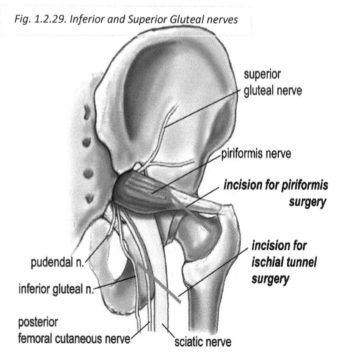

Fig. 1.2.29. Inferior and Superior Gluteal nerves

# CLINICAL RELEVANCE:

## 1. TENDON REFLEXES OF THE LOWER LIMB

- Skeletal muscles receive a segmental innervation.
- Most muscles are innervated by two, three, or four spinal nerves and therefore by the same number of segments of the spinal cord.
- The segmental innervation of the following muscles in the lower limb should be known because it is possible to test them by eliciting simple muscle reflexes in the patient.
  - **Patellar tendon reflex** (knee jerk) **L2, 3, and 4** (extension of the knee joint on tapping the patellar tendon)
  - **Achilles tendon reflex** (ankle jerk) **S1 and S2** (plantar flexion of the ankle joint on tapping the Achilles tendon)

## 2. FEMORAL NERVE INJURY

- The **femoral nerve (L2, 3, and 4)** enters the thigh from behind the inguinal ligament, at a point midway between the anterior superior iliac spine and the pubic tubercle; it lies about a fingerbreadth lateral to the femoral pulse.
- About 2 inches (5 cm) below the inguinal ligament, the nerve splits into its terminal branches.
- The femoral nerve can be injured in **stab or gunshot wounds**, but a complete division of the nerve is rare.
- The following clinical features are present when the nerve is completely divided:
  - **Motor:** The quadriceps femoris muscle is paralyzed, and the knee cannot be extended. In walking, this is compensated for to some extent by use of the adductor muscles.
  - **Sensory:** Skin sensation is lost over the anterior and medial sides of the thigh, over the medial side of the lower part of the leg, and along the medial border of the foot as far as the ball of the big toe; this area is normally supplied by the saphenous nerve.

## 3. SCIATIC NERVE INJURY

- The **sciatic nerve (L4 and 5 and S1, 2, and 3)** curves laterally and downward through the gluteal region, situated at first midway between the posterosuperior iliac spine and the ischial tuberosity, and lower down, midway between the tip of the greater trochanter and the ischial tuberosity.
- The nerve then passes downward in the midline on the posterior aspect of the thigh and divides into the common peroneal and tibial nerves, at a variable site above the popliteal fossa.
- The nerve is sometimes injured by **penetrating wounds, fractures of the pelvis, or dislocations of the hip joint**.
- It is most frequently injured by **badly placed intramuscular injections in the gluteal region**. To avoid this injury, injections into the gluteus maximus or the gluteus medius should be made well forward on the upper outer quadrant of the buttock.
- Most nerve lesions are incomplete, and in 90% of injuries, the common peroneal part of the nerve is the most affected.
- This can probably be explained by the fact that the common peroneal nerve fibers lie most superficial in the sciatic nerve.
- The following clinical features are present:
  - **Motor:** The hamstring muscles are paralyzed, but weak flexion of the knee is possible because of the action of the Sartorius (femoral nerve) and gracilis (obturator nerve). All the muscles below the knee are paralyzed, and the weight of the foot causes it to assume the plantar-flexed position, or **footdrop.**
  - **Sensory:** Sensation is lost below the knee, except for a narrow area down the medial side of the lower part of the leg and along the medial border of the foot as far as the ball of the big toe, which is supplied by the saphenous nerve (femoral nerve). The result of operative repair of a sciatic nerve injury is poor. It is rare for active movement to return to the small muscles of the foot, and sensory recovery is rarely complete. Loss of sensation in the sole of the foot makes the development of trophic ulcers inevitable.

## 3. SCIATICA

- Sciatica describes the condition in which patients have pain along the sensory distribution of the sciatic nerve.
- Thus, the pain is experienced in the posterior aspect of the thigh, the posterior and lateral sides of the leg, and the lateral part of the foot.
- Sciatica can be caused by prolapse of an intervertebral disc, with pressure on one or more roots of the lower lumbar and sacral spinal nerves, pressure on the sacral plexus or sciatic nerve by an intrapelvic tumor, or inflammation of the sciatic nerve or its terminal branches.

## 4. COMMON PERONEAL NERVE INJURY

- The common peroneal nerve (Fig. 10.16) is in an exposed position as it leaves the popliteal fossa and winds around the neck of the fibula to enter the peroneus longus muscle. It is commonly injured in fractures of the neck of the fibula and by pressure from casts or splints. The following clinical features are present:
  - **Motor:** The muscles of the anterior and lateral compartments of the leg are paralyzed, namely, the tibialis anterior, the extensor digitorum longus and brevis, the peroneus tertius, the extensor hallucis longus (supplied by the deep peroneal nerve), and the peroneus longus and brevis (supplied by the superficial peroneal nerve).
  - As a result, the opposing muscles, the plantar flexors of the ankle joint and the invertors of the subtalar and transverse tarsal joints, cause the foot to be plantar flexed **(foot drop)** and inverted, an attitude referred to as **equinovarus.**

○ **Sensory:** Loss of sensation occurs down the anterior and lateral sides of the leg and dorsum of the foot and toes, including the medial side of the big toe. The lateral border of the foot and the lateral side of the little toe are virtually unaffected (sural nerve, mainly formed from tibial nerve). The medial border of the foot as far as the ball of the big toe is completely unaffected (saphenous nerve, a branch of the femoral nerve). When the injury occurs distal to the site of origin of the lateral cutaneous nerve of the calf, the loss of sensibility is confined to the area of the foot and toes.

## 5. TIBIAL NERVE INJURY

- The tibial nerve leaves the popliteal fossa by passing deep to the gastrocnemius and soleus muscles. Because of its deep and protected position, it is rarely injured.
- Complete division results in the following clinical features:
  - ○ **Motor:** All the muscles in the back of the leg and the sole of the foot are paralyzed. The opposing muscles dorsiflex the foot at the ankle joint and evert the foot at the subtalar and transverse tarsal joints, an attitude referred to as **calcaneovalgus.**
  - ○ **Sensory:** Sensation is lost on the sole of the foot; later, trophic ulcers develop.

## 6. OBTURATOR NERVE INJURY

- The **obturator nerve (L2, 3, and 4)** enters the thigh as anterior and posterior divisions through the upper part of the obturator foramen. The anterior division descends in front of the obturator externus and the adductor brevis, deep to the floor of the femoral triangle.
- The posterior division descends behind the adductor brevis and in front of the adductor magnus.
- It is rarely injured in penetrating wounds, in anterior dislocations of the hip joint, or in abdominal hernia through the obturator foramen. It may be pressed on by the fetal head during parturition.
- The following clinical features occur:
  - ○ **Motor:** All the adductor muscles are paralyzed except the hamstring part of the adductor magnus, which is supplied by the sciatic nerve.
  - ○ **Sensory:** The cutaneous sensory loss is minimal on the medial aspect of the thigh.

# PAST ASKED QUESTIONS

| **Which of the following are true regarding tibialis posterior?** | |
|---|---|
| It is found in the posterior compartment of the lower leg | T |
| It is innervated by the deep peroneal nerve | F |
| It causes inversion of foot | T |
| Its tendon passes deep to the inferior extensor retinaculum of the ankle | F |
| **Regarding the ankle joint:** | |
| Its more stable in dorsiflexion than plantarflexion | T |
| Ankle sprain is usually an inversion injury | T |
| An eversion injury may rupture the Deltoid ligament | T |
| Violent eversion may avulse the tuberosity of the 5th metatarsal | F |
| **In relation to the anatomy of the knee:** | |
| The suprapatellar bursa communicates with the synovial cavity of the knee | T |
| The fibres of the medial collateral ligament are firmly attached to the medial meniscus and fibrous capsule of the knee joint | T |
| The anterior cruciate ligaments maintain lateral stability of the knee | F |
| The posterior cruciate ligament is attached to the posterior aspect of the medial condyle of the femur | F |
| **Which tendons traverse the extensor retinaculum of the ankle:** | |
| Tibialis anterior | T |
| Extensor Digitorum longus | T |
| Flexor Hallucis longus | F |
| Peroneus Longus | F |
| **Regarding the anatomy of the ankle and foot:** | |
| The tendon of peroneus longus inserts into the base of the 1st metatarsal | T |
| The long saphenous vein passes posterior to the medial malleolus | F |
| Bohler's angle should be less than 40degrees | T |
| Extension of the big toe is mediated by the L5 and S1 | F |
| The tendon of the peroneus brevis inserts into the base of the 5th metatarsal | T |

| | |
|---|---|
| The distal fibula is not bound to the calcaneum by ligaments | F |
| Tibialis anterior inserts into the medial cuneiform | T |
| The ankle jerk is primarily a test of L5 | F |
| In the subtalar joint, the navicular is bound to the talus | F |
| Tibialis anterior is an inverter of the ankle | T |
| The most injured ligament in an ankle sprain is the ant talofibular ligament | T |

### Which of the following is true regarding ankle joint?

| | |
|---|---|
| The posterior talofibular ligament is stronger than anterior talofibular ligament | T |
| The deltoid ligament has three parts | F |
| The ankle joint is more stable when in dorsiflexion than plantarflexion | T |
| Eversion of the foot at the ankle is caused by tibialis anterior | F |

### Regarding the muscles of the lateral compartment of the leg

| | |
|---|---|
| Their tendons pass posteriorly to the lateral malleolus | T |
| Peroneus longus attaches to the medial cuneiform and base of the first metatarsal | T |
| When the base of the fifth metatarsal is fractured, peroneus brevis pulls on and displaces the proximal fragment | T |
| They act together to invert the foot | F |

### Which statements are true regarding the muscles which adduct the thigh at the hip?

| | |
|---|---|
| The thigh adductor muscles are found in the medial compartment of the inner thigh | T |
| The femoral nerve is the primary nerve supplying the hip adductors | F |
| Adductor longus both adducts and laterally rotates the thigh | F |
| Obturator externus is an adductor muscle of the thigh | T |

### The Femoral artery:

| | |
|---|---|
| Is lateral to the Femoral vein in the inguinal canal | T |
| Is a continuation of the internal Iliac artery | F |
| Crosses the femur beneath the Sartorius | F |
| Runs midway between ASIS and pubic tubercle | T |

### With respect to the content of the femoral triangle:

| | |
|---|---|
| The long Saphenous vein joins the femoral vein | T |
| The femoral artery covers the Sartorius | F |
| The adductor longus forms part of the floor | T |
| The inguinal ligament is its superior limit | T |

### The following are true of peripheral nerves in the lower limb:

| | |
|---|---|
| Sciatic nerve lesions cause paralysis of the knee flexion but preservation of the knee jerk/reflex | T |
| Weak dorsiflexion of the foot may result from tibial nerve damage | F |
| Sciatic nerve injury causes complete loss of sensation below the knee | F |
| The sural nerve supplies sensation to the medial aspect of the foot | F |

### Regarding the anatomy of the lower limb:

| | |
|---|---|
| Adductor magnus attaches to the Ischial tuberosity | T |
| Psoas inserts onto the greater trochanter of the femur | F |
| Meralgia paresthetica results from damage to the medial cutaneous nerve of the thigh | F |
| Iliopsoas is an external rotator of the hip | F |

### Regarding the anatomy of the common peroneal nerve:

| | |
|---|---|
| It receives fibres from both lumbar and sacral nerve routes | T |
| Supplies sensation to the skin of the posterior and lateral aspects of the lower leg | F |
| The common peroneal nerve is closely related to the head of the fibula | T |
| Injury causes weakness of foot plantar flexion | F |

### Which of the following statements regarding the knee joint are true?

| | |
|---|---|
| The medial meniscus is more often injured than the lateral meniscus | T |
| The anterior cruciate ligament is attached to medial femoral condyle | F |
| The anterior cruciate ligament prevents hyperextension of the knee | T |
| Popliteus unlocks the knee by medial rotation of the tibia on a fixed femur | T |

# SECTION 3: THORAX

# I. THORACIC WALL

## 1. OVERVIEW

- The thorax (or chest) is the region of the body between the neck and the abdomen. It is flattened in front and behind but rounded at the sides. The framework of the walls of the thorax, which is referred to as the **thoracic cage,** is formed by the vertebral column behind, the ribs and intercostals spaces on either side, and the sternum and costal cartilages in front.
- Superiorly, the thorax communicates with the neck, and inferiorly it is separated from the abdomen by the diaphragm.
- The thoracic cage protects the lungs and heart and affords attachment for the muscles of the thorax, upper extremity, abdomen, and back. The cavity of the thorax can be divided into a median partition, called the **mediastinum,** and the laterally placed pleurae and lungs. The lungs are covered by a thin membrane called the **visceral pleura,** which passes from each lung at its root (i.e., where the main air passages and blood vessels enter) to the inner surface of the chest wall, where it is called the **parietal pleura.**
- In this manner, two membranous sacs called the **pleural cavities** are formed, one on each side of the thorax, between the lungs and the thoracic walls. The thoracic wall is covered on the outside by skin and by muscles attaching the shoulder girdle to the trunk. It is lined with parietal pleura. The thoracic wall is formed posteriorly by the thoracic part of the vertebral column; anteriorly by the sternum and costal cartilages; laterally by the ribs and intercostals spaces; superiorly by the suprapleural membrane; and inferiorly by the diaphragm, which separates the thoracic cavity from the abdominal cavity.

## 2. STERNUM

- The sternum lies in the midline of the anterior chest wall. It is a flat bone that can be divided into three parts: manubrium sterni, body of the sternum, and xiphoid process. The **manubrium** is the upper part of the sternum.
- It articulates with the body of the sternum at the manubriosternal joint, and it also articulates with the clavicles and with the 1st costal cartilage and the upper part of the 2nd costal cartilages on each side. It lies opposite the 3rd and 4th thoracic vertebrae.
- The **body of the sternum** articulates above with the manubrium at the **manubriosternal joint** and below with the xiphoid process at the **xiphisternal joint.** On each side, it articulates with the 2nd to the 7th costal cartilages.
- The **xiphoid process** is a thin plate of cartilage that becomes ossified at its proximal end during adult life. No ribs or costal cartilages are attached to it.
- The **sternal angle** (angle of Louis), formed by the articulation of the manubrium with the body of the sternum, can be recognized by the presence of a transverse ridge on the anterior aspect of the sternum. The transverse ridge lies at the level of the 2nd costal cartilage, the point from which all costal cartilages and ribs are counted. The sternal angle lies opposite the intervertebral disc between the 4th and 5th thoracic vertebrae.
- The **xiphisternal joint** lies opposite the body of the ninth thoracic vertebra.

## 3. RIBS

- There are 12 pairs of ribs, all of which are attached posteriorly to the thoracic vertebrae. The ribs are divided into three categories:
  - **True ribs:** The upper seven pairs are attached anteriorly to the sternum by their costal cartilages.
  - **False ribs:** The 8th, 9th, and 10th pairs of ribs are attached anteriorly to each other and to the 7th rib by means of their costal cartilages and small synovial joints.
  - **Floating ribs:** The 11th and 12th pairs have no anterior attachment.

### A. TYPICAL RIB

- A typical rib is a long, twisted, flat bone having a rounded, smooth superior border and a sharp, thin inferior border. The inferior border overhangs and forms the **costal groove,** which accommodates the intercostals vessels and nerve. The anterior end of each rib is attached to the corresponding costal cartilage.
- A rib has a **head, neck, tubercle, shaft,** and **angle.** The **head** has two facets for articulation with the numerically corresponding vertebral body and that of the vertebra immediately above.
- The **neck** is a constricted portion situated between the head and the tubercle. The **tubercle** is a prominence on the outer surface of the rib at the junction of the neck with the shaft. It has a facet for articulation with the transverse process of the numerically corresponding vertebra. The shaft is thin and flattened and twisted on its long axis. Its inferior border has the costal groove. The angle is where the shaft of the rib bends sharply forward.

### B. ATYPICAL RIB

- The 1st rib is important clinically because of its close relationship to the lower nerves of the brachial plexus and the main vessels to the arm, namely, the subclavian artery and vein. This rib is small and flattened from above downward. The scalenus anterior muscle is attached to its upper surface and inner border. Anterior to the scalenus anterior, the subclavian vein crosses the rib; posterior to the muscle attachment, the subclavian artery and the lower trunk of the brachial plexus cross the rib and lie in contact with the bone.

## C. COSTAL CARTILAGES

- Costal cartilages are bars of cartilage connecting the upper seven ribs to the lateral edge of the sternum and the 8th, 9th, and 10th ribs to the cartilage immediately above. The cartilages of the 11th and 12th ribs end in the abdominal musculature.
- The costal cartilages contribute significantly to the elasticity and mobility of the thoracic walls. In old age, the costal cartilages tend to lose some of their flexibility as the result of superficial calcification.

## D. MOVEMENTS OF THE RIBS & COSTAL CARTILAGES

- The 1st ribs and their costal cartilages are fixed to the manubrium and are immobile. The raising and lowering of the ribs during respiration are accompanied by movements in both the joints of the head and the tubercle, permitting the neck of each rib to rotate around its own axis.

## E. OPENINGS OF THE THORAX

- The chest cavity communicates with the root of the neck through an opening called the **thoracic outlet.**
- It is called an **outlet** because important vessels and nerves emerge from the thorax here to enter the neck and upper limbs. The opening is bounded posteriorly by the 1st thoracic vertebra, laterally by the medial borders of the 1st ribs and their costal cartilages, and anteriorly by the superior border of the manubrium sterni.
- The opening is obliquely placed facing upward and forward. Through this small opening pass the oesophagus and trachea and many vessels and nerves. Because of the obliquity of the opening, the apices of the lung and pleurae project upward into the neck.
- The thoracic cavity communicates with the abdomen through a large opening. The opening is bounded posteriorly by the 12th thoracic vertebra, laterally by the curving costal margin, and anteriorly by the xiphisternal joint. Through this large opening, which is closed by the diaphragm, pass the oesophagus and many large vessels and nerves, all of which pierce the diaphragm.

## 4. THE THORACIC OUTLET SYNDROME

- The brachial plexus of nerves (C5, 6, 7, and 8 and T1) and the subclavian artery and vein are closely related to the upper surface of the 1st rib and the clavicle as they enter the upper limb.
- It is here that the nerves or blood vessels may be compressed between the bones. Most of the symptoms are caused by pressure on the lower trunk of the plexus producing pain down the medial side of the forearm and hand and wasting of the small muscles of the hand.
- Pressure on the blood vessels may compromise the circulation of the upper limb.

## 5. INTERCOSTAL SPACES

- The spaces between the ribs contain three muscles of respiration: the external intercostal, the internal intercostal, and the innermost intercostal muscle. The innermost intercostals muscle is lined internally by the **endothoracic fascia,** which is lined internally by the parietal pleura. The intercostals nerves and blood vessels run between the intermediate and deepest layers of muscles.
- They are arranged in the following order from above downward: intercostal vein, intercostal artery, and intercostal nerve (i.e., VAN).

## 6. INTERCOSTAL MUSCLES

- The **external intercostal muscle** forms the most superficial layer. Its fibers are directed downward and forward from the inferior border of the rib above to the superior border of the rib below.
- The muscle extends forward to the costal cartilage where it is replaced by an aponeurosis, the **anterior (external) intercostal membrane.**
- The **internal intercostal muscle** forms the intermediate layer. Its fibers are directed downward and backward from the subcostal groove of the rib above to the upper border of the rib below. The muscle extends backward from the sternum in front to the angles of the ribs behind, where the muscle is replaced by an aponeurosis, the **posterior (internal) intercostal membrane.**
- The **innermost intercostal muscle** forms the deepest layer and corresponds to the transversus abdominis muscle in the anterior abdominal wall. It is an incomplete muscle layer and crosses more than one intercostal space within the ribs. It is related internally to fascia (endothoracic fascia) and parietal pleura and externally to the intercostals nerves and vessels. The innermost intercostal muscle can be divided into three portions, which are more or less separate from one another.

### ACTION

- When the intercostal muscles contract, they all tend to pull the ribs nearer to one another.
- If the 1st rib is fixed by the contraction of the muscles in the root of the neck, namely, the scaleni muscles, the intercostal muscles raise the 2nd to the 12th ribs toward the 1st rib, as in inspiration.
- If, conversely, the 12th rib is fixed by the quadrates lumborum muscle and the oblique muscles of the abdomen, the 1st to the 11th ribs will be lowered by the contraction of the intercostal muscles, as in expiration.
- In addition, the tone of the intercostal muscles during the different phases of respiration serves to strengthen the tissues of the intercostal spaces, thus preventing the sucking in or the blowing out of the tissues with changes in intrathoracic pressure.
- For further details concerning the action of these muscles.

## NERVE SUPPLY

- The intercostal muscles are supplied by the corresponding intercostal nerves. The intercostal nerves and blood vessels (the neurovascular bundle), as in the abdominal wall, run between the middle and innermost layers of muscles.
- They are arranged in the following order from above downward: intercostals vein, intercostal artery, and intercostal nerve (i.e., VAN).

## INTERCOSTAL ARTERIES AND VEINS

- Each intercostal space contains a large single posterior intercostal artery and two small anterior intercostal arteries.
- The **posterior intercostal arteries** of the first two spaces are branches from the superior intercostal artery, a branch of the costocervical trunk of the subclavian artery. The posterior intercostal arteries of the lower nine spaces are branches of the descending thoracic aorta.
- The **anterior intercostal arteries** of the first six spaces are branches of the internal thoracic artery, which arises from the first part of the subclavian artery. The anterior intercostal arteries of the lower spaces are branches of the musculophrenic artery, one of the terminal branches of the internal thoracic artery. Each intercostal artery gives off branches to the muscles, skin, and parietal pleura. In the region of the breast in the female, the branches to the superficial structures are particularly large.
- The corresponding **posterior intercostal veins** drain backward into the azygos or hemiazygos veins, and the **anterior intercostal veins** drain forward into the internal thoracic and the musculophrenic veins.

## INTERCOSTAL NERVES

- The intercostal nerves are the anterior rami of the first 11 thoracic spinal nerves.
- The anterior ramus of the 12th thoracic nerve lies in the abdomen and runs forward in the abdominal wall as the **subcostal nerve.**
- Each intercostal nerve enters an intercostal space between the parietal pleura and the posterior intercostals membrane.
- It then runs forward inferiorly to the intercostal vessels in the subcostal groove of the corresponding rib, between the innermost intercostals and internal intercostal muscle. The first six nerves are distributed within their intercostal spaces. The 7th to 9th intercostal nerves leave the anterior ends of their intercostals spaces by passing deep to the costal cartilages, to enter the anterior abdominal wall.
- The 10th and 11th nerves, since the corresponding ribs are floating, pass directly into the abdominal wall.

## BRANCHES

- **Rami communicantes** connect the intercostal nerve to a ganglion of the sympathetic trunk. The gray ramus joins the nerve medial at the point at which the white ramus leaves it.
- The **Collateral branch** runs forward inferiorly to the main nerve on the upper border of the rib below.
- The **Lateral cutaneous branch** reaches the skin on the side of the chest. It divides into an anterior and a posterior branch.
  - The **anterior cutaneous branch,** which is the terminal portion of the main trunk, reaches the skin near the midline. It divides into a medial and a lateral branch.
- **Muscular branches** run to the intercostal muscles.
- **Pleural sensory branches** go to the parietal pleura.
- **Peritoneal sensory branches** (7th to 11th intercostals nerves only) run to the parietal peritoneum.
- The **first intercostal nerve** is joined to the brachial plexus by a large branch that is equivalent to the lateral cutaneous branch of typical intercostal nerves. The remainder of the first intercostal nerve is small, and there is no anterior cutaneous branch.

# SKIN INNERVATION OF THE CHEST WALL AND REFERRED PAIN

- Above the level of the sternal angle, the cutaneous innervations of the anterior chest wall is derived from the **supraclavicular nerves** (C3 and 4). Below this level, the anterior and lateral cutaneous branches of the intercostal nerves supply oblique bands of skin in regular sequence. The skin on the posterior surface of the chest wall is supplied by the posterior rami of the spinal nerves.
- An intercostal nerve not only supplies areas of skin, but also supplies the ribs, costal cartilages, intercostals muscles, and parietal pleura lining the intercostal space. Furthermore, the 7th to 11th intercostal nerves leave the thoracic wall and enter the anterior abdominal wall so that they, in addition, supply dermatomes on the anterior abdominal wall, muscles of the anterior abdominal wall, and parietal peritoneum. This latter fact is of great clinical importance because it means that disease in the thoracic wall may be revealed as pain in a dermatome that extends across the costal margin into the anterior abdominal wall. For example, a pulmonary thromboembolism or a pneumonia with pleurisy involving the costal parietal pleura could give rise to abdominal pain and tenderness and rigidity of the abdominal musculature. The abdominal pain in these instances is called **referred pain.**

# HERPES ZOSTER

- Herpes zoster, or shingles, is a relatively common condition caused by the reactivation of the **latent varicella-zoster virus** in a patient who has previously had chickenpox. The lesion is seen as an inflammation and degeneration of the sensory neuron in a cranial or spinal nerve with the formation of vesicles with inflammation of the skin.
- In the thorax, the first symptom is a band of dermatomal pain in the distribution of the sensory neuron in a thoracic spinal nerve, followed in a few days by a skin eruption. The condition occurs most frequently in patients older than 50 years. The **second intercostal nerve** is joined to the medial cutaneous nerve of the arm by a branch called the **intercostobrachial nerve,** which is equivalent to the lateral cutaneous branch of other nerves. The 2nd intercostal nerve therefore supplies the skin of the armpit and the upper medial side of the arm. In **coronary artery disease,** pain is referred along this nerve to the medial side of the arm. With the exceptions noted, the 1st six intercostal nerves therefore supply the skin and the parietal pleura covering the outer and inner surfaces of each intercostal space, respectively, and the intercostal muscles of each intercostal space and the levatores costarum and serratus posterior muscles.

- In addition, the 7th to 11th intercostal nerves supply the skin and the parietal peritoneum covering the outer and inner surfaces of the abdominal wall, respectively, and the anterior abdominal muscles, which include the external oblique, internal oblique, transversus abdominis, and rectus abdominis muscles. Suprapleural Membrane Superiorly, the thorax opens into the root of the neck by a narrow aperture, the **thoracic outlet**. The outlet transmits structures that pass between the thorax and the neck (oesophagus, trachea, blood vessels, etc.) and for the most part lie close to the midline.
- On either side of these structures, the outlet is closed by a dense fascial layer called the **suprapleural membrane**.
- This tent-shaped fibrous sheet is attached laterally to the medial border of the 1st rib and costal cartilage. It is attached at its apex to the tip of the transverse process of the seventh cervical vertebra and medially to the fascia investing the structures passing from the thorax into the neck. It protects the underlying cervical pleura and resists the changes in intrathoracic pressure occurring during respiratory movements.

# 7. DIAPHRAGM

- The diaphragm is a thin muscular and tendinous septum that separates the chest cavity above from the abdominal cavity below.
- It is pierced by the structures that pass between the chest and the abdomen. The diaphragm is the most important muscle of respiration. It is dome shaped and consists of a peripheral muscular part, which arises from the margins of the thoracic opening, and a centrally placed tendon.
- The origin of the diaphragm can be divided into three parts:
  - A **sternal part** arising from the posterior surface of the xiphoid process
  - A **costal part** arising from the deep surfaces of the lower six ribs and their costal cartilages.
  - A **vertebral part** arising by vertical columns or crura and from the arcuate ligaments
- The **right crus** arises from the sides of the bodies of the first three lumbar vertebrae and the intervertebral discs; the **left crus** arises from the sides of the bodies of the first two lumbar vertebrae and the intervertebral disc.
- Lateral to the crura the diaphragm arises from the **medial** and **lateral arcuate ligaments**. The medial arcuate ligament extends from the side of the body of the second lumbar vertebra to the tip of the transverse process of the first lumbar vertebra. The lateral arcuate ligament extends from the tip of the transverse process of the first lumbar vertebra to the lower border of the 12th rib. The medial borders of the two crura are connected by a **median arcuate ligament,** which crosses over the anterior surface of the aorta.
- The diaphragm is inserted into a **central tendon,** which is shaped like three leaves. The superior surface of the tendon is partially fused with the inferior surface of the fibrous pericardium.
- Some of the muscle fibers of the right crus pass up to the left and surround the oesophageal orifice in a slinglike loop. These fibers appear to act as a sphincter and possibly assist in the prevention of regurgitation of the stomach contents into the thoracic part of the oesophagus.

## SHAPE OF THE DIAPHRAGM

- As seen from in front, the diaphragm curves up into **right and left domes,** or cupulae. The right dome reaches as high as the upper border of the 5th rib, and the left dome may reach the lower border of the 5th rib. (The right dome lies at a higher level, because of the large size of the right lobe of the liver.)
- The central tendon lies at the level of the xiphisternal joint. The domes support the right and left lungs, whereas the central tendon supports the heart. The levels of the diaphragm vary with the phase of respiration, the posture, and the degree of distention of the abdominal viscera. The diaphragm is lower when a person is sitting or standing; it is higher in the supine position and after a large meal.
- When seen from the side, the diaphragm has the appearance of an inverted J, the long limb extending up from the vertebral column and the short limb extending forward to the xiphoid process.

## NERVE SUPPLY OF THE DIAPHRAGM

- **Motor nerve supply:** The right and left phrenic nerves (C3, 4, 5).
- **Sensory nerve supply:** The parietal pleura and peritoneum covering the central surfaces of the diaphragm are from the phrenic nerve and the periphery of the diaphragm is from the lower six intercostal nerves.

## ACTION OF THE DIAPHRAGM

- On contraction, the diaphragm pulls down its central tendon and increases the vertical diameter of the thorax.

## FUNCTIONS OF THE DIAPHRAGM

- **Muscle of inspiration:** On contraction, the diaphragm pulls its central tendon down and increases the vertical diameter of the thorax. The diaphragm is the most important muscle used in inspiration.
- **Muscle of abdominal straining:** The contraction of the diaphragm assists the contraction of the muscles of the anterior abdominal wall in raising the intra-abdominal pressure for micturition, defecation, and parturition. This mechanism is further aided by the person taking a deep breath and closing the glottis of the larynx. The diaphragm is unable to rise because of the air trapped in the respiratory tract. Now and again, air is allowed to escape, producing a grunting sound.
- **Weight-lifting muscle:** In a person taking a deep breath and holding it (fixing the diaphragm), the diaphragm assists the muscles of the anterior abdominal wall in raising the intra-abdominal pressure to such an extent that it helps support the vertebral column and prevent flexion. This greatly assists the postvertebral muscles in the lifting of heavy weights. Needless to say, it is important to have adequate sphincteric control of the bladder and anal canal under these circumstances.

- **Thoracoabdominal pump:** The descent of the diaphragm decreases the intrathoracic pressure and at the same time increases the intra-abdominal pressure. This pressure change compresses the blood in the inferior vena cava and forces it upward into the right atrium of the heart. Lymph within the abdominal lymph vessels is also compressed, and its passage upward within the thoracic duct is aided by the negative intrathoracic pressure.
- The presence of valves within the thoracic duct prevents backflow.

## PATHWAYS THROUGH THE DIAPHRAGM

- There are three openings that act as conduit for these structures:

**VOA (Voice Of America at 8:10: 12):**

- **Vena Cava opening (8 letters) = T8 level**
  - Inferior vena cava
  - Right phrenic nerves.

- **Oesophagus opening (10 letters) =T10 level**
  - Oesophagus,
  - Vagus nerves
  - Oesophageal branches of the left gastric vessels.

- **Aortic Hiatus opening (12 letters) = T12 level**
  - Aorta
  - Thoracic duct
  - Azygos vein.

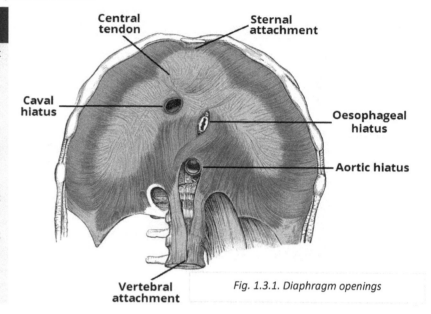

Fig. 1.3.1. Diaphragm openings

## INTERNAL THORACIC ARTERY

- The internal thoracic artery supplies the anterior wall of the body from the clavicle to the umbilicus. It is a branch of the first part of the subclavian artery in the neck. It descends vertically on the pleura behind the costal cartilages, a fingerbreadth lateral to the sternum, and ends in the sixth intercostal space by dividing into the superior epigastric and musculophrenic arteries.

### BRANCHES

- Two **anterior intercostal arteries** for the upper six intercostals spaces
- **Perforating arteries,** which accompany the terminal branches of the corresponding intercostal nerves.
- The **pericardiacophrenic artery,** which accompanies the phrenic nerve and supplies the pericardium
- **Mediastinal arteries** to the contents of the anterior mediastinum (Thymus)
- The **superior epigastric artery,** which enters the rectus sheath of the anterior abdominal wall and supplies the rectus muscle as far as the umbilicus.
- The **musculophrenic artery,** which runs around the costal margin of the diaphragm and supplies the lower intercostal spaces and the diaphragm.

## INTERNAL THORACIC VEIN

- The internal thoracic vein accompanies the internal thoracic artery and drains into the brachiocephalic vein on each side.

## LEVATORES COSTARUM

- There are 12 pairs of muscles. Each levator costa is triangular in shape and arises by its apex from the tip of the transverse process and is inserted into the rib below.
- **Action:** Each raises the rib below and is therefore an inspiratory muscle.
- **Nerve supply:** Posterior rami of thoracic spinal nerves.

## SERRATUS POSTERIOR SUPERIOR MUSCLE

- The serratus posterior superior is a thin, flat muscle that arises from the lower cervical and upper thoracic spines. Its fibers pass downward and laterally and are inserted into the upper ribs.
- **Action:** It elevates the ribs and is therefore an inspiratory muscle.
- **Nerve supply:** Intercostal nerves.

## SERRATUS POSTERIOR INFERIOR MUSCLE

- The serratus posterior inferior is a thin, flat muscle that arises from the upper lumbar and lower thoracic spines. Its fibers pass upward and laterally and are inserted into the lower ribs.
- **Action:** It depresses the ribs and is therefore an expiratory muscle.
- **Nerve supply:** Intercostal nerves.

# 8. NERVES OF THE THORAX

## A. VAGUS NERVES

- The **right vagus nerve** descends in the thorax, first lying posterolateral to the brachiocephalic artery, then lateral to the trachea and medial to the terminal part of the azygos vein. It passes **behind** the root of the right lung and assists in the formation of the **pulmonary plexus.** On leaving the plexus, the vagus passes onto the posterior surface of the oesophagus and takes part in the formation of the **oesophageal plexus.** It then passes through the oesophageal opening of the diaphragm behind the oesophagus to reach the posterior surface of the stomach.

- The **left vagus nerve** descends in the thorax between the left common carotid and the left subclavian arteries. It then crosses the left side of the aortic arch and is itself crossed by the left phrenic nerve. The vagus then turns backward **behind** the root of the left lung and assists in the formation of the **pulmonary plexus.** On leaving the plexus, the vagus passes onto the anterior surface of the oesophagus and takes part in the formation of the **oesophageal plexus.**

- It then passes through the oesophageal opening in the diaphragm in front of the oesophagus to reach the anterior surface of the stomach.

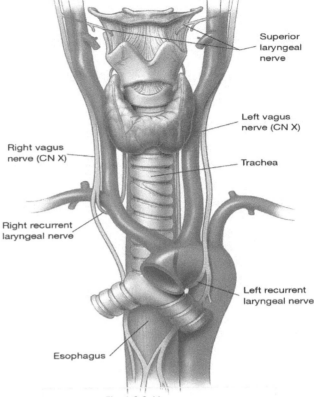

*Fig. 1.3.2. Vagus nerves*

## BRANCHES

- Both vagi supply the lungs and oesophagus. The right vagus gives off cardiac branches, and the left vagus gives origin to the left recurrent laryngeal nerve. (The right recurrent laryngeal nerve arises from the right vagus in the neck and hooks around the subclavian artery and ascends between the trachea and oesophagus.)

- The **left recurrent laryngeal nerve** arises from the left vagus trunk as the nerve crosses the arch of the aorta. It hooks around the ligamentum arteriosum and ascends in the groove between the trachea and the oesophagus on the left side. It supplies all the muscles acting on the left vocal cord (except the cricothyroid muscle, a tensor of the cord, which is supplied by the external laryngeal branch of the vagus).

## B. PHRENIC NERVES

- **Nerve roots:** Anterior rami of C3, C4 and C5.
- **Motor functions:** Innervates the diaphragm.
- **Sensory functions:** Innervates the central part of the diaphragm, the pericardium and the mediastinal part of the parietal pleura.

### ANATOMICAL COURSE

- The phrenic nerve mainly originates from the **C4** spinal root, but it also receives contributions from **C3** and **C5.** It also receives some communicating fibres from the cervical plexus.
- The nerve begins at the lateral border of the **anterior scalene** muscle. It then continues inferiorly over the anterior surface of anterior scalene, deep to the **prevertebral layer** of deep cervical fascia. From here, the course of the phrenic nerve differs between the left and right.

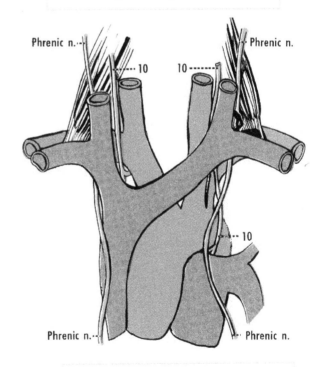

*Fig. 1.3.3. Phrenic nerves*

## RIGHT PHRENIC NERVE

- Passes anteriorly to second part of the subclavian artery, and posteriorly to the subclavian vein. Enters the thorax via the superior thoracic aperture.
- Descends anteriorly to the right lung root, down the right side of the pericardium. Reaches the diaphragm and pieces the muscle to supply the underlying surface.

## LEFT PHRENIC NERVE

- Passes anteriorly to the first part of the subclavian artery, and posteriorly to the subclavian vein. Enters the thorax via the superior thoracic aperture.
- Crosses the aortic arch and vagus nerve, and descends anteriorly to the left lung root, down the left side of the pericardium. Reaches the diaphragm and pieces the muscle to supply the underlying surface.
- **Motor Functions**
  - The phrenic nerve provides motor innervation to the **diaphragm**; the main muscle of respiration.
  - As the phrenic nerve is a bilateral structure, each nerve supplies the **ipsilateral side** of the diaphragm (i.e. the hemi-diaphragm on the same side as itself).
- **Sensory Functions**
  - Sensory fibres from the phrenic nerve supply the central part of the diaphragm, including the surrounding pleura and peritoneum.
  - The nerve also supplies sensation to the **mediastinal pleura** and the **pericardium.**

## 9. AZYGOS SYSTEM OF VEINS

- This venous network drains blood from the body walls and mediastinal viscera, and empties into the **Superior Vena Cava.**
- It consists of three major veins:
  - **Azygos Vein:**
    Formed by the union of the right lumbar vein and the right subcostal vein. It enters the mediastinum via the aortic hiatus and drains into the superior vena cava.
  - **Hemiazygos Vein:**
    Formed by the union of the left lumbar vein and left subcostal vein. It enters the mediastinum through the left crus of the diaphragm, ascending on the left side.
    At the level of **T8,** it turns to the right and combines with the azygos vein.
  - **Accessory Hemiazygos Vein:**
    Formed by the union of the fourth to eighth intercostal veins. It drains into the azygos vein at **T7.**

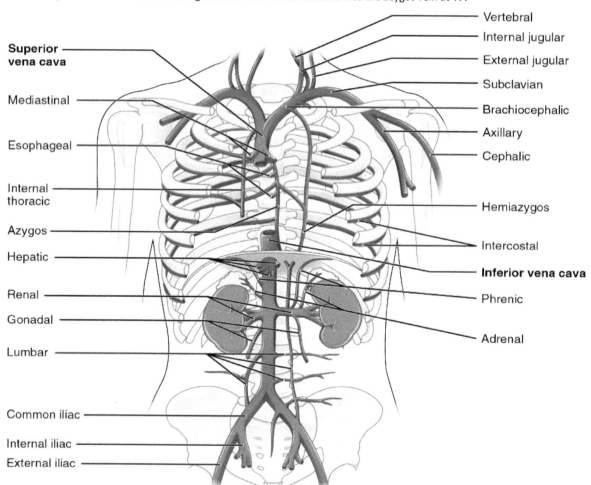

*Fig. 1.3.4. Azygos system of veins*

# CLINICAL RELEVANCE: TRAUMATIC INJURY TO THE THORAX

## FRACTURED STERNUM
o   The sternum is a resilient structure that is held in position by relatively pliable costal cartilages and bendable ribs. For these reasons, fracture of the sternum is not common; however, it does occur in high-speed motor vehicle accidents.
o   Remember that the heart lies posterior to the sternum and may be severely contused by the sternum on impact.

## RIB CONTUSION
o   Bruising of a rib, secondary to trauma, is the most common rib injury. In this painful condition, a small hemorrhage occurs beneath the periosteum.

## RIB FRACTURES
o   Fractures of the ribs are common chest injuries. In children, the ribs are highly elastic, and fractures in this age group are therefore rare. Unfortunately, the pliable chest wall in the young can be easily compressed so that the underlying lungs and heart may be injured. With increasing age, the rib cage becomes more rigid, owing to the deposit of calcium in the costal cartilages, and the ribs become brittle. The ribs then tend to break at their weakest part, their angles.
o   The ribs prone to fracture are those that are exposed or relatively fixed. Ribs 5 through 10 are the most commonly fractured ribs. The first four ribs are protected by the clavicle and pectoral muscles anteriorly and by the scapula and its associated muscles posteriorly. The 11th and 12th ribs float and move with the force of impact.
o   Because the rib is sandwiched between the skin externally and the delicate pleura internally, it is not surprising that the jagged ends of a fractured rib may penetrate the lungs and present as a **pneumothorax.** Severe localized pain is usually the most important symptom of a fractured rib. The periosteum of each rib is innervated by the intercostal nerves above and below the rib. To encourage the patient to breathe adequately, it may be necessary to relieve the pain by performing an intercostal nerve block.

## FLAIL CHEST
o   In severe crush injuries, a number of ribs may break. If limited to one side, the fractures may occur near the rib angles and anteriorly near the costochondral junctions. This causes flail chest, in which a section of the chest wall is disconnected to the rest of the thoracic wall. If the fractures occur on either side of the sternum, the sternum may be flail. In either case, the stability of the chest wall is lost, and the flail segment is sucked in during inspiration and driven out during expiration, producing paradoxical and ineffective respiratory movements.

## TRAUMATIC INJURY TO THE BACK OF THE CHEST
o   The posterior wall of the chest in the midline is formed by the vertebral column. In severe posterior chest injuries, the possibility of a vertebral fracture with associated injury to the spinal cord should be considered. Remember also the presence of the scapula, which overlies the upper seven ribs. This bone is covered with muscles and is fractured only in cases of severe trauma.

## TRAUMATIC INJURY TO THE ABDOMINAL VISCERA AND THE CHEST
o   When the anatomy of the thorax is reviewed, it is important to remember that the upper abdominal organs—namely, the liver, stomach, and spleen—may be injured by trauma to the rib cage. In fact, any injury to the chest below the level of the nipple line may involve abdominal organs as well as chest organs.

## CERVICAL RIB
o   A cervical rib (i.e., a rib arising from the anterior tubercle of the transverse process of the 7th cervical vertebra) occurs in about 0.5% of humans. It may have a free anterior end, may be connected to the 1st rib by a fibrous band, or may articulate with the 1st rib. The importance of a cervical rib is that it can cause pressure on the lower trunk of the brachial plexus in some patients, producing pain down the medial side of the forearm and hand and wasting of the small muscles of the hand.
o   It can also exert pressure on the overlying subclavian artery and interfere with the circulation of the upper limb.

## RIB EXCISION
o   Rib excision is commonly performed by thoracic surgeons wishing to gain entrance to the thoracic cavity. A longitudinal incision is made through the periosteum on the outer surface of the rib, and a segment of the rib is removed.
o   A second longitudinal incision is then made through the bed of the rib, which is the inner covering of periosteum.
o   After the operation, the rib regenerates from the osteogenetic layer of the periosteum.

## PARALYSIS OF THE DIAPHRAGM
o   A single dome of the diaphragm may be paralyzed by crushing or sectioning of the phrenic nerve in the neck.
o   This may be necessary in the treatment of certain forms of lung tuberculosis, when the physician wishes to rest the lower lobe of the lung on one side. Occasionally, the contribution from the fifth cervical spinal nerve joins the phrenic nerve late as a branch from the nerve to the subclavius muscle. This is known as the **accessory phrenic nerve.**
o   To obtain complete paralysis under these circumstances, the nerve to the subclavius muscle must also be sectioned.

## PENETRATING INJURIES OF THE DIAPHRAGM
o   Penetrating injuries can result from stab or bullet wounds to the chest or abdomen. Any penetrating wound to the chest below the level of the nipples should be suspected of causing damage to the diaphragm until proved otherwise.
o   The arching domes of the diaphragm can reach the level of the 5th rib (the right dome can reach a higher level).

# EMERGENCY BEDSIDE THORACOTOMY

- The primary aims of emergency thoracotomy are:
  - Release of cardiac tamponade
  - Control of haemorrhage
  - Allow access for internal cardiac massage
- Secondary manoeuvers include cross-clamping of the descending thoracic aorta.
- Once control is achieved and cardiac activity restored, the patient is transferred rapidly to the operating room for definitive management.

## ANTEROLATERAL THORACOTOMY APPROACH

- A supine anterolateral thoracotomy is the accepted approach for emergency department thoracotomy.
- A left sided approach is used in all patients in traumatic arrest and with injuries to the left chest.
- Patients who are not arrested but with profound hypotension and right sided injuries have their right chest opened first
- The incision is typically made over the **fifth rib into the fourth intercostal space**, beginning at the sternum and extending to the posterior axillary line. The incision should be deep enough to partially transect **the latissimus dorsi muscle.**
- Time should not be taken to count the rib spaces.
- In patients with a suspected left subclavian injury, the incision may be made **in the third intercostal space.**
- A left-sided approach is made in all traumatic arrests and in patients with left-sided chest injuries.
- Division of the sternum results in transection of the **internal mammary arteries.**
- These will start to bleed once blood pressure is restored and will need clipping and ligation subsequently.

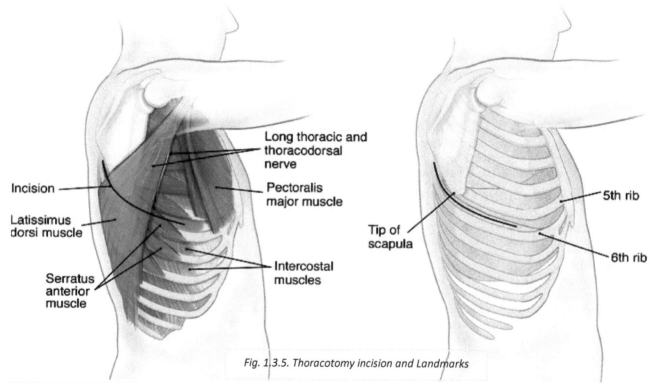

Fig. 1.3.5. Thoracotomy incision and Landmarks

- **RELIEF OF TAMPONADE**
  - The pericardium is opened longitudinally to avoid damage to the phrenic nerve, which runs along its lateral border.
  - It is difficult to visualise the phrenic nerve in the emergency thoracotomy.
  - Make a small incision in the pericardium with scissors and then tear the pericardium longitudinally with your fingers - this will avoid **lacerating the phrenic nerve**. Evacuate any blood and clot from the pericardial cavity.

- **CARDIAC WOUNDS**
  - Cardiac wounds should be controlled initially with direct finger pressure.
  - Large wounds may be controlled temporarily by the insertion of a Foley catheter with inflation of the balloon.
  - The balloon may obstruct inflow or outflow tracts however and it may also lead to extension of the laceration if excessive traction is placed on it. Satinsky clamps can be placed across wounds of the atria to control haemorrhage.
  - With extensive cardiac damage it may be necessary to temporarily obstruct venous inflow to allow repair.
  - Take care also not to miss posterior cardiac wounds.
  - Examination of the posterior surface of the heart requires displacing it anteriorly, which may obstruct venous inflow.

# II. THORACIC INLET & THORACIC PLANE

## THORACIC INLET

**Boundaries**
- o **Posteriorly**   : T1 vertebral body
- o **Laterally**   : First rib and costal cartilage
- o **Anteriorly**   : Manubrium

**Contents:**
➤ **Viscera**
- Lung apices
- Thymus,
- Trachea,
- Oesophagus

➤ *Muscles*
- Sternocleidomastoid muscle
- Anterior and middle scalene muscles
- Sternohyoid muscle
- Sternothyroid muscle

➤ *Vessels, nerves and lymphatics*
- Common carotid arteries
- Confluences of internal jugular and subclavian veins
- Phrenic nerves,
- Vagus nerves,
- Recurrent laryngeal nerves
- Thoracic duct,
- Prevertebral fascia

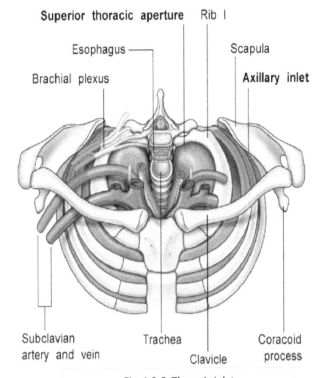

*Fig. 1.3.6. Thoracic inlet*

## THORACIC PLANE

- The thoracic plane, also known as the **Plane of Ludwig** is an artificial horizontal plane used to divide the mediastinum into the superior mediastinum and the inferior mediastinum.
- *It runs from the manubriosternal joint (sternal angle or angle of Louis) to the inferior endplate of T4 (T4-5 disc).*
- **Structures transected by the thoracic plane:**
  - o Bifurcation of the trachea, i.e. The carina
  - o Aortic arch (inner concavity)
  - o Pulmonary trunk bifurcation
  - o Azygos vein drains into the SVC, arching over the right main bronchus
  - o Thoracic duct moves from right to left hand side posterior to the oesophagus
  - o Ligamentum arteriosum
  - o Cardiac plexus (superficial and deep parts)
  - o Termination of the pre-vertebral fascia and pre-tracheal fascia
  - o 2nd rib joins the manubriosternal junction via the costal cartilage

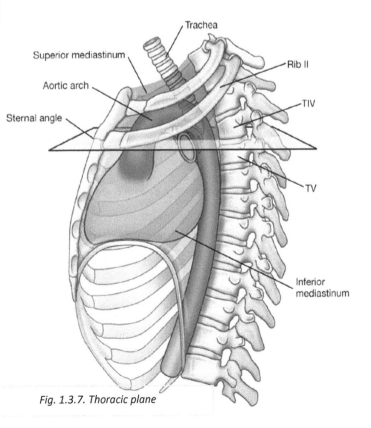

*Fig. 1.3.7. Thoracic plane*

# III. CHEST CAVITY

## OVERVIEW

- The chest cavity is bounded by the chest wall and below by the diaphragm. It extends upward into the root of the neck about one fingerbreadth above the clavicle on each side. The diaphragm, which is a very thin muscle, is the only structure (apart from the pleura and the peritoneum) that separates the chest from the abdominal viscera.
- The chest cavity can be divided into a median partition, called the **mediastinum,** and the laterally placed pleurae and lungs.

## 1. MEDIASTINUM

- The mediastinum, though thick, is a movable partition that extends superiorly to the thoracic outlet and the root of the neck and inferiorly to the diaphragm. It extends anteriorly to the sternum and posteriorly to the vertebral column. It contains the remains of the thymus, the heart and large blood vessels, the trachea and oesophagus, the thoracic duct and lymph nodes, the vagus and phrenic nerves, and the sympathetic trunks.
- The mediastinum is divided into **superior** and **inferior mediastina** by an imaginary plane passing from the sterna angle anteriorly to the lower border of the body of the 4th thoracic vertebra posteriorly.
- The inferior mediastinum is further subdivided into:
  - The **middle mediastinum,** which consists of the pericardium and heart;
  - The **anterior mediastinum,** which is a space between the pericardium and the sternum; and
  - The **posterior mediastinum,** which lies between the pericardium and the vertebral column.

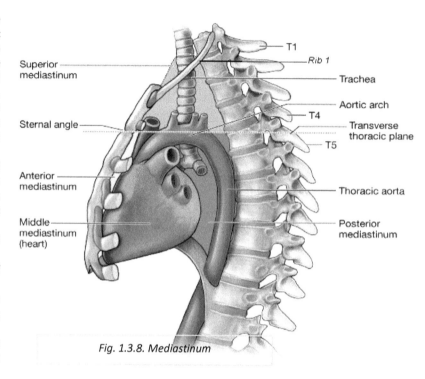

Fig. 1.3.8. Mediastinum

- For purposes of orientation, it is convenient to remember that the major mediastinal structures are arranged in the following order from anterior to posterior.

| | |
|---|---|
| • **Superior Mediastinum**<br>   o Thymus,<br>   o Large veins,<br>   o Large arteries,<br>   o Trachea,<br>   o Oesophagus and thoracic duct, and<br>   o Sympathetic trunks.<br>• The superior mediastinum is bounded in front by the manubrium sterni and behind by the first four thoracic vertebrae. | • **Inferior Mediastinum**<br>   o Thymus,<br>   o Heart within the pericardium with the phrenic nerves on each side,<br>   o Oesophagus and thoracic duct,<br>   o Descending aorta, and<br>   o Sympathetic trunks.<br>• The inferior mediastinum is bounded in front by the body of the sternum and behind by the lower eight thoracic |

## 2. PLEURAE

- The pleurae and lungs lie on either side of the mediastinum within the chest cavity.
- Each pleura has two parts: a **parietal layer,** which lines the thoracic wall, covers the thoracic surface of the diaphragm and the lateral aspect of the mediastinum and extends into the root of the neck to line the undersurface of the suprapleural membrane at the thoracic outlet; and into the neck, lining the undersurface of the suprapleural membrane.
- It reaches a level 1 to 1.5 inches (2.5 to 4 cm) above the medial third of the clavicle.
- The **costal pleura** lines the inner surfaces of the ribs, the costal cartilages, the intercostal spaces, the sides of the vertebral bodies, and the back of the sternum.
- The **diaphragmatic pleura** covers the thoracic surface of the diaphragm. In quiet respiration, the costal and diaphragmatic pleurae are in apposition to each other below the lower border of the lung. In deep inspiration, the margins of the base of the lung descend, and the costal and diaphragmatic pleurae separate.
- This lower area of the pleural cavity into which the lung expands on inspiration is referred to as the **costodiaphragmatic recess.**

- The **mediastinal pleura** covers and forms the lateral boundary of the mediastinum. At the hilum of the lung, it is reflected as a cuff around the vessels and bronchi and here becomes continuous with the visceral pleura. It is thus seen that each lung lies free except at its hilum, where it is attached to the blood vessels and bronchi that constitute the **lung root.** During full inspiration, the lungs expand and fill the pleural cavities. However, during quiet inspiration, the lungs do not fully occupy the pleural cavities at four sites: the right and left costodiaphragmatic recesses and the right and left costomediastinal recesses.
- The **costodiaphragmatic recesses** are slitlike spaces between the costal and diaphragmatic parietal pleurae that are separated only by a capillary layer of pleural fluid. During inspiration, the lower margins of the lungs descend into the recesses. During expiration, the lower margins of the lungs ascend so that the costal and diaphragmatic pleurae come together again.
- The **costomediastinal recesses** are situated along the anterior margins of the pleura. They are slitlike spaces between the costal and mediastinal parietal pleurae, which are separated by a capillary layer of pleural fluid. During inspiration and expiration, the anterior borders of the lungs slide in and out of the recesses.

## NERVE SUPPLY OF THE PLEURA
- **The parietal pleura** is sensitive to **pain, temperature, touch, and pressure** and is supplied as follows:
    o  The costal pleura is segmentally supplied by the **intercostals nerves.**
    o  The mediastinal pleura is supplied by the **phrenic nerve.**
    o  The diaphragmatic pleura is supplied over the **domes by the phrenic nerve** and around the periphery by the lower six intercostal nerves.
- **The visceral pleura** covering the lungs is sensitive to stretch but is **insensitive to common sensations such as pain and touch**. It receives an autonomic nerve supply from the pulmonary plexus.

## 3. TRACHEA
- The trachea is a mobile cartilaginous and membranous tube. It begins in the neck as a continuation of the larynx at the lower border of the cricoid cartilage at the level of the 6th cervical vertebra. It descends in the midline of the neck. In the thorax, the trachea ends below at the **carina** by dividing into right and left principal (main) bronchi at the level of the sternal angle (opposite the disc between the 4th and 5th thoracic vertebrae). During expiration, the bifurcation rises by about one vertebral level, and during deep inspiration may be lowered as far as the 6th thoracic vertebra.
- In adults, the trachea is about 4 1/2 in. (11.25 cm) long and 1 in. (2.5 cm) in diameter. The fibroelastic tube is kept patent by the presence of U-shaped bars (rings) of hyaline cartilage embedded in its wall. The posterior free ends of the cartilage are connected by smooth muscle, the **trachealis muscle.**
- The relations of the trachea in the superior mediastinum of the thorax are as follows:
- **Anteriorly:** The sternum, the thymus, the left brachiocephalic vein, the origins of the brachiocephalic and left common carotid arteries, and the arch of the aorta.
- **Posteriorly:** The oesophagus and the left recurrent laryngeal nerve.
- **Right side:** The azygos vein, the right vagus nerve, and the pleura.
- **Left side:** The arch of the aorta, the left common carotid and left subclavian arteries, the left vagus and left phrenic nerves, and the pleura.

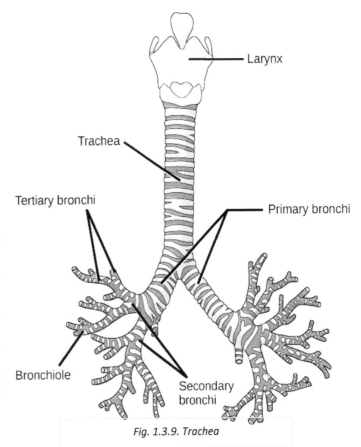

Fig. 1.3.9. Trachea

### BLOOD SUPPLY OF THE TRACHEA
- The upper two thirds are supplied by **the inferior thyroid arteries** and the lower third is supplied by the **bronchial arteries.**

### LYMPH DRAINAGE OF THE TRACHEA
- The lymph drains into the **pretracheal and paratracheal lymph nodes and the deep cervical nodes.**

### NERVE SUPPLY OF THE TRACHEA
- The sensory nerve supply is from the **vagi and the recurrent laryngeal nerves.**
- Sympathetic nerves supply the trachealis muscle.

## 4. THE BRONCHI

- The trachea bifurcates behind the arch of the aorta into the **right and left principal (primary or main) bronchi.**
- The bronchi divide dichotomously, giving rise to several million terminal bronchioles that terminate in one or more respiratory bronchioles. Each respiratory bronchiole divides into 2 to 11 alveolar ducts that enter the alveolar sacs. The alveoli arise from the walls of the sacs as diverticula.

- **PRINCIPAL BRONCHI**
  - ○ **The right principal (main) bronchus** is wider, shorter, and more vertical than the left and is about 1 in. (2.5 cm) long. Before entering the hilum of the right lung, the principal bronchus gives off the **superior lobar bronchus.** On entering the hilum, it divides into a **middle** and an **inferior lobar bronchus**.
  - ○ **The left principal (main) bronchus** is narrower, longer, and more horizontal than the right and is about 2 in. (5 cm) long. It passes to the left below the arch of the aorta and **in front of the oesophagus.** On entering the hilum of the left lung, the principal bronchus divides into a **superior** and an **inferior lobar bronchus.**

## 5. LUNGS

### A. THE APEX (APEX PULMONIS)

- Is rounded, and extends into the root of the neck, reaching from 2.5 to 4 cm above the level of the sternal end of the first rib.

### B. THE BASE (BASIS PULMONIS)

- Is broad, concave, and rests upon the convex surface of the diaphragm, which separates the right lung from the right lobe of the liver, and the left lung from the left lobe of the liver, the stomach, and the spleen. It descends below the medial end of the 12th rib.

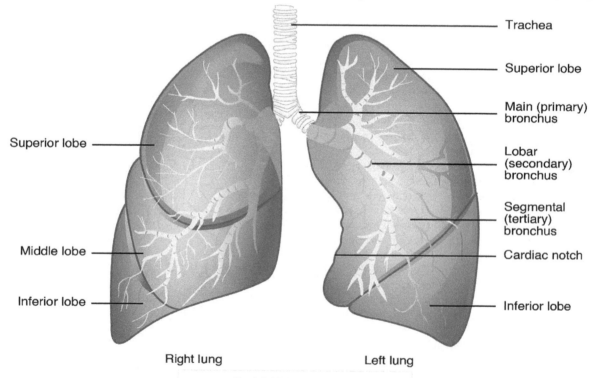

Fig. 1.3.10. Lungs anatomy

### C. SURFACES

- **The costal surface** (facies costalis; external or thoracic surface) is smooth, convex, of considerable extent, and corresponds to the form of the cavity of the chest, being deeper behind than in front.
- **The mediastinal surface** (facies mediastinalis; inner surface) is in contact with the mediastinal pleura.
- *The visceral pleura is sensitive only to stretch and is supplied by autonomic nerves.*
- *The parietal pleura is sensitive to pain and is supplied by somatic nerves*

### D. BORDERS

- **The inferior border (Margo inferior)** is thin and sharp where it separates the base from the costal surface and extends into the phrenicocostal sinus; medially where it divides the base from the mediastinal surface it is blunt and rounded.
- **The posterior border (Margo posterior)** is broad and rounded, and is received into the deep concavity on either side of the vertebral column.
  - ○ It is much longer than the anterior border, and projects, below, into the phrenicocostal sinus.

- The anterior border **(Margo anterior)** is thin and sharp, and overlaps the front of the pericardium.
  - The anterior border of the right lung is almost vertical, and projects into the costomediastinal sinus; that of the left presents, below, an angular notch, the cardiac notch, in which the pericardium is exposed.
  - Opposite this notch the anterior margin of the left lung is situated some little distance lateral to the line of reflection of the corresponding part of the pleura.
  - *The medial ends of the 4th and 5th intercostal spaces are not covered by pleura.*

# E. FISSURES AND LOBES OF THE LUNGS

- The right lung has 3 lobes (upper, middle and lower) while the left lung has only 2 lobes (upper and lower).
- Despite the difference in numbers of lobes, both lungs in general have **10 bronchopulmonary segments.**
- A bronchopulmonary segment is an anatomically discreet section of lung supplied by its own bronchus and artery.
- **Oblique fissures** are found in both lungs:
  - On the left, it separates the left upper from the left lower lobe.
  - In the right lung, the superior part of the oblique fissure separates right upper lobe from the right lower lobe while the inferior part separates the right middle lobe from the right lower lobe.
  - *In both lungs, its surface markings are from the spinous process of T3/T4 round to cross the 5th intercostal space at the mid-axillary line and then follow the oblique contour of the 6th rib anteriorly to join the sternum at the level of the 6th costal cartilage.*
- **The horizontal fissure** (only found in the right lung) separates the right upper lobe from the right middle lobe.
- *Its surface markings arise from the oblique fissure at the level of the 5th intercostal space in the mid-axillary line then roughly follows the course of the 4th rib anteriorly to join the sternum at the level of the 4th costal cartilage.*

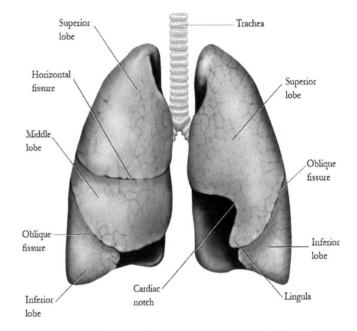

Fig. 1.3.11. Fissures and lobes of the lungs

| INFERIOR BORDER OF RIGHT LUNG: |
- **Posteriorly: at the level of the 10th rib**
- **Mid axillary line: 8th rib**
- **Mid clavicular line: 6th rib**

| INFERIOR BORDER OF PLEURA OF THE RIGHT LUNG: |
- Posteriorly: at the level of the 12th rib
- Mid axillary line: 10th rib
- Mid clavicular line: 8th rib

## F. THE HILUM OF THE LUNG

- The arrangement on the two sides is not symmetrical.
- Right side: (superior to inferior) **"EPHP"**
  - Eparterial bronchus, pulmonary artery, hyparterial bronchus and pulmonary vein
- Left Side: (superior to inferior) **"PBP"**
  - Pulmonary artery, bronchus and pulmonary vein.

## G. VESSELS

- The pulmonary artery conveys the venous blood to the lungs.
- The pulmonary capillaries
- The pulmonary veins commence in the pulmonary capillaries, open into the left atrium of the heart, conveying oxygenated blood to be distributed to all parts of the body by the aorta.

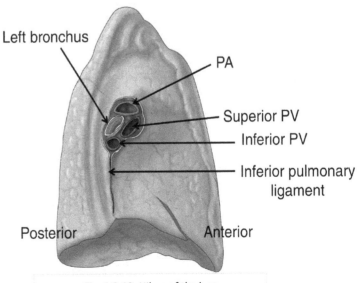

Fig. 1.3.12. Hilum of the lung

- The bronchial arteries supply blood for the nutrition of the lung.
- The bronchial vein is formed at the root of the lung, receiving superficial and deep veins corresponding to branches of the bronchial artery.

## H. NERVES

- The lungs are supplied from the anterior and posterior pulmonary plexuses, formed chiefly by branches from the sympathetic and vagus.

*The Right lung, although shorter by 2.5 cm than the left, in consequence of the diaphragm rising higher on the right side to accommodate the liver, is broader, owing to the inclination of the heart to the left side; its total capacity is greater and it weighs more than the left lung.*

## 6. THE MECHANICS OF RESPIRATION

- Respiration consists of two phases—inspiration and expiration— which are accomplished by the alternate increase and decrease of the capacity of the thoracic cavity.
- The rate varies between 16 and 20 per minute in normal resting patients and is faster in children and slower in the elderly.

## A. INSPIRATION

- Quiet Inspiration
- Compare the thoracic cavity to a box with a single entrance at the top, which is a tube called the **trachea**.
- The capacity of the box can be increased by elongating all its diameters, and this results in air under atmospheric pressure entering the box through the tube.
- Consider now the three diameters of the thoracic cavity and how they may be increased.
  - ➤ **Vertical Diameter** Theoretically, the roof could be raised and the floor lowered. The roof is formed by the suprapleural membrane and is fixed. Conversely, the floor is formed by the mobile diaphragm. When the diaphragm contracts, the domes become flattened and the level of the diaphragm is lowered.
  - ➤ **Anteroposterior Diameter** If the downward-sloping ribs were raised at their sternal ends, the anteroposterior diameter of the thoracic cavity would be increased and the lower end of the sternum would be thrust forward. This can be brought about by fixing the 1st rib by the contraction of the scaleni muscles of the neck and contracting the intercostal muscles. By this means, all the ribs are drawn together and raised toward the first rib.
  - ➤ **Transverse Diameter** The ribs articulate in front with the sternum via their costal cartilages and behind with the vertebral column. Because the ribs curve downward as well as forward around the chest wall, they resemble **bucket handles**. It therefore follows that if the ribs are raised (like bucket handles), the transverse diameter of the thoracic cavity will be increased. As described previously, this can be accomplished by fixing the 1st rib and raising the other ribs to it by contracting the intercostal muscles.

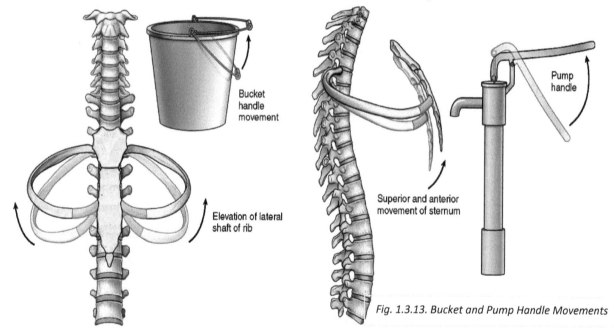

Bucket handle movement

Elevation of lateral shaft of rib

Pump handle

Superior and anterior movement of sternum

*Fig. 1.3.13. Bucket and Pump Handle Movements*

- An additional factor that must not be overlooked is the effect of the descent of the diaphragm on the abdominal viscera and the tone of the muscles of the anterior abdominal wall. As the diaphragm descends on inspiration, intra-abdominal pressure rises. This rise in pressure is accommodated by the reciprocal relaxation of the abdominal wall musculature.
- However, a point is reached when no further abdominal relaxation is possible, and the liver and other upper abdominal viscera act as a platform that resists further diaphragmatic descent. On further contraction, the diaphragm will now have its central tendon supported from below, and its shortening muscle fibers will assist the intercostal muscles in raising the lower ribs. Apart from the diaphragm and the intercostals, other less important muscles also contract on inspiration and assist in elevating the ribs, namely, the **levatores costarum muscles** and the **serratus posterior superior muscles**.

**FORCED INSPIRATION**

- In deep forced inspiration, a maximum increase in the capacity of the thoracic cavity occurs.
- Every muscle that can raise the ribs is brought into action, including the scalenus anterior and medius and the sternocleidomastoid. In respiratory distress, the action of all the muscles already engaged becomes more violent, and the scapulae are fixed by the trapezius, levator scapulae, and rhomboid muscles, enabling the serratus anterior and the pectoralis minor to pull up the ribs.
- If the upper limbs can be supported by grasping a chair back or table, the sterna origin of the pectoralis major muscles can also assist the process.

**LUNG CHANGES ON INSPIRATION**

- In inspiration, the root of the lung descends and the level of the bifurcation of the trachea may be lowered by as much as two vertebrae. The bronchi elongate and dilate and the alveolar capillaries dilate, thus assisting the pulmonary circulation.
- Air is drawn into the bronchial tree as the result of the positive atmospheric pressure exerted through the upper part of the respiratory tract and the negative pressure on the outer surface of the lungs brought about by the increased capacity of the thoracic cavity.
- With expansion of the lungs, the elastic tissue in the bronchial walls and connective tissue are stretched. As the diaphragm descends, the costodiaphragmatic recess of the pleural cavity opens, and the expanding sharp lower edges of the lungs descend to a lower level.

## B. EXPIRATION

- Quiet Expiration Quiet expiration is largely a passive phenomenon and is brought about by the elastic recoil of the lungs, the relaxation of the intercostal muscles and diaphragm, and an increase in tone of the muscles of the anterior abdominal wall, which forces the relaxing diaphragm upward. The **serratus posterior inferior muscles** play a minor role in pulling down the lower ribs.

**FORCED EXPIRATION**

- Forced expiration is an active process brought about by the forcible contraction of the musculature of the anterior abdominal wall. The quadratus lumborum also contracts and pulls down the 12th rib. It is conceivable that under these circumstances some of the intercostal muscles may contract, pull the ribs together, and depress them to the lowered 12th rib.
- The serratus posterior inferior and the latissimus dorsi muscles may also play a minor role.

**LUNG CHANGES ON EXPIRATION**

- In expiration, the roots of the lungs ascend along with the bifurcation of the trachea. The bronchi shorten and contract. The elastic tissue of the lungs recoils, and the lungs become reduced in size. With the upward movement of the diaphragm, increasing areas of the diaphragmatic and costal parietal pleura come into apposition, and the costodiaphragmatic recess becomes reduced in size. The lower margins of the lungs shrink and rise to a higher level.

## C. TYPES OF RESPIRATION

- In babies and young children, the ribs are nearly horizontal. Thus, babies have to rely mainly on the descent of the diaphragm to increase their thoracic capacity on inspiration.
- Because this is accompanied by a marked inward and outward excursion of the anterior abdominal wall, which is easily seen, respiration at this age is referred to as the **abdominal type of respiration.**
- After the second year of life, the ribs become more oblique, and the adult form of respiration is established.
- In the adult, a sexual difference exists in the type of respiratory movements.
- The female tends to rely mainly on the movements of the ribs rather than on the descent of the diaphragm on inspiration. This is referred to as the **thoracic type of respiration.**
- The male uses both the thoracic and abdominal forms of respiration, but mainly the abdominal form.

## CLINICAL RELEVANCE:
### 1. DEFLECTION OF MEDIASTINUM

- In the cadaver, the mediastinum, as the result of the hardening effect of the preserving fluids, is an inflexible, fixed structure.
- In the living, it is very mobile; the lungs, heart, and large arteries are in rhythmic pulsation, and the oesophagus distends as each bolus of food passes through it.
- If air enters the pleural cavity (a condition called **pneumothorax**), the lung on that side immediately collapses and the mediastinum is displaced to the opposite side. This condition reveals itself by the patient's being breathless and in a state of shock; on examination, the trachea and the heart are found to be displaced to the opposite side.

### 2. MEDIASTINITIS

- The structures that make up the mediastinum are embedded in loose connective tissue that is continuous with that of the root of the neck. Thus, it is possible for a deep infection of the neck to spread readily into the thorax, producing a mediastinitis.
- Penetrating wounds of the chest involving the oesophagus may produce a mediastinitis.
- In oesophageal perforations, air escapes into the connective tissue spaces and ascends beneath the fascia to the root of the neck, producing **subcutaneous emphysema.**

## 3. MEDIASTINAL TUMORS OR CYSTS

- Because many vital structures are crowded together within the mediastinum, their functions can be interfered with by an enlarging tumor or organ. A tumor of the left lung can rapidly spread to involve the mediastinal lymph nodes, which on enlargement may compress the left recurrent laryngeal nerve, producing paralysis of the left vocal fold.
- An expanding cyst or tumor can partially occlude the superior vena cava, causing severe congestion of the veins of the upper part of the body. Other pressure effects can be seen on the sympathetic trunks, phrenic nerves, and sometimes the trachea, main bronchi, and oesophagus.

## 4. PLEURAL FLUID

- The pleural space normally contains 5 to 10 mL of clear fluid, which lubricates the apposing surfaces of the visceral and parietal pleurae during respiratory movements. The formation of the fluid results from hydrostatic and osmotic pressures. Since the hydrostatic pressures are greater in the capillaries of the parietal pleura than in the capillaries of the visceral pleura (pulmonary circulation), the pleural fluid is normally absorbed into the capillaries of the visceral pleura.
- Any condition that increases the production of the fluid (e.g., inflammation, malignancy, congestive heart disease) or impairs the drainage of the fluid (e.g., collapsed lung) results in the abnormal accumulation of fluid, called a **pleural effusion.**
- The presence of 300 mL of fluid in the costodiaphragmatic recess in an adult is sufficient to enable its clinical detection. The clinical signs include decreased lung expansion on the side of the effusion, with decreased breath sounds and dullness on percussion over the effusion.

## 5. PLEURISY

- Inflammation of the pleura **(pleuritis** or **pleurisy),** secondary to inflammation of the lung (e.g., **pneumonia**), results in the pleural surfaces becoming coated with inflammatory exudate, causing the surfaces to be roughened.
- This roughening produces friction, and a **pleural rub** can be heard with the stethoscope on inspiration and expiration. Often, the exudate becomes invaded by fibroblasts, which lay down collagen and bind the visceral pleura to the parietal pleura, forming **pleural adhesions.**

## 6. PNEUMOTHORAX, EMPYEMA, AND PLEURAL EFFUSION

- As the result of disease or injury (stab or gunshot wounds), air can enter the pleural cavity from the lungs or through the chest wall (pneumothorax). In the old treatment of tuberculosis, air was purposely injected into the pleural cavity to collapse and rest the lung. This was known as **artificial pneumothorax.**
- A **spontaneous pneumothorax** is a condition in which air enters the pleural cavity suddenly without its cause being immediately apparent. After investigation, it is usually found that air has entered from a diseased lung and a bulla (bleb) has ruptured.
- Stab wounds of the thoracic wall may pierce the parietal pleura so that the pleural cavity is open to the outside air. This condition is called **open pneumothorax.** Each time the patient inspires, it is possible to hear air under atmospheric pressure being sucked into the pleural cavity.
- Sometimes the clothing and the layers of the thoracic wall combine to form a valve so that air enters on inspiration but cannot exit through the wound. In these circumstances, the air pressure builds up on the wounded side and pushes the mediastinum toward the opposite side. In this situation, a collapsed lung is on the injured side and the opposite lung is compressed by the deflected mediastinum. This dangerous condition is called a **tension pneumothorax.**
- Air in the pleural cavity associated with serous fluid is known as **hydropneumothorax,** associated with pus as **pyopneumothorax,** and associated with blood as **hemopneumothorax.**
- A collection of pus (without air) in the pleural cavity is called an **empyema.** The presence of serous fluid in the pleural cavity is referred to as a **pleural effusion.**

## 7. TRACHEITIS OR BRONCHITIS

- The mucosa lining the trachea is innervated by the recurrent laryngeal nerve and, in the region of its bifurcation, by the pulmonary plexus. A tracheitis or bronchitis gives rise to a raw, burning sensation felt deep to the sternum instead of actual pain. Many thoracic and abdominal viscera, when diseased, give rise to discomfort that is felt in the midline.
- It seems that organs possessing a sensory innervation that is not under normal conditions directly relayed to consciousness display this phenomenon. The afferent fibers from these organs traveling to the central nervous system accompany autonomic nerves.

## 8. INHALED FOREIGN BODIES

- Inhalation of foreign bodies into the lower respiratory tract is common, especially in children. Pins, screws, nuts, bolts, peanuts, and parts of chicken bones and toys have all found their way into the bronchi.
- Parts of teeth may be inhaled while a patient is under anaesthesia during a difficult dental extraction.
- Because the right bronchus is the wider and more direct continuation of the trachea, foreign bodies tend to enter the right instead of the left bronchus. From there, they usually pass into the middle or lower lobe bronchi.

# IV. HEART AND PERICARDIUM

## 1. PERICARDIUM

**1. Layers: 3 layers**
- *A superficial*: fibrous pericardium
- *A deep*: two-layer serous pericardium:
    - *The parietal layer* lines the internal surface of the fibrous pericardium
    - *The visceral layer* or *epicardium* lines the surface of the heart
    - They are separated by the *fluid-filled* **pericardial cavity**.

### FIBROUS PERICARDIUM
- Surrounds the heart and forms a protective covering for the cardiac chambers.
- It also acts as an anchor for the heart that keeps it restricted in the chest cavity by binding itself to the adjoining regions.
- It also prevents the overexpansion of the heart when there is a rise in the volume of blood inside the body.

### SEROUS PERICARDIUM
- It is closed sac within fibrous pericardium having Visceral & Parietal layer. The visceral layer of serous pericardium (epicardium) covers the surface of the heart. It also reflects onto the great vessels.
- This transparent membrane surrounds and protects the heart. It also contains a thin film of serous fluid that allows the heart to move and provides it with a frictionless environment to expand as well as contract.

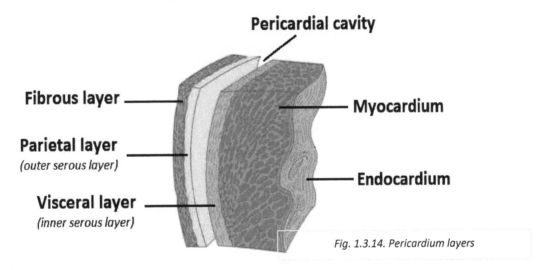

Fig. 1.3.14. Pericardium layers

## 2. BLOOD SUPPLY OF THE PERICARDIUM
- **The visceral pericardium** is supplied and drained by the Coronary System
- **The parietal and fibrous pericardium** receive arterial blood from the following sources:
    - *Pericardiophrenic and Musculophrenic branches* of the Internal Thoracic Artery
    - *Pericardial branches* from Bronchia, Oesophageal and Superior phrenic arteries.
- The veins drain into the Azygos System and Internal Thoracic Veins.

## 3. INNERVATION OF THE PERICARDIUM
- **The visceral pericardium** receives autonomic innervation from the Cardiac Plexus
- **The parietal and fibrous pericardium** are innervated mainly by the Phrenic Nerve.

## 2. THE HEART

### 1. OVERVIEW
- The heart is a myocardial muscular pump consisting of:
    - Four chambers,
    - Two auricles,
    - Four valves and a muscular septum all enclosed within a fluid filled sac, the pericardium
- The heart wall is composed of three distinct layers: The **Epicardium** (outermost layer), the **Myocardium** (middle layer, comprised of muscular fibers), and the **Endocardium** (innermost layer). To pump blood in and out of the chambers, doors are needed. The heart's valves open and shut, regulating the amount of blood that enters and exits. The atrioventricular valves (the tricuspid and mitral valves) control blood flow into the ventricles. They are pulled open by fibrous cords called *chordae tendineae.*
- The pulmonary and aortic valves control the flow of blood out of the heart.

## 2. BORDERS

- The heart has four borders:
  - ○ *The right border*:  right atrium and is in line with the superior and inferior vena cava.
  - ○ *The inferior border*:  the right ventricle, and slightly by the left ventricle near the apex.
  - ○ *The left border*: the left ventricle and very slightly by the left auricle.
  - ○ *The superior border*: is where the great vessels enter and leave the heart. It is formed by both atria.

## 3. HEART WALL

- ○ **Epicardium**: visceral layer of the serous pericardium
- ○ **Myocardium**: cardiac muscle layer forming the bulk of the heart.
- ○ **Fibrous skeleton of the heart**: crisscrossing, interlacing layer of connective tissue.
- ○ **Endocardium**: endothelial layer of the inner myocardial surface

## 5. ATRIA OF THE HEART

- Atria are receiving chambers of the heart. Each atrium has a protruding auricle.
- Pectinate muscles mark atrial walls
- Blood enters right atria from superior and inferior venae cava and coronary sinus.
- Blood enters left atria from pulmonary veins.

## 6. VENTRICLES OF THE HEART

- Ventricles are the discharging chambers of the heart.
- Papillary muscles and trabeculae carinae muscles mark ventricular walls.
- Right ventricle pumps blood into the pulmonary trunk.
- Left ventricle pumps blood into the aorta.

## 7. HEART VALVES

- **Aortic semilunar valve**: lies between left ventricle and aorta.
- **Pulmonary semilunar**:  valve lies between right ventricle and pulmonary trunk.
- Semilunar valves: prevent backflow of blood into ventricles

## 8. GREAT VESSELS

- These are: **SIPPA**
  - Superior vena cava
  - Inferior vena cava
  - Pulmonary arteries
  - Pulmonary veins
  - Aorta

## 9. THE CORONARY VESSELS OF THE HEART

There are two main coronary arteries that branch from the ascending aorta, known as the **Left and Right Coronary Arteries**.

- **The Left Main Coronary Artery supplies:**
  - Left Atrium,
  - Interventricular Septum,
  - Left Ventricle
  - Anterior Wall of the Right Ventricle.
- **The Right Coronary Artery supplies:**
  - Right Atrium,

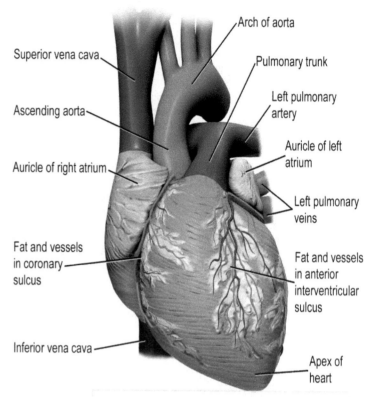

*Fig. 1.3.15. Great vessels of the Heart*

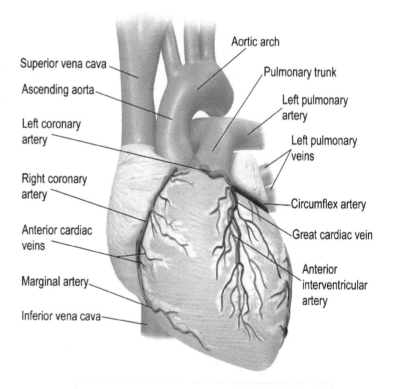

*Fig. 1.3.16. Coronary Vessels of the Heart*

- Right Ventricle
- Sino-Atrial Node.

- Coronary blood flow can be described as a **Phasic Flow.** This is because during systole, extravascular compression occurs; meaning the contraction of the heart squeezes these arteries shut.
- It is only during diastole that these arteries become patent again, allowing blood to flow under aortic pressure into these coronary arteries, capillaries and finally into the coronary veins.
- This is known as *coronary perfusion pressure (CPP)* which is the difference between the diastolic pressure in the aorta and the diastolic pressure in the right atrium creating a pressure gradient, which results in coronary blood flow.
- This is important clinically, as in cases of tachycardia there is less time spent in diastole, implying a reduced time for coronary blood flow to occur and hence increased risk of ischaemia.

### A. LEFT CORONARY ARTERY
- Origin: Arises from Posterior Aortic Sinus
- Left Main or left coronary artery (LCA)
  - **Left anterior descending (LAD)**
    - Diagonal branches
    - Septal branches
  - **Circumflex (Cx)**
    - Marginal branches

### B. RIGHT CORONARY ARTERY
- Origin: arises from the Anterior Aortic Sinus
- Branches:
  - **Acute marginal branch (AM)**
  - **AV node branch**
  - **Posterior descending artery (PDA)**

### C. COMMUNICATION BETWEEN LCA AND RCA
- There are four known communications between the left and right coronary arteries, at different sites within the heart.
- They are:
  - **The artery of the conus**: is a branch of the RCA, with the LAD.
  - **At the interventricular septum**, with **Septal Perforators** between the LAD and PDA.
  - **At the apex of the heart**, with the LAD and PDA.
  - **At the crux**, between the left circumflex and PDA.

### D. CORONARY VEINS
- From: coronary capillaries
- Draining to: the coronary sinus, located on the posterior surface of the heart, emptying into the right atrium. This includes:
  - **The great cardiac vein**, which drains areas of the heart supplied by the left coronary artery and lies in the anterior interventricular sulcus.
  - **The middle cardiac vein**, which drains areas of the heart supplied by the right coronary artery and lies in the posterior interventricular sulcus.
  - **Small cardiac vein** which drains the right atrium and ventricle
  - Other veins: the **oblique vein** draining the left atrium and **Posterior vein** draining the left ventricle.
- Some veins drain directly into the right atrium:
  - The anterior cardiac veins, which drain the right ventricle and the **Venae cordis minime**, also known as the **thesbesian veins.**

## CLINICAL RELEVANCE
## 1. CORONARY ARTERY DISEASE
- The myocardium receives its blood supply through the right and left coronary arteries.
- Although the coronary arteries have numerous anastomoses at the arteriolar level, they are essentially **functional end arteries.**
- A sudden block of one of the large branches of either coronary artery will usually lead to necrosis of the cardiac muscle (myocardial infarction) in that vascular area, and often the patient dies. Most cases of coronary artery blockage are caused by an acute thrombosis on top of a chronic atherosclerotic narrowing of the lumen. Arteriosclerotic disease of the coronary arteries may present in three ways, depending on the rate of narrowing of the lumina of the arteries:
  (1) General degeneration and fibrosis of the myocardium occur over many years and are caused by a gradual narrowing of the coronary arteries.
  (2) **Angina pectoris** is cardiac pain that occurs on exertion and is relieved by rest. In this condition, the coronary arteries are so narrowed that myocardial ischemia occurs on exertion but not at rest.
  (3) **Myocardial infarction** occurs when coronary flow is suddenly reduced or stopped and the cardiac muscle undergoes necrosis. Myocardial infarction is the major cause of death in industrialized nations.

## 2. ANEURYSM AND COARCTATION OF THE AORTA

- The arch of the aorta lies behind the manubrium sterni. A gross dilatation of the aorta (aneurysm) may show itself as a pulsatile swelling in the suprasternal notch. Coarctation of the aorta is a congenital narrowing of the aorta just proximal, opposite, or distal to the site of attachment of the ligamentum arteriosum. This condition is believed to result from an unusual quantity of ductus arteriosus muscle tissue in the wall of the aorta. When the ductus arteriosus contracts, the ductal muscle in the aortic wall also contracts, and the aortic
- lumen becomes narrowed. Later, when fibrosis takes place, the aortic wall also is involved, and permanent narrowing occurs.
- Clinically, the cardinal sign of aortic coarctation is absent or diminished pulses in the femoral arteries of both lower limbs.
- To compensate for the diminished volume of blood reaching the lower part of the body, an enormous collateral circulation develops, with dilatation of the internal thoracic, subclavian, and posterior intercostal arteries. The dilated intercostal arteries erode the lower borders of the ribs, producing characteristic notching, which is seen on radiographic examination. The condition should be treated surgically.

## 3. AORTIC DISSECTION
### CLASSIFICATIONS

### DEBAKEY CLASSIFICATION

- **Type I**: involves ascending and descending aorta (= Stanford A)
- **Type II**: involves ascending aorta only (= Stanford A)
- **Type III**: involves descending aorta only, commencing after the origin of the left subclavian artery (= Stanford B)

### STANFORD CLASSIFICATION

- **Type A**: **A** affects **a**scending **a**orta and arch
  - Accounts for ~60% of aortic dissections
  - Surgical management
  - May result in:
    - Coronary artery occlusion
    - Aortic incompetence
    - Rupture into pericardial sac with resulting cardiac tamponade
- **Type B**: **B** begins **b**eyond **b**rachiocephalic vessels
  - Accounts for ~40% of aortic dissections
  - Dissection commences distal to the left subclavian artery
  - Medical management with blood pressure control

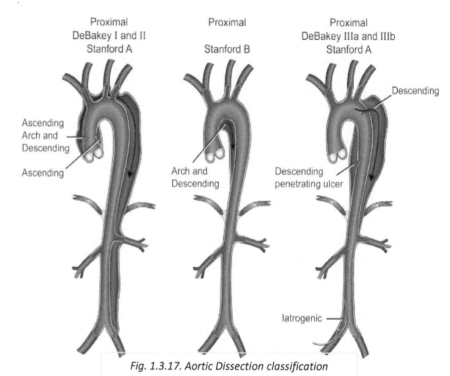

Fig. 1.3.17. Aortic Dissection classification

## CXR SIGNS OF AORTIC DISSECTION

- Widened mediastinum >8cm
- Displaced intimal calcification
- Pleural effusion (left >>> Right)
- Opacification of the AP window
- Left apical pleural cap
- Irregular aortic contour
- NG Tube displacement to the Rt
- Tracheal or oesophageal deviation
- Normal (10-15%)

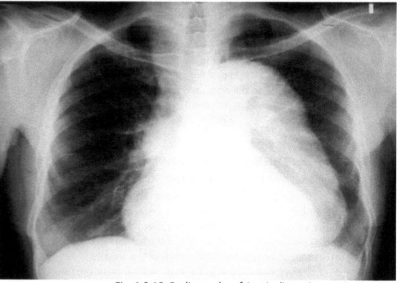

Fig. 1.3.18. Radiography of Aortic dissection

# V. OESOPHAGUS

## OVERVIEW

- The oesophagus is a tubular structure about 25 cm long that is continuous above with the laryngeal part of the pharynx opposite **the 6th cervical vertebra**. It passes through the diaphragm at the level of **the 10th thoracic vertebra** to join the stomach.
- In the neck, the oesophagus lies in front of the vertebral column; laterally, it is related to the lobes of the thyroid gland; and anteriorly, it is in contact with the trachea and the recurrent laryngeal nerves. In the thorax, it passes downward and to the left through the superior and then the posterior mediastinum. At the level of the sternal angle, the aortic arch pushes the oesophagus over to the midline.
- The relations of the thoracic part of the oesophagus from above downward are as follows:
  - **Anteriorly:** The trachea and the left recurrent laryngeal nerve; the left principal bronchus, which constricts it; and the pericardium, which separates the oesophagus from the left atrium.
  - **Posteriorly:** The bodies of the thoracic vertebrae; the thoracic duct; the azygos veins; the right posterior intercostals arteries; and, at its lower end, the descending thoracic aorta.
  - **Right side:** The mediastinal pleura and the terminal part of the azygos vein.
  - **Left side:** The left subclavian artery, the aortic arch, the thoracic duct, and the mediastinal pleura Inferiorly to the level of the roots of the lungs, the vagus nerves leave the pulmonary plexus and join with sympathetic nerves to form the **oesophageal plexus.** The left vagus lies anterior to the oesophagus, and the right vagus lies posterior.
- At the opening in the diaphragm, the oesophagus is accompanied by the two vagi, branches of the left gastric blood vessels, and lymphatic vessels. Fibers from the right crus of the diaphragm pass around the oesophagus in the form of a sling.
- In the abdomen, the oesophagus descends for about 1.3 cm and then enters the stomach. It is related to the left lobe of the liver anteriorly and to the left crus of the diaphragm posteriorly.

## BLOOD SUPPLY OF THE ESOPHAGUS

- The upper third of the oesophagus is supplied by the inferior thyroid artery, the middle third by branches from the descending thoracic aorta, and the lower third by branches from the left gastric artery.
- The veins from the upper third drain into the inferior thyroid veins, from the middle third into the azygos veins, and from the lower third into the left gastric vein, a tributary of the portal vein.

## LYMPH DRAINAGE OF THE ESOPHAGUS

- Lymph vessels from the upper third of the oesophagus drain into the **deep cervical nodes**, from the middle third into the superior and posterior mediastinal nodes, and from the lower third into nodes along the left gastric blood vessels and the celiac nodes.

## NERVE SUPPLY OF THE ESOPHAGUS

- The oesophagus is supplied by parasympathetic and sympathetic efferent and afferent fibers via the vagi and sympathetic trunks.
- In the lower part of its thoracic course, the oesophagus is surrounded by the oesophageal nerve plexus.

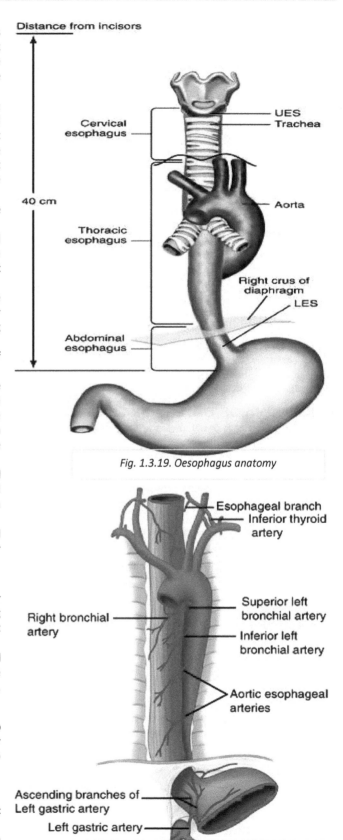

Fig. 1.3.19. Oesophagus anatomy

Fig. 1.3.20. Oesophagus Blood supply

## ESOPHAGEAL CONSTRICTIONS

- The oesophagus has three anatomic and physiologic constrictions.
    - The first is where the pharynx joins the upper end,
    - The second is where the aortic arch and the left bronchus cross its anterior surface, and
    - The third occurs where the oesophagus passes through the diaphragm into the stomach.
- Because a slight delay in the passage of food or fluid occurs at these levels, strictures develop here after the drinking of caustic fluids.
- Those constrictions are also the common sites of carcinoma of the oesophagus. It is useful to remember that their respective distances from the upper incisor teeth are 15 cm, 25 cm, and 41 cm, respectively.

## PORTAL–SYSTEMIC VENOUS ANASTOMOSIS

- At the lower third of the oesophagus is an important portal–systemic venous anastomosis. (For other portal–systemic anastomoses.
- Here, the oesophageal tributaries of the azygos veins (systemic veins) anastomose with the oesophageal tributaries of the left gastric vein (which drains into the portal vein). Should the portal vein become obstructed, as, for example, in **cirrhosis of the liver, portal hypertension** develops, resulting in the dilatation and varicosity of the portal–systemic anastomoses.
- Varicosed oesophageal veins may rupture during the passage of food, causing **hematemesis** (vomiting of blood), which may be fatal.

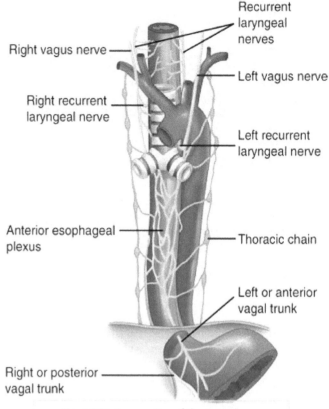

*Fig. 1.3.21. Innervation of the Oesophagus*

## CARCINOMA OF THE LOWER THIRD OF THE ESOPHAGUS

- The lymph drainage of the lower third of the oesophagus descends through the oesophageal opening in the diaphragm and ends in the celiac nodes around the celiac artery.
- A malignant tumor of this area of the oesophagus would therefore tend to spread below the diaphragm along this route.
- Consequently, surgical removal of the lesion would include not only the primary lesion, but also the celiac lymph nodes and all regions that drain into these nodes, namely, the stomach, the upper half of the duodenum, the spleen, and the omentum.
- Restoration of continuity of the gut is accomplished by performing an esophagojejunostomy.

## THE ESOPHAGUS AND THE LEFT ATRIUM OF THE HEART

- The close relationship between the anterior wall of the oesophagus and the posterior wall of the left atrium has already been emphasized. A barium swallow may help a physician assess the size of the left atrium in cases of left-sided heart failure, in which the left atrium becomes distended because of back pressure of venous blood.

## CHEST PAIN

- The presenting symptom of chest pain is a common problem in clinical practice.
- Unfortunately, chest pain is a symptom common to many conditions and may be caused by disease in the thoracic and abdominal walls or in many different thoracic and abdominal viscera.
- The severity of the pain is often unrelated to the seriousness of the cause.
- Myocardial pain may mimic esophagitis, musculoskeletal chest wall pain, and other nonlife-threatening causes.
- Unless the physician is astute, a patient may be discharged with a more serious condition than the symptoms indicate.
- **It is not good enough to have a correct diagnosis only 99% of the time with chest pain.**
- An understanding of chest pain helps the physician in the systematic consideration of the differential diagnosis.

# PAST ASKED QUESTIONS

| **Regarding the lobes and segments of the right lung:** | |
|---|---|
| It has 10 bronchopulmonary segments | T |
| The right middle lobe is separated from the upper lobe by oblique fissure | F |
| Its horizontal fissure lies at the level of 4th intercostal space | T |
| Inferior border of the right lung is at the level of 8th rib in the mid axillary | T |
| **Regarding the vascularization of the thorax:** | |
| The azygos vein drains into the IVC | F |
| The internal thoracic artery arises from the subclavian artery | T |
| The internal thoracic artery runs 1cm lateral to the edge of the sternum | T |
| The thoracic duct joins the Rt internal jugular subclavian junction | F |
| **Regarding to the PA CXR in a normal adult:** | |
| The horizontal fissure runs from the Rt hilum to the 6th rib in the midaxillary line | T |
| The Rt ventricle forms the majority of the Rt heart border | F |
| The Rt middle lobe is adjacent to the Rt heart border | T |
| Consolidation below the hilum on the left, must be in the lower lobe | F |
| **Regarding the anatomy of the chest:** | |
| The visceral pleura is insensitive | T |
| The nipple is the 4th intercostal space in men | T |
| The diaphragm can rise as high as T6 in expiration | T |
| The left main bronchus is more vertical than the right | F |
| **Regarding the aorta in the thorax:** | |
| Has a diameter between 2-3cm | T |
| Does not contribute to spinal cord blood supply | F |
| It is fixed posteriorly beyond the left subclavian artery | T |
| It enters the abdomen at T10 | F |
| **Regarding the anatomy of the thorax:** | |
| The apex of the lungs extends 2cm above the clavicle | T |
| The left lung has 3 lobes | F |
| The lower limit of the pleura ends at the 11th rib posteriorly | F |
| In most people, the right hemidiaphragm is higher than the left | T |
| **Regarding the anatomy of right phrenic nerve:** | |
| It is the sole motor supply to the Rt hemi-diaphragm | T |
| Arises from nerve roots C4, 5 and 6 | F |
| Gives off the recurrent Laryngeal nerve as the only branch | F |
| Has no sensory fibres | F |
| **Regarding the anatomy of the thoracic plane:** | |
| It extends from the manubriosternal angle to the T4-5 disc | T |
| It includes the bifurcation of the trachea | T |
| It includes the attachment of the 3rd costal cartilage to the sternum | F |
| It includes the end of the thoracic arch | T |

# SECTION 4: ABDOMEN

# I. BRIEF EMBRYOLOGY

## A. FORMATION OF THE PRIMITIVE GUT TUBE

- The gut tube is formed from endoderm lining the yolk sac which is enveloped by the developing coelom as the result of cranial and caudal folding. During folding, somatic mesoderm is applied to the body wall to give rise to the parietal peritoneum.
- Visceral (or splanchnic) mesoderm is wraps around the gut tube to form the mesenteries that suspend the gut tube within the body cavity. The mesoderm immediately associated with the endodermal tube also contributes to most of the wall of the gut tube.
- Nerves and neurons found in the wall are derived from neural crest.
- Summary of germ layer contributions:
  - *Endoderm*: mucosal epithelium, mucosal glands, and submucosal glands of the GI tract.
  - *Mesoderm*: lamina propria, muscularis mucosae, submucosal connective tissue and blood vessels, muscularis externa, and adventitia/serosa.
  - *Neural crest*: neurons and nerves of the submucosal and myenteric plexus.

## B. BASIC SUBDIVISIONS OF THE GUT TUBE

- Cranio-caudal and lateral folding cause the opening of the gut tube to the yolk sac to draw closed forming a pocket toward the head end of the embryo called the" anterior (or cranial) intestinal portal" and a "posterior (or caudal) intestinal portal" toward the tail of the embryo.
- These are the future foregut and hindgut, respectively.
- The midgut remains open to the yolk sac.
- Further folding and growth of the embryo causes the communication of the gut with the yolk sac to continue to get smaller and the regions of the gut (foregut, midgut, and hindgut) to become further refined.

## C. DEFINITIVE SUBDIVISIONS OF THE GUT TUBE

- Within the abdominal cavity, the gut is definitively divided into foregut, midgut, and hindgut *based on the arterial supply:*
  - **Foregut** derivatives in the abdomen are supplied by branches of **the Celiac Artery**.
  - **Midgut** derivatives are supplied by branches of **the Superior Mesenteric Artery**.
  - **Hindgut** derivatives are supplied by branches of **the Inferior Mesenteric Artery**.
- The derivatives of the gut regions are as follows:

## 1. FOREGUT

- From oesophagus to D1 and D2
- Gives rise to Oesophagus, stomach, duodenum (D1 and D2), Liver, gallbladder, pancreas (Superior portion)
- Arterial supply: **Caeliac trunk**

## 2. MIDGUT

- from lower D3 to first 2/3 transverse colon
- Gives rise to D3, jejunum, ileum, caecum, appendix, ascending colon and first 2/3 of transverse colon.
- Arterial supply: branches of **Sup. Mesenteric artery**

## 3. HINDGUT

- From last 1/3 of transverse colon to the anal canal
- Gives rises to the 1/3 transverse colon, descending colon, rectum and upper part of the anal canal
- Arterial supply: branches of **Inferior Mesenteric Artery.**

# II. ANTERIOR ABDOMINAL WALL

## A. FUNCTIONS OF THE ABDOMINAL WALL

- Forms a firm, flexible wall which keeps the abdominal viscera in the abdominal cavity.
- Protects the abdominal viscera from injury.
- Maintains the anatomical position of abdominal viscera against gravity.
- Assists in forceful expiration by pushing the abdominal viscera upwards.
- Involved in any action (coughing, vomiting) that increases intra-abdominal pressure.

## B. LAYERS OF THE ABDOMINAL WALL

**(External to internal):**
- Skin
- Fascia:
  - Camper's fascia: Superficial fatty layer
  - Scarpa's fascia: deep fibrous layer
- Muscles
- Transversalis fascia
- Parietal peritoneum.

## A. THE SUPERFICIAL FASCIA

- The superficial fascia consists of fatty connective tissue.
- The composition of this layer depends on its location:
  - *Above the umbilicus*: A single sheet of connective tissue. This continuous with the superficial fascia in other regions of the body.
  - *Below the umbilicus*: It is divided into two layers; the fatty superficial layer (Camper's fascia) and the membranous deep layer (Scarpa's fascia).
  - Superficial vessels and nerves run between these two layers of fascia

## B. MUSCLES OF THE ABDOMINAL WALL

- There are five muscles in the abdominal wall.
- They can be divided into two groups:
  - ➤ *Vertical muscles*:
    - There are two vertical muscles, situated near the mid-line of the body (rectus abdominis and pyramidalis).
  - ➤ *Flat muscles*
    - There are three flat muscles, situated laterally (External oblique, internal oblique and Transversus abdominis).

## 1. EXTERNAL OBLIQUE

- The largest and most superficial flat muscle in the abdominal wall.
- Its fibres run inferomedially.
- As the fibres approach the mid-line, they form an aponeurosis (a broad flat tendon).
- In the mid-line, the aponeuroses of all the flat muscles become entwined, forming the linea Alba.
- This is a fibrous structure that extends from the xiphoid process of the sternum to the pubic symphysis

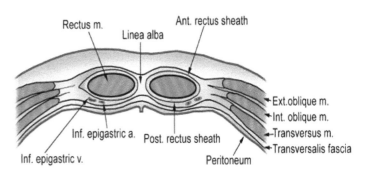

**Above Arcuate Line**

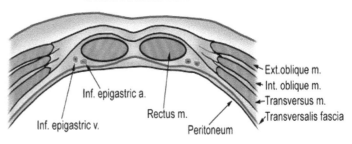

**Below Arcuate Line**

*Fig. 1.4.1. Layers of abdominal wall*

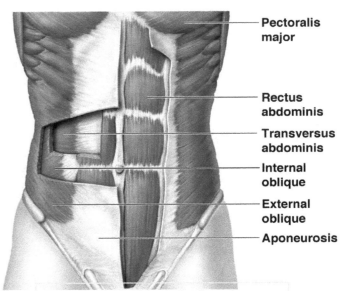

*Fig. 1.4.2. Abdominal wall muscles*

## EXTERNAL OBLIQUE APONEUROSIS.

- The aponeurosis of the external oblique muscle passes anterior to the rectus abdominis.
- Its inferior edge extends from the anterior superior iliac spine to the pubic tubercle and is known as the **inguinal ligament (Poupart's).**
- A part that continues posterior (toward the superior pubic ramus) is termed the **lacunar ligament.**
- A further extension laterally (along the pectin pubis of the superior pubic ramus) is called the **pectineal ligament.**
- Lateral to the pubic tubercle, the aponeurosis of the external oblique muscle divides into medial and lateral crura, which diverge to form the **superficial inguinal ring.**

## 2. INTERNAL OBLIQUE

- This muscle lies deep to the external oblique.
- It is smaller and thinner in structure, with its fibres running superomedially (perpendicular to the fibres of the external oblique).
- Near the midline, it forms aponeurotic fibres which contribute to the linea Alba.

## INTERNAL OBLIQUE APONEUROSIS.

- The aponeurosis of the internal oblique muscle divides into anterior and posterior layers, which pass, respectively, in front of and behind the rectus muscle to reach the linea alba.
- The linea Alba is the median, fibrous intersection of the aponeuroses, extending vertically from the xiphoid process to the pubic symphysis.
- The division into anterior and posterior layers is absent inferiorly, where the aponeuroses of all three muscles pass anterior to the rectus muscles to reach the linea Alba.
- Inferiorly, the medial portion of the fused internal oblique and transversus aponeuroses is termed the **conjoined tendon.**

## 3. TRANSVERSUS ABDOMINIS

- The deepest of the flat muscles, with transversely running fibres.
- Like the other flat muscles, it contributes aponeurotic fibres to the linea Alba.
- Deep to this muscle is a well-formed layer of fascia, called the **transversalis fascia.**

## 4. RECTUS ABDOMINIS

- This is a long, paired muscle, found either side of the midline in the abdominal wall. It is split into two by the linea Alba.
- The lateral border of the two muscles creates a surface marking called **the linea semilunaris.**
- At several places, the muscle is intersected by fibrous strips, known as **tendinous intersections**.
- The tendinous intersections and the linea Alba give rise to the 'six pack' seen in individuals with low body fat.
- As well as assisting the flat muscles in compressing the abdominal viscera, the rectus abdominus also stabilises the pelvis during walking, and depresses the ribs.

## 5. PYRAMIDALIS

- This is a small triangle shaped muscle, found superficially to the rectus abdominus.
- It is located inferiorly, with its base on the pubis bone, and the apex of the triangle attached to the linea Alba.
- It acts to tense the linea Alba.

## 6. RECTUS SHEATH

- The rectus sheath is composed of the aponeuroses of transversus abdominis, external obliqueand internal oblique muscles, which form an anterior and posterior sheath that fuse laterally at the linea semilunaris and in the midline at linea alba.
- Only the middle segment of the rectus abdominis is completely enclosed, with the posterior sheath lacking in parts of the superior and inferior segments:
    - ✓ **Superior to the costal margin** the aponeuroses are deficient because they either do not extend that far superiorly (internal and external oblique muscles) or attach to the costal margin (transversus abdominis)
    - ✓ **Inferior to the arcuate line**, the internal oblique aponeurosis passes anterior to the rectus abdominis and since the other two aponeurosis are fused to it, the posterior surface of rectus abdominis is in contact with the transversalis fascia

## CONTENTS OF RECTUS SHEATH "RECLIS"

- **R**ectus abdominis muscle
- Inferior and superior **E**pigastric vessels
- Fibro fatty **C**onnective tissue
- Occasionally **L**ymph node(s)
- Terminal parts of the lower five **I**ntercostal nerves, and the **S**ubcostal nerve.

# C. BLOOD VESSELS AND LYMPHATIC DRAINAGE

## A. SUPERIOR EPIGASTRIC ARTERY
- Arises from the **internal thoracic artery**, enters the rectus sheath, and descends on the posterior surface the rectus abdominis.
- Anastomoses with the inferior epigastric artery within the rectus abdominis.

## B. INFERIOR EPIGASTRIC ARTERY
- Arises from the **external iliac artery** above the inguinal ligament, enters the rectus sheath, and ascends between the rectus abdominis and the posterior layer of the rectus sheath.
- Anastomoses with the superior epigastric artery, providing collateral circulation between the subclavian and external iliac arteries.
- Gives rise to the **cremasteric artery**, which accompanies the spermatic cord.

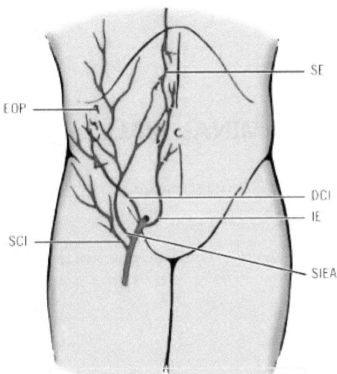

**EOP**- Ext Oblique Perforators

**SCI**- Superficial Circumflex Iliac

**SE**- Superior Epigastric

**DCI**- Deep Circumflex Iliac

**IE**- Deep , inferior Epigastric Artery

**SIEA**- Superficial inferior Epigastric artery

*Fig. 1.4.3. Abdominal wall blood supply*

## C. DEEP CIRCUMFLEX ILIAC ARTERY
- Arises from the **external iliac artery** and runs laterally along the inguinal ligament and the iliac crest between the transverse and internal oblique muscles.
- Forms an ascending branch that anastomoses with the musculophrenic artery.

## D. SUPERFICIAL EPIGASTRIC ARTERIES
- Arise from the **femoral artery** and run superiorly toward the umbilicus over the inguinal ligament.
- Anastomose with branches of the inferior epigastric artery.

## E. SUPERFICIAL CIRCUMFLEX ILIAC ARTERY
- Arises from the **femoral artery** and runs laterally upward, parallel to the inguinal ligament.
- Anastomoses with the deep circumflex iliac and lateral femoral circumflex arteries.

## F. SUPERFICIAL (EXTERNAL) PUDENDAL ARTERIES
- Arise from the **femoral artery**, pierce the cribriform fascia, and run medially to supply the skin above.

## G. THORACOEPIGASTRIC VEINS
- Longitudinal venous connections between the lateral thoracic vein and the superficial epigastric vein.
- Provide a collateral route for venous return if a caval or portal obstruction occurs.

## D. NERVES OF THE ANTERIOR ABDOMINAL WALL

### 1. SUBCOSTAL NERVE (T12)
- Is the ventral ramus of *the twelfth thoracic nerve* and innervates the muscles of the anterior abdominal wall.
- Has a lateral cutaneous branch that innervates the skin of the side of the hip.

### 2. ILIOHYPOGASTRIC NERVE
- **Roots: L1** (with contributions from T12).
- **Motor Functions:** Innervates the internal oblique and transversus abdominis.
- **Sensory Functions:** Innervates the posterolateral gluteal skin in the pubic region.

### 3. ILIOINGUINAL NERVE
- **Roots: L1.**
- **Motor Functions:** Innervates the internal oblique and transversus abdominis.
- **Sensory Functions:**
  - Innervates the skin on the upper middle thigh.
  - **In males:** supplies the skin over the root of the penis and anterior scrotum.
  - **In females:** supplies the skin over mons pubis and labium majus.

# III. POSTERIOR ABDOMINAL WALL

## A. POSTERIOR ABDOMINAL MUSCLES
- There are five muscles: The Iliacus, Psoas Major, Psoas Minor, Quadratus Lumborum and the Diaphragm.

### 1. QUADRATUS LUMBORUM
- **Attachments:**
  - It originates from the iliac crest and iliolumbar ligament.
  - The fibres travel superomedially, inserting onto the transverse processes of L1 – L4 and the inferior border of the 12th rib.
- **Actions:**
  - Lateral flexion of vertebral column, with ipsilateral contraction.
  - Extension of lumbar vertebral column, with bilateral contraction.
  - Fixes the 12th rib during forced expiration
  - Elevates the Ilium (bone), with ipsilateral contraction.
- **Innervation:** Anterior rami of **T12- L4 nerves.**

### 2. PSOAS MAJOR
- **Attachments:**
  - Originates from the transverse processes and vertebral bodies of T12 – L5.
  - It then moves inferiorly and laterally, running deep to the inguinal ligament, and attaching to the lesser trochanter of the femur.
- **Actions:** Flexion of the thigh at the hip and lateral flexion of the vertebral column.
- **Innervation:** Anterior rami of **L1 – L3 nerves.**

### 3. PSOAS MINOR
- The psoas minor muscle is only present in 60% of the population.
- It is located anterior to the psoas major.
  - **Attachments:** Originates from the vertebral bodies of T12 and L1 and attaches to a ridge on the superior ramus of the pubic bone, known as the pectineal line.
  - **Actions:** Flexion of the vertebral column.
  - **Innervation:** Anterior rami of the **L1 spinal nerve.**

### 4. ILIACUS
- **Attachments:**
  - Originates from surface of the iliac fossa and anterior inferior iliac spine.
  - Its fibres combine with the tendon of the psoas major, inserting into the lesser trochanter of the femur.
- Actions: Flexion of the thigh at the hip joint.
- Innervation: **Femoral nerve (L2 – L4).**

## 5. DIAPHRAGM

- The posterior aspect of the diaphragm is considered to be part of the posterior abdominal wall.

## B. FASCIA OF THE POSTERIOR ABDOMINAL WALL

- A layer of fascia lies between the parietal peritoneum and the muscles of the posterior abdominal wall.
- This fascia is continuous with the transversalis fascia of the anterolateral abdominal wall.
- Whilst the fascia is one continuous sheet, it is anatomically correct to name the fascia according to the structure it overlies.

## 1. PSOAS FASCIA

- The psoas fascia covers the psoas major muscle. It is attached to the lumbar vertebrae medially, continuous with the thoracolumbar fascia laterally and continuous with the iliac fascia inferiorly

## 2. THORACOLUMBAR FASCIA

- The thoracolumbar fascia consists of the three layers; posterior, middle and anterior.
- Muscles are enclosed between these layers:
  - Quadratus lumborum – between the anterior and middle layers
  - Deep back muscles – between the middle and posterior layers.
- The posterior layer extends between the 12th rib and the iliac crest posteriorly. Laterally the fascia meets the internal oblique and transversus abdominis muscles, but not the external oblique. As it forms these attachments it covers the latissimus dorsi.
- The anterior layer attaches to the anterior aspect of the transverse processes of the lumbar vertebrae, the 12th rib and the iliac crest.
- Laterally the fascia is continuous with the aponeurotic origin of the transversus abdominis muscle.
- Superiorly the fascia thickens to become the lateral arcuate ligament, which joins the iliolumbar ligaments inferiorly.

## C. POSTERIOR ABDOMINAL BLOOD VESSELS AND LYMPHATICS

### 1. ABDOMINAL AORTA

- Passes through the aortic hiatus in the diaphragm at the level of T12, descends anterior to the vertebral bodies, and bifurcates into the right and left common iliac arteries anterior to L4.
- Gives rise to the following:

### A. INFERIOR PHRENIC ARTERIES

- Arise from the aorta immediately below the aortic hiatus, supply the diaphragm, and give rise to the **Suprarenal Arteries**.
- Diverge across the crus of the diaphragm, with the left artery passing posterior to the oesophagus and right artery passing posterior to the IVC.

**THE SUPERIOR PHRENIC ARTERIES** are small and arise from the lower part of the thoracic aorta; they are distributed to the posterior part of the upper surface of the diaphragm, and anastomose with the **Musculophrenic** and **Pericardiacophrenic Arteries.**

### B. MIDDLE SUPRARENAL ARTERIES

- Arise from the aorta and run laterally on the crus of the diaphragm just superior to the renal arteries.

### C. RENAL ARTERIES

- Arise from the aorta inferior to the origin of the superior mesenteric artery (L1-L2).
- The right artery is longer and a little lower than the left and passes posterior to the IVC; the left artery passes posterior to the left renal vein.
- Give rise to the **Inferior Suprarenal** and **Ureteric Arteries.**
- Divide into the superior, anterosuperior, anteroinferior, inferior, and posterior segmental branches.

### D. TESTICULAR OR OVARIAN ARTERIES

- Descend retroperitoneally and run laterally on the psoas major muscle and across the ureter.
- The testicular artery accompanies the ductus deferens into the scrotum, where it supplies the spermatic cord, epididymis, and testis.
- The ovarian artery enters the suspensory ligament of the ovary, supplies the ovary, and anastomosis with the ovarian branch of the uterine artery.

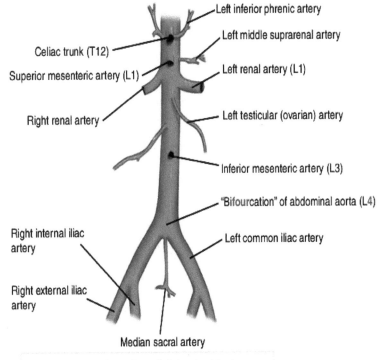

Left inferior phrenic artery

Left middle suprarenal artery

Celiac trunk (T12)

Superior mesenteric artery (L1)

Left renal artery (L1)

Right renal artery

Left testicular (ovarian) artery

Inferior mesenteric artery (L3)

"Bifourcation" of abdominal aorta (L4)

Left common iliac artery

Right internal iliac artery

Right external iliac artery

Median sacral artery

*Fig. 1.4.4. Branches of abdominal Aorta*

### E. LUMBAR ARTERIES
- Consist of four or five pairs that arise from the back of the aorta.
- Run posterior to the sympathetic trunk, the IVC (on the right side), the psoas major muscle and the quadratus lumborum.
- Divide into smaller anterior branches (to supply adjacent muscles) and larger posterior branches, which accompany the dorsal primary rami of the corresponding spinal nerves and divide into spinal and muscular branches.

### F. MIDDLE (MEDIAN) SACRAL ARTERY
- Arises from the back of the aorta, just above its bifurcation; descends on the front of the sacrum; and end at the coccygeal body.
- Supplies the rectum and anal canal, and anastomoses with the lateral sacral and superior and inferior rectal arteries.

### 2. INFERIOR VENA CAVA
- Is formed on the right side of L5 by the union of the two common iliac veins, below the bifurcation of the aorta.
- Is longer than the abdominal aorta and ascends along the right side of the aorta.
- Passes through the opening for the IVC in the central tendon of the diaphragm at the level of T8 and enters the right atrium of the heart.

- **IVC tributaries:** IVC Like **TO R**ise **S**o **H**igh"
  - ✓ **I**liacs
  - ✓ **L**umbar
  - ✓ **T**esticular/ **O**varian (right only)
  - ✓ **R**enal
  - ✓ **S**uprarenal (right only)
  - ✓ **H**epatic vein

### 3. CISTERNA CHILI
- Is the lower dilated end of the thoracic duct and lies just to the right and posterior to the aorta, usually between two crura of the diaphragm.
- Is formed by the intestinal and lumbar lymph trunks

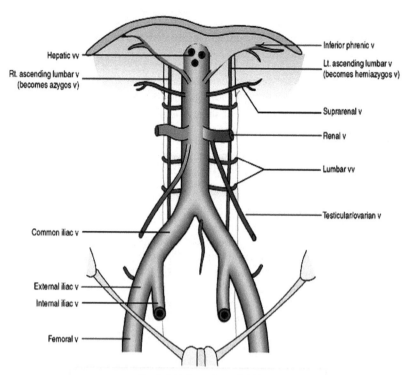

*Fig. 1.4.5. Branches of IVC*

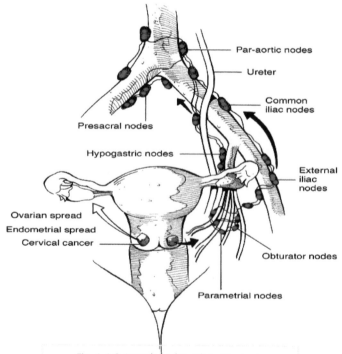

*Fig. 1.4.6. Lymph nodes related to Aorta*

## D. LYMPH NODES RELATED TO THE AORTA

### 1. PREAORTIC NODES
- Include the celiac, superior mesenteric, and inferior mesenteric nodes; drain the lymph from the GI tract, spleen, pancreas, gallbladder, and liver; and their efferent vessels form the intestinal trunk.

### 2. PARA-AORTIC, LUMBAR, OR LATERAL AORTIC LYMPH NODES
- Drain lymph from the kidneys, suprarenal glands, testes or ovaries, uterus, and uterine tubes;
- Receive lymph from the common, internal, or external iliac; and their efferent vessels form the right and left lumbar trunk.

## CLINICAL RELEVANCE

### 1. ABDOMINAL STAB WOUNDS

- Abdominal stab wounds may or may not penetrate the parietal peritoneum and violate the peritoneal cavity and consequently may or may not significantly damage the abdominal viscera. The structures in the various layers through which an abdominal stab wound penetrates depend on the anatomic location. Lateral to the rectus sheath are the following: skin, fatty layer of superficial fascia, membranous layer of superficial fascia, thin layer of deep fascia, external oblique muscle or aponeurosis, internal oblique muscle or aponeurosis, transversus abdominis muscle or aponeurosis, fascia transversalis, extraperitoneal connective tissue (often fatty), and parietal peritoneum.

- Anterior to the rectus sheath are the following: skin, fatty layer of superficial fascia, membranous layer of superficial fascia, thin layer of deep fascia, anterior wall of rectus sheath, rectus abdominis muscle with segmental nerves and epigastric vessels lying behind the muscle, posterior wall of rectus sheath, fascia transversalis, extraperitoneal connective tissue (often fatty), and parietal peritoneum.

- In the midline are the following: skin, fatty layer of superficial fascia, membranous layer of superficial fascia, thin layer of deep fascia, fibrous linea alba, fascia transversalis, extraperitoneal connective tissue (often fatty), and parietal peritoneum. In an abdominal stab wound, washing out the peritoneal cavity with saline solution (**peritoneal lavage**) can be used to determine whether any damage to viscera or blood vessels has occurred.

### 2. ABDOMINAL GUNSHOT WOUNDS

- Gunshot wounds are much more serious than stab wounds; in most patients, the peritoneal cavity has been entered, and significant visceral damage has ensued.

# IV. INGUINAL CANAL & HERNIAS

- The inguinal canal is a short passage that extends inferiorly and medially, through the inferior part of the **abdominal wall**.
- It is superior and parallel to the **inguinal ligament**. It acts as a **pathway** by which structures can pass from the abdominal wall to the **external genitalia**. The inguinal canal also has clinical importance. It is a potential weakness in the abdominal wall, and therefore a common site of **herniation**.
- In the embryological stage, the canal is flanked by an outpocketing of the peritoneum, and the abdominal musculature.
- This outpocketing, the **processes vaginalis**, normally degenerates, but a failure to do so can result in an indirect inguinal hernia.
- The two openings to the inguinal canal are known as rings:
- **The Deep (Internal) Ring:**
  - It is **found above the midpoint of the inguinal ligament** which is lateral to the epigastric vessels.
  - The ring is created by **the transversalis fascia**, which invaginates to form a covering of the contents of the inguinal canal.
- **The Superficial (External) Ring:**
  - Marks the end of the inguinal canal, and lies just **superior to the pubic tubercle.**
  - It is a triangle shaped opening, formed by the evagination of the **external oblique**, which forms another covering of the inguinal canal contents.

**Dissection view showing superficial and deeper features of the scrotum, testes, and related structures**

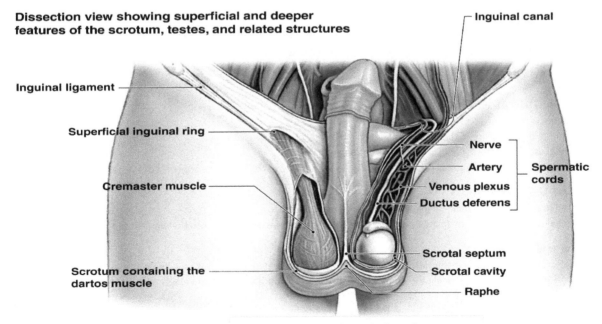

*Fig. 1.4.7. Inguinal canal*

## 'MID-INGUINAL POINT' & 'MIDPOINT OF THE INGUINAL LIGAMENT'

- **The Mid-Inguinal Point:**
  - It is halfway between the pubic symphysis and the anterior superior iliac spine.
  - The **femoral artery** crosses into the lower limb at this anatomical landmark.
- **The Midpoint of the Inguinal Ligament:**
  - The inguinal ligament runs from the pubic tubercle to the ASIS, so the midpoint is halfway between these structures.
  - The opening to the **inguinal canal** is located just above this point.

### Boundaries: MALT (2M, 2A, 2L, 2T) (Salp-Malt)

- **Superior wall (Roof): 2 Muscles**
  - Internal Oblique **M**uscle
  - Transverse Abdominus **M**uscle

- **Anterior wall: 2 Aponeuroses**
  - **A**poneurosis of external oblique
  - **A**poneurosis of internal oblique
- **Lower wall (Floor): 2 Ligaments**
  - Inguinal **L**igament·
  - Lacunar **L**igament
- **Posterior wall: 2Ts**
  - **T**ransversalis fascia
  - Conjoint **T**endon

### Contents

- **Males**
  - ✓ Spermatic cord (**P**iles **D**on't **C**ontribute **T**o **A** **G**ood **S**ex **L**ife)
  - ✓ Genital branch of the Genitofemoral Nerve
- **Females**
  - ✓ Round ligament
  - ✓ Ilioinguinal nerve

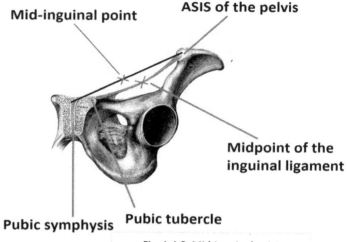

Fig. 1.4.8. Mid-Inguinal point

**Roof**
Transversalis fascia
Internal oblique
Transversus abdominus

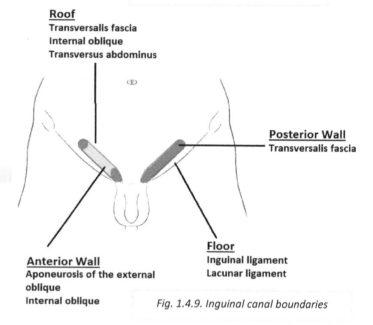

**Posterior Wall**
Transversalis fascia

**Floor**
Inguinal ligament
Lacunar ligament

**Anterior Wall**
Aponeurosis of the external oblique
Internal oblique

Fig. 1.4.9. Inguinal canal boundaries

## CLINICAL RELEVANCE: DIRECT vs INDIRECT INGUINAL HERNIAS

- Hernias involving the inguinal canal can be divided into two main categories:
  - **Indirect**: where the peritoneal sac enters the inguinal canal through the deep inguinal ring.
  - **Direct**: where the peritoneal sac enters the inguinal canal though the posterior wall of the inguinal canal.

### 1. INDIRECT INGUINAL HERNIAS

- More common.
- Has a congenital origin (failure of the processes vaginalis to regress).
- The peritoneal sac enters the inguinal canal via the deep inguinal ring.
- As the sac moves through the inguinal canal, it acquires the same three coverings as the contents of the canal.

### 2. DIRECT INGUINAL HERNIAS

- It is acquired in origin, due to **weakening** in the abdominal musculature.
- The peritoneal sac originates from an area **medial** to the epigastric vessels and bulges into the inguinal canal via the posterior wall.

### 3. FEMORAL HERNIA

- The hernial sac descends through the femoral canal within the femoral sheath, creating a femoral hernia. The femoral sheath is a protrusion of the fascial envelope lining the abdominal walls and surrounds the femoral vessels and lymphatics for about 2.5 cm below the inguinal ligament.
- The **femoral artery,** as it enters the thigh below the inguinal ligament, occupies the lateral compartment of the sheath.
- The **femoral vein,** which lies on its medial side and is separated from it by a fibrous septum, occupies the intermediate compartment.

- The **lymph vessels,** which are separated from the vein by a fibrous septum, occupy the most medial compartment.
- The **femoral canal,** the compartment for the lymphatics, occupies the medial part of the sheath. It is about 1.3 cm long, and its upper opening is referred to as the **femoral ring.** The **femoral septum,** which is a condensation of extraperitoneal tissue, plugs the opening of the femoral ring.
- A femoral hernia is more common in women than in men (possibly because of a wider pelvis and femoral canal). The hernial sac passes down the femoral canal, pushing the femoral septum before it. On escaping through the lower end, it expands to form a swelling in the upper part of the thigh deep to the deep fascia.
- With further expansion, the hernial sac may turn upward to cross the anterior surface of the inguinal ligament.
- The neck of the sac always lies below and lateral to the **pubic tubercle**, which serves to distinguish it from an inguinal hernia. The neck of the sac is narrow and lies at the femoral ring. The ring is related anteriorly to the inguinal ligament, posteriorly to the pectineal ligament and the pubis, medially to the sharp free edge of the lacunar ligament, and laterally to the femoral vein. Because of the presence of these anatomic structures, the neck of the sac is unable to expand.
- Once an abdominal viscus has passed through the neck into the body of the sac, it may be difficult to push it up and return it to the abdominal cavity (**irreducible hernia**).
- Furthermore, after straining or coughing, a piece of bowel may be forced through the neck and its blood vessels may be compressed by the femoral ring, seriously impairing its blood supply (**strangulated hernia**).
- A femoral hernia is a dangerous disease and should always be treated surgically. A femoral hernia can be summarized as follows:
  - It is a protrusion of abdominal parietal peritoneum down through the femoral canal to form the hernial sac.
  - It is more common in women than in men.
  - The neck of the hernial sac lies below and lateral to the pubic tubercle.
  - The neck of the hernial sac lies at the femoral ring and at that point is related anteriorly to the inguinal ligament, posteriorly to the pectineal ligament and the pubis, laterally to the femoral vein, and medially to the sharp free edge of the lacunar ligament.

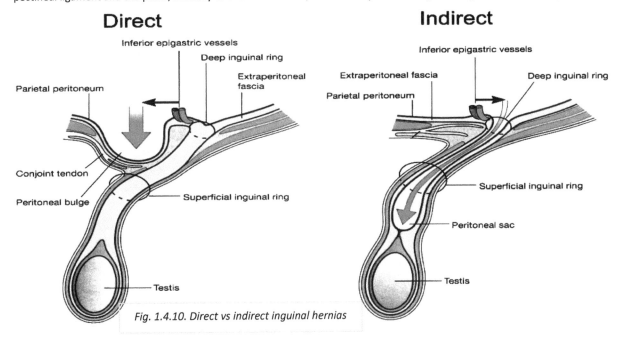

Fig. 1.4.10. Direct vs indirect inguinal hernias

## DIFFERENCE BETWEEN DIRECT AND INDIRECT HERNIA

| FEATURES | INDIRECT HERNIA | DIRECT HERNIA |
|---|---|---|
| Age | Children, young people | Aged people |
| Pathway of protrusion | Coming down the inguinal canal, may enter the scrotum | Pass through the Hesselbach's triangle, rarely enters the scrotum |
| Compress the internal ring after reduction | Controlled | Not controlled |
| Contours of sac | Elliptic, pear-shape | Semispheric, wide base |
| Reduction | Upwards, laterally and backward | Upward and straight backward |
| Relationship between sac neck with inferior Epigastric artery (IEA) | Sac neck is lateral to the IEA | Sac neck is medial to the IEA |
| Incarceration incidence | High | Low |

# V. TESTIS, EPIDIDYMIS AND SPERMATIC CORD

## 1. SPERMATIC CORD

o **Course**
  - The spermatic cord starts at the deep inguinal ring, passes through the inguinal canal and exits at the superficial inguinal ring into the scrotum.

o **Contents:** "Piles Don't Contribute To A Good Sex Life":
  ✓ **P**ampiniform plexus
  ✓ **D**uctus deferens
  ✓ **C**remasteric artery
  ✓ **T**esticular artery
  ✓ **A**rtery of the ductus deferens
  ✓ **G**enital branch of the genitofemoral nerve
  ✓ **S**ympathetic nerve fibers
  ✓ **L**ymphatic vessels

o **Coverings**
  - There are three facial layers; from outermost to innermost:
    o *External spermatic fascia*
  - From external oblique aponeurosis
    o *Cremaster muscle and fascia*
  - From internal oblique muscle and aponeurosis
    o *Internal spermatic fascia*
  - From the transversalis fascia.

o **Relations**
  - *The ilioinguinal nerve runs anterior to the spermatic cord.*
  - *In the scrotum, the spermatic cord terminates at the posteromedial border of the testis.*

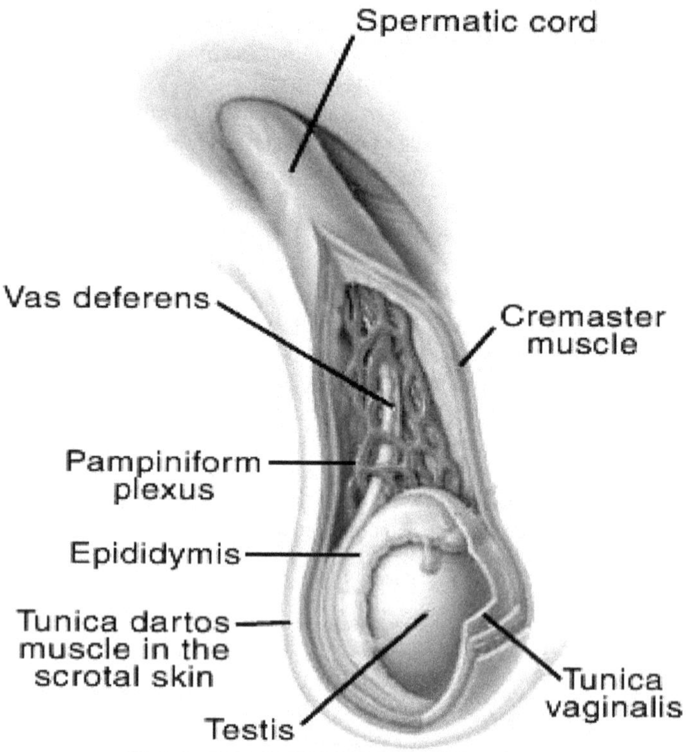

## 2. TESTES

- Located on the posterior abdominal wall.
- During embryonic development, they descend down the abdomen, and through the inguinal canal to reach the scrotum.
- They carry their neurovascular and lymphatic supply with them.
- **Coverings**
  o *The Tunica Vaginalis is situated externally,*
  o *The Tunica Albuginea encloses the testes.*

## LAYERS OF THE SCROTUM:

- **Mnemonic:** Some Damn Englishman Called It The Testes
  ✓ **S:** Skin
  ✓ **D:** Dartos fascia and muscle
  ✓ **E:** External spermatic fascia
  ✓ **C:** Cremasteric fascia
  ✓ **I:** Internal spermatic fascia
  ✓ **T:** Tunica vaginalis
  ✓ **T:** Tunica albuginea

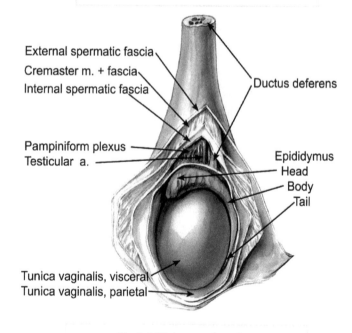

*Fig. 1.4.11. Spermatic cord*

*Fig. 1.4.12. Layers of scrotum*

## 3. EPIDIDYMIS

- Divided into three parts: head, body and tail.
  o **Head:**
    ▪ Most proximal part of the epididymis.
    ▪ Formed by the efferent tubules of the testes, which transport sperm from the testes to the epididymis.

- o **Body:**
  - ▪ Formed by the heavily coiled duct of the epididymis.
- o **Tail:**
  - ▪ Most distal part of the epididymis.
  - ▪ Marks the origin of the vas deferens, which transports sperm to the urethra for ejaculation.

- **INNERVATION:**
  - o The testes and epididymis receive innervation from the Testicular Plexus.

- **VASCULAR SUPPLY:**
  - o **Arterial supply** to the testes and epididymis is via the paired Testicular Arteries, which arise directly from the abdominal aorta.
  - o **Venous drainage** is achieved via the paired Testicular Veins. They are formed from the pampiniform plexus in the scrotum.
  - o *In the abdomen, the Left Testicular Vein drains into the Left Renal Vein, while the Right Testicular Vein drains directly into the IVC.*

- **LYMPHATIC SUPPLY:**
  - o Lymphatic drainage of testes is through lymphatics running with the testicular arteries, draining into Para-Aortic Lymph Nodes.

# VI. PERITONEUM

## 1. STRUCTURE OF THE PERITONEUM

- The peritoneum consists of two layers which are continuous with each other; the parietal peritoneum and the visceral peritoneum.
- They both consist of a layer of simple squamous epithelial cells, called **mesothelium.**

### A. PARIETAL PERITONEUM
- o It is derived from somatic mesoderm in the embryo. It receives the same somatic nerve supply as the region of the abdominal wall that it lines.
- o *Pain from the parietal peritoneum is well localised and it is sensitive to pressure, pain, laceration and temperature.*

### B. VISCERAL PERITONEUM
- o It is derived from splanchnic mesoderm in the embryo. The visceral peritoneum has the same nerve supply as the viscera it invests.
- o *Unlike the parietal peritoneum, pain from the visceral peritoneum is poorly localised and is only sensitive to stretch and chemical irritation.*
- o Pain from the visceral peritoneum is referred to areas of skin (dermatomes) which are supplied by the same sensory ganglia and spinal cord segments as the nerve fibres innervating the viscera.

## 2. PERITONEAL CAVITY
- The peritoneal cavity is a potential space between the parietal and visceral peritoneum.
- It contains a small amount of lubricating fluid.

## 3. RETROPERITONEAL ORGANS
- These organs are only covered in peritoneum on their anterior surface.
- They can be subdivided into two groups:
  - o *Primarily retroperitoneal organs*
  - o *Secondarily retroperitoneal organs.*

## 4. MESENTERY
- o A mesentery is double layer of visceral peritoneum. It connects an intraperitoneal organ to the (usually) posterior abdominal wall.
- o It provides a pathway for nerves, blood vessels and lymphatics from the body wall to the viscera.

### RETROPERITONEAL ORGANS
A useful mnemonic to help in recalling which abdominal viscera are retroperitoneal is: **SAD PUCKER 112 212 111,** this correlating to which ones are Primarily (1) or Secondarily (2) Retroperitoneal:
- ✓ **S** = Suprarenal (adrenal) Glands
- ✓ **A** = Aorta/IVC
- ✓ **D** =Duodenum (except the duodenal cap, first 2cm)
- ✓ **P** = Pancreas (except the tail)
- ✓ **U** = Ureters
- ✓ **C** = Colon (ascending and descending parts)
- ✓ **K** = Kidneys
- ✓ **E** = (O)oesophagus
- ✓ **R** = Rectum

## 5. OMENTUM
- o The omentum is a double layer of peritoneum that extends from the stomach and proximal part of the duodenum to other abdominal organs.

### A. GREATER OMENTUM
- o The greater omentum consists of four layers of peritoneum.
- o It descends from the greater curvature of the stomach and proximal part of the duodenum, then folds back up and attaches to the anterior surface of the transverse colon.
- o It has a role in immunity and is sometimes referred to as the 'abdominal policeman' because it can migrate to infected viscera.

### B. LESSER OMENTUM
- o The lesser omentum is considerably smaller and attaches from the lesser curvature of the stomach and the proximal part of the duodenum to the liver. It consists of two parts: the hepatogastric ligament and the hepatoduodenal ligament.

## 6. PERITONEAL LIGAMENTS
- o A peritoneal ligament is a double fold of peritoneum that connects viscera together or connects viscera to the abdominal wall, for example the hepatogastric ligament which connects the liver to the stomach.

# VII. GASTROINTESTINAL TRACT

## OESOPHAGUS
**Refer to section 3: Thorax**

## A. STOMACH
- Lies between the oesophagus and duodenum in the upper abdomen, on the left side of the abdominal cavity caudal to the diaphragm.
- The stomach (normal volume 45 ml) is divided into distinct regions:
  - o **Cardia**: the area that receives the oesophagus (gastro-oesophageal junction).
  - o **Fundus**: formed by the upper curvature.
  - o **Body (corpus)**: the main central region of the organ.
  - o **Pylorus (antrum)**: the lower section of the stomach that facilitates emptying into the small intestine.
- There are two smooth muscle sphincters, oesophageal and pyloric, that dictate entry into and exit from the stomach.

### RELATIONS
- o **Anteriorly**: left lobe of liver, anterior abdominal wall, left hemidiaphragm.
- o **Posteriorly**: lesser sac, stomach bed.

### BLOOD SUPPLY OF THE STOMACH
- **Arterial Supply**
  - o **Lesser Curvature**: right gastric artery (inferiorly) and left gastric artery(superiorly)
  - o **Cardia**: left gastric artery
  - o **Greater Curvature**: right gastroepiploic artery (inferiorly) and left gastroepiploic artery and short gastric arteries (superiorly)
  - o **Fundus of the Stomach**: short gastric arteries

- **Venous Drainage**
  - o Left and Right Gastric Veins drain to Portal Vein
  - o Short Gastric Vein and Left Gastroepiploic Vein drain to Splenic Vein
  - o Right Gastroepiploic Vein drains to SMA.

- **Lymphatic drainage**
  - o Lymphatics drain with arteries to the coeliac lymph nodes.

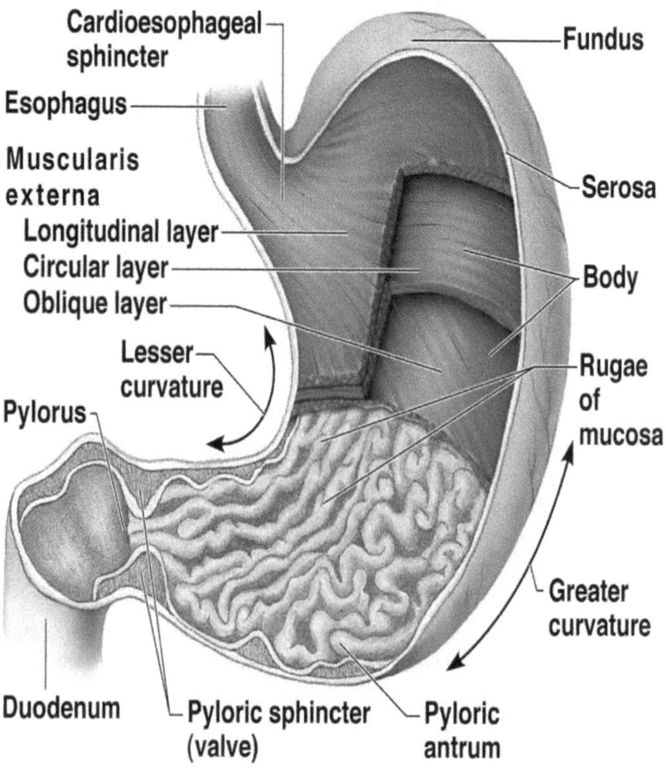

*Fig. 1.4.13. Stomach anatomy*

# THE COELIAC TRUNK

## BRANCHES OF COELIAC TRUNK

- o **Left Gastric Artery**: which branches into:
    - ✓ Oesophageal branch
    - ✓ Hepatic branch
- o **Common Hepatic Artery**: which branches into:
    - ✓ Proper hepatic artery
    - ✓ Right gastric artery
    - ✓ Gastroduodenal artery
    - ✓ Cystic artery
- o **Splenic Artery**: which branches into:
    - ✓ Greater pancreatic artery
    - ✓ Dorsal pancreatic artery
    - ✓ Short gastric arteries
    - ✓ Left gastroepiploic artery

# B. SMALL INTESTINE

## 1. DUODENUM

- o It lies at the level of **L1-3** and the convexity of the duodenum usually encompasses the head of the pancreas. It begins at the duodenal bulb and ends at the ligament of Treitz, where it continues as the jejunum (duodenojejunal or D-J flexure).
- o Segments:
- ▪ **First part (D1) 5cm**
    - • Relations:
        - o Anteriorly - gallbladder, liver
        - o Posteriorly -common bile duct, portal vein, gastroduodenal artery
        - o Superiorly - epiploic foramen
        - o Inferiorly - pancreatic head

- ▪ **Second part (D2) 7.5 cm**
    - • Relations:
        - o Anteriorly - transverse mesocolon
        - o Posteriorly - right kidney, right ureter, right adrenal gland
        - o Superiorly - liver, gallbladder (variable)
        - o Inferiorly - loops of jejunum
        - o Laterally - ascending colon, hepatic flexure, right kidney
        - o Medially - pancreatic head
    - • The pancreatic duct and common bile duct enter the descending duodenum through the major duodenal papilla (ampulla of Vater). This part of the duodenum also contains the minor duodenal papilla, the entrance for the accessory pancreatic duct.
    - • The junction between the embryological foregut and midgut lies just below the major duodenal papilla.

- ▪ **Third part (D3) 10 cm**
    - • Relations:
        - o Anteriorly - small bowel mesentery root
        - o Posteriorly - right psoas muscle, right ureter, gonadal vessels, aorta and IVC
        - o Superiorly - pancreatic head
        - o Inferiorly - loops of jejunum

- ▪ **Fourth part (D4) 2.5 cm**
    - • Relations:
        - o Superiorly – stomach
        - o Inferiorly - loops of jejunum
        - o Posteriorly - left psoas muscle, aorta

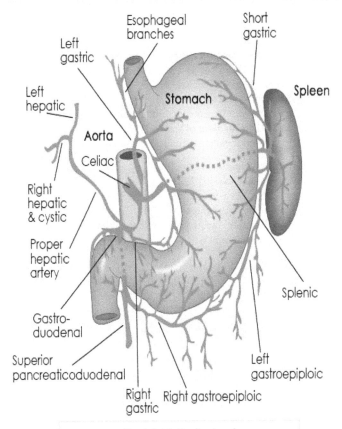

Fig. 1.4.14. Coeliac trunk

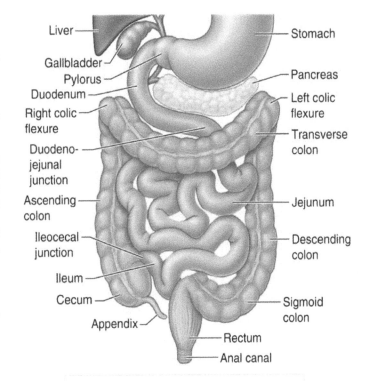

Fig. 1.4.15. Intestines overview

## NEUROVASCULAR SUPPLY OF THE DUODENUM
- From Right gastric, right gastroepiploic, superior and Inferior Pancreaticoduodenal arteries
  - **Arterial Supply:**
    - o **Duodenal cap (first 2.5cm)**
      - Right gastric artery,
      - Right gastroepiploic artery
    - o **Remaining D1 to mid-D2**
      - Superior Pancreaticoduodenal Artery (branch of Gastroduodenal Artery)
    - o **Mid-D2 to ligament of Trietz**
      - Inferior Pancreaticoduodenal Arteries (branch of SMA)

  - **Venous Drainage:**
    - o **Duodenal Cap (First 2.5cm)**
      - Prepyloric Vein (drains to Portal Vein)
    - o **Remaining Duodenum**
      - Superior Pancreaticoduodenal Vein (drains to portal vein) and Inferior Pancreaticoduodenal Vein (drains to Superior Mesenteric Vein)

- **NERVE SUPPLY**
  - o Sympathetic nerve fibres via coeliac and superior mesenteric trunks.
  - o Parasympathetic nerve fibres via anterior and posterior vagal trunks.

- **LYMPHATIC SUPPLY**
  - o Pancreaticoduodenal nodes that drain:
    - Distally to superior mesenteric node
    - Proximally to coeliac nodes

## 2. JEJUNUM VS ILEUM

|  | JEJUNUM | ILEUM |
|---|---|---|
| **Position** | More to the left and above | To the right and below |
| **Appearance** | Redder and wider | Pallor and narrower |
| **feel** | Thicker | Thinner |
|  | Numerous plicae circulares, which can be felt through the bowel wall | Fewer plicae |
| **Aggreged lymphatic follicles** | Fewer and smaller | More and larger |
| **Mesenteric fats** | Less fat in the mesentery of the jejunum near the gut, so that translucent "windows" are visible when the mesentery is held against the light. | Such areas are absent from the mesentery of the terminal ileum. |
| **Arterial arcades** | Jejunal arteries form a greater number of arcades than do the ileal arteries | Ileal arteries form fewer arcades: receive shorter terminal branches from tertiary or quaternary arcades |

### BLOOD SUPPLY OF JEJUNUM AND ILEUM:
- **ARTERIES:**
  - o Both jejunum and ileum are supplied by the **branches of Superior Mesenteric Artery**.
  - o The lowest part of ileum, near the ileocecal junction, is supplied by the **ileocolic artery** in addition to the usual blood supply.
- **VEINS:**
  - o The veins correspond to the arteries and eventually drain into the **Superior Mesenteric Vein**.
- **LYMPH DRAINAGE OF JEJUNUM AND ILEUM:**
  - o The lymphatics from the jejunum and ileum drain into the **Superior Mesenteric Nodes** after passing through a number of intermediate mesenteric nodes.

### NERVE SUPPLY TO JEJUNUM AND ILEUM:
- o Both the sympathetic and parasympathetic fibers come from the **Superior Mesenteric Plexus**.

# C. LARGE INTESTINE
## 1. CAECUM
- Blind-ending sac of bowel that lies below the ileocecal valve, above which the large intestine continues as the ascending colon.
- The caecum measures 6cm in length and can have a maximum diameter of 9cm before it is considered abnormally enlarged.
- ***The appendix typically arises from the posteromedial surface, 2cm inferior to the ileocecal valve***. The caecum is covered in peritoneum, except posteriorly where it has a layer of loose connective tissue and it has a variable mesentery.
- The superior margin of the caecum is defined by the ileocecal ostium.

- Upper and lower flaps consisting smooth muscle protrude into the lumen around the ostium forming the ileocecal valve.
- Its competence (or lack of) is often shown by contrast reflux into the terminal ileum of contrast on contrast enema studies.

**RELATIONS**
- **Anterior** - parietal peritoneum, anterior abdominal wall and loops of small bowel
- **Posterior** - iliacus muscle, psoas muscle, femoral nerve, lateral cutaneous nerve of the thigh and variably appendix
- **Medial** - ileocecal valve and terminal ileum
- **Superior** - ascending colon
- **Inferior** - lateral third of the inguinal ligament

**BLOOD SUPPLY**
- **Arterial Supply** - anterior and posterior caecal arteries from **Colic Artery**, a branch of ileocolic artery from superior mesenteric artery
- **Venous Return** - run with similarly named arteries to the superior mesenteric vein, a tributary of the portal venous system

**NERVE SUPPLY**
- Sympathetic supply via **Superior Mesenteric Plexus**.
- Parasympathetic supply via **Pelvic Splanchnic Nerves (S2 - S4)**.

**LYMPHATIC SUPPLY**
- Lymph travels with the arterial supply to paracolic lymph nodes, which drain to the **Superior Mesenteric Group**.

## 2. APPENDIX
- The appendix or vermiform appendix is a blind muscular tube that arises from the caecum, which is the first part of the large bowel.
- *The appendix arises from the posteromedial surface of the caecum, approximately 2-3 cm inferiorly to the ileocecal valve, where the taeniae coli converge.*
- It is a blind diverticulum, which is variable in length from 2-20 cm.
- The appendix lies on its own mesentery, the mesoappendix.
- The tip of the appendix can have a variable position within the abdominal cavity:
    o **Retro-caecal (65-70%)**
    o **Pelvic (25-30%)**
    o **Pre- or post-ileal (5%)**

**BLOOD SUPPLY**
- **Arterial**: appendicular artery, a branch of the ileocolic artery (a derivative of the superior mesenteric artery)
- **Venous**: similarly named veins draining to the portal venous system

*Nerve supply*: *see caecum*
*Lymphatic supply:* *see caecum*

## 3. COLON
**External Appearance of the Large Intestine**
- Attached to the surface of the large intestine are omental appendices – small pouches of peritoneum, filled with fat.
- Running longitudinally along the surface of the large bowel are three strips of muscle, known as the taeniae coli. They are called the mesocolic, free and omental coli. The taeniae coli contract to shorten the wall of the bowel, producing sacculations known as haustra.
- The colon has four parts; the ascending, transverse, descending and sigmoid. These sections form an arch, encircling the small intestine.

## A. ASCENDING COLON
- Travels superiorly from the cecum.
- When it meets the right lobe of the liver, it turns 90 degrees to the left.
- This turn is known as the right colic flexure (or hepatic flexure), and it marks the start of the transverse colon.

## B. TRANSVERSE COLON
- Crosses the abdomen, running from the right colic flexure to the spleen, where it turns another 90 degrees to point inferiorly.
- This turn is known as the left colic flexure (or splenic flexure).
- The transverse colon is the least fixed part of the colon, and is therefore variable is position, and can dip into the pelvis in tall, thin people.

## C. DESCENDING COLON
o It is a slightly retroperitoneal structure, but is located anteriorly to the left kidney, passing over its lateral border.
o When the colon begins to turn medially, it becomes the sigmoid colon.

## D. SIGMOID COLON
o Has a characteristic 'S' shape, connecting the descending colon to the rectum. Located posteriorly to sigmoid colon are the left ureter and left common iliac artery. Lateral to the ascending and descending colons is a space between the colon and posterior abdominal wall *called the left and right paracolic gutters.*

# BLOOD SUPPLY OF THE INTESTINES

## 1. SUPERIOR MESENTERIC ARTERY

o   *Origin*
- Single vessel arising anteriorly from abdominal aorta at the level of L1.

o   *Course*
- The superior mesenteric vein (SMV) should always lie to the right of the SMA, otherwise malrotation should be suspected.

| BRANCH | SUPPLIES |
| --- | --- |
| Inferior pancreatico-duodenal artery | head of the pancreas and to the ascending and inferior parts of the duodenum |
| Intestinal arteries | branches to ileum, branches to jejunum |
| Ileocolic artery | supplies last part of ileum, cecum, and appendix |
| Right colic artery | Supplies the ascending colon |
| Middle colic artery | Supplies the transverse colon |

## MARGINAL ARTERY OF DRUMMOND

o   *Origin*
- *The terminal branches of the **ileocolic, right colic** and **middle colic arteries** along with the terminal branches of the **left colic artery** and **sigmoid branches of the IMA** form a continuous arterial circle or arcade along the inner border of the colon known as the **Marginal Artery of Drummond.***
- *From this marginal artery, straight vessels (also known as vasa recta) pass to the colon.*

## 2. INFERIOR MESENTERIC ARTERY

o   *Origin*
- Arises from the abdominal aorta anterior to the L3 vertebral body

o   *Course*
- Initially, the inferior mesenteric artery descends anteriorly to the aorta and then passes to the left as it continues inferiorly.

| BRANCH | SUPPLIES |
| --- | --- |
| Left colic artery | Distal 1/3 of the transverse colon and the descending colon:<br>o   **Ascending branch**: supplies the distal 1/3 of the transverse colon, and the upper aspect of the descending colon.<br>o   **Descending branch**: supply the lower part of the descending colon. |
| Sigmoid branches | Supply the descending colon and the sigmoid colon. There are typically 2-4 branches, with the uppermost branch termed the superior sigmoid artery |
| Superior rectal artery | The superior rectal artery is a continuation of the inferior mesenteric artery, supplying the rectum |

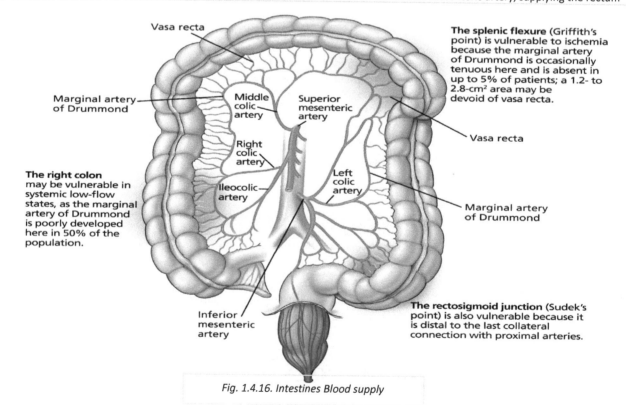

*Fig. 1.4.16. Intestines Blood supply*

## E. RECTUM

- The most distal part of the colon is the rectum, which begins at the level of the **S3 vertebrae.**
- The rectum is a retroperitoneal structure, placed immediately anterior to the sacrum of the vertebral column.
- The distal portion of the rectum is expanded, and is known as the rectal ampulla.
- Macroscopically, the rectum lacks the characteristic features of the large intestine, such as omental appendices and sacculations.
- As the rectal ampulla narrows at the pelvic floor, it gains internal and external anal sphincters, and becomes the anal canal.
- In the pelvis, there is an extension of the peritoneal cavity, which differs in location in men and women:
- In women, it is formed between the posterior wall of the uterus and the colon, and called the **Recto-Uterine Pouch (or Pouch of Douglas)**
- In men, it is between the posterior wall of the bladder and the colon, called the **Recto-Vesical Pouch.**
- In both men and women, the pouch is most inferior portion of peritoneum.

## F. THE ANAL CANAL

| ANAL CANAL | | |
|---|---|---|
| | Above the dentate line | Below the dentate line |
| Arterial supply | • **Superior rectal artery**: from inferior mesenteric artery.<br>• Small contributions from **middle rectal and median sacral arteries.** | • **Inferior rectal artery**: from internal pudendal artery. |
| Venous drainage | • **Superior rectal vein**, draining to inferior mesenteric vein (portal vein). | • **Inferior and middle rectal veins**, draining to internal iliac veins. |
| Nerve supply | • **Sympathetic**: Pelvic Plexus.<br>• **Parasympathetic and afferent sensory:** Pelvic Splanchnic Nerves. | • **Inferior rectal nerve**: branches of the pudendal nerve |
| Lymphatic drainage | • Internal iliac nodes | • Superficial inguinal nodes |
| Epithelium | • Mucus membrane | • Stratified squamous keratinised with hair and sebaceous glands |

## E. BILIARY TRACT
### 1. BILIARY TREE ANATOMY
### A. INTRAHEPATIC BILE DUCTS

- Bile canaliculi unite to form segmental bile ducts, which drain with the following pattern:
  - Segments VI and VII: right posterior duct (RPD), coursing more horizontally.
  - Segments V and VIII: right anterior duct (RAD), coursing more vertically.
  - Right posterior and anterior ducts unite to from the right hepatic duct (RHD).
  - Segmental bile ducts from II-to-IV unite to form the left hepatic duct (LHD).
  - The left and right hepatic ducts unite to form the common hepatic duct (CHD). Bile duct(s) from segment I drain into the angle of their union. The ducts of the left hepatic lobe are more anterior than those of the right lobe; it is important particularly when contrast cholangiogram is performed because contrast may not opacify nondependent ducts.

| 6 + 7 = RPD | 5+8= RAD | 2+3+4=LHD | RPD+RAD=RHD | LHD+RHD= CHD | CHD+CD= CBD |
|---|---|---|---|---|---|

### B. EXTRAHEPATIC BILE DUCTS
- The common hepatic duct is joined by the cystic duct from the gallbladder to form the common bile duct **(CHD+CD=CBD).**
- The common bile duct travels initially in the free edge of the lesser omentum, and then courses posteriorly to the duodenum and pancreas to unite with the main pancreatic duct to form the ampulla of Vater, which drains at the major duodenal papillae on the medial wall of the D2 segment of the duodenum.

### 2. THE LIVER
- During embryological development, the liver is formed within part of the ventral mesentery, which suspends the foregut organs from the anterior abdominal wall. This is useful for remembering the anatomical relations of the liver:
  - **Anterior** to the liver is the anterior abdominal wall and ribcage.
  - **Superior** to the liver is the diaphragm (separating the abdominal cavity from the thoracic cavity)
  - **Posterior** to the liver are the oesophagus, stomach, gallbladder, first part of the duodenum (the foregut-derived organs).

### A. LIVER SURFACES
- There are two liver surfaces – the diaphragmatic and the visceral.
  - **The diaphragmatic surface**
    - Refers to the anterosuperior surface of the liver.
    - It is smooth and convex, fitting snugly beneath the curvature of the diaphragm.
    - A section of this surface is not covered by visceral peritoneum, known as the '***bare area***' of the liver.

o **The visceral surface**
  - Covers the posteroinferior aspect of the liver.
  - It is moulded by the shape of the surrounding organs, making it irregular and flat.
  - It lies in contact with the oesophagus, right kidney, right adrenal gland, right colic flexure, duodenum, gallbladder and the stomach.

## B. LIGAMENTS OF THE LIVER

- **Falciform ligament**
  - Attaches the anterior surface of the liver the anterior abdominal wall.
  - The free edge of this ligament contains the **Ligamentum Teres**, a remnant of the umbilical vein

- **Coronary ligaments** (left and right)
  - Attach the superior surface of the liver to the diaphragm.

- **Triangular ligaments** (left and right)
  - Attach the superior surface of the liver to the diaphragm.

- **Lesser omentum**
  - Consists of the **Hepatoduodenal Ligament** (extends from the duodenum to the liver), and the **Hepatogastric Ligament** (extends from the stomach to the liver).

- In addition to these supporting ligaments, the posterior surface of the liver is secured to the inferior vena cava by hepatic veins and fibrous tissue.

## C. HEPATIC RECESSES

- They are of clinical importance, as infected fluids can collect in these areas, forming an abscess.
  o **Subphrenic spaces** (left and right)
    - Located between the diaphragm and liver, either side of the falciform ligament.
  o **Subhepatic space**
    - Located between the inferior surface of the liver and the transverse colon.
  o **Morison's pouch**
    - The posterosuperior aspect of the right subhepatic space, located between the visceral surface of the liver and the right kidney.

## D. STRUCTURE OF THE LIVER

- The entire liver is covered by a fibrous layer, known as **Glisson's capsule**. The ligaments and surface depressions of the liver divide it into four lobes.
  o It is divided into a right lobe and left lobe by the attachment of the falciform ligament.
  o There are two further 'accessory' lobes that arise from the right lobe, and are located on the visceral surface of liver:
    - **The caudate lobe** is located on the upper aspect of the visceral surface. It lies between the inferior vena cava and a fossa produced by the ligamentum venosum (a remnant of the foetal ductus venosus).
    - **The quadrate lobe** is located on the lower aspect of the visceral surface. It lies between the gallbladder and a fossa produced by the ligamentum teres (a remnant of the foetal umbilical vein).
- Between the caudate and quadrate lobes is a deep fissure, known as the porta hepatis. It transmits all the vessels, nerves and ducts entering or leaving the liver.

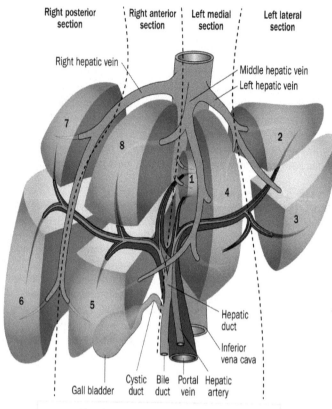

*Fig. 1.4.17. Intrahepatic bile ducts*

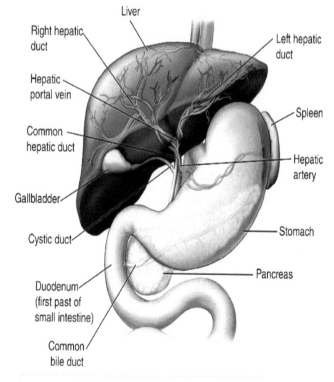

*Fig. 1.4.18. Hepatic blood supply*

## E. ARTERIAL SUPPLY AND VENOUS DRAINAGE

- The liver has a unique dual blood supply:
- **Hepatic artery proper 25%**
  - o Supplies the liver with arterial blood.
  - o It is derived from the coeliac trunk.
- **Hepatic portal vein 75%**
  - o Supplies the liver with deoxygenated blood, carrying nutrients absorbed from the small intestine.
  - o This is the dominant blood supply to the liver parenchyma and allows the liver to perform its gut-related functions, such as detoxification.
- Venous drainage of the liver is achieved through three hepatic veins, which drain into the inferior vena cava.

## F. NERVE SUPPLY

- o The parenchyma of the liver is innervated by *the hepatic plexus,* which contains sympathetic (from the coeliac plexus) and parasympathetic (vagus nerve) nerve fibres.
- o These fibres enter the liver at the porta hepatis and follow the course of branches of the hepatic artery and portal vein.
- o *Glisson's capsule, the fibrous covering of the liver, is innervated by branches of the lower intercostal nerves.*
- o *Distension of the capsule results in a sharp well localised pain.*

## H. LYMPHATIC DRAINAGE

- Drain into hepatic lymph nodes.
- These lie along the hepatic vessels and ducts in the lesser omentum, and empty in the coeliac lymph nodes.

## 3. GALL BLADDER

**STRUCTURE**

- The gallbladder consists of four layers: serosa, muscularis externa, lamina propria and mucosa.
- The gallbladder does not have a submucosa or muscularis mucosae.
- **Hartmann's pouch** lies just proximal to the neck of the gallbladder, a stone may lodge there and become impacted, which can result in a mucocoele.

**Relations**

- **Superiorly**: liver.
- **Inferiorly**: transverse colon, D2 segment of the duodenum (or pylorus of the stomach).
  - o The neck of the gallbladder lies superior to the duodenum.
- **Anteriorly**: transverse colon, 9th costal cartilage.

**BLOOD SUPPLY**

- Arterial supply: **cystic artery.**
- Venous return: there is no single cystic vein, but rather the gallbladder drains directly into the venous system of the liver through the gallbladder fossa and by a number of veins into the right branch of the portal vein.

**NERVE SUPPLY**

- The gallbladder receives both sympathetic and vagal supply:
  - o Sympathetic: via the coeliac plexus
  - o Vagal: via the hepatic branches of anterior vagal trunk

**LYMPHATIC SUPPLY**

- Lymphatics of the gallbladder drain toward the porta hepatis and to portal nodes.

> ### PORTAL TRIAD
> Consists of the following five structures:
> **PHC Like Bachelor**
> ✓ *Portal Vein*
> ✓ *Hepatic artery proper*
> ✓ *Common bile duct*
> ✓ *Lymphatic vessels*
> ✓ *Branch of the vagus nerve*

## 4. PORTAL VEIN

- Portal vein (PV) is the main vessel in the portal venous system and drains blood from the gastrointestinal tract and spleen to the liver.
- Measures approximately 8 cm in adults.
- It originates behind the neck of the pancreas
- Formed by the confluence of the Superior Mesenteric and Splenic Veins, and also receives blood from the Inferior Mesenteric, Gastric, and Cystic Veins. Immediately before reaching the liver, the portal vein divides into left portal vein (supplying liver segments II, III, IV) and the right portal vein, which subsequently divides further into anterior (supplying liver segments V and VIII) and posterior (supplying liver segments VI and VII) portal veins.
- It ramifies further, forming smaller venous branches and ultimately portal venules.
- Each portal venule courses alongside a hepatic arteriole and the two vessels form the vascular components of the portal triad.
- These vessels ultimately empty into the hepatic sinusoids to supply blood to the liver.
- **75% of the blood supplied to the liver comes from the portal vein, but it only supplies 50% of the oxygen supply to the liver**

## F. PANCREAS

### STRUCTURE

- 15 cm (6 in) long. The widest section is called the head. The narrowest part is called the tail.
- The middle section is called the body. Has a series of small tubes that drain into the pancreatic duct.
- The pancreatic duct joins the common bile duct and empties into the duodenum.

### FUNCTION

- **EXOCRINE CELLS (MOST OF CELLS ARE EXOCRINE): Today All Live To See (2C) 3P:**
  - ✓ *Amylase*
  - ✓ *Lipase*
  - ✓ *Trypsinogen,*
  - ✓ *Chymotrypsinogen,*
  - ✓ *Cholesteroesterase*
  - ✓ *Proelastase,*
  - ✓ *Procarboxypeptidase,*
  - ✓ *Phospholipase A2*
  - o Exocrine cells make and release pancreatic juice.
  - o The juice travels through the pancreatic duct into the duodenum. Enzymes in the pancreatic juice help digest fat, carbohydrates and protein in food.

- **ENDOCRINE CELLS (SMALL NUMBER)**
  - o They are arranged in clusters called *Islets or Islets of Langerhans*.
  - o The islets make and release insulin and glucagon into the blood.

### BLOOD SUPPLY

- **Arterial supply**: from the inferior and superior pancreatoduodenal arteries and the splenic artery.
- **Venous return**: The pancreatic and pancreatoduodenal veins drain blood from the pancreas.

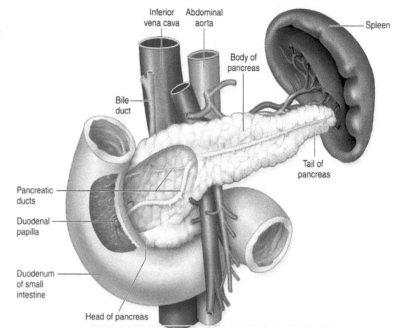

*Fig. 1.4.19. Pancreas Anatomy*

## G. SPLEEN

- Is a wedge-shaped organ lying mainly in the left upper quadrant and is protected by the **left 9th to 11th ribs**.
- It is soft, highly vascular and dark purple in colour. Has two poles (superior and inferior), three borders and two surfaces (diaphragmatic and visceral).
- It is enclosed by a thin capsule, which is easily ruptured. It is completely covered by peritoneum, except at the hilum, and forms a number of ligaments:
  - o **Gastrosplenic Ligament**
    - Attaches the spleen to the greater curvature of the stomach.
    - Contains short gastric and left gastroepiploic arteries.
  - o **Splenorenal Ligament**
    - Attaches the spleen to the left kidney
    - Contains splenic artery and vein and the pancreatic tail.

### RELATIONS

- o Diaphragmatic surface (superoposteriorly): dome of the left hemidiaphragm.
- o Visceral surface (anteromedially)
  - Pancreatic tail
  - Left kidney and adrenal gland and stomach

### BLOOD SUPPLY

- o **Arterial supply:** Splenic artery.
- o **Venous drainage:** Splenic vein.

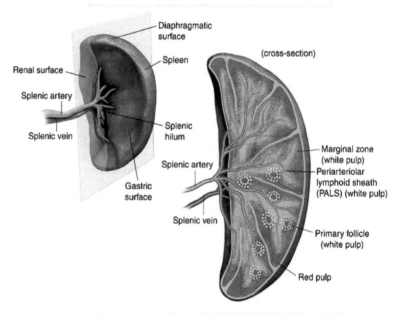

*Fig. 1.4.20. Spleen Anatomy*

# H. KIDNEY

- The kidneys are     paired retroperitoneal organs that lie at the level of the **T12 to L3** vertebral bodies.

## 1. LOCATION

- Located on the posterior abdominal wall, with one on either side of the vertebral column, in the perirenal space.
- The long axis of the kidney is parallel to the lateral border of the psoas muscle.
- *In addition, the kidneys lie at an oblique angle, that is the superior pole is more medial and anterior than the inferior renal pole. Due to the right lobe of the liver, the right kidney usually lies slightly lower than the left kidney*

## 2. STRUCTURE

- In adults, each kidney is normally 10-12 cm in length, 3-5 cm in width and weighs 150-260 g.
- The left kidney is usually slightly larger than the right. Has a fibrous capsule, which is surrounded by pararenal fat.
- The kidney can be divided into renal parenchyma, consisting of renal cortex and medulla, and the renal sinus containing renal pelvis, calyces, renal vessels, nerves, lymphatics and perirenal fat. The renal hilum is the entry to the renal sinus and lies vertically at the anteromedial aspect of the kidney. It contains the renal vessels and nerves, fat and the renal pelvis, which typically emerges posterior to the renal vessels, with the renal vein being anterior to the renal artery.

## 3. RELATIONS OF THE KIDNEY

### A. Right kidney

- o **Anteriorly**
  - ▪ **Superiorly** - right adrenal gland, liver
  - ▪ **Inferiorly** - hepatic flexure, small intestine
- o **Medially** - duodenum
- o **Posteriorly** - diaphragm, posterior abdominal wall

### B. Left kidney

- o **Anteriorly:**
  - ▪ **Superiorly** - left adrenal gland, stomach, spleen
  - ▪ **Inferiorly** - pancreas
- o **Laterally** - splenic flexure, descending colon
- o **Medially** – jejunum
- o **Posteriorly** - diaphragm, posterior abdominal wall

## 4. BLOOD SUPPLY

- o **Arterial supply** - renal arteries (from abdominal aorta)
- o **Venous drainage** - renal veins (to IVC)

## 5. NERVE SUPPLY

- o Sympathetic and parasympathetic Renal Nerve Plexus, which is derived from abdominopelvic splanchnic nerves.

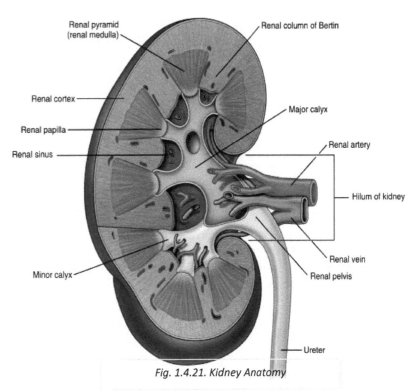

*Fig. 1.4.21. Kidney Anatomy*

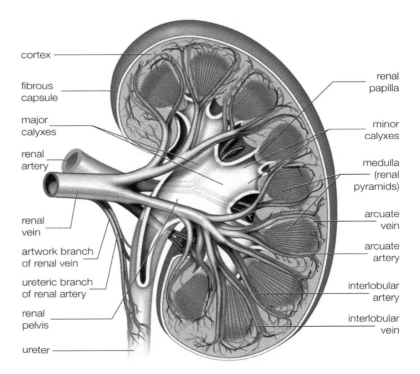

*Fig. 1.4.22. Kidney Blood supply*

## I. URETERS

- The ureter is 25-30cm long and has three parts:
  - **Abdominal Ureter**: from the renal pelvis to the pelvic brim.
  - **Pelvic Ureter**: from the pelvic brim to the bladder.
  - **Intravesical or Intramural Ureter**: within the bladder wall.

## 1. RELATIONS OF URETERS
### A. ABDOMINAL URETER
Following the course of the ureter from superior to inferior:
- **Posteriorly**:
  - Psoas muscle;
  - Genitofemoral nerve;
  - Common iliac vessels;
  - Tips of L2-L5 transverse processes
- **Anteriorly**
  - **Right Ureter**: descending duodenum (D2); gonadal vessels; right colic vessels; ileocolic vessels.
  - **Left Ureter**: gonadal artery; left colic artery; loops of jejunum; sigmoid mesentery and colon.
- **Laterally**
  - Right Ureter: IVC

### B. PELVIC URETER
- **Posteriorly**:
  - Sacroiliac joint, Internal iliac artery
- **Inferiorly**
  - **Male**: Seminal vesicle
  - **Female**: Lateral fornix of the vagina
- **Anteriorly**
  - **Male**: Ductus deferens
  - **Female**: Uterine artery (in the broad ligament)
- **Laterally**
  - **Female**: Cervix

## 2. CONSTRICTIONS
- At the pelvi-ureteric junction (PUJ) of the renal pelvis and the ureter.
- As the ureter enters the pelvis and cross over the common iliac artery bifurcation.
- At the vesicoureteric junction (VUJ) as the ureter enters the bladder wall.
- *The two commonest sites for impaction of kidney stones are at the Pelvic Brim, near the bifurcation of the iliac arteries, and at the Uretovesicular Valve, where the ureter meets the bladder*

### 3. BLOOD SUPPLY
- ***Arterial supply***: from branches of the renal artery, abdominal aorta, superior and inferior vesical arteries
- Some texts also include supply from the gonadal, middle rectal and uterine arteries
- ***Venous drainage***: via similarly named veins but is highly variable.

### 4. LYMPHATIC SUPPLY
- **Abdominal ureter**: aorto-caval and common iliac nodes.
- **Pelvic ureter**: internal and external iliac nodes.

### 5. NERVE SUPPLY
- Derived from renal, aortic and hypogastric autonomic plexuses.
- The ureters have sympathetic innervation via **T11-L1** and parasympathetic innervation via **S2-S4**.
- *Kidney related pain is often referred to the **T11-L1** area.*

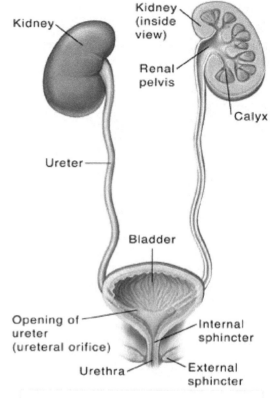

Fig. 1.4.23. Ureters anatomy

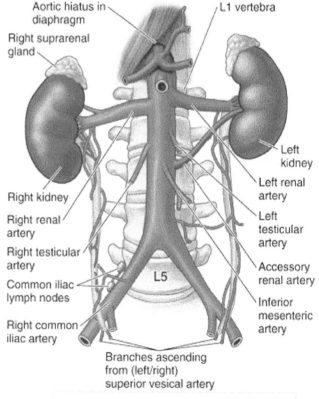

Fig. 1.4.24. Relations of ureters

# CLINICAL RELEVANCE

## TRAUMATIC URETERAL INJURIES

- Because of its protected position and small size, injuries to the ureter are rare.
- Most injuries are caused by gunshot wounds and, in a few individuals, penetrating stab wounds.
- Because the ureters are retroperitoneal in position, urine may escape into the retroperitoneal tissues on the posterior abdominal wall.

## URETERIC STONES

- There are three sites of anatomic narrowing of the ureter where stones may be arrested, namely, the pelviureteral junction, the pelvic brim, and where the ureter enters the bladder. Most stones, although radiopaque, are small enough to be impossible to see definitely along the course of the ureter on plain radiographic examination. An intravenous pyelogram is usually necessary.
- The ureter runs down in front of the tips of the transverse processes of the lumbar vertebrae, crosses the region of the sacroiliac joint, swings out to the ischial spine, and then turns medially to the bladder.

## RENAL COLIC

- The renal pelvis and the ureter send their afferent nerves into the spinal cord at segments T11 and 12 and L1 and 2. In renal colic, strong peristaltic waves of contraction pass down the ureter in an attempt to pass the stone onward.
- The spasm of the smooth muscle causes an agonizing colicky pain, which is referred to the skin areas that are supplied by these segments of the spinal cord, namely, the flank, loin, and groin.
- When a stone enters the low part of the ureter, the pain is felt at a lower level and is often referred to the testis or the tip of the penis in the male and the labium majus in the female. Sometimes, ureteral pain is referred along the femoral branch of the genitofemoral nerve (L1 and 2) so that pain is experienced in the front of the thigh. The pain is often so severe that afferent pain impulses spread within the central nervous system, giving rise to nausea.

# J. URINARY BLADDER

## 1. RELATIONS - MALE
- o Anteriorly - pubic symphysis
- o Posteriorly - rectovesical pouch and rectum
- o Inferiorly - prostate, obturator internus muscle, levator ani muscle.
- o Superiorly - peritoneum
- o Laterally - ischioanal fossa

## 2. RELATIONS - FEMALE
- o Anteriorly - pubic symphysis
- o Posteriorly- vesicouterine pouch, uterus, cervix, vagina.
- o Inferiorly - pelvic fascia, perineal membrane
- o Superiorly - uterus, peritoneum
- o Laterally - ischioanal fossa

## 3. BLOOD SUPPLY
- o **Arterial supply** - superior and inferior vesical arteries (from anterior division of internal iliac artery)
- o **Venous drainage** - vesical venous plexus via similarly named veins to the internal iliac veins

## 4. NERVE SUPPLY
- o Vesical Nerve Plexus

## 5. LYMPHATIC SUPPLY
- o Accompanies blood vessels to the internal iliac lymph and para-aortic node

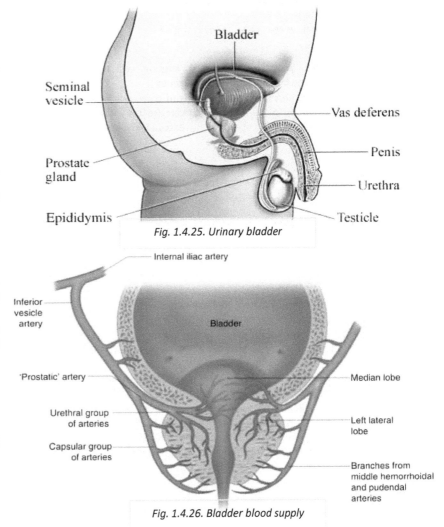

Fig. 1.4.25. Urinary bladder

Fig. 1.4.26. Bladder blood supply

# VIII. MALE INTERNAL GENITALIA

## 1. PROSTATE

o  The prostate is positioned inferiorly to the neck of the **bladder** and superiorly to the **external urethral sphincter**, with the levator ani muscle lying inferolaterally to the gland. Most importantly, posteriorly to the prostate lies the ampulla of the **rectum**: this anatomical arrangement is utilised during Digital Rectal Examinations (DRE) by physicians needing to examine the gland.

o  The prostate is divided into anatomical **lobes** (inferoposterior, inferolateral, superomedial, and anteromedial) by the urethra and the ejaculatory ducts as they pass through the organ. However, more important clinically is histological division of the prostate into zones:

- **Central zone:** Surrounds the ejaculatory ducts, embryologically derived from the Wolffian duct.
- **Transitional zone:** Located centrally and surrounds the urethra, embryologically derived from the urogenital sinus.
- **Peripheral zone:** Makes up the main body of the gland and located posteriorly, embryologically derived from the Urogenital Sinus. **The peripheral zone is the zone felt against the rectum on DRE.**

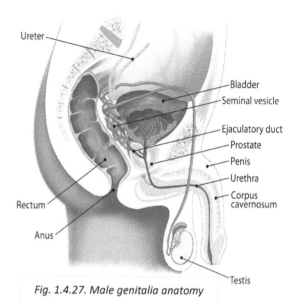

*Fig. 1.4.27. Male genitalia anatomy*

o  **RELATIONS**
- Anteriorly: pubic symphysis
- Inferiorly: urogenital membrane
- Superiorly: bladder
- Posteriorly: rectum
- Laterally: prostatic venous plexus and levator ani

o  **BLOOD SUPPLY**
- **Arterial Supply**: prostatic branch of inferior vesical artery; sometimes supplied by the middle rectal arteries.
- **Venous Drainage**: prostatic venous plexus in communication with the pudendal plexus to the deep dorsal vein (to the internal iliac vein) with some communication to the **Batson vertebral venous plexus.**

o  **NERVE SUPPLY**
- Parasympathetic (**S2-S4**) and sympathetic (**L1-L2**) pelvic nerve plexus

o  **LYMPHATIC SUPPLY**
- Drainage mainly to obturator and internal iliac nodes.
- Some drainage to external iliac, presacral and para-aortic nodes.

## 2. URETHRA

### A. MALE URETHRA

- The male urethra is approximately **15-20cm long.**
- Anatomically, the urethra can be divided into four parts:
  o  **Pre-prostatic (intramural)**: Begins at the internal urethral orifice, located at the neck of the bladder. It passes through the wall of the bladder, and ends at the prostate.
  o  **Prostatic**: Passes through the prostate gland. The ejaculatory ducts and the prostatic ducts drain into the urethra here.
  o  **Membranous**: Passes through the pelvic floor, and the deep perineal pouch. It is surrounded by the external urethral sphincter, which provides voluntary control of micturition.
  o  **Spongy**: Passes through the bulb and corpus spongiosum of the penis, ending at the external urethral orifice.

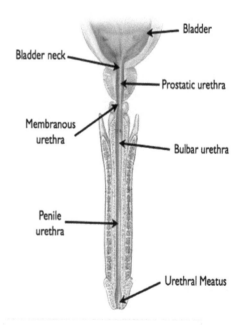

*Fig. 1.4.28. Male urethra parts*

### B. FEMALE URETHRA

- In women, the urethra is relatively short (approximately **4cm**).
- This predisposes women to urinary tract infections.

# IX. FEMALE REPRODUCTIVE SYSTEM

## 1. OVARIES

- They are stabilised by the mesovarium, the ovarian ligament and the infundibulopelvic ligament.
- **Ligaments**
  - Two peritoneal ligaments attach to the ovary:
    - ○ **Suspensory ligament of ovary:** fold of peritoneum extending from the mesovarium to the pelvic wall. Contains neurovascular structures.
    - ○ **Ligament of ovary:** extends from the ovary to the fundus of the uterus. It then continues from the uterus to the connective tissue of the labium majus, as the round ligament of uterus.
- **Arterial supply**
  - **Ovarian artery** - a branch of the abdominal aorta
  - **Uterine artery** - branch internal iliac artery
- **Venous drainage**
  - **Ovarian veins** – these veins are formed from tributaries of the pampiniform plexus which is found in the broad ligament near the ovaries.
  - *The right one drains into the inferior vena cava directly and the left one drains into the left renal vein which in turn drains into the inferior vena cava.*
- **Lymphatic drainage:**
  - Para-aortic nodes.
- **Innervation**
  - **Autonomic** – via the ovarian plexus
  - **Visceral afferents** – accompany the sympathetic fibers to **T10 – T12** level of the spinal cord sensory ganglia.

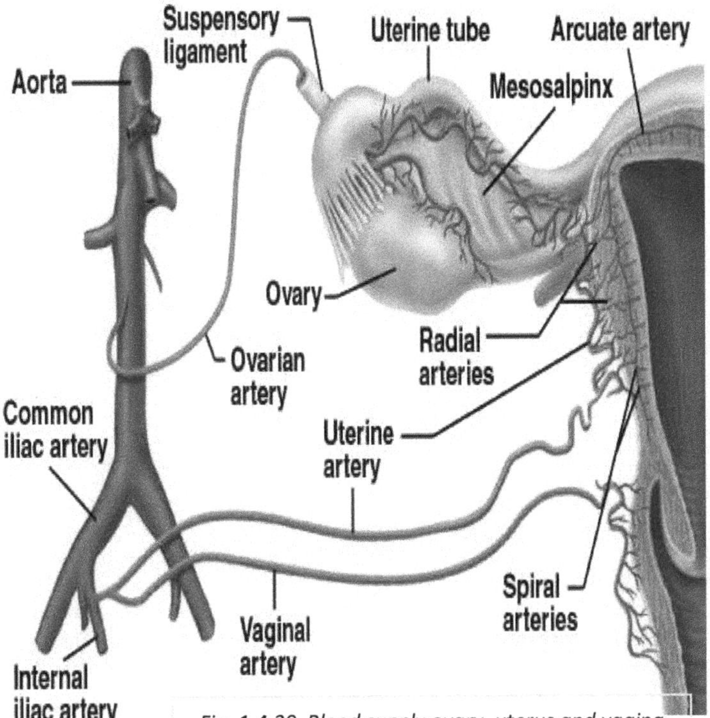

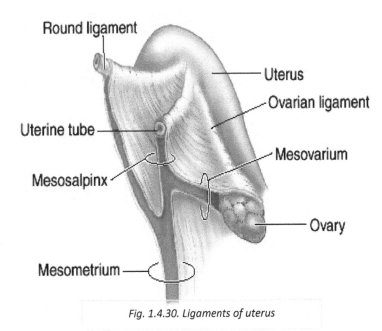

Fig. 1.4.29. Blood supply ovary, uterus and vagina

## 2. UTERUS

- **Anatomical Position**
  - ○ The exact anatomical location of the uterus varies with the degree of distension of the bladder. In the normal adult uterus, it can be described as anteverted with respect to the vagina, and anteflexed with respect to the cervix:
  - ○ **Anteverted:** Rotated forward, towards the anterior surface of the body.
  - ○ **Anteflexed:** Flexed, towards the anterior surface of the body.
  - ○ Thus, the uterus normally lies immediately posterosuperior to the bladder, and anterior to the rectum.

Fig. 1.4.30. Ligaments of uterus

- **Relations**
  - ○ **Anteriorly:** vesicouterine pouch and the urinary bladder
  - ○ **Posteriorly:** rectouterine pouch and the anterior surface of rectum
  - ○ **Laterally:** the broad ligament

- **Ligaments**
  - ○ **Broad Ligament:** This is a double layer of peritoneum attaching the sides of the uterus to the pelvis. It acts as a mesentery for the uterus and contributes to maintaining it in position. It can be divided in 3 parts: **Mesometrium**, **Mesosalpinx** and **Mesovarium**.

- o **Round Ligament**: A remnant of the gubernaculum extending from the uterine horns to the labia majora via the inguinal canal. It functions to maintain the anteverted position of the uterus.
- o **Ovarian Ligament**: Joins the ovaries to the uterus.
- o **Cardinal Ligament**: Located at the base of the broad ligament, the cardinal ligament extends from the cervix to the lateral pelvic walls. It contains the uterine artery and vein in addition to providing support to the uterus.
- o **Uterosacral Ligament**: Extends from the cervix to the sacrum. It provides support to the uterus.

- **Arterial supply**
  - o **Uterine arteries:** a branch of internal iliac artery
  - o **Ovarian arteries:** branch of the abdominal aorta at the level of L1.

- **Venous drainage**
  - o **Uterine veins:** they are formed from the plexus and drain into internal iliac veins

- **Innervation**
  - o **Autonomic:**
    - Hypogastric plexus (sympathetic), **S2-S4** (parasympathetic)
    - **Visceral afferents: T11–T12 and L1**

## 3. VAGINA

- **Relations**
  - o **Anteriorly**: urethral orifice
  - o **Posteriorly**: The rectum

- **Arterial supply**
  - o **Uterine arteries:** supplies the superior portion, a branch of the internal iliac artery
  - o **Vaginal artery** and **internal pudendal arteries**: supply the middle and inferior parts, branches of the internal iliac artery.

- **Venous drainage**
  - o **Uterovaginal plexus**: drains into internal iliac veins

- **Innervation**
  - o **Autonomic:** inferior hypogastric plexus, pelvic splanchnic, pudendal nerve (all provide parasympathetic Innervation from **S2-S4**)
  - o **Visceral afferents** – accompany parasympathetic fibers of inferior hypogastric and pelvic splanchnic nerves to **S2-S4.**
  - o **Somatic afferents** – accompany pudendal nerve to **S2-S4**

## 4. PELVIS

- **The superior portion** of the pelvis is known as **The Greater Pelvis** (or false pelvis).
- It provides support for the lower abdominal viscera (ileum and sigmoid colon), and **has no obstetric relevance.**
- **The inferior portion** of the pelvis is known as **The Lesser Pelvis** (or "true" pelvis).
- Within which resides the pelvic cavity and pelvic viscera.
- The junction between the greater and lesser pelvis is known as the **Pelvic Inlet.**
- The outer bony edges of the pelvic inlet are called the **Pelvic Brim.**

➢ **Pelvic Inlet**
- The pelvic inlet marks the boundary between the greater pelvis and lesser pelvis. Its size is defined by its edge, the **pelvic brim**.
- The pelvic inlet determines the size and shape of the birth canal, with the prominent ridges key areas of muscle and ligament attachment.
- The borders of the pelvic inlet:
  - o **Posterior**: The sacral promontory (the superior portion of the sacrum).
  - o **Lateral**: The arcuate line on the inner surface of the ilium, and the pectineal line on the superior ramus.
  - o **Anterior**: The pubic symphysis.

➢ **Pelvic Outlet**
- The pelvic outlet is located at the end of the lesser pelvis, and the beginning of the pelvic wall.
- Its borders are:
  - o **Posterior**: The tip of the coccyx
  - o **Lateral**: The ischial tuberosities and the inferior margin of the sacrotuberous ligament
  - o **Anterior**: The pubic arch (the inf. border of the ischiopubic rami).
- The angle beneath the pubic arch is known as the **sub-pubic angle** and is of a greater size in women.

## GYNECOID VS ANDROID PELVIS

| GYNECOID PELVIS | ANDROID PELVIS |
|---|---|
| • Is a typical female pelvis<br>• Ideal for vaginal delivery<br>• Rounded or slightly oval inlet<br>• Straight sidewalls with roomy pelvic cavity<br>• Ischial spines are not or less prominent: allowing greater bispinous diameter<br>• Good sacral curve<br>• Subpubic arc is wide (>80-90°) | • Heart shaped or triangular pelvic inlet: due to prominent sacrum<br>• Pelvis funnels from above downwards (convergent sidewalls)<br>• Prominent ischial spines<br>• Oval obturator foramen<br>• Sacrum inclining forward (longer)<br>• Narrow subpubic arch |

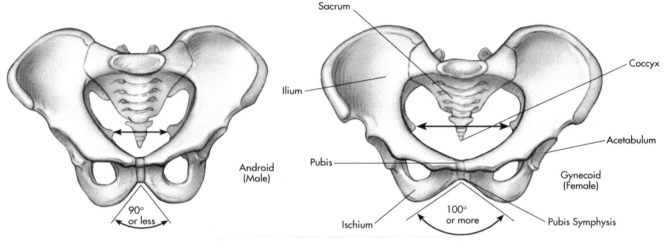

Fig. 1.4.31. Gynecoid and Android pelvis

## 5. PELVIC FLOOR

### PELVIC FLOOR STRUCTURE

- The **Pelvic floor** is a funnel-shaped musculature structure. It attaches to the walls of the lesser pelvis, separating the **pelvic cavity** from the inferior **perineum** (region which includes the genitalia and anus). In order to allow for urination and defecation, there are a few gaps in the structure. There are two 'holes' with clinical significance:
  - **The urogenital hiatus**: An anteriorly situated gap, which allows passage of the urethra (and the vagina in females).
  - **The rectal hiatus**: A centrally positioned gap, which allows passage of the anal canal.
  - Between the urogenital hiatus and the anal canal lies a fibrous node known as the **perineal body** which joins the pelvic floor to the perineum.

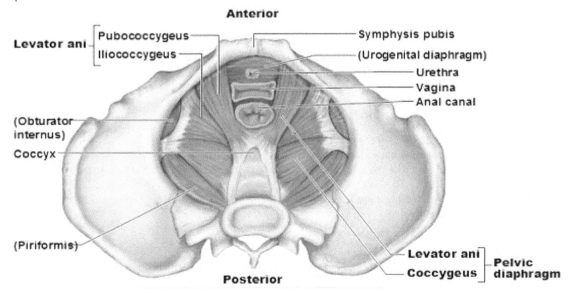

Fig. 1.4.32. Pelvic floor muscles

**FUNCTIONS**
- As the floor of the pelvic cavity, the muscles have important roles to play in the correct functions of the pelvic and abdominal viscera.
- The roles of the pelvic floor muscles are:
  - **Support of abdominopelvic viscera** (bladder, intestines, uterus etc.) through their tonic contraction.
  - **Resistance to increase in intra-pelvic/abdominal pressure** during activities such as coughing or lifting heavy objects.
  - **Urinary and fecal continence.** The muscle fibers have a sphincter action on the rectum and urethra. They relax to allow urination and defecation.

**MUSCLES**
- There are three components of the pelvic floor:
  - Levator ani muscles (largest component).
  - Coccygeus muscle.
  - Fascia coverings of the muscles.

## 1. LEVATOR ANI MUSCLES
  - *Innervated by branches of the **pudendal nerve**, roots **S2, S3 and S4**.*
  - The levator ani is a broad sheet of muscle.
  - It is composed of three separate paired muscles, called the **pubococcygeus**, **puborectalis** and **iliococcygeus**.
  - These muscles have attachments to the pelvis as follows:
    - **Anterior:** The pubic bodies of the hip bone.
    - **Laterally:** Thickened fascia of the obturator internus muscle, known as the tendinous arch.
    - **Posteriorly:** The ischial spines of the hip bone.

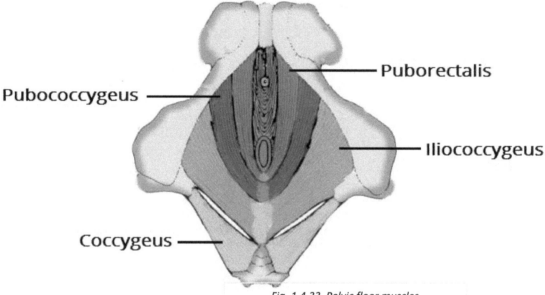

Fig. 1.4.33. Pelvic floor muscles

## A. PUBORECTALIS
  - The puborectalis muscle is a U-shaped sling, extending from the bodies of the pubic bones, past the **urogenital hiatus**, around the anal canal. Its tonic contraction bends the canal anteriorly, creating the anorectal angle (90degrees) at the **anorectal junction** (where the rectum meets the anus).
  - **The main function** of this thick muscle **is to maintain faecal continence** – during defecation this muscle relaxes.

## B. PUBOCOCCYGEUS
  - The muscle fibres of the pubococcygeus are the main constituent of the levator ani.
  - They arise from the body of the **pubic bone** and the anterior aspect of the **tendinous arch**.
  - The fibres travel around the margin of the urogenital hiatus and run posteromedially, attaching at the **coccyx** and **anococcygeal ligament**.
  - As the fibres run inferiorly and medially, some fibres divide and loop around the prostate in males (**levator prostatae**) and around the vagina in females (**pubovaginalis**).
  - Some also terminate in the perineal body.

## C. ILIOCOCCYGEUS
  - The iliococcygeus has thin muscle fibres, which start anteriorly at the **ischial spines** and posterior aspect of the **tendinous arch**.
  - They attach posteriorly to the coccyx and the anococcygeal ligament.

## D. COCCYGEUS
- Innervated by the **anterior rami of S4 and S5**.
- The coccygeus is the smaller, and most posterior, pelvic floor component. The levator ani muscles situated anteriorly.
- It originates from the **ischial spines** and travels to the lateral aspect of the sacrum and coccyx, along the **sacrospinous** ligament

*Obturator internus*

 -makes sharp turn between ischial spine and ischial tuberosity

 -to greater trochanter

*Piriformis*

 -sacrum to greater trochanter

 -key to gluteal region relationships

*Coccygeus*

 -covers sacrospinous ligament

 -good landmark

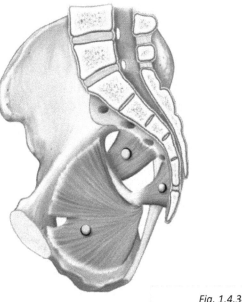
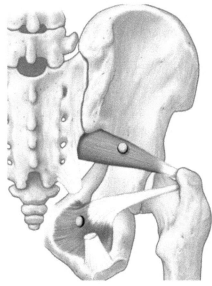

*Fig. 1.4.34. Pelvic floor muscles*

## CLINICAL RELEVANCE

### 1. PELVIC FLOOR DYSFUNCTION
- The pelvic floor acts to support the pelvic viscera, and assist in their functions.
- If the muscles of the floor become damaged, then dysfunction of these viscera can occur.
- The levator ani muscles are involved in supporting the **foetal head** during cervix dilation in childbirth.
- *During the second phase of childbirth, the levator ani muscles and/or the pudendal nerve are at high risk of damage.*
- *Pubococcygeus and puborectalis are the most prone to injury due to them being situated most medially*
- Due to their role in supporting the vagina, urethra and anal canal, injury to these muscles can lead to a number of problems:
  - **Urinary stress incontinence** and **rectal incontinence**: most noticeable during activities where there are increased abdominal pressure (coughing, sneezing and lifting heavy objects).
  - **Prolapse of the pelvic viscera** (bladder and vagina) can occur if there is trauma to the pelvic floor or if the muscle fibres have poor tone.
    - Prolapse of the vagina can also occur if there is damage to the **perineal body** in childbirth.
    - This may be avoided by **episiotomy** which itself can cause damage to the vaginal mucosa and submucosa but helps prevent uncontrolled tearing of the perineal muscles.
  - **Rectal herniation:** If the medial fibres of the puborectalis are torn within the perineal body, then rectal herniation can also occur.
- The pelvic floor can be repaired surgically, however a way to generally strengthen the muscles is to carry out **pelvic floor exercises** on a regular basis (**Kegel exercises).**

### 2. SALPINGITIS
- **Salpingitis** is inflammation of the uterine tubes that is usually caused by bacterial infection. It can cause adhesions of the mucosa which may partially or completely block the lumen of the uterine tubes.
- This can potentially result in **infertility** or an **ectopic pregnancy**.

### 3. ECTOPIC PREGNANCY
- If the lumen of the uterine tube is **partially occluded**, sperm may be able to pass through and fertilise the ovum.
- However, the fertilised egg may not be able to pass into the uterus, and can implant in **the uterine tube**. This is known as an ectopic pregnancy.
- An ectopic pregnancy is a **medical emergency** – if not diagnosed early, the implanted blastocyst can cause rupture and haemorrhage of the affected tube.

# X. LUMBAR AND SACRAL PLEXUSES

## 1. SACRAL PLEXUS BRANCHES: SIX PS

- Nerve to **P**iriformis (S1-S2)
- **Pe**rforating cutaneous nerve (S2-S3)
- **P**osterior femoral cutaneous nerve (S1-S3)
- **P**arasympathetic pelvic splanchnic nerves (S2-S4)
- **P**udendal nerve (S2-S4)
- **Pe**rineal branch of the pudendal nerve (S4)

## 2. LUMBAR PLEXUS BRANCHES

○  IIGLO For Life (IIGLO is used in place of an igloo)
- **I**: iliohypogastric nerve
- **I**: ilioinguinal nerve
- **G**: genitofemoral nerve
- **L**: lateral femoral cutaneous nerve
- **O**: obturator nerve
- **F**: femoral nerve
- **L**: lumbosacral trunk
- The plexus is formed by the anterior rami (divisions) of the lumbar spinal nerves **L1, L2, L3 and L4**.
- Also, receives contributions from thoracic spinal nerve 12.

### A. ILIOHYPOGASTRIC NERVE

- **Roots:** L1 (with contributions from T12).
- **Motor Functions:** Innervates the internal oblique and transversus abdominis.
- **Sensory Functions:** Innervates the posterolateral gluteal skin in the pubic region.

### B. ILIOINGUINAL NERVE

- **Roots:** L1.
- **Motor Functions:** Innervates the internal oblique and transversus abdominis.
- **Sensory Functions:**
  ○ Innervates the skin on the upper middle thigh.
  ○ In males: supplies the skin over the root of the penis and anterior scrotum.
  ○ In females: supplies the skin over mons pubis and labium majus.

### C. GENITOFEMORAL NERVE

- **Roots:** L1-L2.
- **Motor Functions:** The Genital branch innervates the cremasteric muscle.
- **Sensory Functions:**
  ○ The Genital branch innervates the skin of the anterior scrotum (in males) or the skin over mons pubis and labium majus (in females).
  ○ The Femoral branch innervates the skin on the upper anterior thigh.

### D. LATERAL CUTANEOUS NERVE OF THE THIGH

- This nerve has a purely sensory function.
- **Roots:** L2, L3
- **Motor Functions:** None.
- **Sensory Functions:** Innervates the anterior and lateral thigh down to the level of the knee.

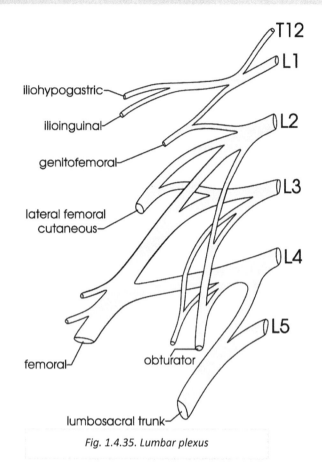

Fig. 1.4.35. Lumbar plexus

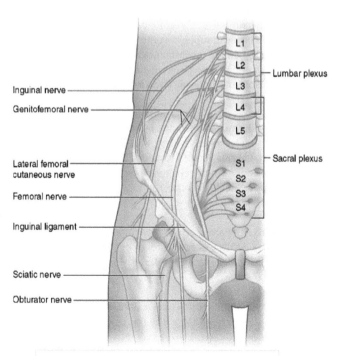

Fig. 1.4.36. Branches of the Lumbar plexus

# PAST ASKED QUESTIONS

| **The posterior triangle of the neck** | |
|---|---|
| Contains the accessory nerve | T |
| Contains branches of the cervical plexus | T |
| Contains the internal jugular vein | F |
| Has the anterior margin of the sternocleidomastoid muscle as its posterior border | F |
| **Which statements are true regarding the testis?** | |
| The testicular surface is covered with tunica vaginalis | T |
| The testicular arteries branch from the abdominal aorta at the level of L2 | T |
| Both testicular veins drain into inferior vena cava | F |
| Lymphatics drain into internal iliac lymph nodes | F |
| **Lymphatic vessels from the anal canal below the dentate line drain into:** | |
| Paraaortic Nodes | F |
| Superior Mesenteric Nodes | F |
| Internal Iliac Nodes | F |
| Superficial Inguinal nodes | T |
| Inferior Mesenteric Nodes | F |
| **Regarding the anatomical position of the Appendix:** | |
| In most people is located anterior a medial to the caecum | F |
| Is typically 4-6cm in length | F |
| Sensory innervation comes from T10 | T |
| McBurney's point describes the location of the tip of the appendix | F |
| **In a stab wound at L1 level, the following structures may be damaged** | |
| Superior mesenteric artery | T |
| Pylorus of stomach | T |
| Body of pancreas | T |
| Left renal artery | T |
| **With Regard to the ovary:** | |
| Ovarian arteries are branches of the internal iliac artery | F |
| Lymph from the ovaries drains into para aortic lymph nodes | T |
| Ligament of the ovary contains neurovascular structures | F |
| The left ovarian vein drains into the inferior vena cava | F |
| **In men during digital rectal examination, the following structures can be palpated:** | |
| Prostate | T |
| Sacrum and coccyx | F |
| Ductus deferent | F |
| Ischial tuberosity | F |
| **The following are true of Levator Ani** | |
| Coccygeus muscle is an important component | F |
| Innervated by Pudendal nerve | T |
| Puborectalis plays a role in fecal continence | T |
| During child birth, iliococcygeus is most likely to be damage | F |
| **Regarding Focus Abdominal Sonography in Trauma (FAST):** | |
| Fluid in the pericardial sac can be seen in left loin views | F |
| The superior mesenteric artery is typically seen perpendicular to the aorta | F |
| Morrison's pouch is between the right kidney and the liver | T |
| Sagittal suprapubic views may show common iliac artery injuries | F |
| **The following are true of the abdominal aorta** | |
| It gives off the testicular artery | T |
| Its maximum diameter is 4cm | F |
| Divides into iliac arteries at L4 level | T |
| Its only separated from lumbar spine by anterior longitudinal ligament | T |

| In a seat-belt injury at L4 level, the following structures may be injured | |
|---|---|
| Liver | F |
| Left kidney | F |
| Left common iliac artery | T |
| Inferior mesenteric artery | F |

| The broad ligament of the uterus is a double layer of the peritoneum which encloses: | |
|---|---|
| Ureter | F |
| Ovarian and round ligament | T |
| Uterine tube | T |
| Uterine artery | T |

| With regards to the sphincters of the anal canal: | |
|---|---|
| Internal sphincter is voluntary | F |
| External sphincter relaxes in response to distension of the rectal ampulla | F |
| Internal sphincter has 3 parts | T |
| External sphincter is a continuation of the circular muscles layers | T |

| Regarding the anatomical relationship of the adult ureters: | |
|---|---|
| On x-ray, they overlie the transverse process of lumbar vertebrae | F |
| They are retroperitoneal for most of their course | T |
| The vesicoureteric junction is located on the anteromedial aspect of the urinary bladder | F |
| The ureters pass posterior to the common iliac veins | F |

| Regarding the Prostate: | |
|---|---|
| Has lateral lobes which are main site of prostatic hypertrophy | F |
| Stores Sperm | F |
| Has venous drainage to the vertebral venous plexus | T |
| Has a membranous urethra passing through it | F |

| The following are true of the bony pelvis | |
|---|---|
| Piriformis muscle passes through the lesser sciatic foramen | F |
| Anterior superior iliac spine provides attachment to the inguinal ligament | T |
| Male pelvis has a wide subpubic angle compared to females | F |

| Lymph drainage in pelvis includes the: | |
|---|---|
| Ovaries to the lateral pelvic nodes | F |
| Uterine cervix to deep inguinal nodes | F |
| Vagina to the lateral pelvic nodes | T |
| Fallopian tubes to the paraaortic nodes | T |

# SECTION 5: HEAD & NECK

## I. STRUCTURES OF THE NECK

### A. MAJOR DIVISIONS AND BONES

### 1. POSTERIOR TRIANGLE

| POSTERIOR TRIANGLE | | |
|---|---|---|
| **Borders** | o | Posterior border of the sternocleidomastoid muscle |
| | o | Anterior border of the trapezius muscle |
| | o | Superior border of the clavicle |
| **Roof** | o | Platysma and the investing (superficial) layer of the deep cervical fascia. |
| **Contents:** | | |
| **Muscles: "LOSS"** | o | **L**evator scapulae. |
| | o | Inferior belly of **O**mohyoid. |
| | o | The **S**calenes (ant/post/middle) |
| | o | **S**plenius |
| **Veins:** | o | Terminal part of **E**xternal **J**ugular **V**ein. |
| **Arteries:** | o | Third part of subclavian artery. |
| | o | Transverse cervical |
| | o | Suprascapular arteries. |
| **Nerves:** | o | Accessory nerve (CN XI), |
| | o | Phrenic nerve |
| | o | Branches of cervical plexus, |
| | o | Root and trunks of brachial plexus, |
| **lymph nodes** | o | Occipital |
| | o | Supraclavicula |

*The internal jugular vein lies in the anterior triangle of the neck. The posterior triangle is further divided into the occipital and subclavian (supraclavicular or omoclavicular) triangles by the omohyoid posterior belly.*

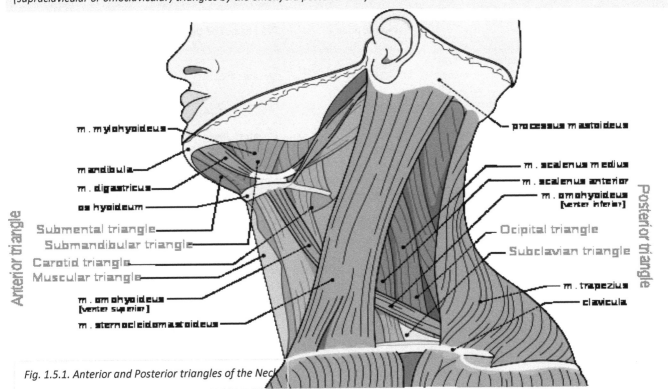

Fig. 1.5.1. Anterior and Posterior triangles of the Neck

## 2. ANTERIOR TRIANGLE
**BORDERS**
- Anterior border of the sternocleidomastoid
- Anterior midline of the neck
- Inferior border of the mandible.

**ROOF**
- Platysma and the investing layer of the deep cervical fascia.
- It is further divided by the omohyoid anterior belly and the digastric anterior and posterior bellies into 4 Triangles:
  o **Digastric (submandibular):** submandibular gland.
  o **Submental (suprahyoid):** Submental Lymph Nodes.
  o **Carotid:** 3C (CNXII, ansa cervicalis & carotid sheath)
  o **Muscular (inferior carotid):** Thyroid and Parathyroid Glands.

**CONTENTS**

| Muscles | Veins | Arteries | Nerves | Bones | Glands | Other structures |
|---|---|---|---|---|---|---|
| Digastric, Stylohyoid, Mylohyoid, Geniohyoid, Sternohyoid, Omohyoid, Thyrohyoid, Sternothyroid Platysma | Internal jugular, Anterior jugular external jugular  Facial and Retromandibular veins | Carotid sheath and  Branches of external carotid artery | Nerve to mylohyoid, CN XII  Ansa cervicalis | Hyoid Larynx bones | Thyroid Parathyroids | Lymph nodes, Submandibular gland Trachea Oesophagus. |

# B. MUSCLES OF THE NECK

| Muscles | Origin | Insertion | Action | Innervation |
|---|---|---|---|---|
| **1. Cervical muscles** | | | | |
| *Platysma* | Upper part of deltoid and pectoralis major | Mandible and angle of mouth | Depresses lower jaw and lip and angle of mouth; wrinkles skin of neck | Facial nerve |
| *Sternocleidomastoid* | Sternum and clavicle | Mastoid process of temporal bone | Singly turns face toward opposite side; together flex head, raise thorax | Accessory nerve C2-8 (sensory) |
| **2. Suprahyoid muscles** | | | | |
| *Digastric* | Ant. belly from digastric fossa of mandible; posterior belly from mastoid notch | Hyoid bone | Elevates hyoid  Opens mouth | Trigeminal nerve (ant. Belly)  Facial n. (Post. Belly) |
| *Mylohyoid* | Inf. Border mandible | Hyoid bone | Elevates hyoid bone & floor mouth, depresses mandible | Trigeminal nerve (mylohyoid n.) |
| *Stylohyoid* | Styloid process | Body of Hyoid bone | Elevates hyoid | Facial nerve |
| *Geniohyoid* | Genial tubercle of mandible | Body of hyoid | Elevates hyoid & floor of mouth | C1 via hypoglossal n. |
| **3. Infrahyoid muscles** | | | | |
| *Sternohyoid* | Manibrium | Body of hyoid bone | Depresses hyoid and larynx | Ansa cervicalis |
| *Sternothyroid* | Manibrium | Oblique line of thyroid cartilage | Depresses hyoid and larynx | Ansa cervicalis |
| *Thyrohyoid* | Thyroid cartilage | Body and greater horn of hyoid | Depresses hyoid and elevates larynx | C1 via hypoglossal nerve |
| *Omohyoid* | Inferior belly from medial lip of suprascapular notch & suprascapular ligament; sup. belly from intermediate tendon | Inferior belly to intermediate tendon; superior belly to body of hyoid | Depresses and retracts hyoid and larynx | Ansa cervicalis |

## C. NERVES OF THE NECK

### 1. ACCESSORY NERVE /CN XI
- It is formed by the union of cranial and spinal roots.
- Traditionally, the accessory nerve is divided into spinal and cranial parts.

#### SPINAL PART
- The spinal portion arises from neurones of the upper spinal cord, specifically **C1-C5/C6** spinal nerve roots.
- These fibres coalesce to form the spinal part of the accessory nerve, which then runs superiorly to enter the cranial cavity via the **foramen magnum.**
- The nerve traverses the posterior cranial fossa to reach the **jugular foramen.**
- It briefly meets the cranial portion of the accessory nerve, before exiting the skull (along with the glossopharyngeal and vagus nerves).
- Outside the cranium, the spinal part descends along the **internal carotid artery** to reach the sternocleidomastoid muscle, which it innervates.
- It then moves across the posterior triangle of the neck to supply motor fibres to the trapezius.
- *The extracranial course of the accessory nerve is relatively superficial (it runs between the investing and prevertebral layers of* fascia*), and thus leaves it vulnerable to damage.*

#### CRANIAL PART
- The cranial portion is much smaller, and arises from the lateral aspect of the **medulla oblongata.**
- It leaves the cranium via the **jugular foramen**, where it briefly contacts the spinal part of the accessory nerve.
- Immediately after leaving the skull, cranial part combines with the **vagus nerve** (CN X) at the inferior ganglion of vagus nerve.
- The fibres from the cranial part are then distributed through the **vagus nerve**.
- For this reason, the cranial part of the accessory nerve is considered as part of the vagus nerve.

#### MOTOR FUNCTION:
- The spinal accessory nerve innervates two muscles:
  - Sternocleidomastoid
  - Trapezius.

### 2. CERVICAL PLEXUS
- It is formed by the ventral primary rami of C1 to C4.

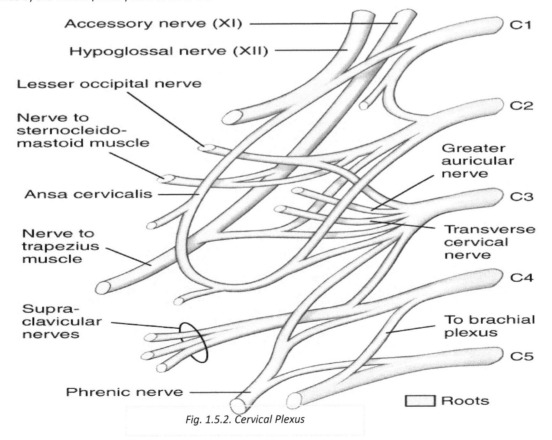

*Fig. 1.5.2. Cervical Plexus*

## 2.1. CUTANEOUS BRANCHES
- ○   *Lesser occipital nerve (C2)*
- ○   *Great auricular nerve (C2 to C3)*
- ○   *Transverse cervical nerve (C2 to C3)*
- ○   *Supraclavicular nerve (C3 to C4)*

## 2.2. MOTOR BRANCHES
### A. ANSA CERVICALIS
- Formed by the union of the superior root (C1 or C1 and C2);

*Innervates the infrahyoid (or strap) muscles, such as the omohyoid, sternohyoid, and sternothyroid muscles, with the exception of the thyrohyoid muscle, which is innervated by C1 via the hypoglossal nerve.*

### B. PHRENIC NERVE (C3 TO C5)
- Provides the motor supply to the diaphragm and sensation to its central part.
- Innervates sensory fibers to these structures.

### C. TWIGS FROM THE PLEXUS
- Innervates the longus capitis and cervicis or coli, sternocleidomastoid, trapezius, levator scapulae, and scalene muscles.

### D. ACCESSORY PHRENIC NERVE (C5)
- Occasionally arises as a contribution of C5 to the phrenic
- Innervates the diaphragm.

## 3. BRACHIAL PLEXUS
- Is formed by the union of the ventral primary rami of C5 to T1 and passes between the anterior scalene and middle scalene muscles.

1) Its roots give rise to the:
### A. DORSAL SCAPULAR NERVE (C5)
- Innervating the levator scapulae and rhomboid muscles.

### B. LONG THORACIC NERVE (C5 TO C7)
- Innervates the serratus anterior.

2) Its upper trunk gives rise to the:
### A. SUPRASCAPULAR NERVE (C5 TO C6)
- Supplies the supraspinatus and infraspinatus muscles.

### B. NERVE TO THE SUBCLAVIUS MUSCLE (C5)
- Innervates the subclavius.
- Communicates with the phrenic nerve as the accessory phrenic nerve in many cases.

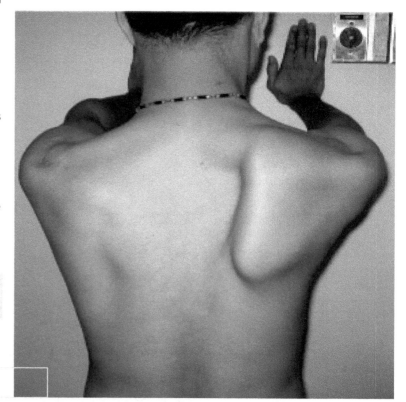

## WINGING OF SCAPULA:
- **Nerve**: *long thoracic nerve*
- **Root**: *C5-C7*
- **Muscle**: *serratus anterior*

*Fig. 1.5.3. Winging of Scapula*

# D. ARTERIES OF THE NECK
## A. SUBCLAVIAN ARTERY

*Mnemonic*:
**V**ery **T**ired **I**ndividuals **S**ip **T**hailand **C**offee **S**erved **D**ouble **D**aily.

- **V**: Vertebral Artery
- **T**: Thyrocervical Trunk Artery:
  - o **I**: Inferior Thyroid Artery
  - o **S**: Suprascapular Artery
  - o **T**: Transverse Cervical Artery
- **C**: Costocervical Trunk:
  - o **S**: Superior Intercostal Artery
  - o **D**: Deep Cervical Artery
- **D**: Dorsal Scapular Artery

## B. COMMON CAROTID ARTERIES

- Have different origins on the right and left sides:
  - o ***The right common carotid artery***, *which begins at the bifurcation of the brachiocephalic artery*
  - o ***The left common carotid artery***, *which arises from the aortic arch*
- Ascend within the carotid sheath and divide at the level of the upper border of the thyroid cartilage into the external and internal carotid arteries.

## 1. RECEPTORS
## a. CAROTID BODY

- Lies at the bifurcation of the common carotid artery as an ovoid body.
- It is a chemoreceptor that is stimulated by chemical changes in the circulating blood that help control respiration.
- It is innervated by the nerve to the carotid body, which arises from the pharyngeal branch of the vagus nerve, and by the carotid sinus branch of the glossopharyngeal nerve.

## b. CAROTID SINUS

- Located at the origin of the internal carotid artery.
- It is a baroreceptor that is stimulated by changes in blood pressure
- When stimulated, it causes a slowing of the heart rate, vasodilation, and a decrease in blood pressure.
- Is innervated primarily by the carotid sinus branch of the glossopharyngeal nerve but is also innervated by the nerve to the carotid body of the vagus nerve.

## 2. INTERNAL CAROTID ARTERY

- ***Has no branches in the neck***, ascends within the carotid sheath in company with the vagus nerve and the internal jugular vein, and enters the cranium through the **carotid canal** in the petrous part of the temporal bone.
- In the middle cranial fossa, gives rise to the *ophthalmic artery* and *the anterior and middle cerebral arteries* and participates in the formation of the circulus arteriosus *(circle of Willis)*.

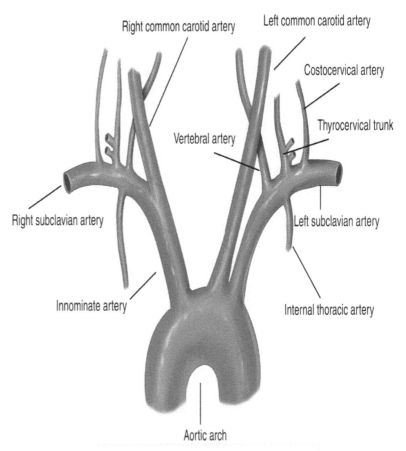

*Fig. 1.5.4. Arteries of the Neck*

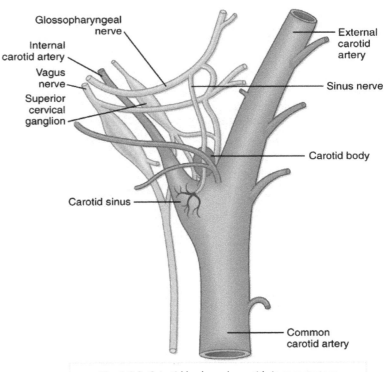

*Fig. 1.5.5. Carotid body and carotid sinus receptors*

## 3. EXTERNAL CAROTID ARTERY

- Extends from the level of the upper border of the thyroid cartilage to the neck of the mandible, where it ends in the parotid gland by dividing into the maxillary and superficial temporal arteries.

- Has eight named branches: SALFO PMS
  - ✓ **S**: superior thyroid artery.
  - ✓ **A**: ascending pharyngeal artery.
  - ✓ **L**: lingual artery.
  - ✓ **F**: facial artery.
  - ✓ **O**: occipital artery.
  - ✓ **P**: posterior auricular artery.
  - ✓ **M**: maxillary artery.
  - ✓ **S**: superficial temporal artery.

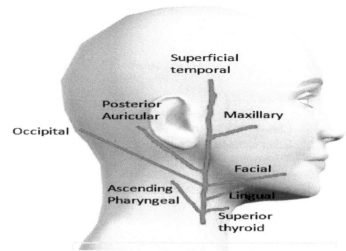

Fig. 1.5.6. Branches of the external carotid artery

## C. INTERNAL JUGULAR VEIN

- ✓ Formed by union of the **Inferior petrosal and Sigmoid Sinus.**
- ✓ Leaves through **jugular foramen**
- ✓ Drains **facial, lingual and retromandibular veins**
- ✓ It descends in the carotid sheath with the internal carotid artery.
- ✓ **Lateral** to Internal and Common carotid artery.
- ✓ **The vagus nerve (CN X)** lies between the two. Drains into **subclavian vein** to form the brachiocephalic vein

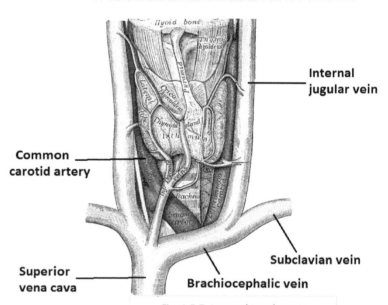

Fig. 1.5.7. Internal Jugular vein

## NERVES FROM THE SKULL

| LOCATION | NERVE | |
|---|---|---|
| **CRIBRIFORM PLATE** | Olfactory nerve | (I) |
| **OPTIC FORAMEN** | Optic nerve | (II) |
| **SUPERIOR ORBITAL FISSURE** | Oculomotor | (III) |
| | Trochlear | (IV) |
| | Abducens | (VI) |
| | Trigeminal V1 *(ophthalmic)* | |
| **FORAMEN ROTUNDUM** | Trigeminal V2 *(maxillary)* | |
| **FORAMEN OVALE** | Trigeminal V3 *(mandibular)* | |
| **INTERNAL AUDITORY CANAL** | Facial | (VII) |
| | Vestibulocochlear | (VIII) |
| **JUGULAR FORAMEN** | Glossopharyngeal | (IX) |
| | Vagus | (X) |
| | Accessory | (XI) |
| **HYPOGLOSSAL CANAL** | Hypoglossal | (XII) |

# CLINICAL RELEVANCE:

## PENETRATING WOUNDS OF THE INTERNAL JUGULAR VEIN

- The hemorrhage of low-pressure venous blood into the loose connective tissue beneath the investing layer of deep cervical fascia may present as a large, slowly expanding hematoma. Air embolism is a serious complication of a lacerated wall of the internal jugular vein.
- Because the wall of this large vein contains little smooth muscle, its injury is not followed by contraction and retraction (as occurs with arterial injuries). Moreover, the adventitia of the vein wall is attached to the deep fascia of the carotid sheath, which hinders the collapse of the vein. Blind clamping of the vein is prohibited because the vagus and hypoglossal nerves are in the vicinity.

## INTERNAL JUGULAR VEIN CATHETERIZATION

- The internal jugular vein is remarkably constant in position. It descends through the neck from a point halfway between the tip of the mastoid process and the angle of the jaw to the sternoclavicular joint.
- Above, it is overlapped by the anterior border of the sternocleidomastoid muscle, and below, it is covered laterally by this muscle. Just above the sternoclavicular joint, the vein lies beneath a skin depression between the sterna and clavicular heads of the sternocleidomastoid muscle. In the posterior approach, the tip of the needle and the catheter are introduced into the vein about two fingerbreadths above the clavicle at the posterior border of the sternocleidomastoid muscle.
- In the anterior approach, with the patient's head turned to the opposite side, the triangle formed by the sternal and clavicular heads of the sternocleidomastoid muscle and the medial end of the clavicle are identified. A shallow skin depression usually overlies the triangle. The needle and catheter are inserted into the vein at the apex of the triangle in a caudal direction.

## SUBCLAVIAN VEIN THROMBOSIS

- Spontaneous thrombosis of the subclavian and/or axillary veins occasionally occurs after excessive and unaccustomed use of the arm at the shoulder joint. The close relationship of these veins to the 1st rib and the clavicle and the possibility of repeated minor trauma from these structures are probably factors in its development.
- Secondary thrombosis of subclavian and/or axillary veins is a common complication of an indwelling venous catheter.
- Rarely, the condition may follow a radical mastectomy with a block dissection of the lymph nodes of the axilla. Persistent pain, heaviness, or edema of the upper limb, especially after exercise, is a complication of this condition.

## CLINICAL SIGNIFICANCE OF THE CERVICAL LYMPH NODES

- Knowledge of the lymph drainage of an organ or region is of great clinical importance.
- Examination of a patient may reveal an enlarged lymph node. It is the physician's responsibility to determine the cause and be knowledgeable about the area of the body that drains its lymph into a particular node.
- For example, an enlarged submandibular node can be caused by a pathologic condition in the scalp, the face, the maxillary sinus, or the tongue. An infected tooth of the upper or lower jaw may be responsible.
- Often, a physician has to search systematically the various areas known to drain into a node to discover the cause.

## EXAMINATION OF THE DEEP CERVICAL LYMPH NODES

- Lymph nodes in the neck should be examined from behind the patient.
- The examination is made easier by asking the patient to flex the neck slightly to reduce the tension of the muscles.
- The groups of nodes should be examined in a definite order to avoid omitting any.
- After the identification of enlarged lymph nodes, possible sites of infection or neoplastic growth should be examined, including the face, scalp, tongue, mouth, tonsil, and pharynx.

## CARCINOMA METASTASES IN THE DEEP CERVICAL LYMPH NODE

- In the head and neck, all the lymph ultimately drains into the deep cervical group of nodes.
- Secondary carcinomatous deposits in these nodes are common.
- The primary growth may be easy to find.
- On the other hand, at certain anatomic sites, the primary growth may be small and overlooked, for example, in the larynx, the pharynx, the cervical part of the oesophagus, and the external auditory meatus.
- The bronchi, breast, and stomach are sometimes the site of the primary tumor.
- In these cases, the secondary growth has spread far beyond the local lymph nodes.
- When cervical metastases occur, the surgeon usually decides to perform a block dissection of the cervical nodes.
- This procedure involves the removal en bloc of the internal jugular vein, the fascia, the lymph nodes, and the submandibular salivary gland. The aim of the operation is removal of all the lymph tissues on the affected side of the neck.
- The carotid arteries and the vagus nerve are carefully preserved.
- It is often necessary to sacrifice the hypoglossal and vagus nerves, which may be involved in the cancerous deposits.
- In patients with bilateral spread, a bilateral block dissection may be necessary.
- An interval of 3 to 4 weeks is necessary before removing the second internal jugular vein.

# FORAMEN OF THE SKULL & STRUCTURES

## 1. Foramen Magnum:
'Spinal Meninges Make A Special Vertical Sheath'

- **S**pinal Cord
- **S**pinal **M**eninges
- **M**eningeal lymphatics
- **A**ccessory nerves (spinal roots)
- **S**ympathetic plexus on vertebral arteries
- **V**ertebral arteries
- **S**pinal branches of vertebral arteries

## 2. Foramen Ovale: MALE
- **M**andibular Nerve (CN V3)
- **A**ccessory meningeal nerve
- **L**esser petrosal nerve
- **E**missary vein (Cavernous sinus to pterygoid plexus)
- Occasionally anterior trunk of middle meningeal artery

## 3. Foramen Spinosum: MEN
- **M**iddle meningeal artery and vein (posterior trunk)
- **E**missary vein.
- **N**ervus spinosus (Meningeal branch of mandibular nerve).

## 4. Foramen Lacerum: MEIG
- Structures passing whole length:
- **M**eningeal branch of Ascending pharyngeal artery
- **E**missary vein
- Other structures partially traversing:
- **I**nternal carotid artery
- **G**reater petrosal nerve

## 5. Carotid Canal:

- Internal carotid artery (ICA) and venous and sympathetic plexus around it.

## 6. Stylomastoid Foramen:
- Facial nerve (CN VII)
- Posterior Auricular artery (Stylomastoid branch)

## 7. Greater Palatine Foramen:
GAP **(Greater and Anterior Palatine Vessels)**
- **G**reater Palatine vessels
- **A**nterior Palatine vessels

## 8. Lesser Palatine Foramen: MPP
- **M**iddle and **P**osterior **P**alatine nerve

## 9. Superior Orbital Fissure: SOFT LAN
- **S**uperior ophthalmic vein
- **O**culomotor nerve/**O**phthalmic nerve (V1)
- **F**rontal nerve
- **T**rochlear nerve
- **L**acrimal nerve
- **A**bducent nerve
- **N**asociliary nerve

## 10. Jugular Foramen

- **Anterior part:**
  - Inferior Petrosal Sinus
- **Middle part: 9,10,11 MAP**
  - CN IX (Glossopharyngeal nerve)
  - CN X (Vagus nerve)
  - CN XI (Accessory nerve)
  - Meningeal branch of Ascending Pharyngeal Artery
- **Posterior part:**
- Internal Jugular vein (IJV) – Sigmoid sinus junction
- Emissary vein (Sigmoid sinus to occipital vein)
- Occipital artery

## 11. Hypoglossal canal: HMME
- **H**ypoglossal nerve
- **M**eningeal branch of Hypoglossal nerve
- **M**eningeal branch of Ascending Pharyngeal artery (MAP)
- **E**missary vein (Sigmoid sinus to internal jugular vein)

## 12. Internal Acoustic Meatus:
- Facial nerve (CN VII)
- Vestibulo-cochlear nerve (CN VIII)
- Nerves intermedius or pars intermedia of wrisberg
- Labyrinthe vessels

## 13. Foramen Rotundum:
- Situated in the sphenoid bone.
- It connects the middle cranial fossa and the pterygopalatine fossa.
- Maxillary nerve (CN V2)

## 14. Mastoid canaliculus (entry) and Tympanomastoid fissure (exit):
- Auricular branch of vagus nerve
- 

## 15. Tympanic Canaliculus
- Tympanic branch of CN IX (Glossopharyngeal nerve)

## 16. Incisive Foramen

- Greater palatine vessels
- Nasopalatine nerves

## 17. Inferior Orbital Fissure: ZIME
- **Z**ygomatic nerve
- **I**nfraorbital vessels
- **M**axillary nerve
- **E**missary vein

# II. DEEP NECK & PREVERTEBRAL REGION STRUCTURES

## A. DEEP STRUCTURES OF THE NECK

### 1. TRACHEA
SEE SECTION 3, THORAX

### 2. ESOPHAGUS
SEE SECTION 3, THORAX

### 3. THYROID GLAND

**RELATIONS**
- **Anteriorly:** strap muscles
- **Posteriorly:** thyroid cartilage, cricoid cartilage, trachea
- **Posteromedially:** tracheo-oesophageal groove (containing lymph nodes, recurrent laryngeal nerve, parathyroid glands)
- **Posterolaterally:** carotid space

**ARTERIAL SUPPLY**
- **Superior thyroid artery** (from external carotid artery)
- **Inferior thyroid artery** (from thyrocervical trunk)
- If the **inferior thyroid artery** arises from the subclavian artery it is referred to as an accessory inferior thyroid artery

**VENOUS DRAINAGE**
- **Superior thyroid vein** (drains to internal jugular vein)
- **Middle thyroid vein** (drains to internal jugular vein)
- **Inferior thyroid vein** (drains to brachiocephalic vein)

**LYMPHATIC DRAINAGE**
- Is multi-directional and initial lymph drainage is to peri-thyroid lymph nodes then onto prelaryngeal, pretracheal and paratracheal nodes (Level 6 lymph nodes)

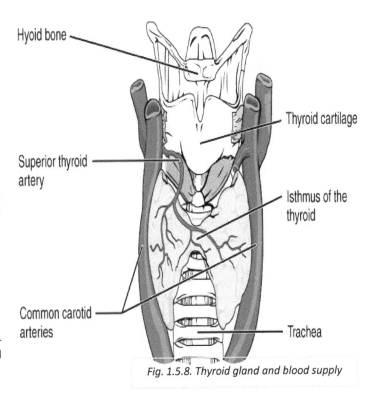

Fig. 1.5.8. Thyroid gland and blood supply

### 4. PARATHYROID GLANDS
- Usually consist of four (two to six) small ovoid bodies that lie against the dorsum of the thyroid under its sheath but with their own capsule.
- Are supplied chiefly by the inferior thyroid artery.

### 5. THYROID CARTILAGES
- It is a hyaline cartilage that forms a laryngeal prominence known as the *Adam's apple*, which is particularly apparent in males.
- Has a superior horn that is joined to the tip of the greater horn of the hyoid bone by the lateral thyroid ligament and an inferior horn that articulates with the cricoid cartilage.

### 6. VAGUS NERVE (CN X)
- **ANATOMICAL COURSE**
  - The vagus nerve has the longest course of all the cranial nerves, extending from the head to the abdomen.
  - Its name is derived from the Latin **'vagary'** – meaning wandering. It is sometimes referred to as the wandering nerve.
- **IN THE HEAD**
  - The vagus nerve originates from the medulla of the brainstem.
  - It exits the cranium via the **jugular foramen,** with the glossopharyngeal and accessory nerves (CN IX and XI respectively).
  - **Branch arising in the head:**
    - **Auricular Branch (Alderman's nerve or Arnold's nerve):** supplies sensation to the posterior part of the external auditory canal and external ear.

- **IN THE NECK**
  - o In the neck, the vagus nerve passes into **the carotid sheath**, travelling inferiorly with the internal jugular vein and common carotid artery.
  - o *At the base of the neck, the right and left nerves have differing pathways:*
  - o *The **Right Vagus Nerve** passes anterior to the subclavian artery and posterior to the sternoclavicular joint, entering the thorax.*
  - o *The **Left Vagus Nerve** passes inferiorly between the left common carotid and left subclavian arteries, posterior to the sternoclavicular joint, entering the thorax.*
    - o **Branches arising in the neck:**
      - ▪ **Pharyngeal branches**: Provides motor innervation to the majority of the muscles of the pharynx and soft palate.
      - ▪ **Superior Laryngeal Nerve:** Splits into internal and external branches.
        - ✓ The **External Laryngeal Nerve** innervates the cricothyroid muscle of the larynx.
        - ✓ The **Internal Laryngeal Nerve** provides sensory innervation to the laryngopharynx and superior part of the larynx.
      - ▪ **Recurrent Laryngeal Nerve** (right side only): Hooks underneath the right subclavian artery, then ascends towards to the larynx. It innervates the majority of the intrinsic muscles of the larynx.

- **IN THE THORAX**
  - o In the thorax, the right vagus nerve forms the **posterior vagal trunk**, and the left forms the **anterior vagal trunk**.
  - o Branches from the vagal trunks contribute to the formation of the oesophageal plexus, which innervates the smooth muscle of the oesophagus.
  - o **Branches arising in the thorax:**
    - ▪ **Left Recurrent Laryngeal Nerve**: it hooks under the arch of the aorta, ascending to innervate the majority of the intrinsic muscles of the larynx.
    - ▪ **Cardiac branches**: these innervate regulate heart rate and provide visceral sensation to the organ.
  - o The vagal trunks enter the abdomen via the oesophageal hiatus, an opening in the diaphragm.

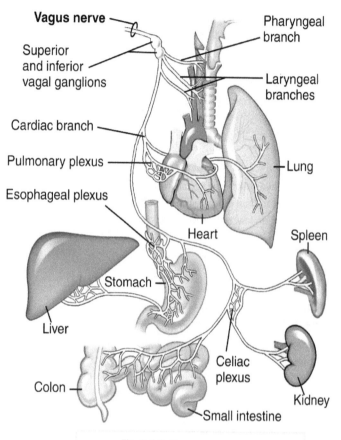

*Fig. 1.5.9. Vagus nerve course*

- **IN THE ABDOMEN**
  - o In the abdomen, the vagal trunks terminate by dividing into branches that supply the oesophagus, stomach and the small and large bowel (up to the splenic flexure).

**SENSORY FUNCTIONS**
- o There are **somatic** and **visceral** components to the sensory function of the vagus nerve.
- o **Somatic** refers to sensation from the skin and muscles. This is provided by the **auricular nerve**.
- o **Viscera sensation** is that from the organs of the body. The vagus nerve innervates:
  - ▪ **Laryngopharynx**: via the internal laryngeal nerve.
  - ▪ **Superior aspect of larynx** (above vocal folds): via the internal laryngeal nerve.
  - ▪ **Heart**: via cardiac branches of the vagus nerve.
  - ▪ **Gastro-intestinal tract** (up to the splenic flexure): via the terminal branches of the vagus nerve.

**SPECIAL SENSORY FUNCTIONS**
- o The vagus nerve has a minor role in taste sensation.
- o It carries afferent fibres from the **root of the tongue** and **epiglottis**. *(This is not to be confused with the special sensation of the glossopharyngeal nerve, which provides taste sensation for the posterior 1/3 of the tongue).*

**MOTOR FUNCTIONS**
- o The vagus nerve innervates the majority of the muscles associated with the pharynx and larynx.
- o These muscles are responsible for the initiation of swallowing and phonation.

o **Muscles of the Pharynx**
  ▪ Most of the muscles of the pharynx are innervated by the **Pharyngeal branches** of the vagus nerve *except the stylopharyngeus which is innervated by the **glossopharyngeal nerve**.*
o **Muscles of the Larynx**
  ▪ Innervation to the intrinsic muscles of the larynx is achieved via the **Recurrent Laryngeal Nerve** and **external branch of the Superior Laryngeal Nerve**.
o In addition to the pharynx and larynx, the vagus nerve also innervates the palatoglossus of the tongue, and the majority of the muscles of the soft palate.

**PARASYMPATHETIC FUNCTIONS**
o In the thorax and abdomen, the vagus nerve is the main parasympathetic outflow to the heart and gastro-intestinal organs.
o **The Heart**
  ▪ Cardiac branches arise in the thorax, conveying parasympathetic innervation to the sino-atrial and atrio-ventricular nodes of the heart. These branches stimulate a reduction in the resting heart rate.
  ▪ They are constantly active, producing a rhythm of 60 – 80 beats per minute.
  ▪ If the vagus nerve was lesioned, the resting heart rate would be around 100 beats per minute.
o **Gastro-Intestinal System**
  ▪ The vagus nerve provides parasympathetic innervation to the majority of the abdominal organs.
  ▪ It sends branches to the oesophagus, stomach and most of the intestinal tract – up to the splenic flexure of the large colon.
  ▪ The function of the vagus nerve is to stimulate smooth muscle contraction and glandular secretions in these organs.
  ▪ For example, in the stomach, the vagus nerve increases the rate of gastric emptying, and stimulates acid production.

## CLINICAL RELEVANCE
### PAROTID SALIVARY GLAND AND LESIONS OF THE FACIAL NERVE
- The parotid salivary gland consists essentially of superficial and deep parts, and the important facial nerve lies in the interval between these parts. A benign parotid neoplasm rarely, if ever, causes facial palsy.
- A malignant tumor of the parotid is usually highly invasive and quickly involves the facial nerve, causing unilateral facial paralysis.

### PAROTID GLAND INFECTIONS
- The parotid gland may become acutely inflamed as a result of retrograde bacterial infection from the mouth via the parotid duct.
- The gland may also become infected via the bloodstream, as in mumps. In both cases, the gland is swollen; it is painful because the fascial capsule derived from the investing layer of deep cervical fascia is strong and limits the swelling of the gland.
- The swollen glenoid process, which extends medially behind the temporomandibular joint, is responsible for the pain experienced in acute parotitis when eating.

### FREY'S SYNDROME
- **Frey's syndrome** is an interesting complication that sometimes develops after penetrating wounds of the parotid gland. When the patient eats, beads of perspiration appear on the skin covering the parotid. This condition is caused by damage to the auriculotemporal and great auricular nerves. During the process of healing, the parasympathetic secretomotor fibers in the auriculotemporal nerve grow out and join the distal end of the great auricular nerve. Eventually, these fibers reach the sweat glands in the facial skin. By this means, a stimulus intended for saliva production produces sweat secretion instead.

## B. DEEP CERVICAL FASCIAE OF THE NECK
Four parts:
- **The investing layer**: Most superficial
  o Encloses the SCM and Trapezius.
- **The carotid sheath**: I See 10 CC's in the IV
  o **I See** (I.C.) = **I**nternal **C**arotid artery
  o **10** = CN **10** (Vagus nerve)
  o **CC** = **C**ommon **C**arotid artery
  o **IV** = **I**nternal Jugular **V**ein
  o NOTE: External jugular vein runs superficially in the neck lying on top of the investing fascia.
- **The pretracheal fascia**:
  o Encloses the visceral region of the neck.
  o **Retropharyngeal space**: Lies in between the pretracheal and prevertebral fascia.
- **The prevertebral fascia**: Encloses the vertebral region of the neck.

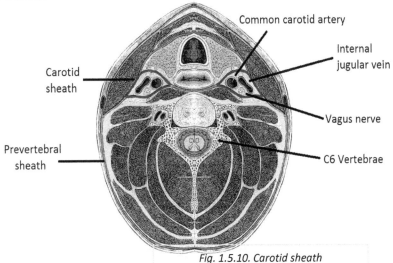

Fig. 1.5.10. Carotid sheath

Labels: Common carotid artery; Internal jugular vein; Carotid sheath; Vagus nerve; Prevertebral sheath; C6 Vertebrae

# CLINICAL SIGNIFICANCE OF THE DEEP FASCIA OF THE NECK

- As previously described, the deep fascia in certain areas forms distinct sheets called the **investing, pretracheal,** and **prevertebral** layers. These fascial layers are easily recognizable to the surgeon at operation.

## FASCIAL SPACES

- Between the more dense layers of deep fascia in the neck is loose connective tissue that forms potential spaces that are clinically important. Among the more important spaces are the visceral, retropharyngeal, submandibular, and masticatory spaces
- The deep fascia and the fascial spaces are important because organisms originating in the mouth, teeth, pharynx, and oesophagus can spread among the fascial planes and spaces, and the tough fascia can determine the direction of spread of infection and the path taken by pus.
- It is possible for blood, pus, or air in the retropharyngeal space to spread downward into the superior mediastinum of the thorax.

## DENTAL INFECTIONS

- Most commonly involve the lower molar teeth. The infection spreads medially from the mandible into the submandibular and masticatory spaces and pushes the tongue forward and upward.
- Further spread downward may involve the visceral space and lead to edema of the vocal cords and airway obstruction.

## LUDWIG'S ANGINA

- It **is** an acute infection of the submandibular fascial space and is commonly secondary to dental infection.

## TUBERCULOUS INFECTION OF THE DEEP CERVICAL LYMPH NODES

- Can result in liquefaction and destruction of one or more of the nodes. The pus is at first limited by the investing layer of the deep fascia. Later, this becomes eroded at one point, and the pus passes into the less restricted superficial fascia. A dumbbell or collar-stud abscess is now present.
- The clinician is aware of the superficial abscess but must not forget the existence of the deeply placed abscess.

| C. NECK ZONES | | |
|---|---|---|
| **ZONE** | **ANATOMY** | **STRUCTURES AT RISK** |
| Zone 1 | Clavicle to cricoid cartilage | • Great vessels: Subclavian vessels, Brachiocephalic veins, common carotid artery, aortic arch and jugular veins<br>• Trachea, oesophagus, Lung apices<br>• Cervical spine, spinal cord, cervical nerve roots. |
| Zone 2 | Cricoid cartilage to angle of Mandible | • Carotid and Vertebral arteries<br>• Jugular veins, pharynx, Larynx, Trachea<br>• Oesophagus, cervical spine, Spinal cord |
| Zone 3 | Angle Mandible to the base of skull | • Salivary and parotid glands<br>• Oesophagus, Trachea, vertebral bodies<br>• Carotid arteries, jugular veins<br>• Spinal cord and other major nerves |

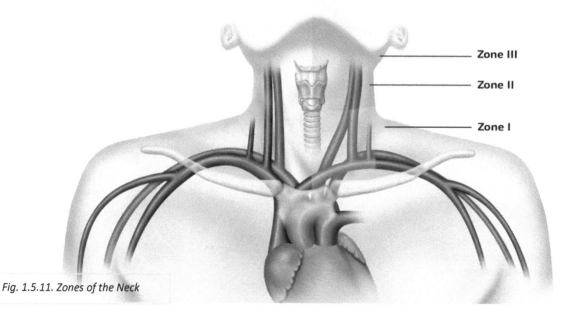

*Fig. 1.5.11. Zones of the Neck*

# III. FACE

## A. MUSCLES

➤ **Orbital Group**
- Has 2 muscles controlling the movements of the eyelids, important in protecting the cornea from damage: Orbicularis oculi & Corrugator supercilii
- They are both innervated by the facial nerve.

➤ **Nasal Group**
- Nasalis, Procerus and Depressor Septi Nasi
- Innervated by the facial nerve

➤ **Oral Group**
- These are the most important group of the facial expressors.
- They are responsible for movements of the mouth and lips.
- The oral group of muscles consists of the orbicularis oris, buccinator, and various smaller muscles.
- Innervated by the facial nerve

➤ **Other Oral Muscles**
- The lower group contains the depressor anguli oris, depressor labii inferioris and the mentalis.
- The upper group contains the risorius, zygomaticus major, zygomaticus minor, levator labii superioris, levator labii superioris alaeque nasi and levator anguli oris.

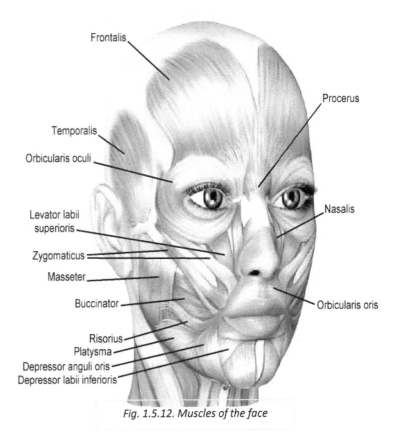

Fig. 1.5.12. Muscles of the face

## B. MOTOR FUNCTION OF FACE: FACIAL NERVE/ CN VII

- **Motor:** Innervates the **muscles of facial expression**, the posterior belly of the digastric, the stylohyoid and the stapedius muscles.
- **Sensory:** None.
- **Special Sensory:** Provides special taste sensation to the anterior 2/3 of the tongue.
- **Parasympathetic:** Supplies many of the glands of the head and neck, including the submandibular, sublingual, nasal, palatine, lacrimal and pharyngeal gland.
- Within the parotid gland, the nerve terminates by splitting into five branches.
- These branches are responsible for innervating the muscles of facial expression: **TEN ZEBRAS BROKE MY CAR:**
  - **T**emporal branch
  - **Z**ygomatic branch
  - **B**uccal branch
  - **M**arginal mandibular branch
  - **C**ervical branch

## C. SENSORY FUNCTIONS OF FACE: TRIGEMINAL NERVE

- The trigeminal nerve, CN V, is also the largest cranial nerve.
- **Sensory**:
  - The three terminal branches of CN V innervate the skin, mucous membranes and sinuses of the face. Their distribution pattern is similar to the dermatome supply of spinal nerves (except there is little overlap in the supply of the divisions).
- **Motor:**
  - **Only the mandibular branch of (CN V3) has motor fibres**.
  - It innervates the muscles of mastication: medial pterygoid, lateral pterygoid, masseter and temporalis. The mandibular nerve also supplies other 1st pharyngeal arch derivatives: anterior belly of digastric, tensor veli palatini and tensor tympani.
- **Parasympathetic Supply**: The post-ganglionic neurones of parasympathetic ganglia travel with branches of the trigeminal nerve.

# DIVISIONS OF TRIGEMINAL NERVE

## 1. OPHTHALMIC NERVE V1

- Ophthalmic nerve gives rise to 3 terminal branches:
- **Frontal, Lacrimal** and **Nasociliary**, which innervate the skin and mucous membrane of:
  - o Forehead and scalp
  - o Frontal and ethmoidal sinus
  - o Upper eyelid and its conjunctiva
  - o Cornea (see clinical relevance)
  - o Dorsum of the nose

**Parasympathetic Supply:**

- **Lacrimal gland**: Post ganglionic fibres from the pterygopalatine ganglion (derived from the facial nerve), travel with the zygomatic branch of V2 and then join the lacrimal branch of V1.
- The fibres supply parasympathetic innervation to the lacrimal gland.

## 2. MAXILLARY NERVE V2

- Maxillary nerve gives rise to 14 terminal branches, which innervate the skin, mucous membranes and sinuses of derivatives of the **maxillary prominence** of the 1st pharyngeal arch:
  - o Lower eyelid and its conjunctiva
  - o Cheeks and maxillary sinus
  - o Nasal cavity and lateral nose
  - o Upper lip
  - o Upper molar, incisor and canine teeth and the associated gingiva
  - o Superior palate
- **Parasympathetic Supply:**
  - o **Lacrimal gland**: Post ganglionic fibres from the pterygopalatine ganglion (derived from the facial nerve), travel with the zygomatic branch of V2 and then join the lacrimal branch of V1. The fibres supply parasympathetic innervation to the lacrimal gland.
  - o **Nasal glands**: Parasympathetic fibres are also carried to the mucous glands of the nasal mucosa. Post-ganglionic fibres travel with the nasopalatine and greater palatine nerves (branches of V2).

## 3. MANDIBULAR NERVE V3

- Mandibular nerve gives rise to 4 terminal branches in the infra-temporal fossa: **"BAIL NERVES"**
  **Buccal** nerve, **Auriculotemporal** nerve, **Inferior alveolar** nerve and **Lingual** nerve.
- These branches innervate the skin, mucous membrane and striated muscle derivatives of the **mandibular prominence** of the 1st pharyngeal arch.

- **Sensory supply:**
  - o Mucous membranes and floor of the oral cavity
  - o External ear
  - o Lower lip
  - o Chin
  - o Anterior 2/3 of the tongue (*only general sensation; special taste sensation supplied by the chorda tympani, a branch of the facial nerve*)
  - o Lower molar, incisor and canine teeth and the associated gingival.

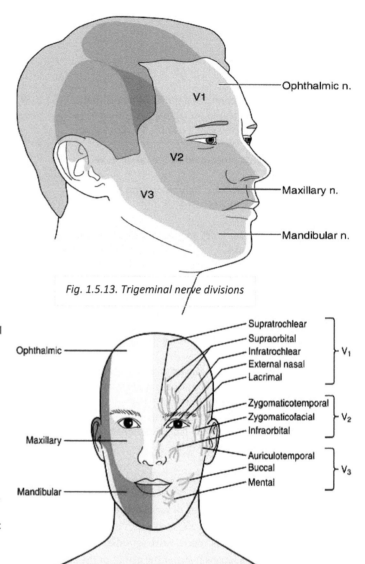

*Fig. 1.5.13. Trigeminal nerve divisions*

*Fig. 1.5.14. Trigeminal nerve Branches*

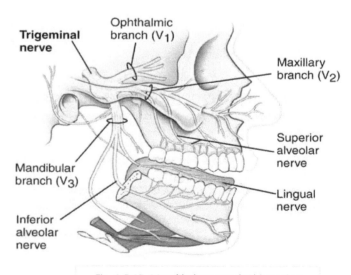

*Fig. 1.5.15. Mandibular nerve (V3) branches*

- **Sensory branches of V3: BAIL**
    - o  **B** - Buccal Nerve (or long buccal n.; not to be confused with the buccal branch of CN VII)
    - o  **A** - Auriculotemporal nerve
    - o  **I** - Inferior Alveolar nerve
    - o  **L** - Lingual nerve

- **Motor Supply:**
    - o  Muscles of mastication: medial pterygoid, lateral pterygoid, masseter, temporalis
    - o  Anterior belly of the digastric muscle and the mylohyoid muscle
    - o  Tensor veli palatini
    - o  Tensor tympani

- **Parasympathetic Supply:**
    - o  **Submandibular and Sublingual glands:** Post-ganglionic fibres from the submandibular ganglion (derived from the facial nerve), travel with the lingual nerve to innervate these glands.
    - o  **Parotid gland:** Post-ganglionic fibres from the otic ganglion (derived from the glossopharyngeal nerve, CN IX), travel with the auriculotemporal branch of the V3 to innervate the parotid gland.

# CLINICAL RELEVANCE:
## CORNEAL REFLEX
- The corneal reflex is the involuntary blinking of the eyelids, stimulated by tactile, thermal or painful stimulation of the cornea.
- In the corneal reflex, the ophthalmic nerve acts as the **afferent limb** – detecting the stimuli.
- The facial nerve is the **efferent limb**, causing contraction of the orbicularis oculi muscle.
- *If the corneal reflex is absent, it is a sign of **damage** to the trigeminal/ophthalmic nerve, or the facial nerve.*

## INFERIOR ALVEOLAR NERVE BLOCK
- The **inferior alveolar nerve**, a branch of V3, travels through the mandibular foramen and mandibular canal.
- Within the mandibular canal, the inferior alveolar nerve forms the inferior dental plexus, which innervates the lower teeth.
- *A major branch of this plexus, the Mental Nerve, supplies the skin and mucous membranes of the lower lip, skin of the chin, and the gingiva of the lower teeth.*
- In some dental procedures, which require a **local anaesthesia**, the inferior alveolar nerve is blocked before it gives rise to the plexus.
- The anaesthetic solution is administered at the **mandibular foramen,** causing numbness of area supplied by the inferior alveolar nerve.
- The anaesthetic fluid also spreads to the **lingual nerve** which originates near the inferior alveolar nerve, causing numbness of the anterior 2/3 of the tongue.

## SENSORY INNERVATION AND TRIGEMINAL NEURALGIA
- The facial skin receives its sensory nerve supply from the three divisions of the trigeminal nerve.
- Remember that a small area of skin over the angle of the jaw is supplied by **the great auricular nerve (C2 and 3).**

## TRIGEMINAL NEURALGIA
- It is a relatively common condition in which the patient experiences excruciating pain in the distribution of the mandibular or maxillary division, with the ophthalmic division usually escaping.
- A physician should be able to map out accurately on a patient's face the distribution of each of the divisions of the trigeminal nerve.

## FACIAL MUSCLE PARALYSIS
- The facial muscles are innervated by the facial nerve.
- Damage to the facial nerve in the internal acoustic meatus (by a tumor), in the middle ear (by infection or operation), in the facial nerve canal (perineuritis, **Bell's palsy**), or in the parotid gland (by a tumor) or caused by lacerations of the face will cause distortion of the face, with drooping of the lower eyelid, and the angle of the mouth will sag on the affected side.
- This is essentially a lower motor neuron lesion. An upper motor neuron lesion (involvement of the pyramidal tracts) will leave the upper part of the face normal because the neurons supplying this part of the face receive corticobulbar fibers from both cerebral cortices.

## INJURY TO THE LINGUAL NERVE
- The lingual nerve passes forward into the submandibular region from the infratemporal fossa by running beneath the origin of the superior constrictor muscle, which is attached to the posterior border of the mylohyoid line on the mandible.
- Here, it is closely related to the last molar tooth and is liable to be damaged in cases of clumsy extraction of an impacted third molar.

## MAXILLARY ARTERY

- Terminal branch of the external carotid artery.
- It is divided into three portions by its relation to the lateral pterygoid muscle:
  - **First (mandibular) part:** posterior to lateral pterygoid muscle (five branches)
  - **Second (pterygoid or muscular) part:** within lateral pterygoid muscle (five branches)
  - **Third (pterygopalatine) part:** anterior to lateral pterygoid muscle (six branches including terminal branch)

## BRANCHES OF MAXILLARY ARTERY

- DAM I AM Piss Drunk But Stupid Drunk I Prefer, Must Phone Alcoholics Anonymous

➤ **First (mandibular) part:**
- **D:** deep auricular artery
- **A:** anterior tympanic artery
- **M:** middle meningeal artery
- **I:** inferior alveolar artery
- **A:** accessory meningeal artery

➤ **Second (pterygoid or muscular) part**
- **M:** masseteric artery
- **P:** pterygoid artery
- **D:** deep temporal artery
- **B:** buccinator artery

➤ **Third (pterygopalatine) part**
- **S:** sphenopalatine artery
- **D:** descending palatine artery
- **I:** infraorbital artery
- **P:** posterior superior alveolar artery
- **M:** middle superior alveolar artery
- **P:** pharyngeal artery
- **A:** anterior superior alveolar artery
- **A:** artery of the pterygoid canal

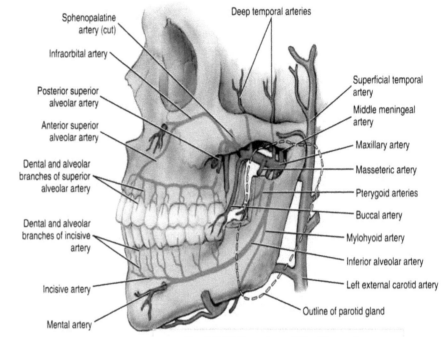

Fig. 1.5.16. Branches of Maxillary artery

# IV. TEMPORAL AND INFRATEMPORAL FOSSAE

## A. INFRATEMPORAL FOSSA
- **Boundaries:**
  - **Anterior:** posterior surface of the maxilla.
  - **Posterior:** styloid process.
  - **Medial:** lateral pterygoid plate of the sphenoid bone.
  - **Lateral:** ramus and coronoid process of the mandible.
  - **Roof:** greater wing of the sphenoid and infratemporal crest.

## B. TEMPORAL FOSSA
- **Boundaries:**
  - **Anterior:** zygomatic process of the frontal bone and the frontal process of the zygomatic bone.
  - **Posterior:** temporal line.
  - **Superior:** temporal line.
  - **Lateral:** zygomatic arch.
  - **Inferior:** infratemporal crest.
  - **Floor:** parts of the frontal, parietal, temporal, and greater wing of the sphenoid bone.

## C. CONTENTS OF THE INFRATEMPORAL FOSSA
  - **Muscles**
    - The infratemporal fossa is associated with the muscles of mastication.
    - The **medial** and **lateral pterygoids** are located within the fossa itself, whilst the **masseter and temporalis muscles** insert and originate into the borders of the fossa.

o **Nerves**
  ▪ **Mandibular nerve**
  ▪ **Buccal, Auriculotemporal, Inferior alveolar and Lingual nerves (BAIL nerves):** sensory branches of the trigeminal nerve.
  ▪ **Chorda tympani:** a branch of the facial nerve (CN VII). It follows the anatomical course of the lingual nerve and provides taste innervation to the anterior 2/3 of the tongue.
  ▪ **Otic ganglion:** a parasympathetic collection of neurone cell bodies. Nerve fibres leaving this ganglion 'hitchhike' along the auriculotemporal nerve to reach the parotid gland.

o **Vasculature**
  ▪ **The Maxillary Artery** (terminal branch of the external carotid artery >> SALFO PMS) travels through the infratemporal fossa.
  ▪ Within the fossa, it gives rise to the **middle meningeal artery**, which travels into the cranial cavity via the **foramen spinosum**.

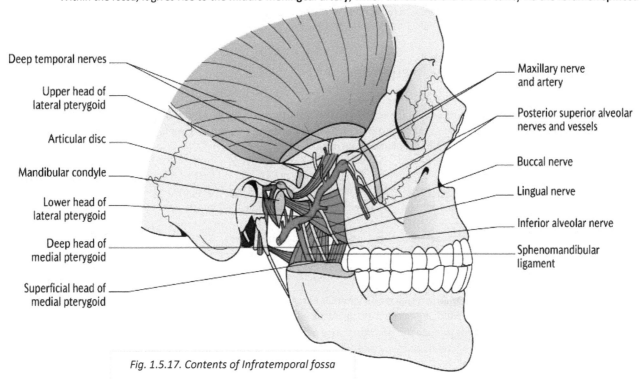

Fig. 1.5.17. Contents of Infratemporal fossa

- Clinically this is important as a site of traumatic bleed as the middle meningeal passes underneath the pterion.
- The middle meningeal artery (MMA) supplies the skull and the dura mater (the outer membranous layer covering the brain). It travels underneath the pterion, thus a fracture of the skull at the pterion can injure or completely lacerate the MMA.
- Blood will then collect in between the dura mater and the skull, causing a dangerous increase in intra-cranial pressure.
- This is known as an Extradural Haematoma.
- **The Pterygoid Venous Plexus** is directly connected to the cavernous sinus, and drains the eye and its locality. Infections of the skin and eye socket are able to track back into the plexus, and on up into the cavernous sinus where meningitis is a substantial risk.
- **Maxillary Vein** and **Middle Meningeal Vein.**

## BOUNDARIES OF TEMPORAL FOSSA

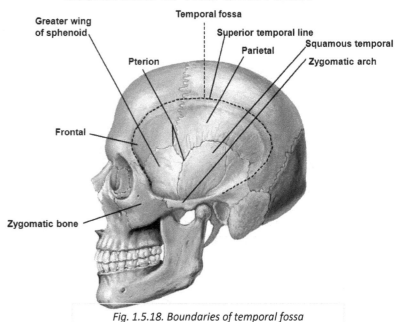

Fig. 1.5.18. Boundaries of temporal fossa

# V. NOSE AND PARANASAL REGION

## 1. PARANASAL SINUSES

- Consist of the ethmoidal, frontal, maxillary, and sphenoidal sinuses.
- Are involved in a reduction of weight and resonance for voice.

### A. ETHMOIDAL SINUS

- Can be subdivided into the following groups:
  - o **Posterior ethmoidal air cells**, which drain into the superior nasal meatus.
  - o **Middle ethmoidal air cells**, which drain into the summit of the ethmoidal bulla of the middle nasal meatus.
  - o **Anterior ethmoidal air cells**, which drain into the anterior aspect of the hiatus semilunaris in the middle nasal meatus.

### B. FRONTAL SINUS

- Is innervated by the supraorbital branch of the ophthalmic nerve.

### C. MAXILLARY SINUS

- Is the largest of the paranasal air sinuses and *is the only paranasal sinus that may be present at birth.*
- Lies in the maxilla on each side, lateral to the lateral wall of the nasal cavity and inferior to the floor of the orbit, and drains into the posterior aspect of the hiatus semilunaris in the middle nasal meatus.

### D. SPHENOIDAL SINUS

- Is innervated by branches from the maxillary nerve and by the posterior ethmoidal branch of the nasociliary nerve.
- The pituitary gland lies above this sinus and can be reached by the transsphenoidal approach, which follows the nasal septum through the body of the sphenoid.
- Care must be taken not to damage the cavernous sinus and the internal carotid artery.

## NERVES, BLOOD VESSELS, AND LYMPHATICS OF THE NOSE

- o **NERVE:**
  - **Nerve to the external nose:** the **infratrochlear and external nasal**, branches of the ophthalmic nerve and the **infraorbital**, branch of the maxillary nerve, both of which are part of the trigeminal nerve.
  - **The olfactory nerves** (CN I) pass through the cribriform plate of the ethmoid bone.
  - General sensory innervation of the nasal cavity and the paranasal sinuses is from the **ophthalmic nerve (CN V1) and maxillary nerve (CN V2).**

- o **Arterial**
  - **External part of the nose:**
    - o Branches of the ophthalmic and maxillary arteries.
  - **The skin of the ala and septum:**
    - o Facial artery.
  - **Walls of the nasal cavity and sinuses:**
    - o Branches of the maxillary artery.
- o There are four arteries anastomosed at **Little's area** to form a vascular plexus called **Kiesselbach's plexus: " LEGS "**
  - ✓ **L** - superior **La**bial artery
  - ✓ **E** - anterior **E**thmoidal artery
  - ✓ **G** - **G**reater palatine artery
  - ✓ **S** - **S**phenopalatine artery

- o **VENOUS**
  - Venous blood is returned from the nasal cavity by veins that accompany the arteries.

- o **LYMPHATIC**
  - Lymph from the nasal cavity drains into the submandibular lymph nodes and vessels that drain into the upper deep cervical lymph nodes.

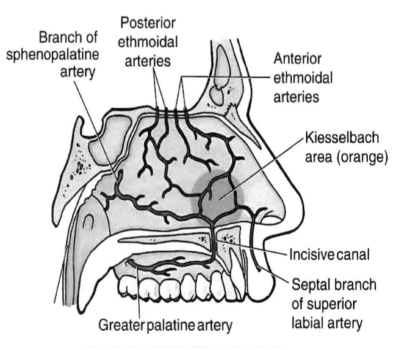

*Fig. 1.5.19. The Little's area*

# VI. MOUTH AND HARD PALATE

## A. INNERVATION OF THE TEETH AND GUMS

➢ **Maxillary teeth**: anterior, middle, and posterior-superior alveolar nerves, branches of the maxillary nerve.

➢ **Mandibular teeth**: inferior alveolar, branch of the mandibular nerve.

➢ **Maxillary gingiva**
- **Outer (buccal) surface:** posterior, middle, and anterior-superior alveolar and Infraorbital nerves.
- **Inner (lingual) surface:** greater palatine and nasopalatine nerves.

➢ **Mandibular gingiva**
- **Outer (buccal) surface:** buccal and mental nerves.
- **Inner (lingual) surface:** lingual nerves.

## B. ORAL CAVITY

- **Roof:**
  o The palate.
- **Floor:**
  o Tongue and the mucosa.
  o Supported by the geniohyoid and mylohyoid muscles.
- **Lateral and anterior walls:**
  o Outer fleshy wall (cheeks and lips).
  o Inner bony wall (teeth and gums).
  o The vestibule is between the walls,
  o The oral cavity proper is the area inside the teeth and gums.

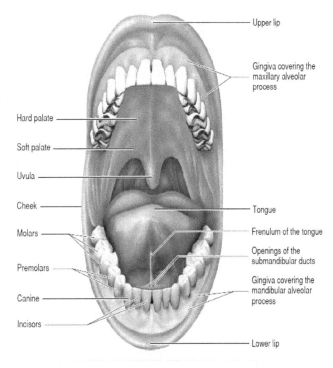

Fig. 1.5.20. Oral cavity anatomy

## C. PALATE

- Forms the roof of the mouth and the floor of the nasal cavity.

### 1. HARD PALATE

- It is the anterior four fifths of the palate and forms a bony framework covered with a mucous membrane between the nasal and oral cavities.
- Consists of the palatine processes of the maxillae and horizontal plates of the palatine bones.
- **Contains:**
  o **Anteriorly:** Incisive foramen in its median plane.
  o **Posteriorly:** greater and lesser palatine foramina.
- **Sensory innervation:**
  o Greater palatine and Nasopalatine nerves.
- **Blood supply:**
  o Greater palatine artery.

### 2. SOFT PALATE

- Is a fibromuscular fold extending from the posterior border of the hard palate and makes up one fifth of the palate.
- Moves posteriorly against the pharyngeal wall to close the oropharyngeal (faucial) isthmus when swallowing or speaking.
- Is continuous with the palatoglossal and palatopharyngeal folds.
- **Blood supply:**
  o The greater and lesser palatine arteries of the descending palatine artery of the maxillary artery,
  o The ascending palatine artery of the facial artery,
  o The palatine branch of the ascending pharyngeal artery.

- **Sensory innervation:**
  o Through the lesser palatine nerves

- **Skeletal motor innervation:**
  o Vagus nerve.
  o ***A lesion of the CN X deviates the uvula to the opposite side.***

## D. TONGUE

- It is attached by muscles to the hyoid bone, mandible, styloid process, palate, and pharynx.
- Is divided by a V-shaped sulcus terminalis into two parts" an anterior two thirds and a posterior one third which differ developmentally, structurally, and in innervation.

➤ **LINGUAL ARTERY**

- Arises from the external carotid artery at the level of the tip of the greater horn of the hyoid bone in the carotid triangle.
- Passes deep to the hyoglossus and lies on the middle pharyngeal constrictor muscle.
- Gives rise to the suprahyoid, dorsal lingual, and sublingual arteries and terminates as the deep lingual artery, which ascends between the genioglossus and inferior longitudinal muscles.

➤ **LINGUAL INNERVATION**

- **Motor:**
  - ○ The extrinsic and intrinsic muscles of the tongue are innervated by the **hypoglossal nerve (CN XII)** except for the palatoglossus, which is innervated by the **vagus nerve.**
  - ○ *A lesion of CN XII deviates the tongue toward the injured side.*

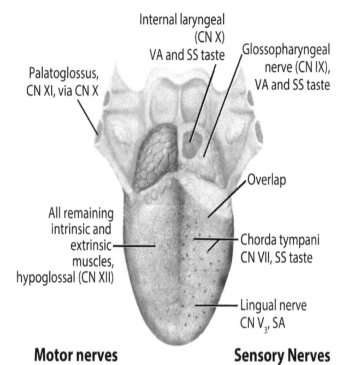

Fig. 1.5.21. Tongue Innervation

- **Sensory:**
  - ○ **The anterior two thirds of the tongue** receives general sensory innervation from the lingual nerve (Trigeminal nerve) and taste sensation from the chorda tympani (Facial nerve).
  - ○ **The posterior one third of the tongue and the vallate papillae** receive both general and taste innervation from the glossopharyngeal nerve (CN IX).
  - ○ **The epiglottic region of the tongue and the epiglottis** receive both general and taste innervation from the internal laryngeal branch of the vagus nerve.

## E. SUBMANDIBULAR GLANDS

- Bilateral salivary glands located in the face.
- Their mixed serous and mucous secretions are important for the lubrication of food during mastication to enable effective swallowing and aid digestion.
- Located within the anterior part of the **submandibular triangle**.

### 1. BOUNDARIES

- **Superiorly:** Inferior body of the mandible.
- **Anteriorly**: Anterior belly of the digastric muscle.
- **Posteriorly:** Posterior belly of the digastric muscle.

### 2. ANATOMICAL STRUCTURE

- The submandibular glands are a pair of elongate, flattened hooks which have two sets of arms; superficial and deep.
- The positioning of these arms is in relation to the **mylohyoid** muscle, which the gland hooks around.
- **Superficial arm**:
  - Comprises the greater portion of the gland and lies partially inferior to the posterior half of the mandible, within an impression on its medial aspect (the submandibular fossa).
  - It is situated outside the boundaries of the oral cavity.
- **Deep arm**:
  - Hooks around the posterior margin of mylohyoid through a triangular aperture to enter the oral cavity proper.
  - It lies on the lateral surface of the **hyoglossus**, lateral to the root of the tongue.

### 3. SUBMANDIBULAR DUCT (WHARTON'S DUCT)

- Secretions from the submandibular glands travel into the oral cavity via the submandibular duct. This is approximately 5cm in length and emerges anteromedially from the deep arm of the gland between the mylohyoid, hypoglossus and genioglossus muscles.
- The duct ascends on its course to open as 1-3 orifices on a small **sublingual papilla** (caruncle) at the base of the lingual frenulum bilaterally.

## 4. Relationship with Nerves

- Both the submandibular gland and duct share an intimate anatomical relationship with three principal nerves:
  - **Lingual nerve** (CN V3)
  - **Hypoglossal nerve** (CN XII)
  - **Facial nerve** (Marginal mandibular branch).

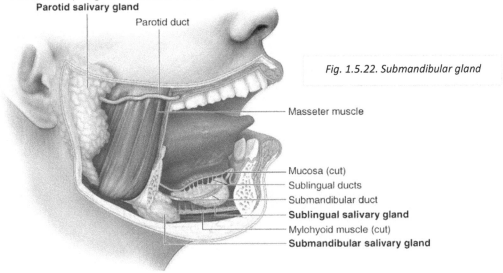

*Fig. 1.5.22. Submandibular gland*

Parotid salivary gland
Parotid duct
Masseter muscle
Mucosa (cut)
Sublingual ducts
Submandibular duct
**Sublingual salivary gland**
Mylohyoid muscle (cut)
**Submandibular salivary gland**

## 5. VASCULATURE

- **Artery: submental arteries** which arise from the facial artery; a branch of the external carotid artery.
- **Venous drainage: submental veins** which drain into the facial vein and then the internal jugular vein.

## 6. INNERVATION

- **Parasympathetic:**
  - Originates from the **superior salivatory nucleus** through pre-synaptic fibres, which travel via the chorda tympani branch of the facial nerve (CNVII).
  - The chorda tympani then unifies with the **lingual branch** of the mandibular nerve (CNV3) before synapsing at the submandibular ganglion and suspending it by two nerve filaments.
  - Post-ganglionic innervation consists of **secretomotor fibres** which directly induce the gland to produce secretions, and vasodilator fibres which accompany arteries to increase blood supply to the gland.
  - *Increased parasympathetic drive promotes saliva secretion.*
- **Sympathetic**
  - Sympathetic innervation originates from the **superior cervical ganglion**, where post-synaptic vasoconstrictive fibres travel as a **plexus** on the internal and external carotid arteries, facial artery and finally the submental arteries to enter each gland.
  - *Increased sympathetic drive reduces glandular blood flow through vasoconstriction and **decreases the volume of salivary secretions, resulting in a more mucus and enzyme-rich saliva.***

## CLINICAL RELEVANCE
### SALIVARY DUCT CALCULI

- A calculus or sialolith is a **calcified deposit** which can block the lumen of a duct.
- The submandibular duct is the most susceptible to calculi out of all the salivary ducts; accounting for approximately 80% of cases.
- The submandibular glands and the patency of the ducts can be examined by direct injection of a contrast medium **(sialogram)**.

### SUBMANDIBULAR GLAND EXCISION

- Submandibular gland excision is a common surgical procedure indicated for conditions such as submandibular gland **neoplasia** or **recurrent calculi**.
- Consequences of the three nerve injuries are:
  - **Lingual nerve:** Beginning lateral to the submandibular duct, this nerve courses anteromedially by looping beneath the duct and then terminating as several medial branches. Immediate post-operative **ipsilateral parasthaesia** and **loss of taste** from the anterior two-thirds of the tongue, which is rarely permanent.
  - **Hypoglossal nerve:** Ipsilateral paresis or paralysis of the intrinsic muscles of the tongue leading to **dysarthria and deviation of tongue to side of the lesion.** This nerve is rarely injured in this procedure to an extent to produce noticeable disability.
  - **Facial nerve (marginal mandibular branch):** Ipsilateral paresis or paralysis of the muscles supplying the lower lip and chin, including depressor labii inferioris, which characteristically presents as **drooping of the lower lip**. This is usually temporary, lasting for 6-12 weeks.

# VII. PHARYNX AND TONSILS

## A. PHARYNX

### 1. Subdivisions of the Pharynx
- The pharynx is a muscular tube that connects the nasal cavities to the larynx and oesophagus.
- It is common to both the gastrointestinal and respiratory tracts.
- It begins at the base of the skull and ends inferiorly to the cricoid cartilage (C6). It is comprised of three parts; the **Nasopharynx, Oropharynx** and **Laryngopharynx** (from superior to inferior).

### A. NASOPHARYNX
- Is situated behind the nasal cavity above the soft palate and communicates with the nasal cavities through the nasal choanae.
- Contains the pharyngeal tonsils in its posterior wall.
- Is connected with the tympanic cavity through the auditory (eustachian) tube, which equalizes air pressure on both sides of the tympanic membrane.

### B. OROPHARYNX
- Extends between the soft palate above and the superior border of the epiglottis below and communicates with the mouth through the oropharyngeal isthmus.
- Contains the palatine tonsils, which are lodged in the tonsillar fossae and are bounded by the palatoglossal and palatopharyngeal folds.

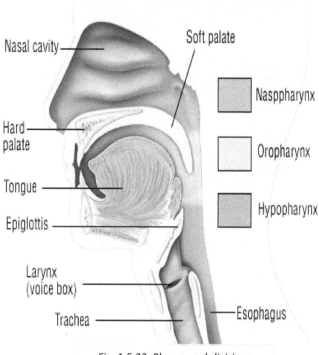

Fig. 1.5.23. Pharynx subdivisions

### C. LARYNGOPHARYNX (HYPOPHARYNX)
- Extends from the upper border of the epiglottis to the lower border of the cricoid cartilage.
- Contains the piriform recesses, one on each side of the opening of the larynx, in which swallowed foreign bodies may be lodged.

### 2. INNERVATION PHARYNX
- Innervation of the majority of the pharynx is achieved by the pharyngeal plexus, which comprises of:
  - Branches of the glossopharyngeal nerve (CN IX)
  - Branches of the vagus nerve (CN X)
  - Sympathetic fibres of the superior cervical ganglion.
- **Sensory:** Each of the three sections of the pharynx have a different innervation:
  - **The nasopharynx** is innervated by the maxillary nerve (CN V2).
  - **The oropharynx** by the glossopharyngeal nerve (CN IX).
  - **The laryngopharynx** by the vagus nerve (CN X).
- **Motor:**
  - All the muscles of the pharynx are innervated by the vagus nerve (CN X), except for the stylopharyngeus, which is innervated by the glossopharyngeal nerve (CN IX).

### 3. BLOOD SUPPLY OF PHARYNX
- **Arterial supply:** is via branches of the external carotid artery: ascending pharyngeal, lingual, facial and maxillary arteries.
- **Venous drainage:** is achieved by the pharyngeal venous plexus, which drains into the internal jugular vein.

## B. LARYNX

### 1. ANATOMICAL POSITION AND RELATIONS
- The larynx is located in the anterior compartment of the neck, suspended from the hyoid bone, and spanning between **C3 and C6.**
- It is a component of the respiratory tract, and has several important functions: **phonation, cough reflex,** and **protection of the lower respiratory tract.**
- It is continuous inferiorly with the trachea, and opens superiorly into the laryngeal part of the pharynx.
- It is covered anteriorly by the infrahyoid muscles, and laterally by the lobes of the thyroid gland.
- The larynx is also closely related to the major blood vessels of neck, which pass either side as they ascend up to the head.

## 2. ANATOMICAL STRUCTURE

- The larynx is formed by a cartilaginous skeleton, which is held together by ligaments and membranes. The laryngeal muscles act to move the components of the larynx for phonation and breathing.
- The internal cavity of the larynx can be divided into three sections:
  - **Supraglottis:** From the inferior surface of the epiglottis to the vestibular folds (false vocal cords).
  - **Glottis:** Contains vocal cords and 1cm below them. The opening between the vocal cords is known as **rima glottidis**, the size of which is altered by the muscles of phonation.
    - *Note that when the vocal cords are fully adducted, the rima glottidis is completely closed, and no air can pass through.*
  - **Subglottis:** From inferior border of the glottis to the inferior border of the cricoid cartilage.

## 3. MUSCLES OF LARYNX

- The muscles of the larynx can be divided into two groups:
  - **The external muscles:** act to elevate or depress the larynx during swallowing.
  - **The internal muscles:** act to move the individual components of the larynx, playing a vital role in breathing and phonation.

➢ **EXTRINSIC MUSCLES**
  - They are comprised of the suprahyoid and infrahyoid groups, and the stylopharyngeus (a muscle of the pharynx).
  - *In general, the suprahyoid muscles and the stylopharyngeus elevate the larynx, whilst the infrahyoid muscles depress the larynx.*

➢ **INTRINSIC MUSCLES**
  - The intrinsic laryngeal muscles act on the individual components of the larynx. They control the shape of the **rima glottidis** and the length and tension of the vocal folds.
  - All the intrinsic muscles of the larynx (except the cricothyroid) are innervated by the **inferior laryngeal nerve**, the terminal branch of the recurrent laryngeal nerve, itself a branch of the vagus nerve.
  - The cricothyroid is innervated by the **external branch of the superior laryngeal nerve**, again derived from the vagus nerve.
  - These muscles are:
    - **Cricothyroid:** Stretches and tenses the vocal ligament.
    - **Thyroarytenoid:** Relaxes the vocal ligament.
    - **Posterior cricoarytenoid:** Abducts vocal folds.
      - The posterior cricoarytenoid muscles are the sole abductors of the vocal folds, and thus the only muscle capable of widening the rima glottidis.
    - **Lateral cricoarytenoid:** Adducts the vocal folds.
      - The lateral cricoarytenoid muscles are the major adductors of the vocal folds. This narrows the rima glottidis, modulating the tone and volume of speech.
    - **Transverse and Oblique Arytenoids:** Adducts the arytenoid cartilages.
      - The transverse and oblique arytenoids muscles adduct the arytenoid cartilages, closing the posterior portion of rima glottidis. This narrows the laryngeal inlet.

## 4. CARTILAGES OF LARYNX

- There are nine cartilages located within the larynx;
  - 3 unpaired
  - 6 paired.

➢ **UNPAIRED CARTILAGES**
- The three unpaired cartilages are the epiglottis, thyroid and cricoid cartilages.
  - **THYROID CARTILAGE**
    - The thyroid cartilage is a large, prominent structure which is easily visible in adult males. It is composed of two sheets (laminae), which join together anteriorly to form the laryngeal prominence (**Adam's apple**).
    - The posterior border of each sheet project superiorly and inferiorly to form the superior and inferior horns (also known as cornu). The superior horns articulate with the hyoid bone, while the inferior horns are in contact with the cricoid cartilage.

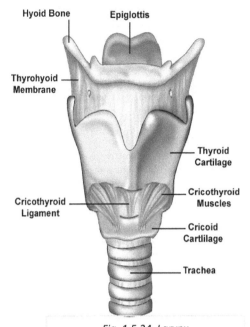

*Fig. 1.5.24. Larynx*

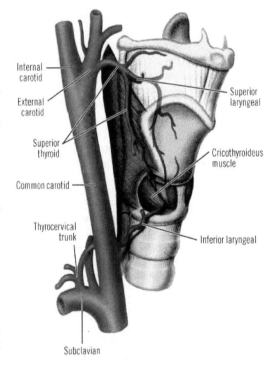

*Fig. 1.5.25. Blood supply of the Larynx*

- o **CRICOID CARTILAGE**
  - The cricoid cartilage is a complete ring of hyaline cartilage, consisting of a broad sheet posteriorly and a much narrower arch anteriorly (said to resemble a signet ring in shape). The cartilage completely encircles the airway, marking the inferior border of the larynx at the level of C6.
  - It articulates with the paired arytenoid cartilages posteriorly, as well as providing an attachment for the inferior horns of the thyroid cartilage.

- o **EPIGLOTTIS**
  - The epiglottis is a leaf shaped plate of elastic cartilage which marks the entrance to the larynx.
  - Its stalk is attached to the posterior aspect of the thyroid cartilage.
  - During swallowing, the epiglottis moves towards the arytenoid cartilages to close off the larynx and prevent aspiration.

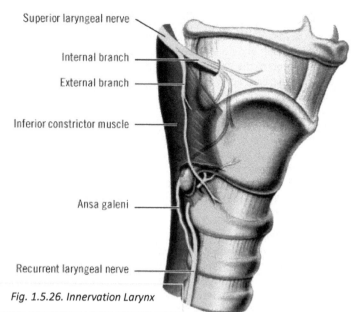

*Fig. 1.5.26. Innervation Larynx*

> **PAIRED CARTILAGES**
- There are three paired cartilages: the arytenoid, corniculate and cuneiform. They are situated bilaterally in the larynx.

  - o **ARYTENOID CARTILAGES**
    - The arytenoid cartilages are pyramidal shaped structures that sit on the cricoid cartilage.
    - They consist of an apex, base, three sides and two processes, and provides an attachment point for various key structures in the larynx:
      - **Apex:** articulates with the corniculate cartilage.
      - **Base:** articulates with the superior border of the cricoid cartilage.

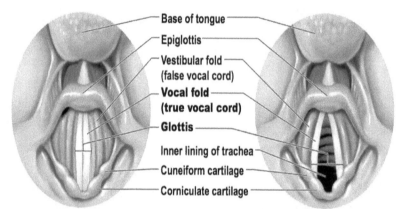

**(a) Vocal folds in closed position; closed glottis**

**(b) Vocal folds in open position; open glottis**

*Fig. 1.5.27. Vocal cords anatomy*

      - **Vocal process:** provides attachment for the vocal ligament.
      - **Muscular process:** provides attachment for the posterior and lateral cricoarytenoid muscles.
  - o **CORNICULATE CARTILAGES**
    - The corniculate cartilages are minor cartilaginous structures. They articulate with the apices of the arytenoid cartilages.
  - o **CUNEIFORM CARTILAGES**
    - The cuneiform cartilages are located within the ary-epiglottic folds. They have no direct attachment, but act to strengthen the folds.

1. **BLOOD VESSELS OF LARYNX**
- **Arterial supply:** via the superior and inferior laryngeal arteries:
  - o **Superior laryngeal artery:** a branch of the superior thyroid artery (derived from the external carotid). It follows the internal branch of the superior laryngeal nerve into the larynx.
  - o **Inferior laryngeal artery:** a branch of the inferior thyroid artery (derived from the thyrocervical trunk). It follows the recurrent laryngeal nerve into the larynx.
- **Venous drainage:** is by the superior and inferior laryngeal veins.
  - o **The superior laryngeal vein:** drains to the internal jugular vein via the superior thyroid.
  - o **The inferior laryngeal vein:** drains to the left brachiocephalic vein via the inferior thyroid vein.

2. **INNERVATION OF LARYNX**
- The larynx receives both motor and sensory innervation via branches of the **vagus nerve:**
  - o **Recurrent laryngeal nerve:** provides sensory innervation to the infraglottis, and motor innervation to all the internal muscles of larynx (except the cricothyroid).
  - o **Superior laryngeal nerve:** the internal branch provides sensory innervation to the supraglottis, and the external branch provides motor innervation to the cricothyroid muscle.

# VIII. EYE

## A. THE EYEBALL

### 1. LAYERS OF THE EYEBALL
- The eyeball can be divided into the **Fibrous, Vascular** and **Inner Layers**.
- **FIBROUS LAYER**
  - The fibrous layer of the eye is the outermost layer.
  - It consists of the **sclera** and **cornea**, which are directly continuous with each other.
  - Their main functions are to provide shape to the eye and support the deeper structures.
- **VASCULAR LAYER**
  - The vascular layer of the eye lies underneath the fibrous layer. It consists of the **choroid, ciliary body** and **iris**:
- **INNER LAYER**
  - The inner layer of the eye consists of the **retina**, the light detecting part of the eye.
  - The retina itself is comprised of two cellular layers:
    - **Neural layer**: Consists of photoreceptors; the light detecting cells of the retina. It is located posteriorly and laterally in the eye.
    - **Pigmented layer**: Lies underneath the neural layer and is attached to the choroid layer. It acts to support the neural layer, and continues around the whole inner surface of the eye.
  - Anteriorly, the pigmented layer continues but the neural layer does not; this is part is known as the **non-visual retina**.
  - Posteriorly and laterally, both layers of the retina are present. This is the **optic part** of the retina.
  - The optic part of the retina can be viewed during ophthalmoscopy. The center of the retina is marked by an area known as the **macula**.
  - It is yellowish in colour, and highly pigmented.
  - The macula contains a depression called the **fovea,** which has a high concentration of light detecting cells. It is the area responsible for high acuity vision.
  - The area that the optic nerve enters the retina is known as the **optic disc** – it contains no light detecting cells.

### 2. OTHER STRUCTURES IN THE EYEBALL
- Within the eyeball, there are structures that are not located in the three layers. These are the **lens and the chambers of the eye**.
  - Lens
    - The lens of the eye is located anteriorly, between the **vitreous humor** and the **pupil**. The shape of the lens is altered by the **ciliary body**, changing its refractive power.
    - In old age, the lens can become opaque, a condition known as a **cataract**.
  - Anterior and Posterior Chambers
    - There are two fluid filled areas in the eye
    - The anterior chamber is located between the **cornea** and the **iris**, and the posterior chamber between the **iris** and **ciliary processes**.
    - The chambers are filled with **aqueous humor**.
    - The aqueous humor is produced constantly, and drains via the trabecular meshwork, an area of tissue at the base of the cornea, near the anterior chamber.
    - If the drainage of aqueous humor is obstructed, the intra-ocular pressure will rise, a condition known as **glaucoma**.

### 3. BLOOD VESSELS
- The eyeball receives arterial blood primarily via the **ophthalmic artery**.
- This is a branch of the internal carotid artery, arising immediately distal to the cavernous sinus.
- The ophthalmic artery gives rise to many branches, which supply different components of the eye.
- The **central artery of the retina** is the most important branch, supplying the internal surface of the retina. Occlusion of this artery will quickly result in blindness.
- Venous drainage of the eyeball is carried out by the **superior** and **inferior ophthalmic** veins. These drain into the cavernous sinus, a dural venous sinus in close proximity to the eye.

## CLINICAL RELEVANCE:
### PAPILLOEDEMA
- *Papilloedema refers to a swelling of the **optic disc**, visible during ophthalmoscopy.*
- *The optic disc is the area of the retina where the optic nerve enters.*
- *The swelling occurs secondary to raised **intra-cranial pressure**.*
- *The high pressure within the cranium resists venous return from the eye.*
- *This causes fluid to collect in the retina, producing a swollen optic disc*

## B. MUSCLES OF THE EYE

- The extraocular muscles are a group of six muscles that regulate the eye movements. Depend on the position of the eye at the time of muscle contraction, these muscles aid in controlling the eye movement.
- The extraocular or extrinsic eye muscles, considering their relatively small size, are incredibly strong and efficient.
- There are the six extraocular muscles, which act to turn or rotate an eye about its vertical, horizontal, and antero-posterior axes:
  - Medial rectus (MR),
  - Lateral rectus (LR),
  - Superior rectus (SR),
  - Inferior rectus (IR),
  - Superior oblique (SO),
  - Inferior oblique (IO).

## EXTRAOCULAR MUSCLES MOVEMENTS:

- Eye muscles work together with other eye muscles, of the same eye and the opposite eye, to move the eyes in various directions.
- However, a given extraocular muscle, if working on its own in isolation (without other extrinsic eye muscles in play), would move the front of an eye in a specific direction or directions, as follows:

### 1. MEDIAL RECTUS (MR),

- Moves the eye inward, toward the nose (adduction)

### 2. LATERAL RECTUS (LR),

- Moves the eye outward, away from the nose (abduction)

### 3. SUPERIOR RECTUS (SR),

- Primarily moves the eye upward (elevation)
- Secondarily rotates the top of the eye toward the nose (intorsion)
- Tertiarily moves the eye inward (adduction)

### 4. INFERIOR RECTUS (IR),

- Primarily moves the eye downward (depression)
- Secondarily rotates the top of the eye away from the nose (extorsion)
- Tertiarily moves the eye inward (adduction)

### 5. SUPERIOR OBLIQUE (SO),

- Primarily rotates the top of the eye toward the nose (intorsion)
- Secondarily moves the eye downward (depression)
- Tertiarily moves the eye outward (abduction)

### 6. INFERIOR OBLIQUE (IO),

- Primarily rotates the top of the eye away from the nose (extorsion)
- Secondarily moves the eye upward (elevation)
- Tertiarily moves the eye outward (abduction)

- The primary muscle that moves an eye in a given direction is known as the **"agonist."**
- A muscle in the same eye that moves the eye in the same direction as the agonist is known as a **"synergist,"** while the muscle in the same eye that moves the eye in the opposite direction of the agonist is the **"antagonist."**
- According to **"Sherrington's Law,"** increased innervation to any agonist muscle is accompanied by a corresponding decrease in innervation to its antagonist muscle(s).

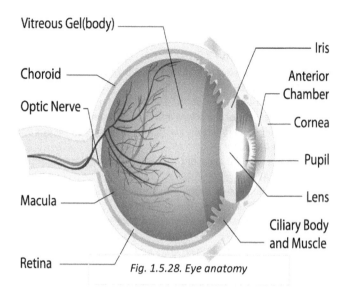

*Fig. 1.5.28. Eye anatomy*

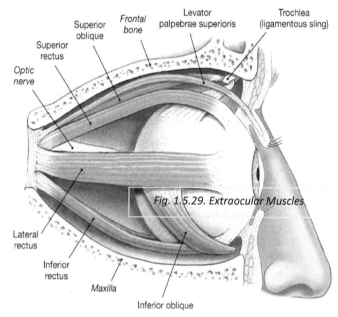

*Fig. 1.5.29. Extraocular Muscles*

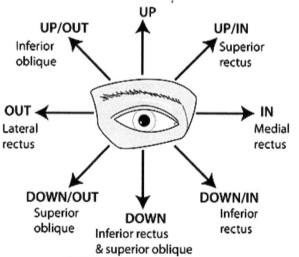

*Fig. 1.5.30. Extraocular muscles movements*

- o The superior rectus moves the eye up and in.
- o The inferior oblique pulls the eye up and out.
- o The inferior rectus pulls the eye down and in.
- o The superior oblique pulls the eye down and out.
- o The lateral rectus is responsible for moving the eye out
- o The medial rectus is responsible for moving the eye in.

## NERVE INNERVATIONS OF THE EXTRAOCULAR MUSCLES: LR6 (SO4) Rest 3

- Extraocular muscles are innervated by a specific cranial nerve (C.N.):
  - o Lateral rectus (LR)—cranial nerve VI (Abducens)
  - o Superior oblique (SO)—cranial nerve IV (Trochlear)
  - o Inferior oblique (IO)—cranial nerve III (Oculomotor)
  - o Superior rectus (SR)—cranial nerve III (Oculomotor)
  - o Inferior rectus (IR)—cranial nerve III (Oculomotor)
  - o Medial rectus (MR)—cranial nerve III (Oculomotor)

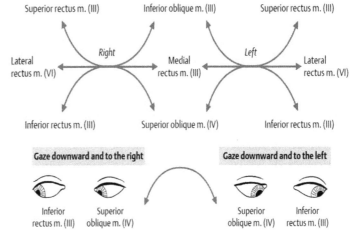

Fig. 1.5.31. Innervation of extraocular muscles

## CLINICAL RELEVANCE: CRANIAL NERVE PALSIES

- **OCULOMOTOR NERVE (CN III)**
  - o A lesion of the oculomotor nerve affects most of the extraocular muscles. The affected eye is displaced laterally by the lateral rectus and inferiorly by the superior oblique.
  - o The eye adopts a position known as **'down and out'**.

- **TROCHLEAR NERVE (CN IV)**
  - o A lesion of CN IV will paralyse the superior oblique muscle.
  - o There is no obvious affect of the resting orientation of the eyeball.
  - o However, the patient will complain of diplopia (double vision), and may develop a head tilt away from the site of the lesion.

- **ABDUCENS NERVE (CN VI)**
  - o A lesion of CN VI will paralyse the lateral rectus muscle.
  - o The affected eye will be adducted by the resting tone of the medial rectus.

## C. BONY ORBIT

### 1. BORDERS AND ANATOMICAL RELATIONS

- o **Roof** (superior wall): Formed by the frontal bone and the lesser wing of the sphenoid. The frontal bone separates the orbit from the anterior cranial fossa.
- o **Floor** (inferior wall): Formed by the maxilla, palatine and zygomatic bones. The maxilla separates the orbit from the underlying maxillary sinus.
- o **Medial wall**: Formed by the ethmoid, maxilla, lacrimal and sphenoid bones. The ethmoid bone separates the orbit from the ethmoid sinus.
- o **Lateral wall**: Formed by the zygomatic bone and greater wing of the sphenoid.
- o **Apex**: Located at the opening to the optic canal, the optic foramen.
- o **Base**: Opens out into the face, and is bounded by the eyelids. It is also known as the orbital rim.

### 2. CONTENTS OF ORBIT

- The bony orbit contains the **eyeballs** and their associated structures:
  - o **Extra-ocular muscles**: These muscles are separate from the eye. They are responsible for the movement of the eyeball and superior eyelid.
  - o **Eyelids**: These cover the orbits anteriorly.
  - o **Nerves**: Several cranial nerves supply the eye and its structures; optic, oculomotor, trochlear, trigeminal and abducens nerves.
  - o **Blood vessels**: The eye receives blood primarily from the ophthalmic artery. Venous drainage is via the superior and inferior ophthalmic veins.
  - o Any space within the orbit that is not occupied is filled with **orbit fat**. This tissue cushions the eye, and stabilises the extraocular muscles.

### 3. PATHWAYS INTO THE ORBIT

- There are three main pathways by which structures can enter and leave the orbit:
  - o The **optic canal**: transmits the optic nerve and ophthalmic artery.
  - o The **superior orbital fissure**: transmits the "SOFT LAN"
  - o The **inferior orbital fissure**: transmits the "ZIME".
- There are other minor openings into the orbital cavity:
  - o **Supraorbital notch or foramen**: supraorbital nerve and vessels.
  - o **Anterior and posterior ethmoidal foramina**: anterior and posterior ethmoidal nerves and vessels, respectively.
  - o **Nasolacrimal canal**: nasolacrimal duct from the lacrimal sac to the inferior nasal meatus.

# ORBITAL BLOW-OUT FRACTURE

## CLINICAL PRESENTATION

- **Orbital blow-out fractures** occur when there is a fracture of one of the walls of orbit but the orbital rim remains intact.
- Typically, this is caused by a direct blow to the central orbit from a fist or ball. *Visual disturbance, limitation of eye movements and a **teardrop sign** on facial x ray are all signs of an orbital blow-out fracture*: Immediate referral to an ophthalmologist or maxillofacial surgeon is essential. There is no evidence to support routine antibiotic prophylaxis in orbital floor fracture.
- Orbital blow-out fractures are usually the result of a direct blow to the orbit.
- This results in a sudden increase in the intraorbital pressure which in turn causes decompression by fracture of one or more of the bounding walls of the orbit. The trauma is usually substantial, but presentation and diagnosis may sometimes be delayed.
- This delay is usually due to intact orbital rim (by definition) and swelling making assessment of diplopia and extra-ocular movement difficult. Associated clinical findings of facial bones injuries may include:

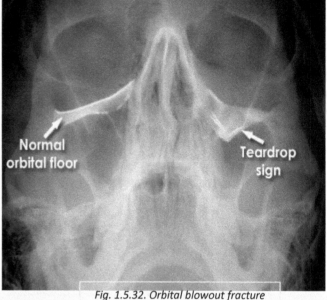

Fig. 1.5.32. Orbital blowout fracture

  o **Enophthalmos and proptosis**: due to increased orbital volume
  o **Diplopia**: due to trapping of the herniated **inferior rectus muscle**
  o **Orbital emphysema**: especially when fracture is into an adjacent **paranasal sinus**
  o **Sensory disturbance to the cheek and upper gum**: a sign of **infraorbital nerve injury**
  o **Restriction of mouth opening in ZMC Fracture**: due to trapping of the **temporalis muscle** or **mandibular condyle**.

## INVESTIGATION

- Radiographs no longer have a real role to play in the assessment of facial trauma. However, if they are obtained, the diagnosis of fractures involving the inferior or medial wall may be suspected by visualisation of fluid with the maxillary sinus and ethmoidal air cells respectively.
- Orbital emphysema may also be visible. Under certain circumstances this may give a **black eyebrow sign**.
- Herniation of orbital fat inferiorly may give a **"tear drop" sign.**
- CT is the modality of choice for assessment of the facial skeleton, and does not require the administration of contrast.

# EYE TRAUMA

- Although the eyeball is well protected by the surrounding bony orbit, it is protected anteriorly only from large objects, such as tennis balls, which tend to strike the orbital margin but not the globe. The bony orbit provides no protection from small objects, such as golf balls, which can cause severe damage to the eye.
- Careful examination of the eyeball relative to the orbital margins shows that it is least protected from the lateral side.

# STRABISMUS

- Many cases of strabismus are nonparalytic and are caused by an imbalance in the action of opposing muscles.
- This type of strabismus is known as **concomitant strabismus** and is common in infancy.

# PUPILLARY REFLEXES

- The pupillary reflexes—that is, the reaction of the pupils to light and accommodation—depend on the integrity of nervous pathways. In the **direct light reflex,** the normal pupil reflex contracts when a light is shone into the patient's eye. The nervous impulses pass from the retina along the optic nerve to the optic chiasma and then along the optic tract. Before reaching the lateral geniculate body, the fibers concerned with this reflex leave the tract and pass to the oculomotor nuclei on both sides via the pretectal nuclei. From the parasympathetic part of the nucleus, efferent fibers leave the midbrain in the oculomotor nerve and reach the ciliary ganglion via the nerve to the inferior oblique. Postganglionic fibers pass to the constrictor pupillae muscles via the short ciliary nerves.
- The **consensual light reflex** is tested by shining the light in one eye and noting the contraction of the pupil in the opposite eye. This reflex is possible because the afferent pathway just described travels to the parasympathetic nuclei of both oculomotor nerves.
- The **accommodation reflex** is the contraction of the pupil that occurs when a person suddenly focuses on a near object after having focused on a distant object. The nervous impulses pass from the retina via the optic nerve, the optic chiasma, the optic tract, the lateral geniculate body, the optic radiation, and the cerebral cortex of the occipital lobe of the brain. The visual cortex is connected to the eye field of the frontal cortex. From here, efferent pathways pass to the parasympathetic nucleus of the oculomotor nerve. From there, the efferent impulses reach the constrictor pupillae via the oculomotor nerve, the ciliary ganglion, and the short ciliary nerves.

# IX. EAR

## I. EXTERNAL EAR

- Consists of the auricle and the external acoustic meatus and receives sound waves.

### A. AURICLE

- Funnels sound waves into the external auditory meatus. Has the following features: Helix, Antihelix, Concha, Tragus and Lobule
- **Sensory nerves:**
  - Branch of the vagus and facial nerves and the greater Auricular nerve,
  - Auriculotemporal branch of the trigeminal nerve, and lesser occipital nerves.
- **Blood supply:**
  - Superficial temporal artery
  - Posterior auricular artery.

### B. EXTERNAL ACOUSTIC (AUDITORY) MEATUS

- It is about 2.5 cm long, extending from the concha to the tympanic membrane. Its external one third is formed by cartilage, and the internal two thirds is formed by bone.
- The cartilaginous portion is wider than the bony portion and has numerous ceruminous glands that produce earwax.
- **Nerve:**
  - Auriculotemporal branch of the trigeminal nerve
  - Auricular branch of the vagus nerve, which is joined by a branch of the facial nerve and the glossopharyngeal nerve.
- **Blood supply:**
  - Superficial temporal, posterior auricular and maxillary arteries (a deep auricular branch).

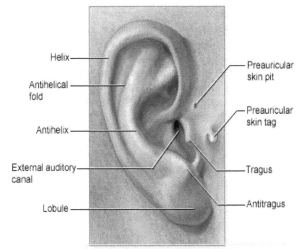

*Fig. 1.5.33. External ear Anatomy*

### C. TYMPANIC MEMBRANE (EARDRUM)

- The **tympanic membrane** is a thin membrane that separates the external ear from the middle ear.
- It acts to transmit sound waves from air in the external auditory canal to the ossicles of the middle ear.
- **The malleus** is the first bone in the ossicular chain that eventually sees the sound wave transmitted to the oval window of the cochlea.
- It consists of three layers (from outside to inside):
  - Cutaneum (skin)
  - Radiatum circulare (collagen fibres)
  - Mucosum (epithelium)
- There are two distinct portions to the membrane:
  - **Pars Tensa:** the tense portion of the membrane is the larger portion and extends from the anterior and posterior malleolar folds at the level of the lateral process of malleus to the inferior edge of the membrane.
  - **Pars Flaccida:** the flaccid portion of the membrane is much smaller and is the portion of the membrane above the anterior and posterior malleolar folds.
- It is anatomically separated into four quadrants:
  - Anterosuperior and anteroinferior
  - Posteroinferior and posterosuperior
- **Innervation**
  - **External surface:**
    - Auriculotemporal nerve (CN V3)
    - Auricular branch of the vagus nerve (CN X)
  - **Internal surface:** glossopharyngeal nerve (CN IX)

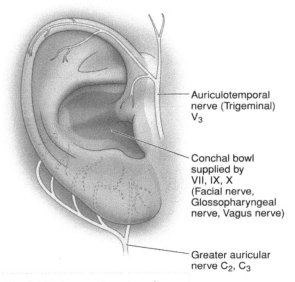

*Fig. 1.5.34. Innervation external ear*

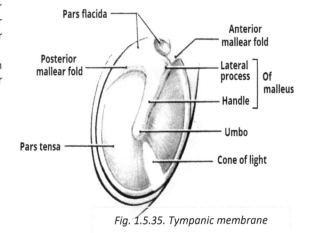

*Fig. 1.5.35. Tympanic membrane*

## II. MIDDLE EAR
o    The middle ear lies within the temporal bone, and extends from the tympanic membrane to the lateral wall of the internal ear.
o    The main function of the middle ear is to transmit vibrations from the tympanic membrane to the inner ear via the three bones of the ear.

### 1. PARTS OF THE MIDDLE EAR
•    The middle ear can be split into two parts; **the tympanic cavity** and **epitympanic recess**.
   o    The tympanic cavity lies medially to the tympanic membrane.
   o    It contains the majority of the bones of the middle ear.
   o    The epitympanic recess is found superiorly, near the mastoid air cells

### 2. BONES
•    The bones of the middle ear are called the auditory ossicles.
•    They are the malleus, incus and stapes.
   o    **The Malleus**
      ▪    The largest and most lateral of the ear bones
      ▪    Attaching to the tympanic membrane, via the handle of malleus.
      ▪    The head of the malleus lies in the epitympanic recess, where it articulates with the next auditory ossicle, the incus.
   o    **The Incus**
      ▪    Consists of a body and two limbs.
      ▪    The body articulates with the malleus,
      ▪    The short limb attaches to the posterior wall of the middle ear.
      ▪    The long limb joins the last of the ossicles; the stapes.

   o    **The Stapes**
      ▪    The smallest bone in the human body.
      ▪    It joins the incus to the oval window of the inner ear.
      ▪    It is stirrup-shaped, with a head, two limbs, and a base.
      ▪    The head articulates with the incus, and the base joins the oval window.

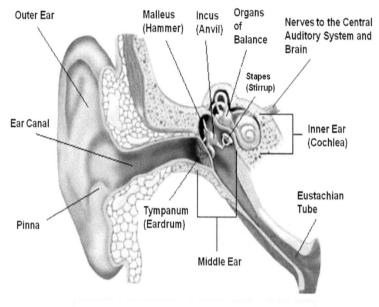

*Fig. 1.5.36. The middle ear anatomy*

### 3. MASTOID AIR CELLS
   o    Located posterior to epitympanic recess. They are a collection of air-filled spaces in the mastoid process of the temporal bone.
   o    The air cells are contained within a cavity called **the mastoid antrum.**
   o    The mastoid antrum communicates with the middle ear via the aditus to mastoid antrum.
   o    The mastoid air cells act as a "buffer system" of air, releasing air into the tympanic cavity when the pressure is too low.

### 4. MUSCLES
   o    There are two muscles which serve a protective function in the middle ear; **the tensor tympani** and **stapedius.**
   o    They contract in response to loud noise, inhibiting the vibrations of the malleus, incus and stapes, and reducing the transmission of sound to the inner ear.
   o    This action is known as the acoustic reflex.
      ▪    **The tensor tympani:** originates from the auditory tube and attaches to the handle of malleus, pulling it medially when contracting. It is innervated by a branch of the mandibular nerve.
      ▪    **The stapedius muscle:** attaches to the stapes, and is innervated by the facial nerve.

### 5. AUDITORY TUBE OR EUSTACHIAN TUBE
   o    The auditory tube is a cartilaginous and bony tube that connects the middle ear to the nasopharynx.
   o    It acts to equalise the pressure of the middle ear to that of the external auditory meatus. Normally, the Eustachian tube is collapsed, but it gapes open both with swallowing and with positive pressure
   o    It extends from the anterior wall of the middle ear, in anterior, medioinferior direction, opening onto the lateral wall of the nasopharynx. *In joining the two structures, it is a pathway by which an upper respiratory infection can spread into the middle ear.*

## III. INNER EAR

### 1. ANATOMICAL POSITION AND STRUCTURE

- The inner ear is located within the petrous part of the temporal bone.
- It lies between the middle ear and the internal acoustic meatus, which lie laterally and medially respectively.
- The inner ear has two main components: the bony labyrinth and membranous labyrinth.
  - **Bony labyrinth:**
    - Consists of a series of bony cavities within the petrous part of the temporal bone. It is comprised of the **cochlea, vestibule** and **three semicircular canals**. All these structures are lined internally with periosteum and contain a fluid called **Perilymph**.
  - **Membranous labyrinth:**
    - Lies within the bony labyrinth. It consists of the **cochlear duct, semicircular ducts, utricle** and **the saccule**.
    - The membranous labyrinth is filled with fluid called **Endolymph**.
- The inner ear has two openings into the middle ear, both covered by membranes:
  - The **oval window** lies between the middle ear and the vestibule
  - The **round window** separates the middle ear from the scala tympani (part of the cochlear duct).

### 2. VASCULATURE

- The bony labyrinth and membranous labyrinth have different arterial supplies.
- The bony labyrinth receives three arteries, which also supply the surrounding temporal bone:
  - **Anterior tympanic branch** (from maxillary artery).
  - **Petrosal branch** (from middle meningeal artery).
  - **Stylomastoid branch** (from posterior auricular artery).
- The membranous labyrinth is supplied by the **labyrinthine artery**, a branch of the inferior cerebellar artery (or, occasionally, the basilar artery). It divides into three branches:
  - **Cochlear branch**: supplies the cochlear duct.
  - **Vestibular branches (x2)**: supply the vestibular apparatus.
- Venous drainage of the inner ear is through the **labyrinthine vein**, which empties into the sigmoid sinus or inferior petrosal sinus.
- **Innervation:** Vestibulocochlear nerve (CN VIII).

## INFECTIONS AND OTITIS MEDIA

- Pathogenic organisms can gain entrance to the middle ear by ascending through the auditory tube from the nasal part of the pharynx. Acute infection of the middle ear **(otitis media)** produces bulging and redness of the tympanic membrane.
- **Complications of Otitis Media**
  - Inadequate treatment of otitis media can result in the spread of the infection into the mastoid antrum and the mastoid air cells **(acute mastoiditis)**. Acute mastoiditis may be followed by the further spread of the organisms beyond the confines of the middle ear. The meninges and the temporal lobe of the brain lie superiorly.
  - A spread of the infection in this direction could produce a meningitis and a cerebral abscess in the temporal lobe.
  - Beyond the medial wall of the middle ear lie the facial nerve and the internal ear. A spread of the infection in this direction can cause a facial nerve palsy and **labyrinthitis** with **vertigo**. The posterior wall of the mastoid antrum is related to the sigmoid venous sinus. If the infection spreads in this direction, a thrombosis in the sigmoid sinus may well take place. These various complications emphasize the importance of knowing the anatomy of this region.

## PAEDIATRIC vs ADULT AIRWAY

There are a number of developmental characteristics that distinguish the Paediatric airway from the adult airway:

- *Size:* The Paediatric airway is smaller in diameter and shorter in length than the adult's.
- *Tongue:* The young child's tongue is relatively larger in the oropharynx than the adult's.
- *Larynx:* The larynx in infants and young children is located more anteriorly compared with the adult's.
- *Epiglottis:* The epiglottis in infants and young children is relatively long, floppy, and narrow
- In children, younger than 10 years of age, the narrowest portion of the airway is below the glottis at the level of the cricoid cartilage.

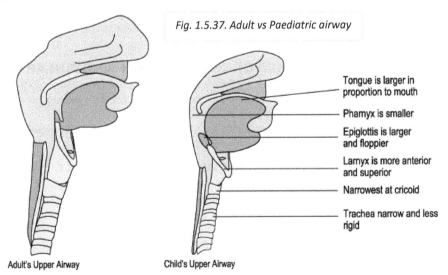

Fig. 1.5.37. Adult vs Paediatric airway

Tongue is larger in proportion to mouth

Pharynx is smaller

Epiglottis is larger and floppier

Larnyx is more anterior and superior

Narrowest at cricoid

Trachea narrow and less rigid

Adult's Upper Airway          Child's Upper Airway

# X. TEMPOROMANDIBULAR JOINT

## 1. BONY SURFACES

- The TMJ consists of articulations between **3** surfaces: the mandibular fossa and articular tubercle (from the squamous part of the **temporal bone**), and the head of **mandible**.
- This joint has a unique mechanism; the articular surfaces of the bones never come into contact with each other, they are separated by an **articular disk**.
- The presence of such a disk splits the joint into **two** synovial joint cavities, each lined by a synovial membrane.
- *The articular surface of the bones are covered by fibrocartilage, not hyaline cartilage.*

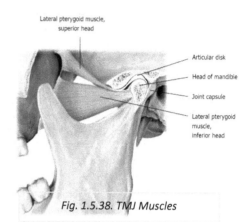

Fig. 1.5.38. TMJ Muscles

## 2. LIGAMENTS

The ligaments give passive stability to the TMJ.

- **The temporomandibular ligament** is the thickened lateral portion of the capsule, and it has two parts, an outer oblique portion and an inner horizontal portion.
- **The stylomandibular ligament** runs from the styloid process to the angle of the mandible.
- **The sphenomandibular ligament** runs from the spine of the
- sphenoid bone to the lingula of mandible.
- **The oto-mandibular ligaments** are the **discomalleolar ligament** (DML), which arises from the malleus (one of the ossicles of the middle ear) and runs to the medial retrodiscal tissue of the TMJ, and the **anterior malleolar ligament** (AML), which arises from the malleus and connects with the lingula of the mandible via the sphenomandibular ligament.

## 3. MOVEMENTS OF THE TMJ JOINT

- Traumatic impact is transmitted around the ring, causing a single fracture or multiple fractures of the mandible, often far removed from the point of impact. The jaw can move forward and back, side to side and can open and close. Each of these movements are performed by a number of muscles working together to perform the movement while controlling the position of the condyle within the mandibular fossa. Chewing and talking require a combination of jaw movements in a number of directions.
- **Opening** – inferior head of lateral pterygoid, anterior digastric, mylohyoid. Opening is also controlled by eccentric contraction of the closing muscles against gravity. Opening is a complex movement consisting of an early rotary component in the first 2-3cms of movement with a forward glide towards the end of range. The articular disc moves forward with the condyle as it glides forward, effectively extending the superior articular surface of the mandibular fossa.
- **Closing** – masseter, anterior and middle temporalis, medial pterygoid, superior head lateral pterygoid.
- **Protrusion** – bilateral contraction of the lateral pterygoid.
- **Retrusion** – middle and posterior temporalis, possibly helped by deep posterior portion of masseter
- **Laterotrusion** (side to side) – ipsilateral middle and posterior temporalis, contralateral inferior head lateral pterygoid.

## CLINICAL RELEVANCE

### FRACTURES OF THE MANDIBLE

- The mandible is horseshoe shaped and forms part of a bony ring with the two temporomandibular joints and the base of the skull.
- Traumatic impact is transmitted around the ring, causing a single fracture or multiple fractures of the mandible, often far removed from the point of impact.

### CLINICAL SIGNIFICANCE OF THE TEMPOROMANDIBULAR JOINT

- The temporomandibular joint lies immediately in front of the external auditory meatus.
- The great strength of the lateral temporomandibular ligament prevents the head of the mandible from passing backward and fracturing the tympanic plate when a severe blow falls on the chin.
- The **articular disc** of the temporomandibular joint may become partially detached from the capsule, and this results in its movement becoming noisy and producing an audible click during movements at the joint.

### DISLOCATION OF THE TEMPOROMANDIBULAR JOINT

- Dislocation sometimes occurs when the mandible is depressed. In this movement, the head of the mandible and the articular disc both move forward until they reach the summit of the articular tubercle.
- In this position, the joint is unstable, and a minor blow on the chin or a sudden contraction of the lateral pterygoid muscles, as in yawning, may be sufficient to pull the disc forward beyond the summit. In bilateral cases, the mouth is fixed in an open position, and both heads of the mandible lie in front of the articular tubercles.
- Reduction of the dislocation is easily achieved by pressing the gloved thumbs downward on the lower molar teeth and pushing the jaw backward. The downward pressure overcomes the tension of the temporalis and masseter muscles, and the backward pressure overcomes the spasm of the lateral pterygoid muscles.

# XI. VERTEBRAL COLUMN

## 1. FUNCTIONS

- **Protection**: it encloses the spinal cord, shielding it from damage.
- **Support**: it carries the weight of the body above the pelvis (below the pelvis, the lower limbs take over).
- **Axis**: the vertebral column forms the central axis of the body.
- **Movement**: it has roles in both posture and movement.

## 2. VERTEBRAL STRUCTURE

Each vertebra consists of a **vertebral body anteriorly**, and a **vertebral arch posteriorly**.

### A. VERTEBRAL BODY

- The vertebral body is the anterior part of the vertebrae. It is the **weight-bearing** component, and its size increases as the vertebral column descends (having to support increasing amounts of weight each time).
- The superior and inferior aspects of the vertebral body are lined with **hyaline cartilage**.
- Adjacent vertebral bodies are separated by a fibrocartilaginous **intervertebral disc**.

### B. VERTEBRAL ARCH

- The vertebral arch refers to the lateral and posterior parts of the vertebrae.
- With the vertebral body, the vertebral arch forms an enclosed hole, called a **vertebral foramen.**
- The foramina of the all vertebrae line up to form the **vertebral canal**, which encloses the spinal cord.
- The vertebral arches have a number of bony prominences, which act as attachment sites for muscles and ligaments:
  - **Pedicles**: There are two of these, one left and one right. They point posteriorly, meeting the flatter laminae.
  - **Lamina**: The bone between the transverse and spinal processes.
  - **Transverse processes**: These extend laterally and posteriorly away from the pedicles. In the thoracic vertebrae, the transverse processes articulate with the ribs.
  - **Articular processes**: At the junction of the lamina and the pedicles, superior and inferior processes arise. These articulate with the articular processes of the vertebrae above and below.
  - **Spinous processes**: Posterior and inferior projection of bone, a site of attachment for muscles and ligaments.

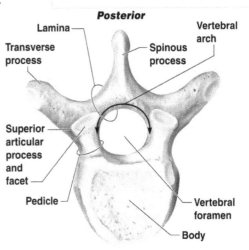

*Fig. 1.5.39. Vertebral structure*

## 3. CLASSIFICATIONS OF VERTEBRAE

### A. CERVICAL VERTEBRAE

- **CHARACTERISTICS OF A TYPICAL CERVICAL VERTEBRA**
- A typical cervical vertebra has the following characteristics:
  - The transverse processes possess a **foramen transversarium** for the passage of the vertebral artery and veins (note that the vertebral artery passes through the transverse processes C1 to 6 and not through C7).
  - The spines are small and bifid.
  - The body is small and broad from side to side.
  - The vertebral foramen is large and triangular.
  - The superior articular processes have facets that face posteriorly and superiorly; the inferior processes have facets that face inferiorly and anteriorly.

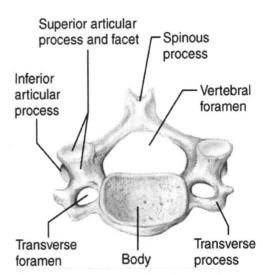

*Fig. 1.5.40. Cervical vertebra*

- **CHARACTERISTICS OF THE ATYPICAL CERVICAL VERTEBRAE**
  - The 1st, 2nd, and 7th cervical vertebrae are atypical.
  - The **1ˢᵗ cervical vertebra,** or **atlas**, does not possess a body or a spinous process. It has an anterior and posterior arch. It has a lateral mass on each side with articular surfaces on its upper surface for articulation with the occipital condyles **(atlanto-occipital joints)** and articular surfaces on its inferior surface for articulation with the axis **(atlantoaxial joints).**
  - The **2ⁿᵈ cervical vertebra,** or **axis**, has a peglike **odontoid process (dens)** that projects from the superior surface of the body (representing the body of the atlas that has fused with the body of the axis).

o The **7th cervical vertebra,** or **vertebra prominens,** is so named because it has the longest spinous process, and the process is not bifid. The transverse process is large, but the foramen transversarium is small and transmits the vertebral vein or veins.

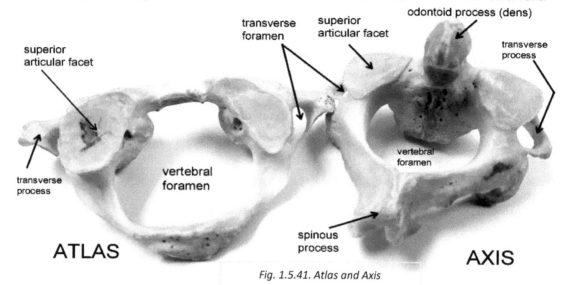

Fig. 1.5.41. Atlas and Axis

## B. THORACIC VERTEBRA

- A typical thoracic vertebra has the following characteristics:
  o The body is medium size and heart shaped.
  o The vertebral foramen is small and circular.
  o The spines are long and inclined downward.
  o Costal facets are present on the sides of the bodies for articulation with the heads of the ribs.
  o Costal facets are present on the transverse processes for articulation with the tubercles of the ribs (T11 and 12 have no facets on the transverse processes).
  o The superior articular processes bear facets that face posteriorly and laterally, whereas the facets on the inferior articular processes face anteriorly and medially.
  o The inferior articular processes of the 12th vertebra face laterally, as do those of the lumbar vertebrae.

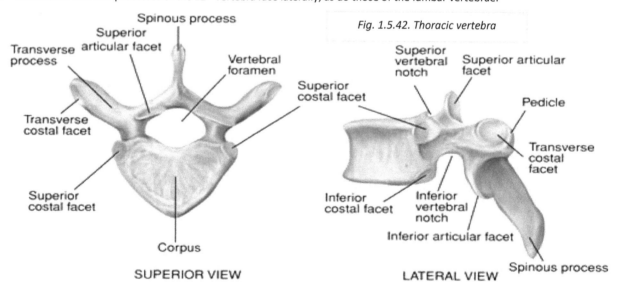

Fig. 1.5.42. Thoracic vertebra

SUPERIOR VIEW                    LATERAL VIEW

## C. LUMBAR VERTEBRA

- A typical lumbar vertebra has the following characteristics:
  o The body is large and kidney shaped.
  o The pedicles are strong and directed backward.
  o The laminae are short in a vertical dimension (important when performing a spinal tap).
  o The vertebral foramina are triangular.
  o The transverse processes are long and slender.
  o The spinous processes are short, flat, and quadrangular and project posteriorly.
  o The articular surfaces of the superior articular processes face medially, and those of the inferior articular processes face laterally.

- Note that the lumbar vertebrae have no facets for articulation with ribs and no foramina in the transverse processes.

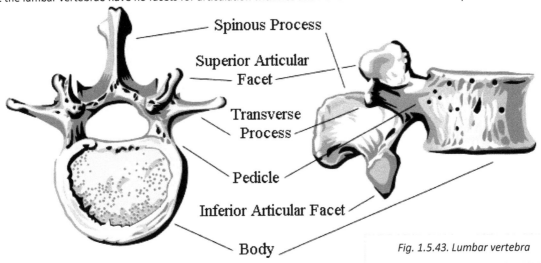

*Fig. 1.5.43. Lumbar vertebra*

## D. SACRUM

- The sacrum consists of five rudimentary vertebrae fused together to form a wedge-shaped bone, which is concave anteriorly.
- The upper border, or base, of the bone articulates with the 5th lumbar vertebra.
- The narrow inferior border articulates with the coccyx. Laterally, the sacrum articulates with the two iliac bones to form the sacroiliac joints.
- The anterior and upper margin of the first sacral vertebra bulges forward as the posterior margin of the pelvic inlet and is known as the **sacral promontory.**
- The sacral promontory in the female is of considerable obstetric importance and is used when measuring the size of the pelvis.
- The vertebral foramina are present and form the **sacral canal.**
- The laminae of the 5th sacral vertebra, and sometimes those of the 4th also, fail to meet in the midline, forming the **sacral hiatus**.
- The sacral canal contains the anterior and posterior roots of the sacral and coccygeal spinal nerves, the filum terminale, and fibrofatty material. It also contains the lower part of the subarachnoid space down as far as the lower border of the second sacral vertebra.
- The anterior and posterior surfaces of the sacrum each have four foramina on each side for the passage of the anterior and posterior rami of the upper four sacral nerves.

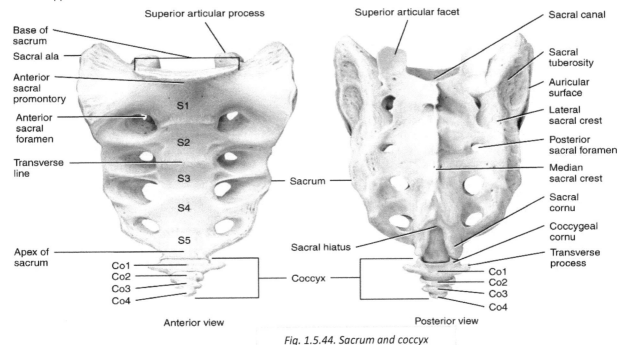

*Fig. 1.5.44. Sacrum and coccyx*

## E. COCCYX

- The coccyx consists of four vertebrae fused together to form a single, small triangular bone that articulates at its base with the lower end of the sacrum.
- The first coccygeal vertebra is usually not fused or is incompletely fused with the second vertebra

## IMPORTANT VARIATIONS IN THE VERTEBRAE

- The number of cervical vertebrae is constant, but the seventh cervical vertebra may possess a **cervical rib**.
- The thoracic vertebrae may be increased in number by the addition of the 1st lumbar vertebra, which may have a rib.
- The 5th lumbar vertebra may be incorporated into the sacrum; this is usually incomplete and may be limited to one side.
- The 1st sacral vertebra may remain partially or completely separate from the sacrum and resemble a 6th lumbar vertebra.
- A large extent of the posterior wall of the sacral canal may be absent because the laminae and spines fail to develop.
- The coccyx, which usually consists of four fused vertebrae, may have three or five vertebrae. The 1st coccygeal vertebra may be separate. In this condition, the free vertebra usually projects downward and anteriorly from the apex of the sacrum.

## 3. JOINTS OF THE VERTEBRAL COLUMN

### A. ATLANTO-OCCIPITAL JOINTS

- The atlanto-occipital joints are synovial joints that are formed between the occipital condyles, which are found on either side of the foramen magnum superiorly and the facets on the superior surfaces of the lateral masses of the atlas inferiorly.
- They are enclosed by a capsule.
- **LIGAMENTS**
  - ○ **Anterior atlanto-occipital membrane:** This is a continuation of the anterior longitudinal ligament, which runs as a band down the anterior surface of the vertebral column. The membrane connects the anterior arch of the atlas to the anterior margin of the foramen magnum.
  - ○ **Posterior atlanto-occipital membrane:** This membrane is similar to the ligamentum flavum and connects the posterior arch of the atlas to the posterior margin of the foramen magnum.
- **MOVEMENTS**
  - ○ Flexion, extension, and lateral flexion. No rotation is possible.

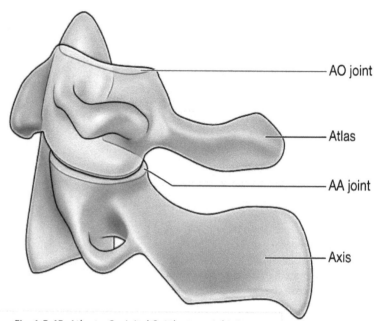

*Fig. 1.5.45. Atlanto-Occipital & Atlanto-axial Joints*

### B. ATLANTOAXIAL JOINTS

- The atlantoaxial joints are three synovial joints: one is between the odontoid process and the anterior arch of the atlas, and the other two are between the lateral masses of the bones. The joints are enclosed by capsules.
- **LIGAMENTS**
  - ○ **Apical ligament:** This median-placed structure connects the apex of the odontoid process to the anterior margin of the foramen magnum.
  - ○ **Alar ligaments:** These lie one on each side of the apical ligament and connect the odontoid process to the medial sides of the occipital condyles.
  - ○ **Cruciate ligament:** This ligament consists of a transverse part and a vertical part. The transverse part is attached on each side to the inner aspect of the lateral mass of the atlas and binds the odontoid process to the anterior arch of the atlas. The vertical part runs from the posterior surface of the body of the axis to the anterior margin of the foramen magnum.
  - ○ **Membrana tectoria:** This is an upward continuation of the posterior longitudinal ligament. It is attached above to the occipital bone just within the foramen magnum. It covers the posterior surface of the odontoid process and the apical, alar, and cruciate ligaments.
- **MOVEMENTS**
  - ○ There can be extensive rotation of the atlas and thus of the head on the axis.

### C. JOINTS OF THE VERTEBRAL COLUMN BELOW THE AXIS

- With the exception of the first two cervical vertebrae, the remainder of the mobile vertebrae articulates with each other by means of cartilaginous joints between their bodies and by synovial joints between their articular processes.

### D. JOINTS BETWEEN TWO VERTEBRAL BODIES

- The superior and inferior surfaces of the bodies of adjacent vertebrae are covered by thin plates of hyaline cartilage.
- Sandwiched between the plates of hyaline cartilage is an intervertebral disc of fibrocartilage. The collagen fibers of the disc strongly unite the bodies of the two vertebrae. In the lower cervical region, small synovial joints are present at the lateral sides of the intervertebral disc between the upper and lower surfaces of the bodies of the vertebrae.

## E. INTERVERTEBRAL DISCS

- The intervertebral discs are the main structures that bind together the vertebral bodies, and they extend from C2 to the sacrum (C1 has no vertebral body). The discs are responsible for one quarter of the length of the vertebral column below the level of C2.
- They are thickest in the cervical and lumbar regions, where the movements of the vertebral column are greatest.
- They may be regarded as semielastic discs, which lie between the rigid bodies of adjacent vertebrae.
- Their physical characteristics permit them to serve as shock absorbers when the load on the vertebral column is suddenly increased, as when one is jumping from a height. Their elasticity allows the rigid vertebrae to move one on the other.
- Unfortunately, their resilience is gradually lost with advancing age.
- Each disc consists of a peripheral part, the anulus fibrosus, and a central part, the nucleus pulposus.
- The **anulus fibrosus** is composed of fibrocartilage, in which the collagen fibers are arranged in concentric layers or sheets.
- The collagen bundles pass obliquely between adjacent vertebral bodies, and their inclination is reversed in alternate sheets.
- The more peripheral fibers are strongly attached to the anterior and posterior longitudinal ligaments of the vertebral column.
- The **nucleus pulposus** in children and adolescents is an ovoid mass of gelatinous material containing a large amount of water, a small number of collagen fibers, and a few cartilage cells. It is normally under pressure and situated slightly nearer to the posterior than to the anterior margin of the disc.
- The superior and inferior surfaces of the bodies of adjacent vertebrae that abut onto the disc are covered with thin plates of hyaline cartilage. No discs are found between the first two cervical vertebrae or in the sacrum or coccyx.

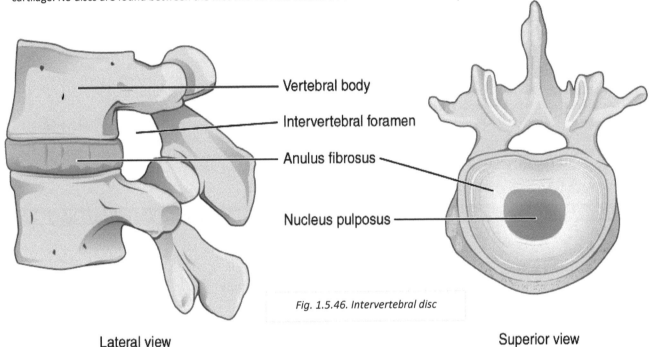

Vertebral body

Intervertebral foramen

Anulus fibrosus

Nucleus pulposus

*Fig. 1.5.46. Intervertebral disc*

Lateral view

Superior view

### FUNCTION OF THE INTERVERTEBRAL DISCS

- The semifluid nature of the nucleus pulposus allows it to change shape and permits one vertebra to rock anteriorly or posteriorly on another, as in flexion and extension of the vertebral column.
- A sudden increase in the compression load on the vertebral column causes the semifluid nucleus pulposus to become flattened. The outward thrust of the nucleus is accommodated by the resilience of the surrounding annulus fibrosus. Sometimes, the outward thrust is too great for the anulus fibrosus and it ruptures, allowing the nucleus pulposus to herniate and protrude into the vertebral canal, where it may press on the spinal nerve roots, the spinal nerve, or even the spinal cord.
- With advancing age, the water content of the nucleus pulposus diminishes and is replaced by fibrocartilage. The collagen fibers of the anulus degenerate and, as a result, the anulus cannot always contain the nucleus pulposus under stress. In old age, the discs are thin and less elastic, and it is no longer possible to distinguish the nucleus from the anulus.
- **LIGAMENTS**
  o The **anterior** and **posterior longitudinal ligaments** run as continuous bands down the anterior and posterior surfaces of the vertebral column from the skull to the sacrum.
  o The anterior ligament is wide and is strongly attached to the front and sides of the vertebral bodies and to the intervertebral discs. The posterior ligament is weak and narrow and is attached to the posterior borders of the discs.
  o These ligaments hold the vertebrae firmly together but at the same time permit a small amount of movement to take place between them.

## F. JOINTS BETWEEN TWO VERTEBRAL ARCHES

- The joints between two vertebral arches consist of synovial joints between the superior and inferior articular processes of adjacent vertebrae. The articular facets are covered with hyaline cartilage, and the joints are surrounded by a capsular ligament.
- **Ligaments**
  - o **Supraspinous ligament**: This runs between the tips of adjacent spines.
  - o **Interspinous ligament**: This connects adjacent spines.
  - o **Intertransverse ligaments**: These run between adjacent transverse processes.
  - o **Ligamentum flavum:** This connects the laminae of adjacent vertebrae.
- In the cervical region, the supraspinous and interspinous ligaments are greatly thickened to form the strong **Ligamentum nuchae.**
- The latter extends from the spine of the 7th cervical vertebra to the external occipital protuberance of the skull, with its anterior border being strongly attached to the cervical spines in between.

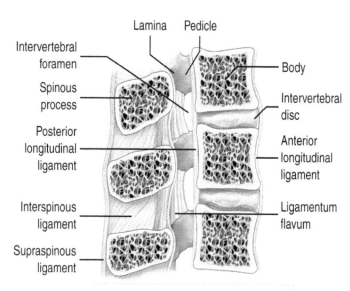

Fig. 1.5.47. Intervertebral ligaments

## 4. NERVE SUPPLY OF VERTEBRAL JOINTS

- The joints between the vertebral bodies are innervated by the small meningeal branches of each spinal nerve.
- The nerve arises from the spinal nerve as it exits from the intervertebral foramen.
- It then re-enters the vertebral canal through the intervertebral foramen and supplies the meninges, ligaments, and intervertebral discs.
- The joints between the articular processes are innervated by branches from the posterior rami of the spinal nerves.
- It should be noted that the joints of any particular level receive nerve fibers from two adjacent spinal nerves.

## 5. VERTEBRAL LEVEL OF MAJOR HUMAN STRUCTURES

| HUMAN STRUCTURES | VERTEBRAL LEVEL | HUMAN STRUCTURES | VERTEBRAL LEVEL |
|---|---|---|---|
| • Larynx | C3-C6 | | |
| • Oesophagus | C6-Rib11, (25-40cm) | • Abdominal Aorta | |
| | | • Top of left kidney | T12 |
| | | • Inferior phrenic artery | |
| • Trachea | C6 | • Caeliac Trunk | T12-L1 |
| • Superior angle scapula | T2 | • Cauda Equina | Below L1 |
| • Thoracic Aorta lower border | T4 | • Renal Arteries | L1-L2 |
| • Bifurcation Trachea | T4/5 | • Gonadal Arteries | L2 |
| • Bronchus | T5 | • Inferior Mesenteric Artery | L3 |
| | | • Psoas Muscles | |
| • Xiphisternal joint | T9 | • Bifurcation to Common Iliac | L4 |
| • Diaphragm | Xiphoid process-L2 | • Beginning of Duodenum | |
| | T8 | • Pancreas (Body and tail) | |
| o IVC Foramina | T10 | • Superior Mesenteric Artery | |
| o Oesophagus Hiatus | T12 | • Portal vein | L1 |
| | | • Transpyloric plane of Addison. | |
| o Aortic Hiatus | | • Fundus of the gallbladder. | |
| | | • Hila of the Kidney | |
| • Upper liver and Spleen | T11 | • IVC | L5 |
| • Kidneys | T12-L3 | • Rectum | S3 |

# PAST ASKED QUESTIONS

### Regarding the anatomy of the internal jugular vein

| | |
|---|---|
| It is a continuation of the transverse sinus | F |
| It joins the external carotid vein | F |
| Runs medial to the internal carotid artery | F |
| Drains the floor of the mouth via the lingual vein | T |

### Regarding the sensory supply of the face

| | |
|---|---|
| The mandibular nerve supplies the skin over the angle of the mandible | F |
| Damage to the infraorbital nerve can result in numbness to the canine tooth | T |
| The lingual nerve carries taste fibres from the posterior 1/3 of the tongue | F |
| The mental nerve supplies the lateral border of the tongue with sensation | F |

### Which statements regarding facial anatomy are true?

| | |
|---|---|
| Orbicularis oculi muscle is supplied by facial nerve | T |
| Skin of upper lip is supplied by infraorbital nerve | T |
| The facial artery is a branch of common carotid artery | F |
| There is no deep fascia in the face | T |

### Regarding the facial nerve:

| | |
|---|---|
| It emerges through the stylomastoid foramen | T |
| It lies deep to the parotid gland | F |
| It has bilateral cortical innervation | T |
| Infranuclear lesions may cause reduced hearing due to paralysis of stapedius | F |

### The following statements are in relation to the floor of the mouth

| | |
|---|---|
| The submandibular duct lies superior to the lingual nerve as it opens into the floor of the mouth | T |
| The superficial and deep parts of the submandibular gland are separated by the genioglossus muscle | F |
| Mylohyoid makes up the floor of the sublingual space | T |
| Cancerous lesions in the anterior 2/3 of the floor of the mouth carry a poorer prognosis than those in the anterior third | F |

### Regarding epistaxis

| | |
|---|---|
| The majority of nose bleeds arise from the anterior part of the nasal mucosa | T |
| Local trauma around Little's area is the most common cause for nosebleeds | T |
| The leakage of clear fluid from the nose post head injury may indicate damage to the sella tursica | F |

### True or False

| | |
|---|---|
| The Eustachian tube is usually open | F |
| The incus connects to the oval window of the tympanic membrane | F |
| C2-C3 contribute to the sensation of the skin of the ear | T |
| The S shaped curvature of the ear canal can be straightened by pulling the ear in posterior and superior direction during otoscopy | T |

### The Paediatric airway differs from the adult in that

| | |
|---|---|
| The narrowest part is at the level of the glottis | F |
| The epiglottis is more floppy | T |
| The tongue is relatively smaller | F |
| The larynx is more anterior | T |

### The following statements are true of the orbit

| | |
|---|---|
| The lesser wing of the sphenoid forms the medial wall of the orbit | F |
| The infraorbital foramen arises from a part of the zygomatic bone | F |
| The roof of the maxillary sinus is made up of a single bone | F |
| The bony landmark for the supraorbital foramen is the lateral third of the supraorbital margin | F |

### The following statements are true about the openings within the orbit

| | |
|---|---|
| There is a rich anastomosis between the superior ophthalmic vein and the pterygopalatine plexus | F |
| The superior orbital fissure can be anatomically divided into the three parts | T |
| The ophthalmic artery and vein run together in the optic canal | F |
| The trochlea nerve is within the common tendinous ring within the superior orbital fissure | F |

### Regarding the zones of the neck during a penetrating injury

| | |
|---|---|
| Zone I is defined as the area from the clavicles to the tip of the thyroid cartilage | F |
| Oesophageal damages is likely in Zone 3 injuries | F |
| Asymptomatic Zone 2 injuries do not require any investigations | F |
| A pneumothorax is a known complication of a penetrating neck injury | T |

### Regarding the nasal anatomy

| | |
|---|---|
| The majority of the nasal septum is bony in origin | F |
| A septal haematoma is best managed conservatively | F |
| The nasolacrimal duct drains into the middle meatus | F |
| Obstruction of the middle meatus may present with symptoms of toothache | T |

# SECTION 6: CENTRAL NERVOUS SYSTEM

## I. SCALP

- The scalp consists of 5 layers: **S**kin, **C**onnective tissue, epicranial **A**poneurosis, **L**oose areolar tissue, and **P**ericranium.

## 1. ARTERIAL SUPPLY

- The scalp has a rich vascular supply.
- The blood vessels traverse the connective tissue layer, which receives vascular contribution from **the internal and external carotid arteries**.
- The blood vessels anastomose freely in the scalp.
- From the midline, anteriorly, the arteries present as follows:
  - **Supratrochlear artery** (or frontal artery): branch of ophthalmic artery
  - **Supraorbital artery:** branch of ophthalmic artery
  - **Superficial temporal artery:** branch of ECA
  - **Posterior auricular artery**: branch of ECA
  - **Occipital artery**: branch of ECA

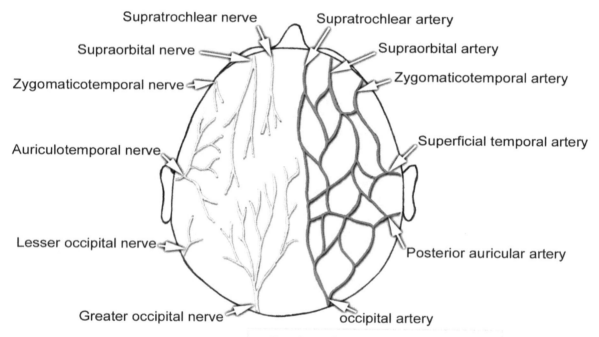

Fig. 1.6.1. Scalp Innervation and Blood supply

## 2. VENOUS DRAINAGE

- The veins of the scalp freely anastomose with one another and are connected to the diploic veins of the skull bones and the intracranial dural sinuses through several emissary veins.
- The emissary veins are valveless.
- The scalp veins accompany the arteries and have similar names.

## 3. LYMPHATIC DRAINAGE

- The part of the scalp that is anterior to the auricles is drained to the Parotid, Submandibular, and Deep Cervical Lymph Nodes.
- The posterior part of the scalp is drained to the posterior auricular (mastoid) and occipital lymph nodes.

## 4. INNERVATION OF SCALP

- **Sensory**
  - **Supratrochlear nerve (CN V1):** A branch of the ophthalmic division of the trigeminal nerve; this nerve supplies the scalp in the medial plane at the frontal region, up to the vertex
  - **Supraorbital nerve (CN V1):** Also, a branch of the ophthalmic division of the trigeminal nerve; this nerve supplies the scalp at the front, lateral to the supratrochlear nerve distribution, up to the vertex
  - **Zygomaticotemporal nerve (CN V2):** A branch of the maxillary division of the trigeminal nerve; it supplies the scalp over the temple region

- o **Auriculotemporal nerve (CN V3):** A branch of the mandibular division of the trigeminal nerve; it supplies the skin over the temporal region of the scalp
- o **Lesser occipital nerve (C2-C3):** A branch of the cervical plexus; it supplies the scalp over the lateral occipital region
- o **Greater occipital nerve (C2):** A branch of the posterior ramus of the second cervical nerve; it supplies the scalp in the median plane at the occipital region, up to the vertex.

- **Motor supply**
  - o **The frontal branch of the facial nerve** supplies the frontal bellies of the occipitofrontalis muscle.
  - o **The auricular branch of the facial nerve** supplies the occipital bellies of the muscle.

# II. SKULL

- Divided into two types of bones:
  - o **8 cranial bones** (unpaired frontal, occipital, ethmoid, and sphenoid bones and paired parietal and temporal bones), which can be seen in the cranial cavity
  - o **14 facial bones** (paired lacrimal, nasal, palatine, inferior turbinate, maxillary, and zygomatic bones and unpaired vomer and mandible).

## 1. CRANIUM
- Restricted to the skull without the mandible.

## 2. CALVARIA
- It is the skull cap, which is the vault of the skull without the facial bones. It consists of the superior portions of the frontal, parietal, and occipital bones.
- Its highest point on the sagittal suture is the vertex.

## 3. SUTURES OF THE SKULL
- o **Coronal suture:** lies between the frontal bone and the 2 parietal bones.
- o **Sagittal suture:** lies between the two parietal bones.
- o **Squamous (squamoparietal) suture:** lies between the parietal bone and the squamous part of the temporal bone.
- o **Lambdoid suture:** lies between the two parietal bones and the occipital bone.

## 4. JUNCTIONS OF THE CRANIAL SUTURES
- o **Lambda:** intersection of the lambdoid and sagittal sutures.
- o **Bregma:** intersection of the sagittal and coronal sutures.

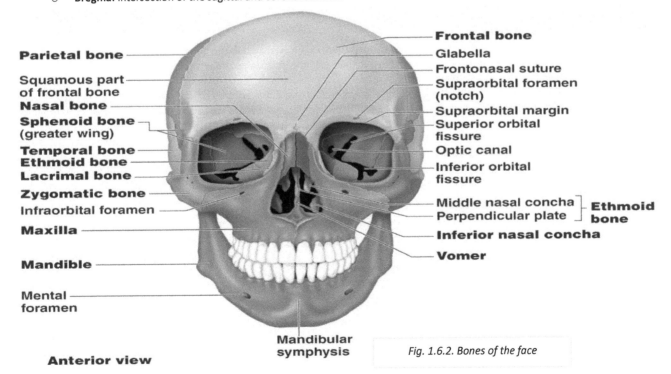

Fig. 1.6.2. Bones of the face

**Anterior view**

CLINICAL RELEVANCE
## CLINICAL SIGNIFICANCE OF THE SCALP STRUCTURE
- It is important to realize that the skin, the subcutaneous tissue, and the epicranial aponeurosis are closely united to one another and are separated from the periosteum by loose areolar tissue. The skin of the scalp possesses numerous sebaceous glands, the ducts of which are prone to infection and damage by combs. For this reason, **sebaceous cysts** of the scalp are common.

## LACERATIONS OF THE SCALP
- The **scalp has a profuse blood supply** to nourish the hair follicles. Even a small laceration of the scalp can cause severe blood loss.
- It is often difficult to stop the bleeding of a scalp wound because the arterial walls are attached to fibrous septa in the subcutaneous tissue and are unable to contract or retract to allow blood clotting to take place.
- Local pressure applied to the scalp is the only satisfactory method of stopping the bleeding. In automobile accidents, it is common for large areas of the scalp to be cut off the head as a person is projected forward through the windshield.
- Because of the profuse blood supply, it is often possible to replace large areas of scalp that are only hanging to the skull by a narrow pedicle. Suture them in place, and necrosis will not occur.
- The tension of the **epicranial aponeurosis,** produced by the tone of the occipitofrontalis muscles, is important in all deep wounds of the scalp. If the aponeurosis has been divided, the wound will gape open.
- For satisfactory healing to take place, the opening in the aponeurosis must be closed with sutures.
- Often, a wound caused by a blunt object such as a baseball bat closely resembles an incised wound.
- This is because the scalp is split against the unyielding skull, and the pull of the occipitofrontalis muscles causes a gaping wound.
- This anatomic fact may be of considerable forensic importance.

## LIFE-THREATENING SCALP HEMORRHAGE
- Anatomically, it is useful to remember in an emergency that all the superficial arteries supplying the scalp ascend from the face and the neck. Thus, in an emergency situation, encircle the head just above the ears and eyebrows with a tie, shoelaces, or even a piece of string and tie it tight.
- Then, insert a pen, pencil, or stick into the loop and rotate it so that the tourniquet exerts pressure on the arteries.

## SCALP INFECTIONS
- Infections of the scalp tend to remain localized and are usually painful because of the abundant fibrous tissue in the subcutaneous layer.
- Occasionally, an infection of the scalp spreads by the emissary veins, which are valveless, to the skull bones, causing osteomyelitis. Infected blood in the diploic veins may travel by the emissary veins farther into the venous sinuses and produce venous sinus thrombosis.
- Blood or pus may collect in the potential space beneath the epicranial aponeurosis. It tends to spread over the skull, being limited in front by the orbital margin, behind by the nuchal lines, and laterally by the temporal lines. On the other hand, subperiosteal blood or pus is limited to one bone because of the attachment of the periosteum to the sutural ligaments.

## FRACTURES OF THE SKULL
- They are common in the adult but much less so in the young child. In the infant skull, the bones are more resilient than in the adult skull, and they are separated by fibrous sutural ligaments. In the adult, the inner table of the skull is particularly brittle. Moreover, the sutural ligaments begin to ossify during middle age.
- The type of fracture that occurs in the skull depends on the age of the patient, the severity of the blow, and the area of skull receiving the trauma. The **adult skull** may be likened to an eggshell in that it possesses a certain limited resilience beyond which it splinters. A severe, localized blow produces a local indentation, often accompanied by splintering of the bone. Blows to the vault often result in a series of linear fractures, which radiate out through the thin areas of bone. The petrous parts of the temporal bones and the occipital crests strongly reinforce the base of the skull and tend to deflect linear fractures.
- In the **young child,** the skull may be likened to a table-tennis ball in that a localized blow produces a depression without splintering.
- This common type of circumscribed lesion is referred to as a **"pond" fracture.**

## FRACTURES OF THE ANTERIOR CRANIAL FOSSA
- In fractures of the anterior cranial fossa, the cribriform plate of the ethmoid bone may be damaged. This usually results in tearing of the overlying meninges and underlying mucoperiosteum. The patient will have bleeding from the nose **(epistaxis)** and leakage of cerebrospinal fluid into the nose **(cerebrospinal rhinorrhoea).**
- Fractures involving the orbital plate of the frontal bone result in hemorrhage beneath the conjunctiva and into the orbital cavity, causing **exophthalmos.** The frontal air sinus may be involved, with hemorrhage into the nose.

## FRACTURES OF THE MIDDLE CRANIAL FOSSA
- Fractures of the middle cranial fossa are common, because this is the weakest part of the base of the skull. Anatomically, this weakness is caused by the presence of numerous foramina and canals in this region; the cavities of the middle ear and the sphenoidal air sinuses are particularly vulnerable. The leakage of cerebrospinal fluid and blood from the external auditory meatus is common. The 7th and 8th cranial nerves may be involved as they pass through the petrous part of the temporal bone.
- The 3rd, 4th, and 6th cranial nerves may be damaged if the lateral wall of the cavernous sinus is torn. Blood and cerebrospinal fluid may leak into the sphenoidal air sinuses and then into the nose.

# FRACTURES OF THE POSTERIOR CRANIAL FOSSA

- In fractures of the posterior cranial fossa, blood may escape into the nape of the neck deep to the postvertebral muscles. Some days later, it tracks between the muscles and appears in the posterior triangle, close to the mastoid process. The mucous membrane of the roof of the nasopharynx may be torn, and blood may escape there. In fractures involving the jugular foramen, the 9th, 10th, and 11th cranial nerves may be damaged. The strong bony walls of the hypoglossal canal usually protect the hypoglossal nerve from injury.

# FRACTURES OF FACIAL BONES

- **Bone Injuries and Skeletal Development**
  - The developing bones of a child's face are more pliable than an adult's, and fractures may be incomplete or greenstick.
  - In adults, the presence of well-developed, air-filled sinuses and the mucoperiosteal surfaces of the alveolar parts of the upper and lower jaws means that most facial fractures should be considered to be open fractures, susceptible to infection, and requiring antibiotic therapy.
- **ANATOMY OF COMMON FACIAL FRACTURES**
  - Automobile accidents, fisticuffs, and falls are common causes of facial fractures. Fortunately, the upper part of the skull is developed from membrane (whereas the remainder is developed from cartilage); therefore, this part of the skull in children is relatively flexible and can absorb considerable force without resulting in a fracture.
  - Signs of fractures of the facial bones include deformity, ocular displacement, or abnormal movement accompanied by crepitation and malocclusion of the teeth. Anaesthesia or paraesthesia of the facial skin will follow fracture of bones through which branches of the trigeminal nerve pass to the skin.
  - The muscles of the face are thin and weak and cause little displacement of the bone fragments. Once a fracture of the maxilla has been reduced, for example, prolonged fixation is not needed. However, in the case of the mandible, the strong muscles of mastication can create considerable displacement, requiring long periods of fixation.
  - The most common facial fractures involve the nasal bones, followed by the zygomatic bone and then the mandible. To fracture the maxillary bones and the supraorbital ridges of the frontal bones, an enormous force is required.

# NASAL FRACTURES

- Fractures of the nasal bones, because of the prominence of the nose, are the most common facial fractures. Because the bones are lined with mucoperiosteum, the fracture is considered open; the overlying skin may also be lacerated. Although most are simple fractures and are reduced under local anaesthesia, some are associated with severe injuries to the nasal septum and require careful treatment under general anaesthesia.

# MAXILLOFACIAL FRACTURES

- Maxillofacial fractures usually occur as the result of massive facial trauma. There is extensive facial swelling, midface mobility of the underlying bone on palpation, malocclusion of the teeth with anterior open bite, and possibly leakage of cerebrospinal fluid (cerebrospinal rhinorrhoea) secondary to fracture of the cribriform plate of the ethmoid bone.
- **Double vision (diplopia)** may be present, owing to orbital wall damage. Involvement of the infraorbital nerve with anaesthesia or paraesthesia of the skin of the cheek and upper gum may occur in fractures of the body of the maxilla. Nose bleeding may also occur in maxillary fractures. Blood enters the maxillary air sinus and then leaks into the nasal cavity. The sites of the fractures were classified by Le Fort as type I, II, or III.

# BLOWOUT FRACTURES OF THE MAXILLA

- A severe blow to the orbit (as from a baseball) may cause the contents of the orbital cavity to explode downward through the floor of the orbit into the maxillary sinus.
- Damage to the infraorbital nerve, resulting in altered sensation to the skin of the cheek, upper lip, and gum, may occur.

# FRACTURES OF THE ZYGOMA OR ZYGOMATIC ARCH

- The zygoma or zygomatic arch can be fractured by a blow to the side of the face. Although it can occur as an isolated fracture, as from a blow from a clenched fist, it may be associated with multiple other fractures of the face, as often seen in automobile accidents.

# III. BRAIN

- The brain is made of three main parts:
  - o  Forebrain,
  - o  Midbrain,
  - o  Hindbrain.
- **The forebrain** consists of the cerebrum, thalamus, and hypothalamus (part of the limbic system).
- **The midbrain** consists of the tectum and tegmentum.
- **The hindbrain** is made of the cerebellum, pons and medulla.
- Often the midbrain, pons, and medulla are referred to together as the **brainstem.**

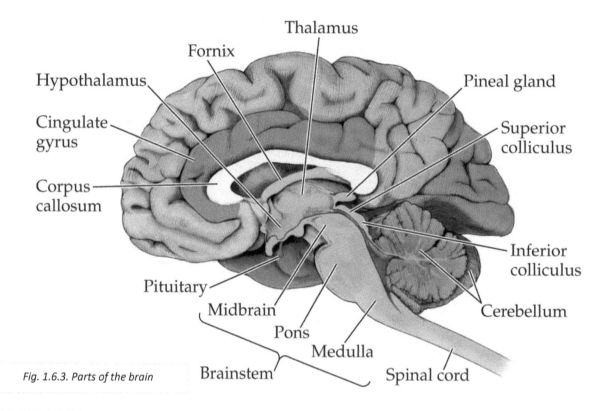

*Fig. 1.6.3. Parts of the brain*

## A. FOREBRAIN

### 1. THE CEREBRUM

- o  This is the largest brain structure in humans and accounts for about two-thirds of the brain's mass.
- o  It is divided into two sides (the left and right hemispheres) that are separated by a deep groove down the center from the back of the brain to the forehead.
- o  These two halves are connected by long neuron branches called the ***corpus callosum*** which is relatively larger in women's brains than in men's.
- o  The cerebrum is positioned over and around most other brain structures, and its four lobes are specialized by function but are richly connected.
- o  The outer 3 millimeters of "gray matter" is the ***cerebral cortex*** which consists of closely packed neurons that control most of the body functions, including the mysterious state of consciousness, the senses, the body's motor skills, reasoning and language.
- o  Each of the cerebral hemispheres is divided into four lobes and are name for the cranial (skull) bones that lie over them:

### a. THE FRONTAL LOBE

- o  The most recently-evolved part of the brain and the last to develop in young adulthood.
- o  Functions: see above
- **Frontal lobe syndromes:**
  - o  **Broca's area** is a region of the frontal operculum (inferior frontal gyrus), which overlaps with Brodmann area 44 and 45, which is responsible for speech production.
  - o  Patients with left frontal operculum lesions may demonstrate **Broca aphasia** and defective verb retrieval, whereas patients with exclusively right opercular lesions tend to develop **expressive aprosodia.**

o  Patients with orbitofrontal lesions tend to have difficulty with disinhibition, emotional lability, and memory disorders. Patients are said to have an *orbital* **personality.**

o  Patients with superior mesial lesions affecting the cingulate cortex typically develop **akinetic mutism.**

o  Patients with inferior mesial (basal forebrain) lesions tend to manifest **anterograde and retrograde amnesia and confabulation.**

# Functional Areas of the Brain

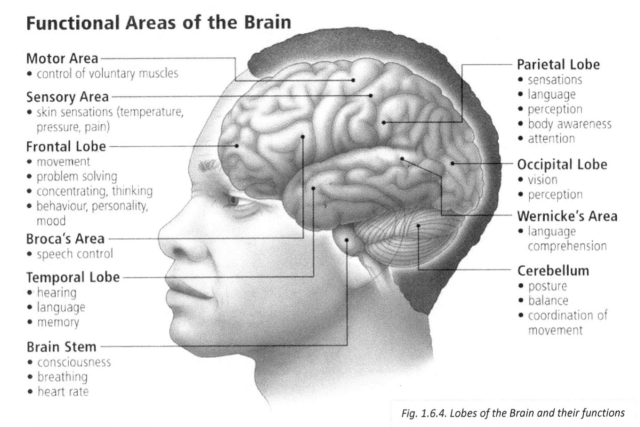

**Motor Area**
• control of voluntary muscles

**Sensory Area**
• skin sensations (temperature, pressure, pain)

**Frontal Lobe**
• movement
• problem solving
• concentrating, thinking
• behaviour, personality, mood

**Broca's Area**
• speech control

**Temporal Lobe**
• hearing
• language
• memory

**Brain Stem**
• consciousness
• breathing
• heart rate

**Parietal Lobe**
• sensations
• language
• perception
• body awareness
• attention

**Occipital Lobe**
• vision
• perception

**Wernicke's Area**
• language comprehension

**Cerebellum**
• posture
• balance
• coordination of movement

*Fig. 1.6.4. Lobes of the Brain and their functions*

## b. THE TEMPORAL LOBE
o  Controls memory storage area, emotion, hearing, and, on the left side, language.

o  **Prosopagnosia**, also called **face blindness**, is impairment in the recognition of faces and it is associated with damage to the temporal lobe.

o  **Wernicke's area** refers to the posterior aspect of the superior temporal gyrus, which overlaps with Brodmann area 22.

o  This region is generally responsible for speech comprehension, and selective injury to it can lead to impaired understanding with preserved speech production **(Wernicke's aphasia)**.

## c. THE PARIETAL LOBE
o  Receives and processes sensory information from the body including calculating location and speed of objects.

o  It is involved in sensory functions of the skin including pain, temperature, and touch.

o  It also interprets size, shape, vibrations and texture.

o  Other areas are also important in cognitive and intellectual processes.

## d. THE OCCIPITAL LOBE
o  Processes visual data and routes it to other parts of the brain for identification and storage.

o  Lesions to ventral occipital cortex can produce severe deficits in color vision, a syndrome known as cerebral **achromatopsia.**

## 2. THE LIMBIC SYSTEM
o  Includes these structures: cingulate gyrus, corpus callosum, mammillary body, olfactory tract, amygdala, and hippocampus.

## a. HIPPOCAMPUS
o  Located deep within the brain, it processes new memories for long-term storage.

o  It is among the first functions to falter in Alzheimer's.

## b. AMYGDALA
o  Lying deep in the center of the limbic emotional brain, this powerful structure is constantly alert to the needs of basic survival including sex, emotional reactions such as anger and fear.

o  Consequently, it inspires aversive cues, such as sweaty palms, and has recently been associated with a range of mental conditions including depression to even autism.

o  It is larger in male brains, often enlarged in the brains of sociopaths and it shrinks in the elderly.

### 3. HYPOTHALAMUS

- o Located at the base of the brain where signals from the brain and the body's hormonal system interact, the hypothalamus maintains the body's status quo.
- o It monitors numerous bodily functions such as blood pressure and body temperature, as well as controlling body weight and appetite.

### 4. THALAMUS

- o Located at the top of the brain stem, the thalamus acts as a two-way relay station, sorting, processing, and directing signals from the spinal cord and mid-brain structures up to the cerebrum, and, conversely, from the cerebrum down the spinal cord to the nervous system.

## B. BRAINSTEM

### 1. MEDULLA OBLONGATA

- o The medulla oblongata, or simply medulla, is continuous with and superior to the cervical spinal cord. The medulla oblongata joins the spinal cord at the foramen magnum.
- o It influences heart, breathing and circulation.
- o It's the center for vomiting, coughing and hiccuping
- o Controls our digestive, respiratory and circulatory systems.

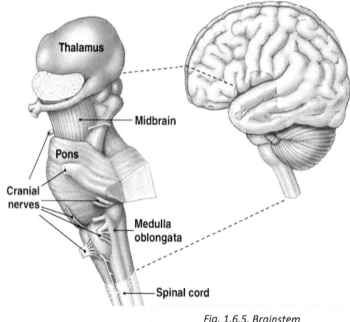

Fig. 1.6.5. Brainstem

### 2. PONS

- o Superior to the medulla lies the pons, the ventral surface of which has a characteristic band of horizontal fibers.
- o It connects the cerebellum with the cerebrum and links the midbrain to the medulla oblongata. **The pons is the reflex center for cranial nerves V through VIII.**
- o The pons is involved in chewing, taste, saliva, hearing and equilibrium. The pons interacts with the cerebellum, motor control and respiration. Helps regular breathing.
- o Other structures in the pons control sleep and excitement. The pons also relays information between the brain and the spinal cord. *Dorsally, the pons forms the floor of the fourth ventricle.*

### 3. MIDBRAIN

- o The midbrain, also termed the mesencephalon, is the superiormost aspect of the brainstem.
- o **Is the reflex center for cranial nerves III and IV and is involved in eye reflexes and movements.** *Between the cerebral peduncles, the third cranial nerve (oculomotor) can be seen exiting. The fourth cranial nerve (trochlear) exits dorsally and is unique in this regard.*

### 4. CEREBELLUM

- o The cerebellum occupies the posterior fossa, dorsal to the pons and medulla.
- o It is involved primarily in modulating motor control to enable precisely coordinated body movements.
- o Similar to the cerebrum, which has gyri and sulci, the cerebellum has finer folia and fissures that increase the surface area.
- o The cerebellum consists of 2 hemispheres, connected by a midline structure called the **vermis**.
- o In contrast to the neocortex of the cerebrum, the cerebellar cortex has 3 layers: **Molecular, Purkinje, and Granular.**
- o There are 4 deep cerebellar nuclei: The Fastigial, Globose, Emboliform, and Dentate Nuclei, in sequence from medial to lateral.
- o *The cerebellum contributes to the posterior wall of the IVth ventricle.*
- o The dendate nucleus is located within the deep white matter of each cerebellar hemisphere.
- o The afferent and efferent pathways to and from the cerebellum exist within the 3 cerebellar peduncles.

**CRANIAL NERVES ORIGIN FROM PARTS OF BRAIN:**
- • Midbrain            : CN I-IV (1-4)
- • Pons                : CN V-VIII (5-8)
- • Medulla             : CN IX-XII (9-12)

**TYPE OF CRANIAL NERVES:**
- • Pure motor          : CN IV, VI, XI, XII (4 6 11 12)
- • Purse sensory       : CN I, II, VIII (1 2 8)
- • Mixed               : III, V, VII, IX, X (3 5 7 9 10)

# IV. MENINGES OF THE BRAIN

- The meninges refer to the membranous coverings of the brain and spinal cord.
- There are three layers of meninges, known as the Dura Mater, Arachnoid Mater and Pia Mater.

## 1. DURA MATER

- It is the outermost layer of the meninges, lying directly underneath the bones of the skull and vertebral column.
- It is thick, tough and inextensible.
- Within the cranial cavity, the dura contains two connective tissue sheets:
  - **Endosteal layer**: Lines the inner surface of the bones of the cranium.
  - **Meningeal layer**: Lines the endosteal layer inside the cranial cavity. *It is the only layer present in the vertebral column.*
- Between these two layers, the dural venous sinuses are located.
- They are responsible for the venous vasculature of the cranium, draining into the internal jugular veins.

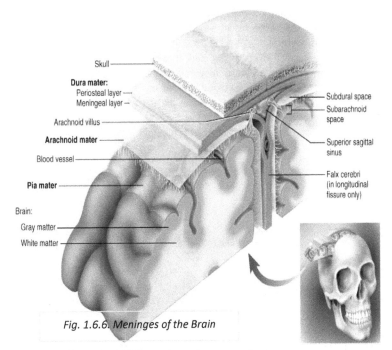

Fig. 1.6.6. Meninges of the Brain

- **Blood supply:** The dura mater receives its own vasculature; primarily from **the middle meningeal artery and vein**.
- **Innervation:** Trigeminal nerve (V1, V2 and V3).

## 2. ARACHNOID MATER

- The arachnoid mater is the middle layer of the meninges, lying directly underneath the dura mater.
- **It consists of layers of connective tissue, is avascular, and does not receive any innervation.**
- Underneath the arachnoid is a space known as the **Sub-Arachnoid Space:**
  - It contains cerebrospinal fluid, which acts to cushion the brain.
  - Small projections of arachnoid mater into the dura (known as **arachnoid granulations**) allow CSF to re-enter the circulation via the dural venous sinuses.

## 3. PIA MATER

- The pia mater is located underneath the sub-arachnoid space.
- It is very thin, and tightly adhered to the surface of the brain and spinal cord. It is the only covering to follow the contours of the brain (the gyri and fissures).
- Like the dura mater, it is highly vascularised, with blood vessels perforating through the membrane to supply the underlying neural tissue.

## CLINICAL RELEVANCE

- There are two types of hematomas involving the dura mater: extradural (Epidural) and Subdural hematomas.

### INTRACRANIAL HEMORRHAGE

- Intracranial hemorrhage may result from trauma or cerebral vascular lesions. Four varieties are considered here: extradural, subdural, subarachnoid, and cerebral.

### EXTRADURAL HAEMORRHAGE

- Results from injuries to the meningeal arteries or veins. The most common artery to be damaged is the anterior division of the middle meningeal artery. A comparatively minor blow to the side of the head, resulting in fracture of the skull in the region of the anteroinferior portion of the parietal bone, may sever the artery.
- The arterial or venous injury is especially liable to occur if the artery and vein enter a bony canal in this region. Bleeding occurs and strips up the meningeal layer of dura from the internal surface of the skull. The intracranial pressure rises, and the enlarging blood clot exerts local pressure on the underlying motor area in the precentral gyrus. Blood may also pass outward through the fracture line to form a soft swelling under the temporalis muscle.
- To stop the hemorrhage, the torn artery or vein must be ligated or plugged. The burr hole through the skull wall should be placed about 2.5 to 4 cm above the midpoint of the zygomatic arch.

## SUBDURAL HEMORRHAGE

- Results from tearing of the superior cerebral veins at their point of entrance into the superior sagittal sinus. The cause is usually a blow on the front or the back of the head, causing excessive anteroposterior displacement of the brain within the skull. This condition, which is much more common than middle meningeal hemorrhage, can be produced by a sudden minor blow. Once the vein is torn, blood under low pressure begins to accumulate in the potential space between the dura and the arachnoid. In about half the cases, the condition is bilateral.
- Acute and chronic forms of the clinical condition occur, depending on the speed of accumulation of fluid in the subdural space. For example, if the patient starts to vomit, the venous pressure will rise as a result of a rise in the intrathoracic pressure. Under these circumstances, the subdural blood clot will increase rapidly in size and produce acute symptoms. In the chronic form, over a course of several months, the small blood clot will attract fluid by osmosis so that a haemorrhagic cyst is formed, which gradually expands and produces pressure symptoms.
- In both forms, the blood clot must be removed through burr holes in the skull.

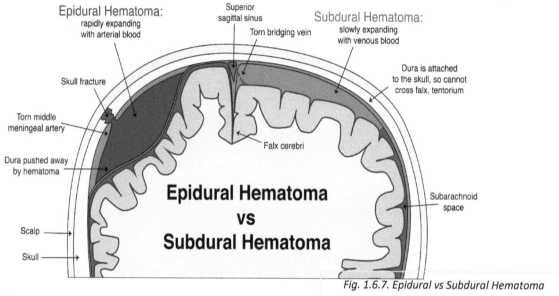

Fig. 1.6.7. Epidural vs Subdural Hematoma

## SUBARACHNOID HEMORRHAGE

- Results from leakage or rupture of a congenital aneurysm on the circle of Willis or, less commonly, from an angioma. The symptoms, which are sudden in onset, include severe headache, stiffness of the neck, and loss of consciousness.
- The diagnosis is established by withdrawing heavily blood-stained cerebrospinal fluid through a lumbar puncture (spinal tap).

## CEREBRAL HEMORRHAGE

- It is generally caused by rupture of the thin-walled lenticulostriate artery, a branch of the middle cerebral artery. The hemorrhage involves the vital corticobulbar and corticospinal fibers in the internal capsule and produces hemiplegia on the opposite side of the body. The patient immediately loses consciousness, and the paralysis is evident when consciousness is regained.

## INTRACRANIAL HEMORRHAGE IN THE INFANT

- Intracranial hemorrhage in the infant may occur during birth and may result from excessive molding of the head. Bleeding may occur from the cerebral veins or the venous sinuses. Excessive anteroposterior compression of the head often tears the anterior attachment of the falx cerebri from the tentorium cerebelli.
- Bleeding then takes place from the **great cerebral veins,** the **straight sinus,** or the **inferior sagittal sinus.**

## BRAIN INJURIES

- Injuries of the brain are produced by displacement and distortion of the neuronal tissues at the moment of impact. The brain may be likened to a log soaked with water floating submerged in water. The brain is floating in the cerebrospinal fluid in the subarachnoid space and is capable of a certain amount of anteroposterior movement, which is limited by the attachment of the superior cerebral veins to the superior sagittal sinus.
- Lateral displacement of the brain is limited by the falx cerebri. The tentorium cerebelli and the falx cerebelli also restrict displacement
- of the brain. It follows from these anatomic facts that blows on the front or back of the head lead to displacement of the brain, which may produce severe cerebral damage, stretching and distortion of the brainstem, and stretching and even tearing of the commissures of the brain. The terms concussion, contusion, and laceration are used clinically to describe the degrees of brain injury.
- Blows on the side of the head produce less cerebral displacement, and the injuries to the brain consequently tend to be less severe.

# V. BLOOD SUPPLY OF THE BRAIN

## A. INTERNAL CAROTID ARTERY

- The internal carotid arteries (ICA) *originate at the bifurcation of the left and right common carotid arteries*, at the level of the fourth cervical vertebrae (C4).
- They move superiorly within the carotid sheath, and enter the brain via the **carotid canal** of the temporal bone. They do not supply any branches to the face or neck.
- Once in the cranial cavity, the internal carotids pass anteriorly through the cavernous sinus.
- Distal to the cavernous sinus, each ICA gives rise to:
  - **Ophthalmic artery**: Supplies the structures of the orbit.
  - **Posterior communicating artery**: Acts as an anastomotic 'connecting vessel' in the Circle of Willis.
  - **Anterior cerebral artery**: Supplies part of the cerebrum.
  - The internal carotids then continue as the **Middle Cerebral Artery** (MCA), which supplies the lateral portions of the cerebrum.

## B. VERTEBRAL ARTERY

- The right and left vertebral arteries *arise from the subclavian arteries*, medial to the anterior scalene muscle.
- They then ascend up the posterior side of the neck, through holes in the transverse processes of the cervical vertebrae, known as **foramen transversarium**.
- The vertebral arteries enter the cranial cavity via the **Foramen Magnum**.
- Within the cranial vault, some branches are given off:
  - **Meningeal branch**: supplies the falx cerebelli, a sheet of dura mater.
  - **Anterior and posterior spinal arteries**: supplies the spinal cord, spanning its entire length.
  - **Posterior inferior cerebellar artery**: supplies the cerebellum.
  - After this, the two vertebral arteries converge to form the **Basilar Artery**. Several branches from the basilar artery originate here, and go onto supply the cerebellum and pons.
  - The basilar artery terminates by bifurcating into the **Posterior Cerebral Arteries**.

### Blood Supply of the Brain

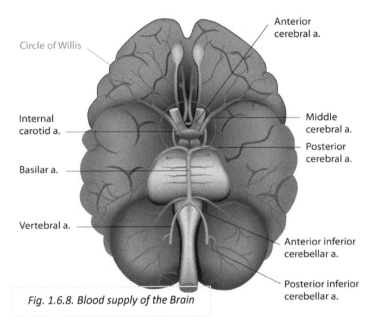

Fig. 1.6.8. Blood supply of the Brain

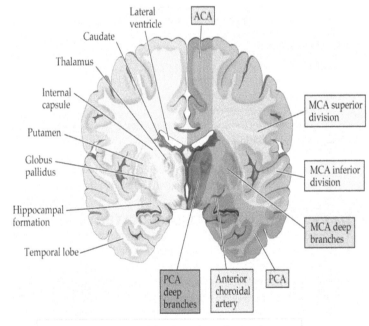

Fig. 1.6.9. Regional blood supply to the Cerebrum

## C. ARTERIAL CIRCLE OF WILLIS

- The terminal branches of the vertebral and internal carotid arteries all anastomose to form a circular blood vessel, called the Circle of Willis.
- There are three main (paired) constituents of the Circle of Willis:
  - **Anterior cerebral arteries**: These are terminal branches of the internal carotids.
  - **Internal carotid arteries**: Present immediately proximal to the origin of the middle cerebral arteries.
  - **Posterior cerebral arteries**: These are terminal branches of the vertebral arteries.
- To complete the circle, two 'connecting vessels' are also present:
  - **Anterior communicating artery:** This artery connects the two anterior cerebral arteries.
  - **Posterior communicating artery**: A branch of the internal carotid, this artery connects the ICA to the posterior cerebral artery.

## D. REGIONAL BLOOD SUPPLY TO THE CEREBRUM

- There are three cerebral arteries; anterior, middle and inferior.
  - o **The Anterior Cerebral Arteries** supply the **anteromedial** portion of the cerebrum.
  - o **The Middle Cerebral Arteries** are situated laterally, supplying the majority of the **lateral** part of the brain.
  - o **The Posterior Cerebral Arteries** supply both the medial and lateral parts of the **posterior** cerebrum.

## CLINICAL RELEVANCES:

### 1. COMPLETE MCA SYNDROMES (MRCEM 09/12/2015)

- Contralateral hemiplegia
- Contralateral hemiparesis
- Contralateral **homonymous hemianopia**
- Gaze preference to the ipsilateral side
- If dominant hemisphere involved:
  - o **Global aphasia**
- If non-dominant hemisphere involved:
  - o Hemispatial neglect
  - o **Anosognosia:** "lack of insight" or "lack of awareness"
  - o Construction apraxia

### 2. ACA SYNDROMES

- Paralysis of the contralateral foot and leg
- Sensory loss in the contralateral foot and leg
- Left sided strokes may develop transcortical motor aphasia
- Akinetic mutism, slowness and lack of spontaneity
- Gait apraxia
- Urinary incontinence which usually occurs with bilateral damage in the acute phase.
- Frontal cortical release reflexes: Contralateral gasp & sucking reflexes

*Note: If stroke occurs prior to the anterior communicating artery, it is usually well tolerated secondary to collateral circulation*

### 3. PCA STROKE

- **Peripheral (cortical):**
  - o Homonymous hemianopia
  - o Memory deficits
  - o Perversion (repeat response)
  - o Several visual deficits: cortical blindness, lack of depth perception, hallucinations.
- **Central (penetrating):**
  - o **Thalamus:** contralateral sensory loss, spontaneous pain
  - o **Cerebral peduncle:** CN III palsy with contralateral hemiplegia
  - o **Brain stem:** CN palsies, Nystagmus, pupillary abnormalities

### 4. DISSECTION OF VERTEBRAL ARTERY (MRCEM 09/12/2015)

- **Ipsilateral facial dysesthesia** (pain and numbness): most common symptom.
- Dysarthria or hoarseness (cranial nerves IX and X)
- Contralateral loss of pain and temperature sensation in the trunk and limbs.
- Ipsilateral loss of taste (nucleus and tractus solitarius).
- Hiccups, Vertigo, Nausea and vomiting
- Diplopia or oscillopsia (image movement experienced with head motion)
- Dysphagia (CN IX and X)
- Disequilibrium, Unilateral hearing loss
- Rarely, patients may manifest the following symptoms of a medial medullary syndrome:
  - o Contralateral weakness or paralysis (pyramidal tract)
  - o Contralateral numbness (medial lemniscus)
- Depending upon which areas of the brainstem or cerebellum are experiencing ischemia, the following signs may be present:
  - o Limb or truncal ataxia
  - o Nystagmus, Ipsilateral Horner syndrome
  - o Ipsilateral hypogeusia or ageusia (diminished or absent sense of taste)
  - o Ipsilateral impairment of fine touch and proprioception
  - o Contralateral impairment of pain and thermal sensation in the extremities (i.e., spinothalamic tract)
  - o Lateral medullary syndrome.

## E. VENTRICLES

- The ventricles are structures that produce cerebrospinal fluid, and transport it around the cranial cavity.
- CSF is produced by the **choroid plexus**, located in the lining of the ventricles.
- It consists of capillaries and loose connective tissue, surrounded by **cuboidal epithelial** cells.
- Plasma is filtered from the blood by the epithelial cells to produce CSF.
- In this way, the exact chemical composition of the fluid can be controlled.
- Drainage of the CFS occurs in the **subarachnoid cisterns** (or space).
- Small projections of arachnoid mater (called arachnoid granulations), protrude into the dura mater.
- They allow the fluid to drain into the **dural venous sinuses**.

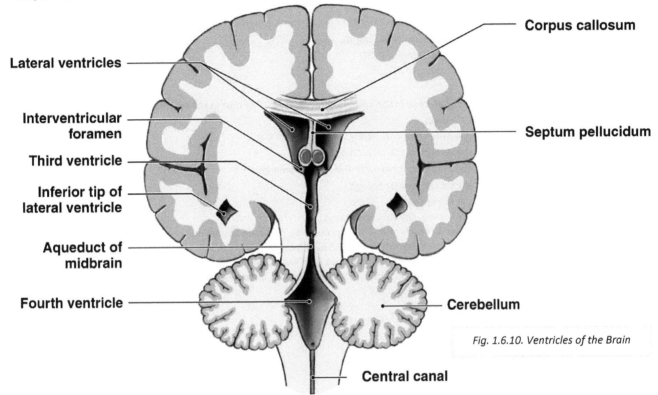

Fig. 1.6.10. Ventricles of the Brain

## A. TWO LATERAL VENTRICLES

- The left and right lateral ventricles are located within their respective hemispheres of the cerebrum.
- They have 'horns' which project into the frontal, occipital and temporal lobes. The volume of the lateral ventricles increases with age.

## B. THIRD VENTRICLE

- The lateral ventricles are connected to the third ventricle by *the foramen of Monro*
- The third ventricle is situated in between the right and the left thalamus.
- The anterior surface of the ventricle contains two protrusions:
  - Supraoptic recess: located above the optic chiasm.
  - Infundibular recess: located above the optic stalk.

## C. FOURTH VENTRICLE

- The fourth ventricle is the last in the system – it receives CSF from the third ventricle via *the Cerebral Aqueduct or Aqueduct of sylvius.*
- It lies within the brainstem, at the junction between the pons and medulla oblongata.
- From the 4th ventricle, the fluid drains into 2 places:
  - Central spinal canal: Baths the spinal cord
  - Subarachnoid cisterns: Baths the brain, between arachnoid mater and pia mater. Here the CSF is reabsorbed back into the circulation.
- **The Lateral apertures** (of Luschka) are two of the foramina in the ventricular system and link the fourth ventricle and the quadrigeminal cistern.
- Together with **the Median aperture** (of Magendie) they comprise two of the three ways that CSF can leave the fourth ventricle and enter the subarachnoid space.

# CEREBROSPINAL FLUID

o    Characteristics of normal spinal fluid are below:

- Total volume: **150 mL**
- Color: Colorless, clear, like water
- Opening pressure: **90-180 mm H$_2$O** (with patient lying in lateral position)
- Osmolarity at 37°C: **281 mOsm/L**
- Specific gravity: 1.006 to 1.008
- Acid-base balance:
  - o    pH: 7.28-7.
  - o    Pc$_{o2}$: 47.9 mmHg
  - o    HCO$_3$-: 22.9 mEq/L
- Sodium: 135-150 mmol/L
- Glutamine: 8-18 mg/dL
- Lactic acid: 1.1-2.8 mmol/L
- Glucose: 45-80 mg/dL

- Potassium: 2.7-3.9 mmol/L
- Chloride: 116-127 mmol/L
- Calcium: 2.0-2.5 mEq/L (4.0 to 5.0 mg/dL)
- Magnesium: 2.0-2.5 mEq/L (2.4 to 3.1 mg/dL)
- Proteins: 20-40 mg/dL
- Prealbumin: 2-7%

  o    ***Note that normal concentration of glucose in CSF samples is 60-80% (2/3) of that in the plasma***

- Lactate dehydrogenase (LDH): <2.0-7.2 U/mL
- o    Absolute activity depends on testing method; approximately 10% of serum value
- **CSF lactate >35 mg/dL** is seen in patients with bacterial meningitis
- **CSF lactate 25-35 mg/dL** is seen in patients with tubercular and fungal meningitis
- **CSF lactate <25 mg/dL** is seen in patients with viral meningitis.
- Conditions associated with changes in the appearance of CSF:
  - o    **Infections meningitis**: Turbid, milky, cloudy CSF samples.
  - o    **Hemorrhage or traumatic tap**: Xantochromic CSF samples with increased hemoglobin.
  - o    **Kernicterus**: Xantochromic CSF samples with increased bilirubin.
  - o    **Meningeal melanosarcoma**: Xantochromic CSF samples with increased melanin.
  - o    **Disorders affecting blood-brain barrier**: Cloudy CSF samples with increased proteins (above 150 mg/dL) and albumin and IgG.

**Layers: Lumbar puncture: SSS I LED AS**
- **S**kin
- **S**uperficial fascia
- **S**upraspinous ligament
- **I**nterspinous ligament
- **L**igamentum flavum
- **E**pidural space
- **D**ura mater
- **A**rachnoid
- **S**ubarachnoid     space     containing cerebrospinal fluid

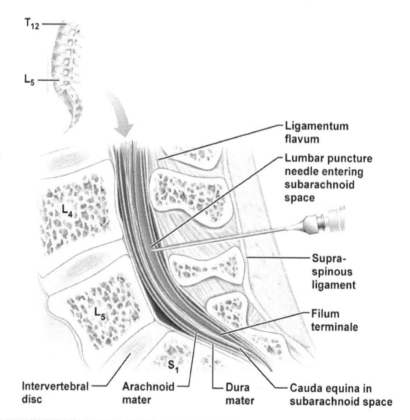

Fig. 1.6.11. Lumbar puncture; Layers penetrated by the spinal needle

# F. CAVERNOUS SINUS

- The cavernous sinuses are a clinically important pair of dural sinuses.
- They are located next to the lateral aspect of the body of the sphenoid bone.
- This sinus receives blood from the **superior and inferior ophthalmic veins**, the **middle superficial cerebral veins**, and from another dural venous sinus; the **sphenoparietal sinus**.
- **OTOM:** Lateral wall components, in order from superior to inferior
- **CA:** the components within the sinus, from medial to lateral
    - **O**: Oculomotor Nerve (III)
    - **T**: Trochlear Nerve (IV)
    - **O**: Ophthalmic Nerve (V1)
    - **M**: Maxillary Nerve (V2)
    - **C**: Carotid Artery (cooling of the blood before it reaches the brain)
    - **A**: Abducent Nerve (VI)
    - **T**: Trochlear Nerve (IV)

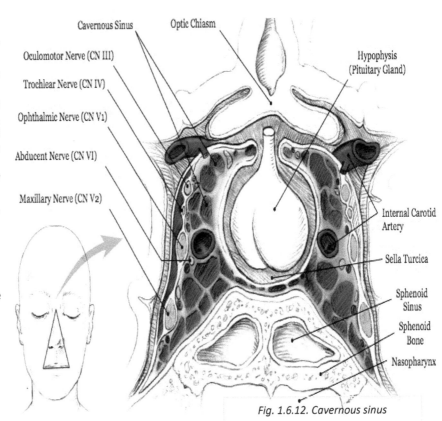

*Fig. 1.6.12. Cavernous sinus*

# CLINICAL RELEVANCE:
## FACIAL INFECTIONS AND CAVERNOUS SINUS THROMBOSIS

- The area of facial skin bounded by the nose, the eye, and the upper lip is a potentially dangerous zone to have an infection.
- For example, a boil in this region can cause thrombosis of the facial vein, with spread of organisms through the inferior ophthalmic veins to the cavernous sinus.
- The resulting cavernous sinus thrombosis may be fatal unless adequately treated with antibiotics

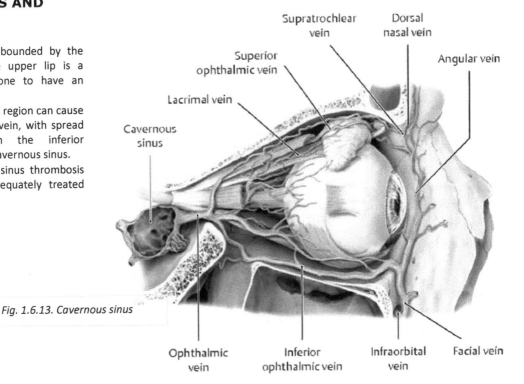

*Fig. 1.6.13. Cavernous sinus*

- *If the cavernous sinus becomes infected, these nerves are at risk of damage.*
- *The facial vein is connected to cavernous sinus via the superior ophthalmic vein.*
- *The facial vein is valveless; blood can reverse direction and flow from the facial vein to the cavernous sinus.*
- *This provides a potential pathway by which infection of the face can spread to the venous sinuses.*

# VI. HEMORRHAGE AND SHOCK CLASSIFICATIONS

- **Hemorrhage is the most common cause of shock in trauma patients.** The trauma patient's response to blood loss is made more complex by shifts of fluids among the fluid compartments in the body— particularly in the extracellular fluid compartment.
- The classic response to blood loss must be considered in the context of fluid shifts associated with soft tissue injury.

**DEFINITION OF HEMORRHAGE**

- Hemorrhage is defined as an acute loss of circulating blood volume.
- Although there is considerable variability, the normal adult blood volume is approximately 7% of body weight. For example, a 70-kg male has a circulating blood volume of approximately 5 L.
- The blood volume of obese adults is estimated based on their ideal body weight, because calculation based on actual weight can result in significant overestimation.
- The blood volume for a child is calculated as 8% to 9% of body weight (80–90 mL/kg).

## 1. DIFFERENT TYPES OF SHOCK

| CAUSES OF SHOCK | |
|---|---|
| **Hypovolaemic** | Haemorrhage<br>Gastroenteritis, stomal losses<br>Intussusception, volvulus<br>Burns<br>Peritonitis |
| **Distributive** | Septicaemia<br>Anaphylaxis<br>Vasodilating drugs<br>Spinal cord injury |
| **Cardiogenic** | Arrhythmias<br>Heart failure (cardiomyopathy, myocarditis)<br>Valvular disease<br>Myocardial contusion |
| **Obstructive** | Congenital cardiac (coarctation, hypoplastic left heart, aortic stenosis)<br>Tension/haemopneumothorax<br>Flail chest<br>Cardiac tamponade<br>Pulmonary embolism |
| **Dissociative** | Profound anaemia<br>Carbon monoxide poisoning<br>Methaemoglobinaemia |

| Class of shock | Class I | Class II | Class III | Class IV |
|---|---|---|---|---|
| **Volume Blood loss (ml)** | Up to 750 | 750-1500 | 1500-2000 | >2000 |
| **Volume of blood loss (%)** | 0-15% | 15-30% | 30-40% | >40% |
| **Heart Rate** | <100 | >100 | >120 | >140 |
| **Blood Pressure** | Normal | Normal | Decreased | Decreased |
| **Pulse Pressure** | Normal or increased | Decreased | Decreased | Decreased |
| **Respiratory Rate** | 14-20 | 20-30 | 30-40 | >35 |
| **Urine output (ml/h)** | >30 | 20-30 | 5-15 | Negligible |
| **Mental State** | Slightly anxious | Mildly anxious | Anxious, confused | Confused, lethargic |
| **Initial fluid replacement** | Crystalloid | Crystalloid | Crystalloid & blood | Crystalloid & blood |

## 2. DIRECT EFFECTS OF HEMORRHAGE

- The classification of hemorrhage into four classes based on clinical signs is a useful tool for estimating the percentage of acute blood loss.
- These changes represent a continuum of ongoing hemorrhage and serve only to guide initial therapy. **Subsequent volume replacement is determined by the patient's response to initial therapy.**
- This classification system is useful in emphasizing the early signs and pathophysiology of the shock state.
  - **Class I hemorrhage** is exemplified by the condition of an individual who has donated a unit of blood.
  - **Class II hemorrhage** is uncomplicated haemorrhage for which crystalloid fluid resuscitation is required.
  - **Class III hemorrhage** is a complicated haemorrhagic state in which at least crystalloid infusion is required and perhaps also blood replacement.
  - **Class IV haemorrhage** is considered a preterminal event; unless very aggressive measures are taken, the patient will die within minutes.
- Hemorrhage control and balanced fluid resuscitation must be initiated when early signs and symptoms of blood loss are apparent or suspected — not when the blood pressure is falling or absent. Bleeding patients need blood!

## 1. CLASS I HEMORRHAGE

- **Up to 15% Blood Volume Loss**
- The clinical symptoms of volume loss with class I haemorrhage are minimal.
- In uncomplicated situations, minimal tachycardia occurs. No measurable changes occur in blood pressure, pulse pressure, or respiratory rate.
- For otherwise healthy patients, **this amount of blood loss does not require replacement**, because transcapillary refill and other compensatory mechanisms will restore blood volume within 24 hours, usually without the need for blood transfusion.

## 2. CLASS II HEMORRHAGE

- **15% to 30% Blood Volume Loss**
- In a 70-kg male, volume loss with class II haemorrhage represents **750 to 1500 mL of blood**.
- Clinical signs include **tachycardia (heart rate above 100 in an adult), tachypnoea, and decreased pulse pressure;** the latter sign is related primarily to a rise in the diastolic component due to an increase in circulating catecholamines.
- These agents produce an increase in peripheral vascular tone and resistance. Systolic pressure changes minimally in early haemorrhagic shock; therefore, it is important to evaluate pulse pressure rather than systolic pressure.
- Other pertinent clinical findings with this amount of blood loss include subtle central nervous system (CNS) changes, such as anxiety, fright, and hostility.
- Despite the significant blood loss and cardiovascular changes, urinary output is only mildly affected. The measured urine flow is usually 20 to 30 mL/hour in an adult. Accompanying fluid losses can exaggerate the clinical manifestations of class II hemorrhage. Some patients in this category may eventually require blood transfusion, but most are stabilized initially with crystalloid solutions.

## 3. CLASS III HEMORRHAGE

- **30% to 40% Blood Volume Loss**
- The blood loss with class III hemorrhage (approximately **1500–2000 mL in an adult**) can be devastating. Patients almost always present with the classic signs of inadequate perfusion, including **marked tachycardia and tachypnoea, significant changes in mental status, and a measurable fall in systolic pressure**. In an uncomplicated case, this is the least amount of blood loss that consistently causes a drop in systolic pressure.
- Patients with this degree of blood loss almost always require transfusion.
- However, the priority of initial management is to stop the hemorrhage, by emergency operation or embolization if necessary.
- Most patients in this category will require packed red blood cells (pRBCs) and blood product resuscitation in order to reverse the shock state. The decision to transfuse blood is based on the patient's response to initial fluid resuscitation.

## 4. CLASS IV HEMORRHAGE

- **More than 40% Blood Volume Loss**
- The degree of exsanguination with class IV haemorrhage is immediately life-threatening. Symptoms include **marked tachycardia, a significant decrease in systolic blood pressure, and a very narrow pulse pressure** (or an unobtainable diastolic pressure). Urinary output is negligible, and mental status is markedly depressed. The skin is cold and pale.
- Patients with class IV hemorrhage frequently **require rapid transfusion and immediate surgical intervention**. Loss of more than 50% of blood volume results in loss of consciousness and decreased pulse and blood pressure.

# VII. VISUAL FIELDS AND PATHWAYS

## 1. OVERVIEW

- The optic nerve (CN II) is the second cranial nerve. It is responsible for transmitting the special sensory information for **sight**. It is one of two nerves that do not join with the **brainstem** (the other being the olfactory nerve, CN I).

- Embryologically, the optic nerve is developed from the **optic vesicle**, an out-pocketing of the forebrain. Thus, the entirety of the nerve can be considered part of the central nervous system and as a consequence, examining the optic nerve (usually performed via ophthalmoscopy) enables an assessment of intra-cranial health to be made. Due to its unique anatomical relation to the brain, the optic nerve is surrounded by **cranial meninges** (not by epi-, peri- and endoneurium like most other nerves).

## 2. ANATOMICAL COURSE

- The anatomical course of the optic nerve describes the transmission of special sensory information from the **retina** of the eye to the **primary visual cortex** of the brain.

- It can be divided into extracranial (outside the cranial cavity), and intracranial parts:

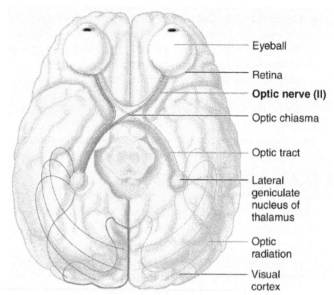

*Fig. 1.6.14. Visual fields and Pathways*

### EXTRACRANIAL

- The optic nerve is formed by the convergence of axons from the **retinal ganglion cells**. These cells in turn receive impulses from the photoreceptors of the eye (the rods and cones).

- After its formation, the nerve leaves the bony orbit via the **optic canal**, a passageway through the sphenoid bone. It enters the cranial cavity, running along the surface of the middle cranial fossa (in close proximity to the pituitary gland)

### INTRACRANIAL (THE VISUAL PATHWAY)

- Within the middle cranial fossa, the optic nerves from each eye unite to form the **optic chiasm**.

- At the chiasm, fibres from the nasal (medial) half of each retina cross over, forming the optic tracts:
  - **Left optic tract** – contains fibres from the left temporal (lateral) retina, and the right nasal (medial) retina.
  - **Right optic tract** – contains fibres from the right temporal retina, and the left nasal retina.

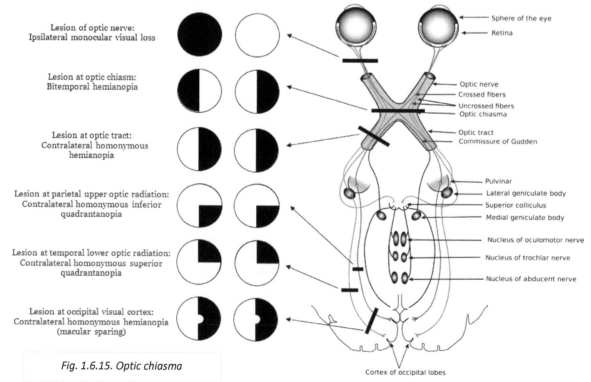

*Fig. 1.6.15. Optic chiasma*

- Each optic tract travels to its corresponding cerebral hemisphere to reach the **Lateral Geniculate Nucleus (LGN)**, a relay system located in the thalamus; the fibres synapse here.
- Axons from the LGN then carry visual information via a pathway known as the **optic radiation**. The pathway itself can be divided into:
  - **Upper optic radiation** – carries fibres from the superior retinal quadrants (corresponding to the inferior visual field quadrants). It travels through the parietal lobe to reach the visual cortex.
  - **Lower optic radiation** – carries fibres from the inferior retinal quadrants (corresponding to the superior visual field quadrants). It travels through the temporal lobe, via a pathway known as Meyers' loop, to reach the visual cortex.
- Once at the visual cortex, the brain processes the sensory data and responds appropriately.
- A pituitary adenoma is a tumour of the pituitary gland. Within the middle cranial fossa, the pituitary gland lies in close proximity to the **optic chiasm**. Enlargement of the pituitary gland can therefore affect the functioning of the optic nerve.
- Compression to the optic chiasm particularly affects the fibres that are crossing over from the nasal half of each retina. This produces visual defect affecting the peripheral vision in both eyes, known as a **bitemporal hemianopia**.
- Surgical intervention is commonly required. To access the gland, the surgeon uses a **transspehenoidal** approach, accessing the gland via the sphenoidal sinus.

## OPTIC CHIASM LESIONS

| LOCATION | VISUAL DEFECT |
| --- | --- |
| Optic nerve | Unilateral central scotoma |
| Optic Chiasm | Bitemporal hemianopsia |
| Anterior chiasm | Junctional defect (ipsilateral central scotoma and a contralateral superior temporal field cut) |
| Posterior chiasm | Central temporal scotomas |
| Optic tract | Incongruous homonymous hemianopsia, afferent pupillary defect, and bow-tie atrophy |
| Lateral geniculate nucleus | Homonymous sectoranopia |
| Lateral geniculate nucleus | Incongruous homonymous hemianopsia |
| Temporal lobe | Upper Homonymous Quadrantanopsia: Homonymous upper quadrant defect "pie in the sky". |
| Parietal lobe | Lower Homonymous Quadrantanopsia: Homonymous defect, denser inferiorly |
| Parietal lobe | **Gerstmann syndrome** and a homonymous defect, denser inferiorly |
| Not well-localized | Complete homonymous hemianopsia |
| Occipital lobe (lower bank) | Homonymous upper quadrantanopsia with macular sparing |
| Occipital lobe (upper bank) | Homonymous lower quadrantanopsia with macular sparing |
| Occipital lobe | Isolated homonymous defect (macular sparing) without other neurologic findings |
| Bilateral occipital lobe lesions | **Anton syndrome** (cortical blindness) |
| Bilateral occipitoparietal lesions | **Balint syndrome** |
| Left occipital lobe and angular gyrus | **Alexia without agraphia** |
| Bilateral occipito-temporal lesions | **Central achromatopsia** |

# VIII. PATHWAYS IN THE CNS

## A. ASCENDING AND DESCENDING TRACTS

| ASCENDING AND DESCENDING TRACTS | | | | Lesions |
|---|---|---|---|---|
| **Ascending Tracts** | **Dorsal Column Medial Lemniscus (DCML)** | Fine touch Vibration Proprioception | | **Ipsilateral** loss of proprioception & fine touch (Vit B12 def. & Tabes dorsalis) |
| | **Anterolateral** | **Anterior Spinothalamic** | Crude touch Pressure | **Contralateral** loss of pain and temperature |
| | | **Lateral spinothalamic** | Pain Temperature | |
| | **Spinocerebellar** unconscious sensation: Pain, Touch & Temperature | **Posterior spinocerebellar** **Anterior spinocerebellar** | Sensation from lower limb to ipsilateral cerebellum | **Ipsilateral** loss of muscles coordination |
| | | **Cuneocerebellar** **Rostral spinocerebellar** | Sensation from upper limb to ipsilateral cerebellum | |
| **Descending Tracts** | **Pyramidal** | Originates from **Cerebral cortex** | **Corticospinal** | Supplies muscle BODY |
| | | Voluntary control of muscles of body and face | **Corticobulbar** | Supplies muscle HEAD & NECK |
| | **Extrapyramidal** | Originates from **Brainstem** Involuntary and autonomic of all muscles: Muscles Tone, Balance, locomotion & Posture | **Vestibulospinal & Reticulospinal tracts** | Do not decussate, providing **ipsilateral** innervation. |
| | | | **Ruprospinal & Tectospinal tracts** | Do decussate, and therefore provide **contralateral** innervation |

## NEUROGENIC SHOCK & SPINAL SHOCK

- *Neurogenic shock* results from impairment of the descending sympathetic pathways in the cervical or upper thoracic spinal cord. This condition results in the loss of vasomotor tone and in sympathetic innervation to the heart. Neurogenic shock is rare in spinal cord injury below the level of T6; if shock is present in these patients, an alternative source should be strongly suspected.

- Loss of vasomotor tone causes vasodilation of visceral and lower-extremity blood vessels, pooling of blood, and, consequently, hypotension. Loss of sympathetic innervation to the heart may cause the development of bradycardia or at least a failure of tachycardia in response to hypovolemia. In this condition, the blood pressure may not be restored by fluid infusion alone, and massive fluid resuscitation may result in fluid overload and pulmonary edema. The blood pressure may often be restored by the judicious use of vasopressors after moderate volume replacement. Atropine may be used to counteract hemodynamically significant bradycardia.

- *Spinal shock* refers to the flaccidity (loss of muscle tone) and loss of reflexes seen after spinal cord injury. The "shock" to the injured cord may make it appear completely nonfunctional, although the cord may not necessarily be destroyed. The duration of this state is variable.

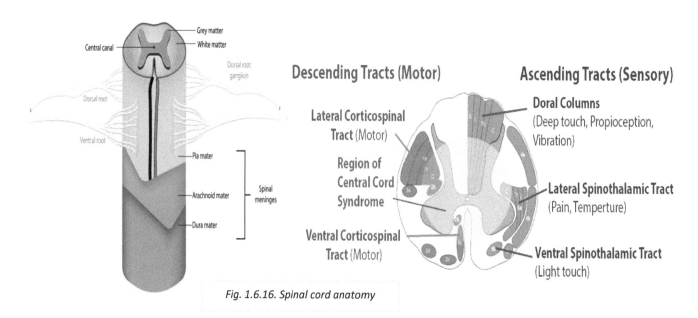

*Fig. 1.6.16. Spinal cord anatomy*

# SPINAL CORD SYNDROMES

- Certain characteristic patterns of neurologic injury are frequently encountered in patients with spinal cord injuries, such as central cord syndrome, anterior cord syndrome, and Brown-Séquard syndrome. These patterns should be recognized so they do not confuse the examiner.

## 1. CENTRAL CORD SYNDROME

- It is characterized by a disproportionately greater loss of motor strength in the upper extremities than in the lower extremities, with varying degrees of sensory loss. Usually this syndrome occurs after a hyperextension injury in a patient with preexisting cervical canal stenosis (often due to degenerative osteoarthritic changes), and the history is commonly that of a forward fall that resulted in a facial impact.
- Central cord syndrome is thought to be due to vascular compromise of the cord in the distribution of the anterior spinal artery. This artery supplies the central portions of the cord.
- Because the motor fibers to the cervical segments are topographically arranged toward the center of the cord, the arms and hands are the most severely affected.
- Central cord syndrome may occur with or without cervical spine fracture or dislocation. Recovery usually follows a characteristic pattern, with the lower extremities recovering strength first, bladder function next, and the proximal upper extremities and hands last.
- The prognosis for recovery in central cord injuries is somewhat better than with other incomplete injuries.

## 2. ANTERIOR CORD SYNDROME

- It is characterized by paraplegia and a dissociated sensory loss with a loss of pain and temperature sensation.
- Dorsal column function (position, vibration, and deep pressure sense) is preserved.
- Usually, anterior cord syndrome is due to infarction of the cord in the territory supplied by the anterior spinal artery. This syndrome has the poorest prognosis of the incomplete injuries.

## 3. BROWN-SÉQUARD SYNDROME

- Results from hemisection of the cord, usually as a result of a penetrating trauma. Although this syndrome is rarely seen, variations on the classic picture are not uncommon.
- In its pure form, the syndrome consists of ipsilateral motor loss (corticospinal tract) and loss of position sense (dorsal column), associated with contralateral loss of pain and temperature sensation beginning one to two levels below the level of injury (spinothalamic tract).
- Even when the syndrome is caused by a direct penetrating injury to the cord, some recovery is usually seen.

**BROWN-SÉQUARD SYNDROME**

- o *Refers to a **hemisection** (one sided lesion) of the spinal cord. This is most often due to traumatic injury, and involves both the anterolateral system and the DCML pathway:*
- o *DCML pathway: **ipsilateral loss of tactile sensation and proprioception***
- o *Anterolateral system: **contralateral loss of pain and temperature sensation.***
- o *It will also involve the descending motor tracts, causing **ipsilateral hemiparesis.***

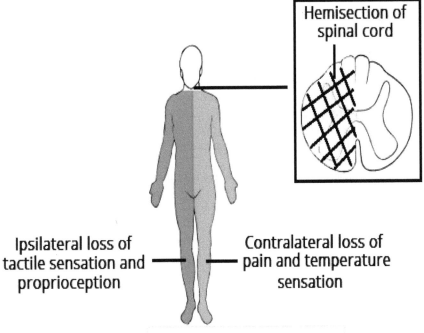

*Fig. 1.6.17. Brown-Séquard syndrome*

# PAST ASKED QUESTIONS

## True or False:

| | |
|---|---|
| The CSF is produced in the arachnoid granulations | F |
| Autoregulation maintains constant cerebral flow between MAP about 50 to 150 mmHg | T |
| The oculomotor nerve III is the only nerve passing through the cavernous sinus | F |
| Superior oblique internally rotates and depresses the eye | T |
| The retina and optic disk are supplied by branches of ophthalmic artery | T |
| Homonymous hemianopia indicates a lesion prior to the optic chiasm | F |
| Proximal branches of the Middle cerebral artery supply the internal capsule | T |
| The anterior cerebral circulation supplies the region of the motor cortex involved in movement of the face and arms | F |
| Lateral hemisection of the cord (Brown-Séquard) causes contralateral paralysis and ipsilateral loss of pain and temperature sensation below the level of the lesion | F |

## A 50 yr old patient with head injury and a deep laceration to the Scalp:

| | |
|---|---|
| Profuse bleeding indicates an injury involving the aponeurosis layer | F |
| The epicranial aponeurosis has no bony insertion anteriorly | T |
| There is a good anastomosis between blood vessels supplying the scalp | T |
| The patient is likely to develop black eyes | T |

## The following are true of palsies affecting the eye:

| | |
|---|---|
| The characteristic features of the 3rd nerve palsy is a small pupil with the pupil looking down and out | F |
| 4th nerve palsy results in loss of function of inferior oblique and a head tilt towards the side of the lesion | F |
| 4th nerve palsy is characterized of diplopia in the vertical gaze | T |
| 6th nerve palsy involves action of the lateral rectus | T |

## Which statements regarding cranial nerves are true?

| | |
|---|---|
| The maxillary division of trigeminal nerve exits the skull through foramen rotundum | T |
| The nucleus of the abducens nerve is located in the pons | T |
| The trochlear nerve is pure motor nerve | T |
| The facial nerve carries only sensory fibres | F |

## Normal cerebrospinal fluid has the following properties

| | |
|---|---|
| Opening pressure of 30-40cmH2O | F |
| CSF glucose concentration less than 1/3rd of serum glucose | F |
| Less than 5 leukocytes/mm3 | T |
| No red cells | T |

## True or False:

| | |
|---|---|
| Pyramidal tract upper motor neurons synapse with the lower motor neurons of the peripheral nerves in the ventral horns of the spinal cord T | T |
| Nerves fibres called A Delta fibre transmit the sharp immediate sensation of pain | T |
| Pain afferents terminate in the dorsal horn of the spinal column | T |
| Neurogenic shock is classified as a form of hypovolemic shock | F |

## The following statements are true:

| | |
|---|---|
| The transverse processes of the L5 are level with iliac crests | T |
| The lower pole of the right kidney is higher than the left | F |
| The spinal cord terminates at L2/3 in adults | F |
| The umbilicus is typically in the same plane as the L3/4 junction | T |

# SECTION 7: CRANIAL NERVE LESIONS

## 1. OLFACTORY NERVE (CRANIAL NERVE I)
o  **Special somatic sensory**: Olfaction (sense of smell)
o  **Damage**:
- Anosmia (loss of the sense of smell),
- hyposmia (a decreased sense of smell),
- parosmia (a perversion of the sense of smell), or
- Cacosmia (awareness of a disagreeable or offensive odor that does not exist) are common.

## 2. OPTIC NERVE (CRANIAL NERVE II)
o  **Special somatic sensory**: Vision
o  **Damage**:
- Immediate monocular blindness (partial or complete).
- Damage affects specific aspects of vision that depend on the location of the lesion.
- A person may not be able to see objects on their left or right sides (homonymous hemianopsia), or may have difficulty seeing objects on their outer visual fields (bitemporal hemianopsia) if the optic chiasm is involved.

## 3. OCULOMOTOR NERVE (CRANIAL NERVE III)
o  **Somatic motor** - Control of levator palpebrae superioris and the medial rectus, inferior oblique, superior and inferior rectus muscles for eye movement.
o  **Parasympathetic** - innervation of the ciliary ganglion controlling the sphincter pupillae and ciliary muscles.
o  **Damage**:
- Double vision (**diplopia**)
- Inability to coordinate the movements of both eyes (**strabismus**)
- Eyelid drooping (**ptosis**) and pupil dilation (**mydriasis**).
- Lesions may also lead to **inability to open the eye** due to paralysis of *the levator palpebrae muscle*.
- Individuals suffering from a lesion to the oculomotor nerve may compensate by tilting their heads to alleviate symptoms due to paralysis of one or more of the eye muscles it controls. The eye adopts a position known as '**down and out**'.

## 4. TROCHLEAR NERVE (CRANIAL NERVE IV)
o  **Somatic motor** - Control of the superior oblique muscle leading to depression and intorsion (inward rotation of the upper pole) of the eye.
o  **Damage**:
- A lesion of CN IV will paralyse the superior oblique muscle. There is no obvious affect of the resting orientation of the eyeball.
- However, the patient will complain of diplopia (double vision), and may develop a head tilt away from the site of the lesion.

## 5. TRIGEMINAL NERVE (CRANIAL NERVE V)
o  **General somatic sensory** - Sensation of touch, pain, proprioception and temperature for the face, mouth, nasal passages, anterior 2/3 of the tongue (posterior 1/3 CN IX) and part of the meninges (supratentorial dura mater).
o  **Branchial motor** - It also innervates the muscles of mastication (masseter, temporalis, lateral pterygoid, and medial pterygoid) and tensor tympani.
o  **Damage**:
- Conditions affecting the trigeminal nerve (CN V) include trigeminal neuralgia, cluster headache, and trigeminal zoster.
- Trigeminal neuralgia occurs later in life, from middle age onwards, most often after age 60, and is a condition typically associated with very strong pain distributed over the area innervated by the maxillary or mandibular nerve divisions of the trigeminal nerve ($V_2$ & $V_3$)
- Corneal drying, abrasions, and/or pain, decreased salivation, and, especially, anaesthesia of the forehead, eyebrow, and/or nose.

## 6. ABDUCENS NERVE (CRANIAL NERVE VI)
o  **Somatic motor** - Controls the lateral rectus, leading to abduction of the eye.
o  **Damage**:
- Damage to the abducens nerve (CN VI) can also result in diplopia.
- This is due to impairment in the lateral rectus muscle, which is innervated by the abducens nerve
- **In a complete injury** of the abducens nerve, the affected eye is turned medially.
- **In an incomplete injury,** the affected eye is seen at midline at rest, but the patient cannot deviate the eye laterally.

## 7. FACIAL NERVE (CRANIAL NERVE VII)
○ **Branchial motor** - Innervates the muscles of facial expression as well as the stapedius and digastric muscle.
○ **Parasympathetic** - Stimulates the lacrimal, sublingual, submandibular and other salivary glands (except parotid).
○ **Special visceral sensory** - Senses taste on the anterior 2/3 of the tongue (posterior 1/3 CN IX).
○ **Damage:**
  • Complete or partial paralysis of the face,
  • Hyperacusis, and/or an unusual or impaired sense of taste can occur.
  • The **"disinhibition syndrome"**, in which there is an increase in cochlear amplifier gain, can occur subsequent to head injury.

## 8. VESTIBULOCOCHLEAR NERVE (CRANIAL NERVE VIII)
○ **Special somatic sensory** - Controls the sensation of hearing and balance.
○ **Damage:**
  • When damaged, the vestibular nerve may give rise to the sensation of spinning and dizziness.
  • Damage to the cochlear nerve will cause partial or complete deafness in the affected ear.
  • Damage to the nerve endings can also cause tinnitus.
  • Damage to the vestibulocochlear nerve can also present as repetitive and involuntary eye movements (nystagmus), particularly when looking in a horizontal plane.

## 9. GLOSSOPHARYNGEAL NERVE (CRANIAL NERVE IX)
○ **Branchial motor** - innervates the stylopharyngeus
○ **Parasympathetic** - stimulates the parotid gland
○ **General somatic sensory** - detects sensation from the middle ear, near the External acoustic meatus (EAM), pharynx and posterior 1/3 of the tongue (anterior 2/3 CN V).
○ **Special visceral sensory** - sensation of taste on the posterior 1/3 of the tongue (anterior 2/3 CN VII).
○ **General visceral sensory** - innervates chemo and baroreceptors on the carotid bodies
○ **Damage:**
  • Unilateral absence of a gag reflex suggests a lesion of the glossopharyngeal nerve (CN IX), and perhaps the vagus nerve (CN X).

## 10. VAGUS NERVE (CRANIAL NERVE X)
○ **Branchial motor** - Innervates the muscles of the pharynx and larynx for swallowing and speech.
○ **Parasympathetic** - innervation of the heart, lungs and digestive tract down to the splenic flexure.
○ **General somatic sensory** - provides general sensation to the pharynx, meninges (posterior fossa) and a small region around the EAM.
○ **Special visceral sensory** - taste from the epiglottis and pharynx
○ **General visceral sensory** - chemo and baroreceptors of the aortic arch.
○ **Damage:**
  • Loss of function of the vagus nerve (X) will lead to a loss of parasympathetic innervation to a very large number of structures.
  • Major effects of damage to the vagus nerve may include a **rise in blood pressure and heart rate**.
  • Isolated dysfunction of only the vagus nerve is rare, but can be diagnosed by a hoarse voice, due to dysfunction of one of its branches, **the recurrent laryngeal nerve.**
  • Damage to this nerve may result in difficulties swallowing.

## 11. SPINAL ACCESSORY NERVE (CRANIAL NERVE XI)
○ **Branchial motor** - innervation of the sternocleidomastoid and upper part of trapezius muscle.
○ **Damage:**
  • Damage to the accessory nerve (CN XI) will lead to ipsilateral weakness in the trapezius muscle.
  • This can be tested by asking the subject to raise their shoulders or shrug, upon which the shoulder blade (scapula) will protrude into a winged position.
  • Additionally, if the nerve is damaged, weakness or an inability to elevate the scapula may be present because the levator scapulae muscle is now solely able to provide this function.
  • Depending on the location of the lesion there may also be weakness present in the sternocleidomastoid muscle, which acts to turn the head so that the face points to the opposite side.

## 12. HYPOGLOSSAL NERVE (CRANIAL NERVE XII)
○ **Somatic motor** - The intrinsic muscles of the tongue.
○ **Damage:**
  • The hypoglossal nerve (CN XII) is unique in that it is innervated from both the motor cortex of both hemispheres of the brain.
  • Damage to the nerve at **lower motor neuron** level may lead to fasciculations or atrophy of the muscles of the tongue.
  • **Upper motor neuron** damage will not lead to atrophy or fasciculations, but only weakness of the innervated muscles.

# Part Two: Physiology

Compiled and Edited by:
**Dr Moussa Issa**
MBChB MRCEM
Senior ED Registrar

# SECTION I: BASIC CELLULAR PHYSIOLOGY

## I. HOMEOSTASIS

### A. INTRODUCTION

- Homeostasis in a general sense refers to stability, balance or equilibrium.
- It is the body's attempt to maintain a constant internal environment.
- Homeostatic regulation involves three parts or mechanisms: 1) the receptor, 2) the control center and 3) the effector.
- *The receptor* or **detectors** receives information that something in the environment is changing.
- *The control center* or **comparators** or **integration center** receives and processes information from the receptor.
- *The effector* responds to the commands of the control center by either opposing or enhancing the stimulus.

### B. POSITIVE AND NEGATIVE FEEDBACK

### 1. NEGATIVE FEEDBACK

- A reaction in which the system responds in such a way as to reverse the direction of change.
- Since this tends to keep things constant, it allows the maintenance of homeostasis.
  - For instance, when the concentration of carbon dioxide in the human body increases, the lungs are signalled to increase their activity and expel more carbon dioxide.
  - Thermoregulation is another example of negative feedback. When body temperature rises, receptors in the skin and the hypothalamus sense a change, triggering a command from the brain. This command, in turn, effects the correct response, in this case a decrease in body temperature.
  - The negative feedback system operates around a narrow range of variables called "**set point**", which can vary throughout life.

### 2. POSITIVE FEEDBACK

- A response is to amplify the change in the variable.
- This has a destabilizing effect, so does not result in homeostasis.
- Positive feedback is less common in naturally occurring systems than negative feedback, but it has its applications.
  - For example, in nerves, a threshold electric potential triggers the generation of a much larger action potential.
  - Blood clotting in which the platelets process mechanisms to transform blood liquid to solidify is an example of positive feedback loop.
  - Another example is the secretion of oxytocin which provides a pathway for the uterus to contract, leading to child birth.

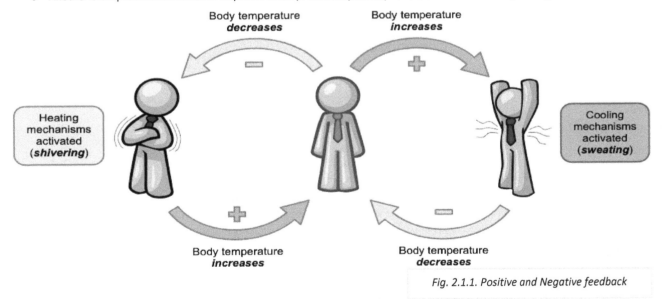

Fig. 2.1.1. Positive and Negative feedback

### 3. HARMFUL POSITIVE FEEDBACK

- Although Positive Feedback is needed within Homeostasis it also can be harmful at times.
- When you have a high fever it causes a metabolic change that can push the fever higher and higher.
- In rare occurrences the body temperature reaches 113 degrees Fahrenheit / 45 degrees Celsius and the cellular proteins stop working and the metabolism stops, resulting in death.

# II. COMPARTMENTS AND FLUID SPACES

## A. INTRODUCTION
- The human body may be conceptually divided into two major fluid compartments:
  - The intracellular compartment
  - The extracellular compartment.

### 1. THE INTRACELLULAR COMPARTMENT
- Is the space within the organism's cells; it is separated from the extracellular compartment by cell membrane.
- About two thirds of the human body's water is held in its cells and the remainder is found in the extracellular compartment.
- Intracellular fluid is contained by the cell's plasma membrane, and is the matrix in which cellular organelles are suspended, and chemical reactions take place.
- In humans, the intracellular compartment contains on average about **28 litres of fluid,** and under ordinary circumstances remains in osmotic equilibrium.
- *It contains moderate quantities of magnesium and sulphate ions.*

### 2. THE EXTRACELLULAR FLUIDS
- May be divided into three types:
  - Interstitial fluid in the "interstitial compartment" (surrounding tissue cells and bathing them in a solution of nutrients and other chemicals),
  - Blood plasma in the "intravascular compartment" (the blood vessels), and small amounts of transcellular fluid such as ocular and cerebrospinal fluids in the "transcellular compartment".

## COMPARTMENTS AND FLUID SPACES

| | | TOTAL BODY WEIGHT 70 KG 60% REPRESENT TOTAL BODY FLUID= 42 LITERS | | |
|---|---|---|---|---|
| **COMPARTMENTS** | | **FROM BODY WEIGHT (70Kg)** | | **IF 42L = 100% BODY FLUID (approx.)** |
| **INTRACELLULAR** | | 40% | 28L | 65% |
| **EXTRACELLULAR** | **PLASMA** | 5% | 3.5L | 13% |
| | **INTERSTITIAL** | 15% | 10.5L | 22% |
| **TOTAL BODY FLUID** | | 60% | 42L | 100% |

## IONS IN BODY FLUIDS

| ELECTROLYTES | ECF (35% TOTAL BODY FLUID) | | ICF (65% TBF) |
|---|---|---|---|
| | INTERSTITIAL (22% TBF) | PLASMA (13% TBF) | |
| **SODIUM** | 143 | 143 | 10 |
| **POTASSIUM** | 4 | 4 | 140 |
| **CALCIUM** | 3 | 3 | < 0.01 |
| **CHLORIDE** | 129 | 108 | 3-30 |
| **BICARBONATE** | 29 | 29 | 9 |

- The interstitial and intravascular compartments readily exchange water and solutes but the third extracellular compartment, *the transcellular*, is thought of as separate from the other two and not in dynamic equilibrium with them.
- The interstitial, intravascular and transcellular compartments comprise the extracellular compartment

### A. INTERSTITIAL COMPARTMENT
- The interstitial compartment (also called "tissue space") surrounds tissue cells. It is filled with interstitial fluid. Interstitial fluid provides the immediate microenvironment that allows for movement of ions, proteins and nutrients across the cell barrier.
- This fluid is not static, but is continually being refreshed and recollected by lymphatic channels.
- In the average male (70 kg) human body, the interstitial space has *approximately 10.5 liters of fluid*.

### B. INTRAVASCULAR COMPARTMENT (PLASMA)
- The main intravascular fluid in mammals is blood, a complex fluid with elements of a suspension (blood cells), colloid (globulins) and solutes (glucose and ions). The average volume of plasma in the average (70 kg) male is approximately *3.5 liters*.
- The volume of the intravascular compartment is regulated in part by hydrostatic pressure gradients and by reabsorption by the kidneys.

## C. TRANSCELLULAR COMPARTMENT

- The third extracellular compartment, the transcellular, consists of those spaces in the body where fluid does not normally collect in larger amounts, or where any significant fluid collection is physiologically nonfunctional.
- Examples of transcellular spaces include the eye, the central nervous system, and the peritoneal and pleural cavities.
- A small amount of fluid does exist normally in such spaces.

## B. FLUID SHIFTS

- It occurs when the body's fluids move between the fluid compartments. Physiologically, this occurs by a combination of hydrostatic pressure gradients and osmotic pressure gradients. Water will move from one space into the next passively across a semi permeable membrane until the hydrostatic and osmotic pressure gradients balance each other.

### 1. THIRD SPACING

- Third spacing is the unusual accumulation of fluid in a transcellular space.
- In medicine, the term is most commonly used with regard to burns, but also can refer to ascites and pleural effusions
- The actual volume of fluid in a patient's third space is difficult to accurately quantify.
- Third spacing conditions may include peritonitis, pyometritis, and pleural effusions.

### 2. OSMOSIS AND DIFFUSION

- **Osmosis** is the diffusion of water through a semi-permeable membrane from a hypotonic solution to a hypertonic solution (osmosis is passive).
- **Diffusion** is the passive random movement of molecules or particles in a fluid (liquid or gas) from a region in which they are in higher concentration to regions of lower concentration.
- Diffusion stops when a uniform concentration is established.

### 3. COMPARING SOLUTIONS

- o **Isotonic**: the solutions have the same concentration of solutes.
- o **Hypotonic:** a hypotonic solution has a lower solute concentration than the other.
- o **Hypertonic:** a hypertonic solution has a higher solute concentration than the other.
- o **Solute:** dissolved substances.
- o **Solvent:** the substance in which the solute dissolves.
- o **Flux:** the amount of solute that crosses a given area in a given amount of time, in millimoles /cm²sec.
- Remember
  - o Water is the solvent of life.
  - o The higher the solute concentration the lower the water concentration.
  - o A semi-permeable membrane is a partition that permits the passage of some substances but not others.
  - o Cell membranes are semi-permeable, typically allowing the passage of water more readily than the dissolved substances.

## C. MEMBRANE PERMEABILITY

- Small ions (Na⁺ and K⁺) have very limited permeability through the membrane directly, i.e. through small, transient, water-filled holes in the membrane. They are not completely impermeable.

### 1. SECONDARY ACTIVE TRANSPORT

- The **Na/K ATPAse** creates the concentration gradient: three Na+ out for every two K+ in.
- The Na gradient thus created; there is a **Na/Glucose symport** into the cell, to transport glucose into the cell, against glucose's concentration gradient.

### 2. Na⁺/K⁺ ATPASE PUMP MECHANISM

- The pump, after binding ATP, binds 3 intracellular Na+ ions.
- ATP is hydrolysed, leading to phosphorylation of the pump and subsequent release of ADP.
- A conformational change in the pump exposes the Na+ ions to the outside.
- ***The phosphorylated form of the pump has a low affinity for Na+ ions, so they are released.*** The pump binds 2 extracellular K+ ions.

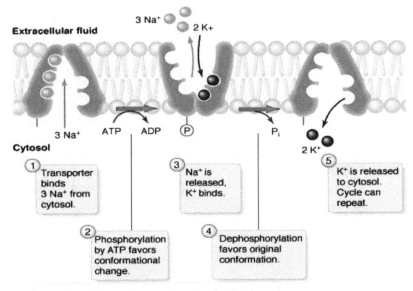

*Fig. 2.1.1. Positive and Negative feedback*

- This causes the dephosphorylation of the pump, reverting it to its previous conformational state, transporting the K+ ions into the cell.
- ***The unphosphorylated form of the pump has a higher affinity for Na+ ions than K+ ions, so the two bound K+ ions are released.***
- ATP binds, and the process starts again.

## 3. CELL VOLUME REGULATION:

- In the absence of active transport, cells tend to swell, due to impermeable solutes in the cell.
- The Sodium pump makes sodium behave as though it were an impermeable solute, as it constantly restores any small amounts of Na+ that leak into the cell. This effect is important to maintain fluid / volume homeostasis.

## 4. OSMOLES

- Both osmolarity and osmolality are defined in terms of osmoles.
- **An osmole** is a unit of measurement that describes the number of moles of a compound that contribute to the osmotic pressure of a chemical solution.
- The osmole is related to osmosis and is used in reference to solution where osmotic pressure is important, such as blood and urine.

## OSMOLARITY

- **Osmolarity** is defined as the number of osmoles of solute per liter (L) of solution. It is expressed in terms of **osmol/L or Osm/L.**
- A 1 mol/L NaCl solution has an osmolarity of 2 osmol/L. A mole of NaCl dissociates fully in water to yield two moles of particles: Na+ ions and Cl- ions. Each mole of NaCl becomes two osmoles in solution.

## OSMOLALITY

- **Osmolality** is defined as the number of osmoles of solute per kilogram of solvent. It is expressed in terms of **osmol/kg or Osm/kg.**
- The normal reference range is **275-295 mOSm per kg.**
- Since the amount of solvent will remain constant regardless of changes in temperature and pressure, osmolality will not be affected by these changes and is easier to evaluate and is more commonly used.
- Osmolality is measured using an osmometer, which works on the method of depression of the **freezing point.**

## Serum Osmolality = 2(Na + K) + Urea + Glucose

**Plasma contents**

- Three important proteins found in plasma are:
  - ○ Albumin,
  - ○ Clotting (coagulation) factors,
  - ○ Immunoglobulins

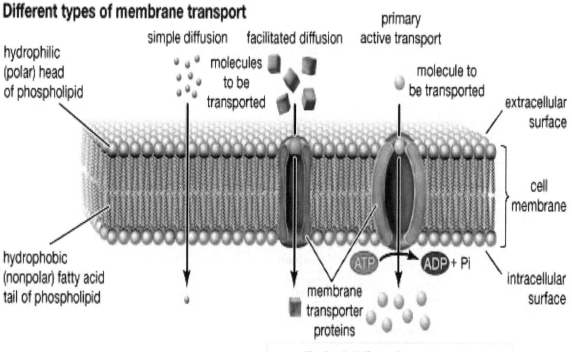

*Fig. 2.1.3. Cell membrane transports*

# III. KEY ASPECTS OF CELL STRUCTURE & FUNCTION

## 1. CELL MEMBRANES

- This membrane is very selective about what it allows to pass through; this characteristic is referred to as **"selective permeability."**
- For example, it allows oxygen and nutrients to enter the cell while keeping toxins and waste products out.
- The plasma membrane is a **double phospholipid membrane**, or a **lipid bilayer**, with the nonpolar hydrophobic tails pointing toward the inside of the membrane and the polar hydrophilic heads forming the inner and outer surfaces of the membrane.

### A. PROTEIN AND CHOLESTEROL

- There are a variety of membrane proteins that serve various functions:
- *Channel proteins:* Proteins that provide passageways through the membranes for certain hydrophilic or water-soluble substances such as polar and charged molecules. No energy is used during transport; hence this type of movement is called **facilitated diffusion.**
- *Transport proteins:* Proteins that spend energy (ATP) to transfer materials across the membrane. When energy is used to provide passageway for materials, the process is called *active transport*.
- *Recognition proteins:* Proteins that distinguish the identity of neighbouring cells. These proteins have oligosaccharide or short polysaccharide chains extending out from their cell surface.
- *Adhesion proteins:* Proteins that attach cells to neighbouring cells or provide anchors for the internal filaments and tubules that give stability to the cell.
- *Receptor proteins:* Proteins that initiate specific cell responses once hormones or other trigger molecules bind to them.
- *Electron transfer proteins:* Proteins that are involved in moving electrons from one molecule to another during chemical reactions.

### B. ACTIVE TRANSPORT ACROSS THE CELL MEMBRANE

- Active transport is the movement of solutes against a gradient and requires the expenditure of energy, usually in the form of ATP.
- Active transport is achieved through one of these two mechanisms:

#### PROTEIN PUMPS

- Transport proteins in the plasma membrane transfer solutes such as small ions ($Na^+$, $K^+$, $Cl^-$, $H^+$), amino acids, and monosaccharides.
- The proteins involved with active transport are also known as ion pumps.
- The protein binds to a molecule of the substance to be transported on one side of the membrane, and then it uses the released energy (ATP) to change its shape, and releases it on the other side.
- The protein pumps are specific; there is a different pump for each molecule to be transported.
- *Protein pumps are catalysts in the splitting of ATP $\rightarrow$ ADP + phosphate, so they are called ATPase enzymes.*
  - ○ *The sodium-potassium pump* (also called the $Na^+/K^+$-ATPase enzyme) actively moves sodium out of the cell and potassium into the cell. These pumps are found in the membrane of virtually every cell, and are essential in transmission of nerve impulses and in muscular contractions.
  - ○ Cystic fibrosis is a genetic disorder that results in a mutated chloride ion channel. By not regulating chloride secretion properly, water flow across the airway surface is reduced and the mucus becomes dehydrated and thick.

#### VESICULAR TRANSPORT

- Vesicles or other bodies in the cytoplasm move macromolecules across the plasma membrane. Types of vesicular transport include:
  - ○ *Exocytosis,* which describes the process of vesicles fusing with the plasma membrane and releasing their contents to the outside of the cell. This process is common when a cell produces substances for export.
  - ○ *Endocytosis,* which describes the capture of a substance outside the cell when the plasma membrane merges to engulf it. The substance subsequently enters the cytoplasm enclosed in a vesicle.
- **There are three kinds of endocytosis:**
  - ○ *Phagocytosis* or cellular eating occurs when the dissolved materials enter the cell. The plasma membrane engulfs the solid material, forming a phagocytic vesicle.
  - ○ *Pinocytosis* or cellular drinking occurs when the plasma membrane folds inward to form a channel allowing dissolved substances to enter the cell. When the channel is closed, the liquid is encircled within a pinocytic vesicle.
  - ○ *Receptor-mediated endocytosis* occurs when specific molecules in the fluid surrounding the cell bind to specialized receptors in the plasma membrane. As in pinocytosis, the plasma membrane folds inward and the formation of a vesicle follow.

## 2. CYTOPLASM

- The gel-like material within the cell membrane is referred to as the cytoplasm.
- It is a fluid matrix, the cytosol, which consists of 80% to 90% water, salts, organic molecules and many enzymes that catalyse reactions, along with dissolved substances such as proteins and nutrients.

Role:

- The cytoplasm plays an important role in a cell, serving as a "molecular soup" in which organelles are suspended and held together by a fatty membrane.

- It plays a mechanical role by moving around inside the membrane and pushing against the cell membrane helping to maintain the shape and consistency of the cell and again, to provide suspension to the organelles.
- It is also a storage space for chemical substances indispensable to life, which are involved in vital metabolic reactions, such as anaerobic glycolysis and protein synthesis.

## 3. CYTOSKELETON

- It helps cells maintain their shape and allows cells and their contents to move.
- The cytoskeleton allows certain cells such as neutrophils and macrophages to make amoeboid movements.
- The network is composed of three elements: microtubules, actin filaments, and intermediate fibers.

## 4. ORGANELLES

- Organelles are also known as cell compartments.
- Eukaryotic cells have membrane bound compartments in which specific metabolic activities takes place.
- The organelles of the prokaryotes are not membrane bound and are simpler structures.

### A. EUKARYOTIC ORGANELLES

- The cells of eukaryotic organelles are structurally complex and have organized interior compartments that are enclosed by lipid membranes. The list of organelles are as follows:

**Eukaryotic Organelles and their Functions**

| ORGANELLES | MAIN FUNCTION |
|---|---|
| Cytoplasm | • Transports substances and has many metabolic pathways |
| Nucleus | • Location of replication of genetic information in the form of DNA |
| Endoplasmic reticulum<br><br>Smooth ER= no ribosomes<br><br>Rough ER= with ribosomes | • Synthesis of lipids (smooth ER)<br><br>• Translation and folding of new proteins (rough ER) |
| Golgi apparatus | • Modification, sorting, stockage and transport of proteins and lipids<br><br>• Also forms lysosomes and Peroxisomes |
| Endosome | • Sorting and transport of substances into the cell |
| Lysosome | • Digestion of substances inside the cell |
| Peroxisome | • Oxidation of molecules |
| Ribosome | • Synthesis of proteins |
| Mitochondria | • Synthesis of ATP (Energy) by aerobic respiration |
| Chloroplast | • ATP synthesis by photosynthesis, and nitrogen fixation |

### B. PROKARYOTIC ORGANELLES

- Do not have compartmentalized organelles.
- Are not complex structurally as the eukaryotes
- The DNA of the prokaryotic cells are free floating in the cytosol and is surrounded by a cell membrane.
  - *Nucleoid, Pilli* (fimbria), *Flagellum, Plasmid, Ribosome (70S) and Mesosomes*

## 5. CELL METABOLISM

- *Catabolism:* The energy releasing process in which a chemical or food is used (broken down) by degradation or decomposition, into smaller pieces.
- *Anabolism:* Anabolism is just the opposite of catabolism. In this portion of metabolism, the cell consumes energy to produce larger molecules via smaller ones.

**ATP**

- ATP is the currency of the cell. The total quantity of ATP in the human body at any one time is about 0.1 Mole.
- The energy used by human cells requires the hydrolysis of 200 to 300 moles of ATP daily. ATP cannot be stored; hence its consumption must closely follow its synthesis. On a per-hour basis, 1 kilogram of ATP is created, processed and then recycled in the body.
- Looking at it another way, a single cell uses about 10 million ATP molecules per second to meet its metabolic needs, and recycles all of its ATP molecules about every 20-30 seconds.

# 6. CELLULAR RESPIRATION

- Cellular respiration is the energy releasing process by which sugar molecules are broken down by a series of reactions and the chemical energy gets converted to energy stored in ATP molecules. *The reactions that convert the fuel (glucose) to usable cellular energy (ATP) are Glycolysis, the Krebs cycle (sometimes called the citric acid cycle), and the Electron transport chain*
- Altogether these reactions are referred to as "cellular respiration" or "aerobic respiration." Oxygen is needed as the final electron acceptor, and carrying out cellular respiration is the very reason we breathe and the reason we eat.

## A. GLYCOLYSIS

- The glycolytic pathway (glycolysis) is where glucose, the smallest molecule that a carbohydrate can be broken into during digestion, gets oxidized and broken into two *3-carbon molecules (pyruvates)*, which are then fed into the Krebs's Cycle.
- *Glycolysis is the beginning of cellular respiration and takes place in the cytoplasm.*
- *2 molecules of ATP are required for glycolysis, but 4 are produced so there is a net gain of 2 ATP per glucose molecule*
- Two NADH molecules transfer electrons (in the form of hydrogen ions) to the electron transport chain in the mitochondria, where they will be used to generate additional ATP.
- During physical exertion when the mitochondria are already producing the maximum ATP possible with the amount of oxygen available, glycolysis can continue to produce an additional 2 ATP per glucose molecule without sending the electrons to the mitochondria.
- However, during this anaerobic respiration lactic acid is produced, which may accumulate and lead to temporary muscle cramping.

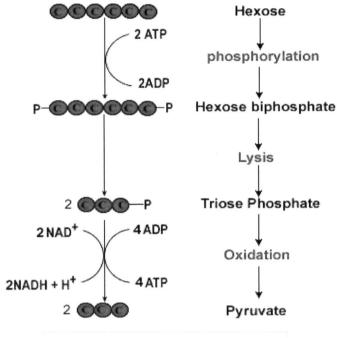

*Fig. 2.1.4. Glycolysis*

## B. KREBS CYCLE (SUMMARY)

- This is also called the *tricarboxylic acid cycle*.
- When oxygen is present, acetyl-CoA is produced from the pyruvate molecules created from glycolysis.
- When oxygen is present, the mitochondria will undergo aerobic respiration which leads to the Krebs cycle.
- However, if oxygen is not present, fermentation of the pyruvate molecule will occur. In the presence of oxygen, when acetyl-CoA is produced, the molecule then enters the citric acid cycle (Krebs cycle) inside the mitochondrial matrix, and is oxidized to $CO_2$ while at the same time reducing NAD to NADH. NADH can be used by the electron transport chain to create further ATP as part of oxidative phosphorylation. To fully oxidize the equivalent of one glucose molecule, two acetyl-CoA must be metabolized by the Krebs cycle. Two waste products, $H_2O$ and $CO_2$, are created during this cycle.
- The citric acid cycle is an 8-step process involving different enzymes and co-enzymes. During the cycle, acetyl-CoA (2 carbons) + oxaloacetate (4 carbons) yields citrate (6 carbons), which is rearranged to a more reactive form called isocitrate (6 carbons).
- Isocitrate is modified to become α-ketoglutarate (5 carbons), succinyl-CoA, succinate, fumarate, malate, and, finally, oxaloacetate.
- The net gain of high-energy compounds from one cycle is 3 Nicotinamide adenine dinucleotide (NADH), 1 Flavin adenine dinucleotide (FADH₂), and 1 Guanosine Triphosphate (GTP); the GTP may subsequently be used to produce ATP.
- *Therefore, at the end of two cycles, the products are:*
  - *2 ATP,*
  - *6 NADH₂*
  - *2 FADH₂*
  - *2 QH₂ (ubiquinol) and*
  - *4 CO₂.*

## C. THE ELECTRON TRANSPORT CHAIN

- The electron transport chain is the stepwise process of cellular respiration that is responsible for producing:
  - Water (with the help of oxygen we breathe)
  - up to 34 ATP (thanks to the proton gradient)
  - NAD and FAD (which are recycled to be used again in the Citric acid cycle and glycolysis)
- This process happens in the mitochondria of Eukaryotes and cell membrane of Prokaryotes.
- This only happens in aerobic conditions (oxygen present). If there is a shortage of oxygen cellular respiration will take an alternative pathway at the end of glycolysis resulting in the production of lactic acid and ATP.

# IV. VESSEL FLUID DYNAMICS

## 1. BLOOD COMPOSITION

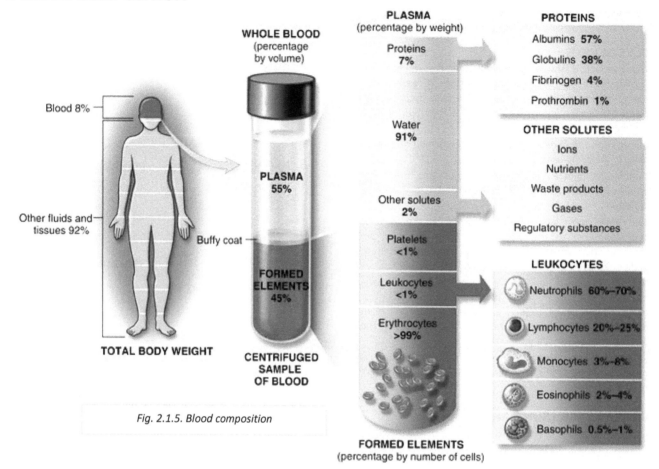

Fig. 2.1.5. Blood composition

## 2. CLOTTING PROTEINS

- Are mainly produced in the liver as well.
- There are at least 12 "clotting factors" that participate in the clotting process.
- One important clotting protein that is part of this group is *fibrinogen*, one of the main components in the formation of blood clots.
- In response to tissue damage, fibrinogen makes fibrin threads, which serve as adhesive in binding platelets, red blood cells, and other molecules together, to stop the blood flow.
- Plasma also carries Respiratory gases; CO2 in large amounts (about 97%) and O2 in small amounts (about 3%), various nutrients (glucose, fats), and wastes of metabolic exchange (urea, ammonia), hormones, and vitamins.

## 3. RED BLOOD CELLS (ERYTHROCYTES)

- RBCs are formed in the *myeloid tissue* or most commonly known *as red bone marrow*, although when the body is under severe conditions the yellow bone marrow, which is also in the fatty places of the marrow in the body will also make RBCs.
- The formation of RBCs is called **erythropoiesis**. Red blood cells lose nuclei upon maturation, and take on a **biconcave, dimpled, shape.**
- They are about 7-8 micrometers in diameter. There are about 1000x more red blood cells than white blood cells.
- RBCs live about **120 days** and do not self-repair. RBCs contain hemoglobin which transports oxygen from the lungs to the rest of the body, such as to the muscles, where it releases the oxygen load. The hemoglobin gets its red color from their respiratory pigments.
- RBCs lack a nucleus (no DNA) and no organelles, meaning that these cells cannot divide or replicate themselves like the cells in our skin and muscles.
- **Main Component:** The main component of the RBC is hemoglobin protein, of which there are about 250 million per cell.
- *Hemoglobin* is composed of four protein subunits: polypeptide globin chains that contain anywhere from 141 to 146 amino acids.
- Hemoglobin is responsible for the cell's ability to transport oxygen and carbon dioxide.
- Hemoglobin, iron, and oxygen interact with each other, forming the RBCs' bright red color. You can call this interaction by product **oxyhaemoglobin.**

- **Carbon Monoxide** binds with hemoglobin faster than oxygen, and stays bound for several hours, making hemoglobin temporarily unavailable for oxygen transport.
- **Carbaminohemoglobin** is a compound of hemoglobin and carbon dioxide, and is one of the forms in which carbon dioxide exists in the blood.
- **Destruction:**
  - Erythrocytes are removed by the reticulo-endothelial system.
  - *The globin* part of the hemoglobin is broken down into amino acid components, which in turn are recycled by the body.
  - *The iron* is recovered and returned to the bone marrow to be reused.
  - *The heme* portion of the molecule experiences a chemical change and then gets excreted as bile pigment (bilirubin) by the liver.
  - Heme portion after being broken down contributes to the color of feces and skin color changing after being bruised.

- **Types of Hb:**
  - **Hb F to Hb A switch at 3-6 months**
  - **Hb A ($\alpha2\beta2$)**        **: 96-98%**
  - **Hb A2 ($\alpha2\delta2$)**       **: 1.5-3.2%**
  - **Hb F ($\alpha2\gamma2$)**        **: 0.5-0.8%**

- **Normal values range:**
  - Reticulocytes     : 0.5-2% (50-100 $10^9$/L)
  - RBC             : 4.5-5.3 million (Female 4.1- 5.1millions)
  - Hb              : 13-18 (11.5-16.5)
  - Hct             : 39-50 (36-44)
  - MCV           : 80-98

## 4. WHITE BLOOD CELLS (LEUKOCYTES)

- **Shape**: White blood cells are different from red cells in the fact that they are usually larger in size 10-14 micrometers in diameter.
- White blood cells also have nuclei that are somewhat segmented and are surrounded by electrons inside the membrane.
- **Functions**: White blood cells are made in the bone marrow but they also divide in the blood and lymphatic systems.
- Types of WBC's: Basophils, Eosinophils, Neutrophils, Monocytes, B- and T-cell lymphocytes.
- Neutrophils, Eosinophils, and Basophils are all granular leukocytes.
- Lymphocytes and Monocytes are agranular leukocytes.
  - **Basophils** store and synthesize histamine which is important in allergic reactions. They enter the tissues and become "**Mast Cells**" which help blood flow to injured tissues by the release of histamine.
  - **Eosinophils** are chemotoxic and kill parasites.
  - **Neutrophils** are the first to act when there is an infection and are also the most abundant white blood cells. Neutrophils fight bacteria and viruses by phagocytosis. The life span of a Neutrophil is only about **12-48 hours.**
  - **Monocytes** are the biggest of the white blood cells and are responsible for rallying the cells to defend the body. Monocytes carry out phagocytosis and are also called **Macrophages**.
  - **Lymphocytes** help with our immune response. There are two Lymphocytes: the B- and T- cell:
    - B-Lymphocytes produce antibodies that find and mark pathogens for destruction.
    - T-Lymphocytes kill anything that they deem abnormal to the body.
- Neutrophils make up 50-70% of Granular cells; Eosinophils make up 2-4%, and Basophils 0-1%. Monocytes make up 2-8% of Agranular cells. B and T Lymphocytes make up 20-30%.

- **Normal Rage:**
  - WBC            : 4.0 - 11 $10^9$/L
  - Neutrophils     : 1.7-7.5 $10^9$/L
  - Lymphocytes    : 1.5-4.5 $10^9$/L
  - Monocytes      : 0.2-1.0 $10^9$/L
  - Eosinophils     : 0.0-0.5 $10^9$/L
  - Basophils       : 0.0 -0.1 $10^9$/L

## 5. PLATELETS (THROMBOCYTES)

- Platelets are membrane-bound cell fragments.
- Normal Value: *150-450 $10^9$/L*
- Platelets have no nucleus, they are between one to two micrometers in diameter, and are about 1/10th to 1/20th as abundant as white blood cells. *Platelets express HLA class 1 antigens on surface.*
- Less than 1% of whole blood consists of platelets.
- They result from fragmentation of large cells called ***Megakaryocytes***, which are cells derived from stem cells in the bone marrow.

- Platelets are produced at a rate of 200 billion per day.
- Their production is regulated by the hormone called **Thrombopoietin**.
- The circulating life of a platelet is **8–10 days.**
- The sticky surface of the platelets allows them to accumulate at the site of broken blood vessels to form a clot. This aids in the process of haemostasis.
- Platelets secrete factors that increase local platelet aggregation (e.g., Thromboxane A), enhance vasoconstriction (e.g., Serotonin), and promote blood coagulation (e.g., Factor 3 or tissue factor or tissue thromboplastin).

## 6. HEMOSTASIS

- When vessels are damaged, there are three mechanisms that promote hemostasis:
- **Vasoconstriction**: there is an immediate reflex, following damage that promotes reducing blood loss.
- **Platelet adhesion**: Collagen exposed from the damaged site will promote adhesion of platelets.
  - When platelets adhere to the damaged vessel, they undergo degranulation and release cytoplasmic granules, which contain serotonin, ADP and Thromboxane $A_2$.
    - Serotonin: vasoconstrictor
    - ADP: attracts more platelets to the area
    - Thromboxane $A_2$: promotes platelet aggregation, degranulation, and vasoconstriction.
- Thus, ADP and thromboxane A2 promote more platelet adhesion and therefore more ADP and thromboxane.
- **Formation of platelet plug**: by the *positive feedback mechanism*. The process of coagulation can now start:
  - *Damaged tissue releases factor III (tissue factor or tissue thromboplastin), which with the aid of $Ca^{++}$ will activate factor VII, thus initiating the Extrinsic Mechanism.*
  - *Factor XII from active platelets will activate factor XI, thus initiating the Intrinsic Mechanism.*
  - Both active factor VII and active factor XI will promote cascade reactions, eventually activating factor X.
  - Active factor X, along with factor III, factor V, $Ca^{++}$, and platelet thromboplastic factor ($PF_3$), will activate prothrombin activator.
  - *Prothrombin activator converts prothrombin to thrombin.*
  - *Thrombin converts fibrinogen to fibrin.*
  - Fibrin initially forms a loose mesh, but then factor XIII causes the formation of covalent cross links, which convert fibrin to a dense aggregation of fibers.
  - Platelets and red blood cells become caught in this mesh of fiber, thus the formation of a blood clot.

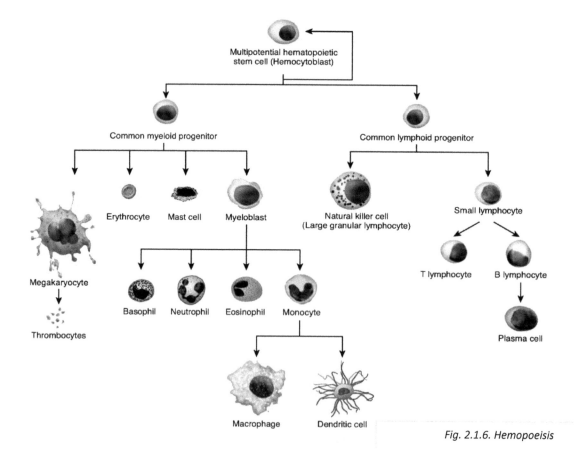

*Fig. 2.1.6. Hemopoeisis*

# V. NEUROLOGICAL ACTION POTENTIAL

## 1. OVERVIEW

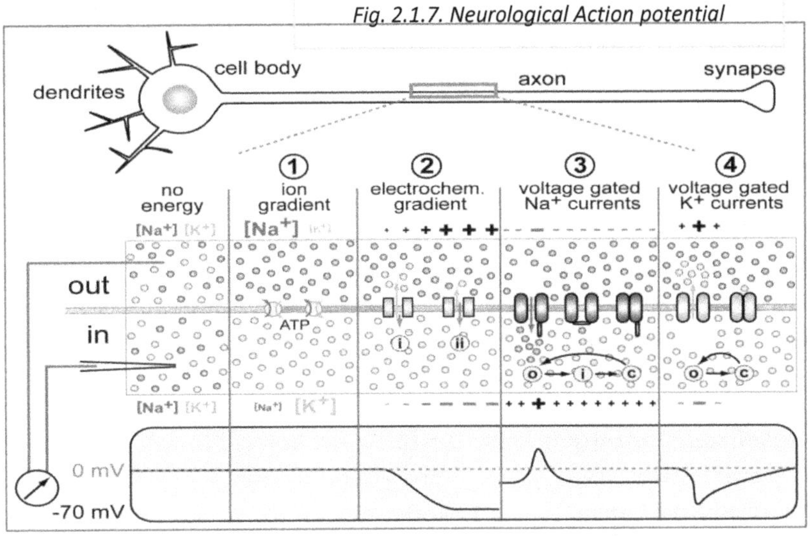

- When a neuron is inactive, just waiting for a nerve impulse to come along, *the neuron is polarized*; that is, the cytoplasm inside the cell has a negative electrical charge, and the fluid outside the cell has a positive charge. The electrical difference across the membrane of the neuron is called its *resting potential*. The resting potential is created by a transport protein called *the sodium-potassium pump*.

- This protein moves large numbers of sodium ions ($Na^+$) outside the cell, creating the positive charge. At the same time, the protein moves some potassium ($K^+$) ions into the cell's cytoplasm. Because the number of $Na^+$ ions moved outside the cell is greater than the number of $K^+$ ions moved inside, *the cell is more positive outside than inside*.

*Fig. 2.1.7. Neurological Action potential*

- When a stimulus reaches a resting neuron, the neuron transmits the signal as an impulse called an action potential.

- During an action potential, ions cross back and forth across the neuron's membrane, causing electrical changes that transmit the nerve impulse: The stimulus causes sodium channels in the neuron's membrane to open, allowing the $Na^+$ ions that were outside the membrane to rush into the cell. The sodium channels are *called gated ion channels* because they can open and close in response to signals like electrical changes.

- When the $Na^+$ ions enter the neuron, the cell's electrical potential becomes more positive. If the signal is strong enough and the voltage reaches a threshold, it triggers the action potential. More gated ion channels open, allowing more $Na^+$ ions inside the cell, and the cell depolarizes so that the charges across the membrane completely reverse: The inside of the cell becomes positively charged and the outside becomes negatively charged.

- The peak voltage of the action potential causes the gated sodium channels to close and potassium channels to open. Potassium ions move outside the membrane, and sodium ions stay inside the membrane, *repolarising the cell*.

- The result is a polarization that's opposite of the initial polarization that had $Na^+$ ions on the outside and $K^+$ ions on the inside.

- The neuron becomes hyperpolarized when more potassium ions are on the outside than sodium ions are on the inside.

- When the $K^+$ gates finally close, the neuron has slightly more $K^+$ ions on the outside than it has $Na^+$ ions on the inside.

- This causes the cell's potential to drop slightly lower than the resting potential. The neuron enters a refractory period, which returns potassium to the inside of the cell and sodium to the outside of the cell.

---

- ○ *Resting membrane potentials of neurons is -70mV.*
- ○ *Opening of voltage gated Na+ channels depolarise the nerve cell membrane causing the swift upstroke of the nerve cell action potential. After around 1ms the voltage gated Na+ channels close and the nerve cell membrane is repolarised by delayed opening of voltage gated K+ channels. The duration of a typical nerve cell action potential is 1-2 ms.*
- ○ *The value of the resting membrane potential varies from cell to cell, and ranges from about –20 mV to –100 mV:*
  - ▪ *Typical neuron, its value is –70 mv*
  - ▪ *Typical skeletal muscle cell, its value is –90 mv,*
  - ▪ *Typical epithelial cell, its value is closer to –50 mv.*
- ○ *Wrapping of the nerve cell membrane in layers of lipid rich electrically insulating myelin (myelination) allows action potentials to pass by direct conduction through the cytoplasm of myelinated regions of axon.*
- ○ *Direct conduction is much faster than membrane transmission of the all-or-nothing action potential and consequently myelinated axons conduct action potentials up to 50 times faster than unmyelinated nerves.*

---

## 2. EFFECT OF LIDOCAINE ON ACTION POTENTIALS

- Lidocaine, and most local anesthetics, block the sodium channels that are involved in the onset of an action potential.
- So, these drugs will reduce the probability that an action potential fires. Given that it alters signal conduction in neurons.
- At high enough concentrations, they inhibit the action potential altogether. With sufficient blockade, the membrane of the postsynaptic neuron will not depolarize and so fail to transmit an action potential, leading to its anaesthetic effects.
- That is why they are good at relieving pain. The pain stimulus is there, but the message never gets to the spinal cord and you don't react.

# VI. SYMPATHETIC & PARASYMPATHETIC NERVOUS SYSTEMS

|  | PARASYMPATHETIC NERVOUS SYSTEM | SYMPATHETIC NERVOUS SYSTEM |
|---|---|---|
| Introduction | Its general function is to control homeostasis and the body's **rest-and-digest** response. | Its general action is to mobilize the body's **fight-or-flight** response. |
| Function | Control the body's response while at rest. | Control the body's response during perceived threat. |
| Originates in | Spinal cord, medulla | Spinal cord, thoracic and lumbar spinal cord |
| Activates response of | Rest and digest | Fight-or-flight |
| Neuron Pathways | Longer pathways, slower system | Very short neurons, faster system |
| General Body Response | Counterbalance; restores body to state of calm. | Body speeds up, tenses up, and becomes more alert. Functions not critical to survival shut down. |
| Cardiovascular System (HR) | Decreases heart rate | Increases contraction, heart rate |
| Pulmonary System (lungs) | Bronchial tubes constrict | Bronchial tubes dilate |
| Musculoskeletal System | Muscles relax | Muscles contract |
| Pupils | Constrict | Dilate |
| Gastrointestinal System | Increases stomach movement and secretions | Decreases stomach movement and secretions |
| Salivary Glands | Saliva production increases | Saliva production decreases |
| Adrenal Gland | No involvement | Releases adrenaline |
| Glycogen to Glucose Conversion | No involvement | Increases; converts glycogen to glucose for muscle energy |
| Urinary Response | Increase in urinary output | Decrease in urinary output |

# VII. RECEPTORS

## A. ADRENERGIC RECEPTORS

- Useful generalizations concerning these are:
    - Activation of alpha 1 and beta 1 receptors cause stimulatory responses.
    - Activation of alpha 2, beta 2 & beta 3 receptors cause inhibitory responses.
    - Norepinephrine causes a greater response than Epinephrine when activating $\alpha1$ receptors ($\alpha1$: NE>E).
    - E causes a greater or equal response than NE when activating $\alpha 2$ receptors ($\alpha2$: E≥NE).
    - Both cause equal responses when activating beta 1 receptors ($\beta1$: E=NE).
    - Epinephrine causes a significantly greater response than Norepinephrine when activating $\beta2$ receptors ($\beta2$: E>NE).

| | | | |
|---|---|---|---|
| Adrenoreceptors | α1 | • Vasoconstriction<br>• Increased Peripheral resistance<br>• Increased BP | • Mydriasis<br>• Increased closure of internal sphincter of bladder |
| | α2 | Inhibition of:<br>• Norepinephrine release<br>• Ach release<br>• Insulin release | |
| | β1 | • Increased heart rate.<br>• Increased myocardia contractility<br>• Increased release of renin | • Increased lipolysis<br>• Increased platelet aggregation |
| | β2 | • Vasodilation<br>• Bronchodilation<br>• Slightly decreased Peripheral resistance | • Increased muscles and liver glycogenolysis<br>• Increased release glucagon<br>• Relax uterine smooth muscles |
| | β3 | • Lipolysis | |

# B. DOPAMINE RECEPTORS

- **Roles of Dopamine**
  - Role in movement
  - Role in pleasure and motivation
  - Controls the flow of information from other areas of the brain
- There are five types of dopamine receptors: D1 to D5. Categorized in two main subtypes:
  - **D1 like receptor family**:
    - The Gs protein is involved and adenylyl cyclase would be activated.
    - The action of the enzyme causes the conversion of adenosine triphosphate to cyclic adenosine monophosphate (cAMP).
  - **D2 like receptor family**:
    - Which is the receptor combining with the Gi protein and its activated alpha subunit then inhibits adenylyl cyclase so that the concentration of cAMP is reduced.
- **Dopamine Receptors**
  - The D1 and D5 receptors are closely related, and couple to Gs alpha and stimulate adenylyl cyclase activity.
  - In contrast, the D2, D3 and D4 receptors couple to Gi alpha and inhibit the formation of cAMP.
- **Therapeutic uses of DA1 Receptor Agonists**
  - Decreases peripheral resistance
  - Inducing lowering of arterial blood pressure;
  - Increases in heart rate and increases in sympathetic tone
  - Increases in activity of the renin aldosterone system
- **Therapeutic uses of DA2 receptor agonists**
  - Used for treating Parkinson's disease
  - Inhibits prolactin release (which decreases tumor size)

# C. ACH RECEPTORS

- Acetylcholine is released from a presynaptic neuron into the synaptic cleft. Once in the synaptic gap, acetylcholine can:
  - **Bind to presynaptic receptors:** presynaptic activation or inhibition leads to automodulation of the presynaptic cholinergic neuron.
  - **Be degradated by acetylcholinesterase**: activity of this enzyme on acetylcholine triggers its degradation into choline and acetyl coenzyme A, thus terminating its effect.
  - **Bind to postsynaptic receptors:** activation of these receptors by acetylcholine leads to cholinergic response.
- There are two types of acetylcholine receptors: **Muscarinic ad Nicotinic,** which are named after the agonist muscarine and nicotine, respectively. These receptors are functionally different, the muscarinic type being **G-protein coupled receptors (GPCRs)** that mediate a slow metabolic response via second messenger cascades, while the nicotinic type are **ligand-gated ion channels** that mediate a fast-synaptic transmission of the neurotransmitter.

## 1. MUSCARINIC CHOLINERGIC RECEPTORS

- Muscarinic receptors bind both acetylcholine and muscarine, an alkaloid present in certain poisonous mushrooms (it was first isolated in Amanita muscaria).
- Cholinergic transmission (acetylcholine-mediated) that activates muscarinic receptors occurs mainly at autonomic ganglia, organs innervated by the parasympathetic division of the autonomic nervous system and in the central nervous system.
- All muscarinic receptors are G-protein coupled receptors. There are five subtypes of muscarinic AChRs based on pharmacological activity: M1-M5.
  - **M1, M4 and M5 receptors: CNS**. These receptors are involved in complex CNS responses such as memory, arousal, attention and analgesia.
  - **M1 receptors** are also found at gastric parietal cells and autonomic ganglia.
  - **M2 receptors: heart.** Activation of M2 receptors lowers conduction velocity at sinoatrial and atrioventricular nodes, thus lowering HR.
  - **M3 receptors: smooth muscle.** Activation of M3 receptors at the smooth muscle level produces responses on a variety of organs that include: bronchial tissue, bladder, exocrine glands, among others.

## 2. NICOTINIC CHOLINERGIC RECEPTORS

- When bound to acetylcholine, these receptors undergo a conformational change that allows the entry of **sodium ions**, resulting in the depolarization of the effector cell.
- $N_1$ or $N_M$ **receptors:** these receptors are located at **the neuromuscular junction**; acetylcholine receptors of the $N_M$ subtype are the only acetylcholine receptors that can be found at the neuromuscular junction.
- $N_2$ or $N_N$ **receptors:** as mentioned before, nicotinic receptors play a key role in the transmission of cholinergic signals in the autonomic nervous systems. Nicotinic receptors of the $N_N$ subtype can be found both at cholinergic and adrenergic ganglia, but not at the target tissues (e.g., heart, bladder, etc). These receptors are also present in the CNS and adrenal medulla.

## NICOTINIC AND MUSCARINIC RECEPTORS AND THEIR ACTIONS

| MUSCARINIC | NICOTINIC |
|---|---|
| Bind muscarine | Bind nicotine |
| Blocked by **atropine (inhibits Vagus nerve)** | Blocked by **curare** (tubocurarine) |
| Linked to 2nd messenger systems through G proteins | Linked to ionic channels |
| Response is slow and prolonged | Response is brief and fast |
| Found on myocardial muscle, certain smooth muscle, and in discrete CNS regions | Located at neuromuscular junctions, autonomic ganglia, and to a small extent in the CNS |
| Mediate inhibition and excitation in target cells | Mediate excitation in target cells |
| Both pre- and postsynaptic | Postsynaptic |

## D. CELL SURFACE RECEPTORS

- Cell surface receptors are integral membrane proteins and, as such, have regions that contribute to three basic domains:
  - *Extracellular domains:* Some of the residues exposed to the outside of the cell interact with and bind the hormone - another term for these regions is the *ligand-binding domain*.
  - *Transmembrane domains:* Hydrophobic stretches of amino acids are "comfortable" in the lipid bilayer and serve to anchor the receptor in the membrane.
  - *Cytoplasmic or intracellular domains:* Tails or loops of the receptor that are within the cytoplasm react to hormone binding by interacting in some way with other molecules, leading to generation of second messengers. Cytoplasmic residues of the receptor are thus the *effector region* of the molecule.

## E. CYCLIC ADENOSINE MONOPHOSPHATE

- Cyclic adenosine monophosphate (cAMP, cyclic AMP, or 3',5'-cyclic adenosine monophosphate) *is a second messenger*, used for intracellular signal transduction, such as transferring into cells the effects of hormones like glucagon and Epinephrine, which cannot pass through the plasma membrane.
- Cyclic adenosine monophosphate (cAMP) is a nucleotide generated from ATP through the action of the enzyme adenylate cyclase.
- One prominent and important effect of elevated concentrations of cAMP is activation of a cAMP-dependent protein kinase called **protein kinase A.** Protein kinase A is nominally in a catalytically-inactive state, but becomes active when it binds cAMP.
- Upon activation, protein kinase A phosphorylates a number of other proteins, many of which are themselves enzymes that are either activated or suppressed by being phosphorylated. Such changes in enzymatic activity within the cell clearly alter its state. Adenylate cyclase is activated by a range of signalling molecules through the activation of adenylate cyclase stimulatory G (G$_s$)-protein-coupled receptors. *Adenylate cyclase* is inhibited by agonists of adenylate cyclase inhibitory G (G$_i$)-protein-coupled receptors.
- *Liver adenylate cyclase responds more strongly to glucagon, and muscle adenylate cyclase responds more strongly to adrenaline.*
- cAMP decomposition into AMP is catalysed by the *enzyme phosphodiesterase.*

## F. SECOND MESSENGER SYSTEMS

- Currently, four second messenger systems are recognized in cells, as summarized in the table below. *Note that not only do multiple hormones utilize the same second messenger system, but a single hormone can utilize more than one system.*

| Second Messenger | Examples of Hormones Which Utilize This System |
|---|---|
| *Cyclic AMP*<br><br>"PAGE-C" | - PTH<br>- All pituitary hormones except GH and Prolactin<br>- Glucagon<br>- Epinephrine and Norepinephrine<br>- Calcitonin |
| *Protein kinase activity*<br><br>"POEGGI" | - Prolactin & Oxytocin<br>- Erythropoietin<br>- GH<br>- Several Growth factors<br>- Insulin |
| *Calcium and/or phosphoinositides*<br><br>"AGATE" | - ADH<br>- GRH<br>- Angiotensin II<br>- TRH<br>- Epinephrine and Norepinephrine, |
| *Cyclic GMP*<br>"AN" | - Atrial natriuretic hormone<br>- Nitric oxide |

# VIII. MUSCLE PHYSIOLOGY

## 1. MUSCLES STRUCTURE

- Muscles are covered in a fibrous connective tissue, known as **Endomysium** which insulates each muscle fiber.
- Muscle fibers can range from 10 to 80 micrometers in diameter and may be up to 35cm long.
- Beneath the Endomysium and surrounding the muscle fibre is the **Sarcolemma** which is the fibres cell membrane.
- Beneath this is the **Sarcoplasm,** which is the cells cytoplasm, a gelatinous fluid which fills most cells. This contains Glycogen and Fats for energy and also Mitochondria which are the cells powerhouses, inside which the cells energy is produced.
- Each muscle fiber itself contains cylindrical organelles known as **Myofibrils.** Each muscle fiber contains hundreds to thousands of Myofibrils. These are bundles of **Actin and Myosin proteins** which run the length of the muscle fiber and are important in muscle contraction. Surrounding the Myofibril there is a network of tubules and channels called the **Sarcoplasmic Reticulum** in which Calcium is stored which is important in muscle contraction.
- Transverse tubules pass inwards from the Sarcolemma throughout the Myofibril, through which nerve impulses travel.
- Each Myofibril can then be broken down into functional repeating segments called **Sarcomeres.**

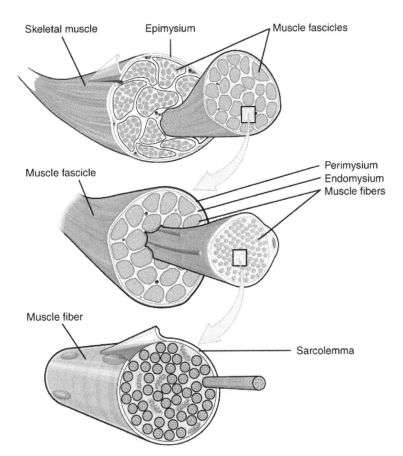

Fig. 2.1.8. Muscle structure

## 2. TYPES OF MUSCLES

- There are three types of muscles:
  - ○ **Smooth muscle or "involuntary muscle"**
  - ○ **Cardiac muscle is also an "involuntary muscle"**
  - ○ **Skeletal muscle or "voluntary muscle"**

| MUSCLES | LOCATION | FUNCTION | APPEARANCE | CONTROL |
|---|---|---|---|---|
| **SKELETAL** | Skeleton | Movement, heat, Posture | **Striated** Multinucleated Parallel fibers | **Voluntary** |
| **CARDIAC** | Heart | Pump blood continuously | **Striated** One central nucleus | **Involuntary** |
| **VISCERAL** | GIT Uterus, eyes Blood vessels | Peristalsis Blood pressure Pupil size Erects hairs | **No striations** One central nucleus | **Involuntary** |

| Which of the following statements are true regarding skeletal muscle contraction? | |
|---|---|
| A motor unit is composed of a single motor neuron and the one or more skeletal muscle fibres it supplies | T |
| Acetylcholine binds with muscarinic receptors at neuromuscular junction to initiate action potential | F |
| The resting membrane potential of muscle cells is -90mV | T |
| Ca2+ binds with Troponin T to initiate muscle contraction | F |
| **Which statement regarding nerve conduction are true** | |
| The resting membrane potential of neurons is 0Mv | F |
| Opening of voltage gated Na+ channels depolarise the nerve cell membrane | T |
| The nerve cell action potential lasts 100-200ms in duration | F |
| Myelination increases speed of action potential conduction | T |

# SECTION 2: RESPIRATORY PHYSIOLOGY
## I. THE RESPIRATORY CENTER (RC)

- Respiratory center is divided into four major cliques:

## RESPIRATORY CENTERS

### INSPIRATORY CENTER (DORSAL RESPIRATORY GROUP)

- o **Location:** Dorsal portion of medulla
- o **Nucleus:** Nucleus tractus solitarius
- o **Functions:**
  - Appears to be the physiologically most important brainstem center responsible for coordinating respiration.
  - In the absence of any afferent input, networks of neurons within the inspiratory center intrinsically display a rhythmic pattern of discharge that is transmitted to the diaphragm via the phrenic nerve and *is responsible for normal, quiet breathing.*
  - However, the Inspiratory Center is also the primary locus that receives sensory afferents from the chemoreceptors as well as lung receptors such as the pulmonary stretch receptors, irritant receptors, and J receptors

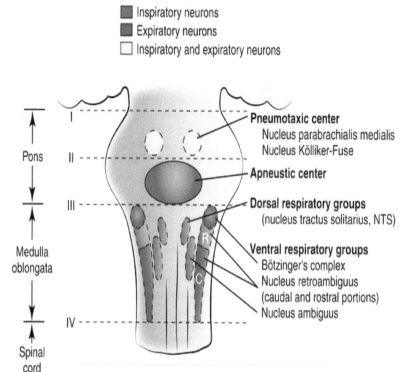

■ Inspiratory neurons
■ Expiratory neurons
□ Inspiratory and expiratory neurons

**Pneumotaxic center**
Nucleus parabrachialis medialis
Nucleus Kölliker-Fuse

**Apneustic center**

**Dorsal respiratory groups**
(nucleus tractus solitarius, NTS)

**Ventral respiratory groups**
Bötzinger's complex
Nucleus retroambiguus
(caudal and rostral portions)
Nucleus ambiguus

Pons I, II, III
Medulla oblongata
Spinal cord IV

*Fig. 2.2.1. Respiratory centers*

### EXPIRATORY CENTER (VENTRAL RESPIRATORY GROUP)

- o **Location:** Antero- lateral part of medulla, about 5 mm anterior and lateral to dorsal respiratory group.
- o **Nucleus:** Nucleus ambiguous and nucleus retro ambiguous.
- o **Function:**
  - Primarily activate the rectus abdominus and other expiratory muscles.
  - The expiratory center is normally quiescent during quiet breathing but can be activated by intense stimulation of the inspiratory center, thus providing active expiration of the lungs when inspiration is highly stimulated.
  - *It sends inhibitory impulse to the apneustic center.*

### PNEUMOTAXIC CENTER

- o **Location:** Pons (upper part)
- o **Nucleus:** Nucleus parabrachialis
- o **Function:**
  - Primarily acts to inhibit the length of ramping by the inspiratory center.
  - Pneumotaxic inhibition of inspiratory center ramping time results *in shallower and more frequent breaths, thus raising the respiratory rate but reducing inspiratory volume.*

### APNEUSTIC CENTER

- o **Location:** Pons (lower part)
- o **Functions:**
  - It discharges stimulatory impulse to the inspiratory center causing inspiration.
  - It receives inhibitory impulse from pneumotaxic center and from stretch receptor of lung.
  - It discharges inhibitory impulse to expiratory center.

### PRE BOTZINGER'S COMPLEX:

- *Located near the upper end of the medullary respiratory centre. Plays an important role in controlling breathing and responding to hypoxia. The BötC consists primarily of glycinergic neurons which inhibit respiratory activity.*
- *It contains pacemaker cells and nonpacemaker cells that initiate spontaneous breathing*

# II. RESPIRATORY CONTROL

## A. OVERVIEW

- The respiratory pattern profoundly influences the rate of alveolar ventilation which in turn determines the partial pressures of arterial oxygen and carbon dioxide and in turn the blood pH.
- These values reciprocally influence the pattern of respiration, allowing for a negative feedback control circuit that helps maintain relatively stable values of arterial oxygen, carbon dioxide, and pH.
- In the absence of derangements in arterial oxygen, carbon dioxide, and pH; the inspiratory center of the brainstem respiratory centers independently maintains the relatively stable respiratory pattern of normal, quiet breathing.

### 1. CHANGES IN ARTERIAL OXYGEN

- *The peripheral chemoreceptors are the only sensory component which can directly sense and respond to changes in the partial pressure of arterial oxygen* When hypoxemia ensues, the peripheral chemoreceptors are strongly activated and increase respiratory drive by activating the inspiratory brainstem respiratory centers.
- The resultant increase in alveolar ventilation thus aids in restoring arterial oxygen tension.
- Increased oxygen tensions may reduce afferent stimuli from the peripheral chemoreceptors, this does little to suppress respiration.

### 2. CHANGES TO CARBON DIOXIDE

- ***Changes to the partial pressure of arterial carbon dioxide are sensed by both the central and peripheral chemoreceptors*** However, modulation of the central chemoreceptors is by far more important in coordinating respiratory changes in response to changing in arterial $CO_2$ tension. Increased arterial partial pressures of $CO_2$ strongly stimulate the central chemoreceptors which send afferent signals to the inspiratory brainstem respiratory centers that increase respiratory drive.

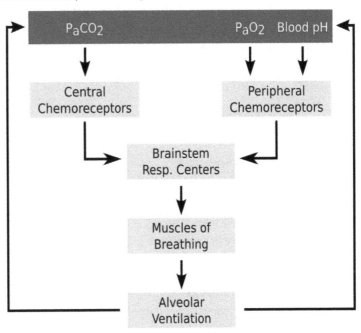

*Fig. 2.2.2. Respiratory control*

- The resultant increase in alveolar ventilation results in pulmonary elimination of carbon dioxide and thus restoration of lower arterial carbon dioxide levels. Conversely, decreased arterial partial pressures of $CO_2$ strongly suppress respiratory drive and thus reduce alveolar ventilation, allowing for build-up of arterial carbon dioxide levels.

### 3. CHANGES TO pH

- Changes to blood pH can profoundly modify the respiratory drive.
- Acidosis increases respiratory drive, thus increasing alveolar ventilation which helps increase the blood pH by breathing off of carbon dioxide. Conversely, alkalosis decreases respiratory drive, thus decreasing alveolar ventilation which helps reduce the blood pH by slowing elimination of carbon dioxide.
- *Changes to the pH of blood are likely sensed by both the central chemoreceptors as well as the aortic bodies of the peripheral chemoreceptors.* The peripheral chemoreceptors are likely the dominant afferent sensory stimulus for pH changes whereas the contribution of the central chemoreceptors displays slower kinetics given the extensive time required for free hydrogen ions to cross the relatively impermeable blood brain barrier.
- These sensors modulate the inspiratory brainstem respiratory centers to coordinate appropriate changes in respiratory drive.

## B. BARORECEPTORS AND CHEMORECEPTORS
### 1. BARORECEPTORS
- Baroreceptors (mechanoreceptors), sense changes in arterial pressure
- Pressure sensors are located in walls of **carotid sinus** and **aortic arch**

### a. Carotid sinus

- Responds to ↑ and ↓ in arterial pressure (BP)
- Nerve: **Glossopharyngeal nerve (CN IX)**
- Nucleus: Nucleus tractus solitarius of medulla

## b. Aortic arch

- Respond **ONLY** to ↑ in arterial pressure (BP)
- Nerve: **Vagus nerve (CN X)**
- Nucleus: Nucleus tractus solitarius of medulla

### BARORECEPTOR REFLEX

- e.g., **Hypotension and Hemorrhage:** ↓ arterial pressure
- ↓ arterial pressure → ↓ stretch → ↓ afferent baroreceptor firing → ↑ efferent sympathetic firing and ↓ efferent parasympathetic firing → vasoconstriction → ↑ HR → ↑ contractility → ↑ BP
- e.g., **Carotid Massage**
- ↑ pressure on carotid artery → ↑ stretch → ↑ afferent baroreceptor firing → ↓ HR

## 2. CHEMORECEPTORS
### a. Peripheral chemoreceptors

- Receptors in carotid and aortic bodies sense ↓ $PO_2$, ↑ $PCO_2$, ↓ pH
- **Carotid Bodies**
  - Nerve: **Glossopharyngeal nerve (CN IX)**
  - Nucleus: Nucleus tractus solitarius of medulla
- **Aortic Bodies**
  - Nerve: **Vagus nerve (CN X)**
  - Nucleus: Nucleus tractus solitarius of medulla

| Baroreceptors | | Carotid sinus | CN IX |
|---|---|---|---|
| | | Aortic Arch | CN X |
| Chemoreceptors | Peripheral | Carotid bodies | CN IX |
| | | Aortic bodies | CN X |
| | Central | Changes in PCO2 and pH only | |

### b. Central chemoreceptors

- Receptors in medulla sense ↑/↓ PCO2, ↑/↓ pH **(NOT ↑/↓ PO2)** in brain fluid
- PCO2, pH influenced by arterial CO2

# C. RESPIRATORY REFLEXES
## 1. CHEMORECEPTOR REFLEXES
- Detect changes in the chemical composition of the blood and CSF.

### a. CENTRAL CHEMORECEPTORS
- **Location:** On the ventrolateral surface of the medulla oblongata.
- **Stimulation:** changes in pco2 (pH) and in the cerebrospinal fluid.

### b. PERIPHERAL CHEMORECEPTORS
- **Location:**
  - **In the Carotid Bodies**: At the bifurcation of carotid arteries, innervated by the glossopharyngeal (IX) nerve.
  - **In the Aortic Bodies:** Above and below the aortic arch, innervated by the vagus (X) nerve.
- **Stimulation:** Detect a decrease in PO2 (hypoxia) and pH.
*NB: PCO2 affects pH so peripheral chemoreceptors will indirectly respond to increased PCO2 (hypercapnea).*

## 2. HERING-BREUER REFLEXES
- The Hering-Breuer reflexes function in controlling the inflation and deflation of the lungs during forced breathing.
- They are activated by either a stretching or a non-stretching and compression of the lung.
- Impulses are transmitted from the receptor sites through the **vagus nerve** to the brainstem and then to the respiratory center.
- **The Inflation Reflex**
  - Prevents the lungs from overinflating, which regulates tidal volume of the lungs. This inhibits the dorsal respiratory group and stimulates the expiratory center of the ventral respiratory group leading to active exhalation.
- **The Deflation Reflex**
  - Inhibits the expiratory centres and stimulates the inspiratory centres during a forced exhalation.

## 3. J RECEPTORS (JUXTAPULMONARY-CAPILLARY RECEPTORS)
- Located in, or near, the walls of pulmonary microvessels.
- They appear to be stimulated by vascular emboli, interstitial edema, and certain chemicals (phenyldiguanide or capsaicin).
- Information from the J-receptors is also delivered via the **vagus nerve** to the brain stem.
- Their stimulation results in rapid shallow breathing (tachypnoea).
- These receptors are thought to be responsible for the psychological sensation of "air hunger", also known as dyspnoea.

# III. LUNG VOLUME AND CAPACITY

## 1. SPIROMETRY

- Spirometry is the most commonly employed lung function test and can measure both the amount (volume) and speed (flow) of air that can be inhaled and exhaled. In asthma/COPD (obstructive lung disorders) the forced expiratory volume in 1 second (FEV1) is usually decreased, the forced vital capacity (FVC) is usually normal and the ratio FEV1/FVC is decreased.
- In restrictive disorders the FEV1 and FVC are both decreased, leaving a normal FEV1/FVC.
- Common measurements obtained by spirometry include:
  - **Vital capacity (VC) or forced vital capacity (FVC)** - the maximum amount of air that can be expelled from the lungs after a full inhalation
  - **Forced expiratory volume in 1 second (FEV1)**, volume of air which can be forcibly exhaled in one second
  - **Tidal volume (TV)** - the volume of air inhaled and exhaled during restful breathing.

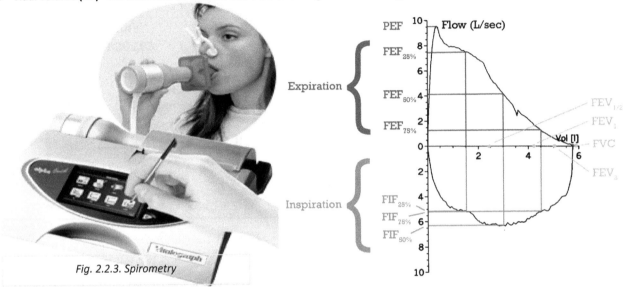

*Fig. 2.2.3. Spirometry*

## 2. WHOLE BODY PLETHYSMOGRAPHY OR HELIUM DILUTION.

- Spirometry cannot be used to measure residual volume (**RV**= the volume of air present in the lungs after a forced expiration) or any capacities which incorporate the residual volume such as functional residual capacity (**FRC**) and total lung capacity (**TLC**).
- Volumes and capacities which include the FRC are estimated using alternative techniques such as whole-body plethysmography or helium dilution.

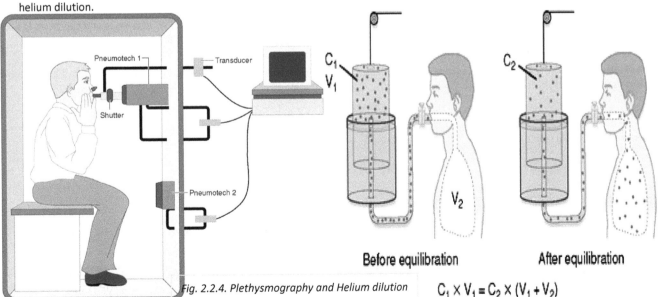

*Fig. 2.2.4. Plethysmography and Helium dilution*    $C_1 \times V_1 = C_2 \times (V_1 + V_2)$

*Body box (Plethysmography) measures all thoracic gas (including any bullae, pneumothorax, etc) while the Helium dilution can underestimate lung volumes in airway obstruction (bullae, pneumothorax don't receive helium).*

*Volume measured by body box is > Helium dilution*

## 3. LUNG VOLUMES

- *Tidal Volume (VT):* is the normal volume moved in or out of the lungs during quiet breathing. It is about **500ml.**

- *Vital capacity (VC):* is the maximum amount of air a person can expel from the lungs after a maximum inhalation. It is equal to the sum of inspiratory reserve volume, tidal volume, and expiratory reserve volume.

- *Forced vital capacity (FVC):* This measures the amount of air you can exhale with force after you inhale as deeply as possible. (3.7L females, 4.8L males).

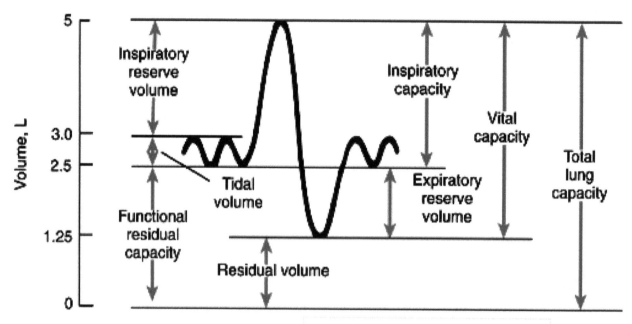

Fig. 2.2.5. Lung Volumes

- *Forced expiratory volume (FEV):*
  - This measures the amount of air you can exhale with force in one breath.
  - The amount of air you exhale may be measured at 1 second (FEV1), 2 seconds (FEV2), or 3 seconds (FEV3).
- *The FEV1 is reduced in both obstructive and restrictive lung disease.*
- *The FEV1 is reduced in obstructive lung disease because of increased airway resistance.*
- *It is reduced in restrictive lung disease because of the low vital capacity.*
- **FEV1/FVC:** This is the percentage of the vital capacity which is expired in the first second of maximal expiration. In healthy patients the FEV1/FVC is usually around 70%.
- Restrictive disorders have a near normal FEV1/FVC. In patients with obstructive lung disease FEV1/FVC decreases and can be as low as 20-30% in severe obstructive airway disease. $FEV_1$/FVC ratio <70% predicted is required for a diagnosis of COPD.
- *Forced expiratory flow 25% to 75%.* This measures the air flow halfway through an exhale.
- *Peak expiratory flow (PEF).* This measures how much air you can exhale when you try your hardest. It is usually measured at the same time as your forced vital capacity (FVC).

## 4. STAGES OF COPD

| Stage I | Mild COPD | FEV1/FVC<0.70 | $FEV_1 \geq$ 80% normal |
|---|---|---|---|
| Stage II | Moderate COPD | FEV1/FVC<0.70 | $FEV_1$ 50-79% normal |
| Stage III | Severe COPD | FEV1/FVC<0.70 | $FEV_1$ 30-49% normal |
| Stage IV | Very Severe COPD | FEV1/FVC<0.70 | $FEV_1$ <30% normal, or <50% normal with chronic respiratory failure present |

| COPD | RESTRICTIVE LUNG DISEASE |
|---|---|
| • FEV1/FVC <75%<br>• Raised FRC, TLC, RV, RV/TLC ratio (normal is 20%)<br>• Reduced KCO<br>KCO: CO Breath_Hold | • FEV1/FVC > 75% (with reduced FEV1 and FVC values)<br>• Reduced FRC, TLC, RV, VC, FEV1<br>• Reduced KCO: interstitial Lung disease<br>• Raised KCO: respiratory muscles weakness |

- *Maximum voluntary ventilation (MVV).* This measures the greatest amount of air you can breathe in and out during 1 minute.
- *Slow vital capacity (SVC).* This measures the amount of air you can slowly exhale after you inhale as deeply as possible.
- *Total lung capacity (TLC).* This measures the amount of air in your lungs after you inhale as deeply as possible. (4.7L females, 6L males).
- *Functional residual capacity (FRC).* This measures the amount of air in your lungs at the end of a normal exhaled breath.
- *Residual volume (RV).* This measures the amount of air in your lungs after you have exhaled completely. This is about **1000 ml.**
- *Expiratory reserve volume (ERV).* This measures the difference between the amount of air in your lungs after a normal exhale (FRC) and the amount after you exhale with force (RV). This is about **1400 ml of air.**
- **Diffusing Capacity of the Lung for Carbon Monoxide (DLCO):** Carbon monoxide can be used to measure the diffusing capacity of the lung.

- **Respiratory Minute Volume (or Minute Ventilation or Expired Minute Volume):** Volume of air moved into the lungs per minute. The normal tidal volume of a person is around 8- 10 ml per kg of weight. That is for a 70-kg person the tidal volume would be 700 ml.
- The normal respiratory rate is about 14- 18 breaths per minute. Hence,
- **Minute ventilation = Tidal Volume X Respiratory Rate.**
- *Minute ventilation for a 70-kg person would be 500 X 15 which would be approximately 7500ml.*

- Alveolar Ventilation: Volume of air available for gas exchange per minute.
*Alveolar Ventilation = (Tidal Volume - Dead Space) x (Respiratory Rate)*
*Normal alveolar ventilation value for a 70Kg person = (500 ml - 150 ml / breath) x (15 breaths / minute) = 5250 ml / minute*

   o **Dead Space Is 30% of Tidal Volume**: 150mls

> *Fig. 2.2.6. Lung volumes and capacities*

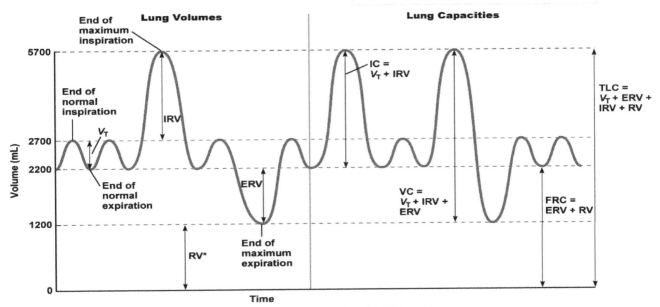

Normal lung volumes and capacities for a healthy 70-kg male

| Lung Volumes | Lung Capacities |
|---|---|
| $V_T$ = Tidal volume = 500 mL | IC = Inspiratory capacity = $V_T$ + IRV = 3500 mL |
| IRV = Inspiratory reserve volume = 3000 mL | VC = Vital capacity = $V_T$ + IRV + ERV = 4500 mL |
| ERV = Expiratory reserve volume = 1000 mL | FRC = Functional residual capacity = ERV + RV = 2200 mL |
| RV = Residual volume* = 1200 mL | TLC = Total lung capacity = $V_T$ + ERV + IRV + RV = 5700 mL |
| *Cannot be measured by spirometry | |

| Typical lung volumes and capacities of an adult male (70 Kg) would be: | |
|---|---|
| • Tidal volume | 500ml |
| • Inspiratory reserve volume | 2.0L |
| • Expiratory reserve volume | 1.0L |
| • Residual volume | 1.3L |
| • Total lung capacity | 5.0L |
| • Vital capacity | 4.8L |
| • Inspiratory capacity | 2.5L |
| • Functional residual capacity | 2.5L |

# IV. PNEUMOCYTES, SURFACTANT & COMPLIANCE

## 1. LUNG PNEUMOCYTES

### A. TYPE I PNEUMOCYTES

- De-oxygenated Type I pneumocytes (or squamous alveolar cells) cover approximately 90–95% of the alveolar surface, and are involved in the gas exchange between the alveoli and blood.

### B. TYPE II PNEUMOCYTES

- Type II pneumocytes cover a minority of the alveolar surface.
- Their function is **to secrete surfactant, which decreases surface tension within the alveoli.**
- They are also capable of cellular division, giving rise to more Type I pneumocytes when the lung tissue is damaged.

## 2. PULMONARY SURFACTANT

- Pulmonary surfactant is a **surface-active lipoprotein complex (phospholipoprotein)** formed by type II alveolar cells.
- The proteins and lipids that make up the surfactant have both hydrophilic and hydrophobic regions.

**Function of Surfactant:**
- To increase pulmonary compliance by decreasing the surface tension within the alveoli
- To prevent atelectasis (collapse of the lung) at the end of expiration.
- To facilitate recruitment of collapsed airways.

- Alveoli can be compared to gas in water, as the alveoli are wet and surround a central air space. The surface tension acts at the air-water interface and tends to make the bubble smaller (by decreasing the surface area of the interface).

**Laplace Law:** The gas pressure (P) needed to keep equilibrium between the collapsing force of surface tension (γ) and the expanding force of gas in an alveolus of radius (r) is expressed by the **Law** of Laplace: $P=2\gamma/r$

- The internal surface of the alveolus is covered with a thin coat of fluid. The water in this fluid has a high surface tension, and provides a force that could collapse the alveolus. The presence of surfactant in this fluid breaks up the surface tension of water, making it less likely that the alveolus can collapse inward.
- If the alveolus were to collapse, a great force would be required to open it, meaning that compliance would decrease drastically.
- In premature infants, **Hyaline Membrane Disease** develops because of impaired surfactant synthesis and secretion leading to atelectasis.

## 3. PULMONARY (LUNG) COMPLIANCE

- Compliance is the ability of lungs and thorax to expand. Lung compliance is defined as the volume change per unit of pressure change across the lung. Pulmonary compliance is calculated using the following equation, where ΔV is the change in volume, and ΔP is the change in pleural pressure: $Compliance=\Delta V/\Delta P$
- Pulmonary surfactant thus greatly reduces surface tension, increasing compliance allowing the lung to inflate much more easily, thereby reducing the work of breathing. It reduces the pressure difference needed to allow the lung to inflate.
- In clinical practice it is separated into two different measurements, static compliance and dynamic compliance.
    - **Static compliance** is the compliance measured when there is no gas flow into or out of the lung.
    - **Dynamic lung compliance** is the compliance of the lung at any given time during actual movement of air.
- **Low compliance**
    - Indicates a stiff lung and means extra work is required to bring in a normal volume of air.
    - The lung's compliance decreases and ventilation decreases when lung tissue becomes diseased and fibrotic.
    - This occurs as the lungs lose their distensibility and become stiffer.
- **High compliance (Emphysema)**
    - Higher compliance is the ability of lungs and thorax to expand.
    - The elastic tissue is damaged by enzymes.
    - These enzymes are secreted by leukocytes (white blood cells) in response to a variety of inhaled irritants, such as cigarette smoke.

| FACTORS AFFECTING LUNG COMPLIANCE | |
|---|---|
| **INCREASE** | **DECREASE** |
| o   High standing of a diaphragm | o   Supine position |
| o   Increasing age | o   Laparoscopic surgical interventions |
| o   Hydrothorax | o   Fibrosis: |
| o   Pneumothorax | • Severe restrictive pathologies |
| o   Emphysema/COPD | • Chronic restrictive pathologies (Lung Mesothelioma) |
| o   Acute asthma attacks: Increased compliance also occurs, for an unclear reason. | |

# V. AIRWAY RESISTANCE

- Higher Airway resistance is the opposition to flow caused by the forces of friction.
- It is defined as the ratio of driving pressure to the rate of air flow. *Resistance to flow in the airways depends on whether the flow is laminar or turbulent, on the dimensions of the airway, and on the viscosity of the gas.*

$$R=\Delta P/V$$

- **LAMINAR FLOW**
  - o Resistance is quite low. That is, a relatively small driving pressure is needed to produce a certain flow rate.
  - o Resistance during laminar flow may be calculated via a rearrangement of

    *Poiseuille's Law: $Q=\pi Pr^4/8\eta\iota$*

    - Q: Flow rate
    - P: Pressure
    - R: Radius
    - $\eta$: Fluid viscosity
    - $\iota$: Length of tubing
  - o The most important variable here is the radius, which, by virtue of its elevation to the fourth power, has a tremendous impact on the resistance. **Thus, if the diameter of a tube is doubled, resistance will drop by a factor of sixteen.**

- **TURBULENT FLOW**
  - o Resistance is relatively large. That is, compared with laminar flow, a much larger driving pressure would be required to produce the same flow rate.
  - o Because the pressure-flow relationship ceases to be linear during turbulent flow, no neat equation exists to compute its resistance.
  - o For this reason, the large and particularly the medium-sized airways actually provide greater resistance to flow than do the more numerous small airways.
- *Airway resistance decreases as lung volume increases because the airways distend as the lungs inflate, and wider airways have lower resistance.*

## FACTORS CONTRIBUTING TO AIRWAYS RESISTANCE

- o **Active factors: Autonomic nervous system**
  - Parasympathetic vagal stimulation causes bronchoconstriction and increased glandular secretion of mucus>>> increases resistance.
  - Sympathetic ß2 stimulation causes bronchodilation>>> decreases resistance.

- o **Local responses:**
  - Increased local $PCO_2$ or decrease local $PO_2$ causes dilation of small airways >>> decreases resistance.
  - Decreased local $PCO_2$ causes constriction of small airways >>> increases resistance.

- o **Passive factors:**
  - Airways resistance is inversely related to lung volume: Airways resistance is low at high lung volumes and high at low lung volumes. Raised Respiratory Rate leads to increasing turbulent flow >>> increasing airway resistance.
  - Airway collapse is most likely to occur in small airways with no cartilaginous support.

| Increased airway resistance | Decreased airway resistance |
|---|---|
| • Parasympathetic vagal stimulation | • Sympathetic β2 stimulation |
| • ↓PCO2 or ↑PO2 | • ↑PCO2 or ↓PO2 |
| • ↑RR | • ↓RR |
| • Low lung volumes | • High lung volumes |

## FACTORS AFFECTING PULMONARY VASCULAR RESISTANCE

| Pulmonary vascular Resistance | | Systemic Vascular Resistance | |
|---|---|---|---|
| **Increased by:** | **Decreased by:** | **Increased by:** | **Decreased by:** |
| Hypoxia↓PO2 | High FIO2 | Hyperoxia | Hypoxia |
| Hypercabia ↑PCO2 | Hypocarbia | Hypercabia (moderate) | Hypercabia (severe) |
| Acidosis | Alkalosis | Sympathetic stimulation | Vasodilatation |
| Hypervolemia | Anaemia | α-agonists | α-antagonists |
| Polycythaemia | Vasodilatation | | Calcium Channel Blockers |
| Atelectasis | α-antagonists | | Phosphodiesterase II |
| Increased airway pressure | PG E1 | | inhibitors |
| Sympathetic stimulation | | | |
| α-agonists | | | |
| N2O/ Ketamine | | | |

# VI. GAS TRANSPORT WITHIN THE CIRCULATION

*Atmosphere: The composition remains the same either is at sea level or altitude, but the Atmospheric pressure falls at altitude.*

- **Sea level:**
  - 78% Nitrogen (Partial Pressure = 78 kPa)
  - 21% Oxygen (Partial Pressure = 21 kPa)
  - 1% Argon
  - 0.04% $CO_2$
- **Atmospheric Pressure (sea Level):** 101kPa (760mmHg)
- **Alveolar Oxygen:** 14kPa (107mmHg)
- **Alveolar $CO_2$:** 4.8kPa (40mmHg)
- **Dead Space Is 30% of Tidal Volume:** 150mls

| Classification of respiratory Failure | |
|---|---|
| **Type I: HYPOXEMIC**<br>**Failure of Oxygenation** | **Type II: VENTILATORY**<br>**Respiratory Pump failure** |
| • *Oxygen < 8 KPa (60mmHg)*<br>• *$CO_2$ normal or decreased (<6 KPa/50mmHg)*<br>• *PA-aO2 increases* | • *Oxygen < 8kPa (60mmHg)*<br>• *$CO_2$ > 6kPa (50mmHg)*<br>• *PA-aO2 normal*<br>• *pH decreased (acidosis)* |

- Requirements for O2 delivery:
  - Atmosphere to alveoli
  - Across alveolar capillary membrane
  - Oxygen carrying capacity
  - Blood flow to tissues (Cardiac output)
- **Clinical causes for Hypoxia:**
  - **a. Hypoventilation**
    - $PCO_2$ increases (because Alveolar Ventilation decreases)
    - **Effect of supplementary Oxygen:** corrects hypoxia, (maybe) not Ventilation.
    - **Causes:**
      - ✓ Drugs overdose
      - ✓ Brain injury, Muscle weakness...

    *Pitfall: In Patient with Opiates Overdose or Brain Injury, saturation is not a valuable technique to monitor ventilation.*

  - **b. Diffusion impairment**
    - **Causes:** Thickening of alveolar capillary membrane in certain conditions such as Asbestosis, Sarcoidosis, and Rheumatoid Arthritis...
    - **Effect of supplementary Oxygen:** Hypoxia is easily corrected
  - **c. Shunt**
    - **Causes:** ARDS, AV fistulas, Pneumonia/Pus, Congenital Heart disease...
    - **Effect of supplementary Oxygen:** No amount of O2 will return the Saturation to Normal.
  - **d. Ventilation Perfusion inequality: see V/Q Mismatch**
    - P-V = S >>> perfusion without ventilation =Shunt
    - V-P = D >>> ventilation without perfusion = Dead Space
  - **e. Reduced FiO2: Altitude**

## 1. TRANSPORT OF OXYGEN

- 1.34 mls of oxygen carried per gramme of Hb.
- Each 100mls of blood contains 20mls of O2 (1liter of blood=200ml O2)
- The exchange of oxygen and carbon dioxide takes place in between the lungs and blood.
- The greater part of oxygen diffuses into the blood and at the same time, carbon dioxide diffuses out.

- The most part oxygen (about 97%) is now carried by the erythrocytes. In which it combines with the haemoglobin, the iron containing respiratory pigment under high concentration forming loose chemical compound the oxy-haemoglobin.
- Along the blood stream during circulation, the oxy-haemoglobin reaches the tissues, breaks up releasing most of its oxygen, and regains its normal purple color as haemoglobin, there by the blood acts as an efficient oxygen carrier.
- A small portion of oxygen (about 3%) also dissolves in the plasma and is carried in the form of solution to the tissues blood stream.
- Now this free oxygen, before entering into the tissue proper first passes into the tissue fluid and then enters the tissue by diffusion.
- In return, the carbon dioxide is given out by the tissues, dissolves in the tissue fluid and finally passes into the blood stream and conveyed of blood is 10 to 26 volumes of oxygen per 100 volumes of blood.
- The oxygen transport from lungs to tissues is achieved because haemoglobin has the highest affinity for oxygen at 100 mm Hg $PO_2$ (which is almost present in the alveolar air) and low affinity for oxygen at 40 mm Hg $PO_2$ which is prevalent in the tissues.
- So oxygen readily combines with the reduced haemoglobin of venous blood in the lungs and it is readily given off to the tissues by the arterial blood.
- The release of oxygen from blood is further increased by the fall in pH, increased $CO_2$ tension, and rise in temperature etc.

## 2. TRANSPORT OF CARBON DIOXIDE

- Solubility of CO2 is 20 times more than O2. A small portion of carbon dioxide, about 5 percent, remains unchanged and is transported dissolved in blood. The remainder is found in reversible chemical combinations in red blood cells or plasma.
- Some carbon dioxide binds to blood proteins, principally haemoglobin, to form a compound known as *carbamate*.
- About 88 percent of carbon dioxide in the blood is in the form of bicarbonate ion.
- The distribution of these chemical species between the interior of the red blood cell and the surrounding plasma varies greatly, with the red blood cells containing considerably less bicarbonate and more carbamate than the plasma.
- Less than 10 percent of the total quantity of carbon dioxide carried in the blood is eliminated during passage through the lungs.
- Complete elimination would lead to large changes in acidity between arterial and venous blood. Furthermore, blood normally remains in the pulmonary capillaries less than a second, an insufficient time to eliminate all carbon dioxide.
- Carbon dioxide enters blood in the tissues because its local partial pressure is greater than its partial pressure in blood flowing through the tissues. As carbon dioxide enters the blood, it combines with water to form carbonic acid ($H_2CO_3$), a relatively weak acid, which dissociates into hydrogen ions ($H^+$) and bicarbonate ions ($HCO_3^-$).
- Blood acidity is minimally affected by the released hydrogen ions because blood proteins, especially haemoglobin, are effective buffering agents. (A buffer solution resists change in acidity by combining with added hydrogen ions and, essentially, inactivating them.) The natural conversion of carbon dioxide to carbonic acid is a relatively slow process; however, carbonic anhydrase, a protein enzyme present inside the red blood cell, catalyses this reaction with sufficient rapidity that it is accomplished in only a fraction of a second.
- Because the enzyme is present only inside the red blood cell, bicarbonate accumulates to a much greater extent within the red cell than in the plasma. The capacity of blood to carry carbon dioxide as bicarbonate is enhanced by an ion transport system inside the red blood cell membrane that simultaneously moves a bicarbonate ion out of the cell and into the plasma in exchange for a chloride ion. The simultaneous exchange of these two ions, known as the chloride shift, permits the plasma to be used as a storage site for bicarbonate without changing the electrical charge of either the plasma or the red blood cell.
- Only 26 percent of the total carbon dioxide content of blood exists as bicarbonate inside the red blood cell, while 62 percent exists as bicarbonate in plasma; however, the bulk of bicarbonate ions is first produced inside the cell, and then transported to the plasma. A reverse sequence of reactions occurs when blood reaches the lung, where the partial pressure of carbon dioxide is lower than in the blood. Haemoglobin acts in another way to facilitate the transport of carbon dioxide. Amino groups of the haemoglobin molecule react reversibly with carbon dioxide in solution to yield carbamates.
- A few amino sites on haemoglobin are oxylabile, that is, their ability to bind carbon dioxide depends on the state of oxygenation of the haemoglobin molecule. The change in molecular configuration of haemoglobin that accompanies the release of oxygen leads to increased binding of carbon dioxide to oxylabile amino groups.
- Thus, release of oxygen in body tissues enhances binding of carbon dioxide as carbamate.
- Oxygenation of haemoglobin in the lungs has the reverse effect and leads to carbon dioxide elimination.
- Only 5 percent of carbon dioxide in the blood is transported free in physical solution without chemical change or binding, yet this pool is important, because only free carbon dioxide easily crosses biologic membranes. Virtually every molecule of carbon dioxide produced by metabolism must exist in the free form as it enters blood in the tissues and leaves capillaries in the lung.
- Between these two events, most carbon dioxide is transported as bicarbonate or carbamate.

### HENRY'S LAW

- *When a gas is in contact with the surface of a liquid, the amount of the gas which will go into solution is proportional to the partial pressure of that gas.*
- A simple rationale for Henry's law is that if the partial pressure of a gas is twice as high, then on the average twice as many molecules will hit the liquid surface in a given time interval, and on the average twice as many will be captured and go into solution.

## GRAHM'S LAW

- *States that oxygen and carbon dioxide (and other gases) move independently, at different rates, from an area of high pressure to an area of lower pressure.*

## RED BLOOD CELLS AND HAEMOGLOBIN

- The red blood cells contain a pigment called haemoglobin, each molecule of which binds four oxygen molecules to form Oxyhaemoglobin. The oxygen molecules are carried to individual cells in the body tissue where they are released.
- The binding of oxygen is a reversible reaction.

$$Hb + 4O_2 \rightleftharpoons Hb.4O_2$$

- At high oxygen concentrations oxyhaemoglobin forms, but at low oxygen concentrations oxyhaemoglobin dissociates to haemoglobin and oxygen. *The balance can be shown by an oxygen dissociation curve for oxyhaemoglobin.*

## 3. OXYGEN DISSOCIATION CURVE

- The curve shows that:
  - At relatively low oxygen concentrations there is uncombined haemoglobin in the blood and little or no oxyhaemoglobin, e.g. in body tissue
  - At relatively high oxygen concentrations there is little or no uncombined haemoglobin in the blood; it is in the form of oxyhaemoglobin, e.g. in the lungs.
  - Note Historically oxygen and carbon dioxide concentrations are expressed as partial pressures (measured in kPa), also called oxygen or carbon tension.
- The amount of oxygen held by the haemoglobin, i.e. its saturation level, is normally expressed as a percentage.
- *Oxygen dissociation curves can be used to illustrate Le Chatelier's Principle which states that a system in dynamic equilibrium responds to any stress by restoring the equilibrium.*
- For example, shifts in the position of the curve occur as a result of the concentration of $CO_2$ or changes in pH.

**LIRD** affinity: **L**eft **I**ncreases and **R**ight **D**ecreases affinity

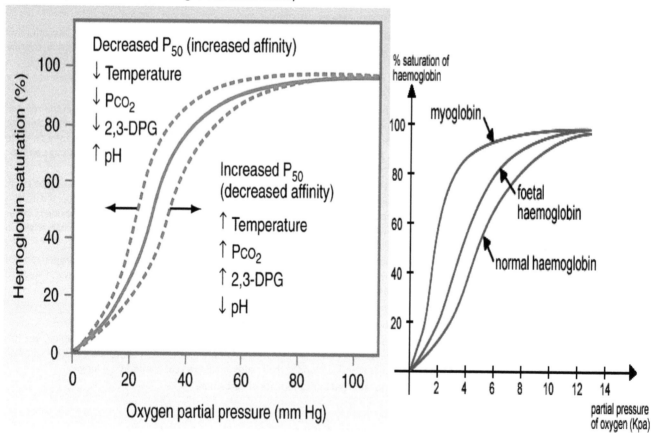

***CO Poisoning, Fetal Hb and Myoglobin have higher affinity to O2 (left shift)***

*Fig. 2.2.7. Oxygen dissociation curve*

## 4. THE EFFECT OF CARBON DIOXIDE IN THE BLOOD

- Haemoglobin can also bind carbon dioxide, but to a lesser extent. Carbaminohaemoglobin forms.
- Some carbon dioxide is carried in this form to the lungs from respiring tissues. *The presence of carbon dioxide helps the release of oxygen from haemoglobin; this is known as the* **Bohr Effect.**
- This can be seen by comparing the oxygen dissociation curves when there is less carbon dioxide present and when there is more carbon dioxide in the blood. When carbon dioxide diffuses into the blood plasma and then into the red blood cells (erythrocytes) in the presence of the catalyst carbonic anhydrase most $CO_2$ reacts with water in the erythrocytes and the following dynamic equilibrium is established

$$H_2O + CO_2 \rightleftharpoons H_2CO_3$$

- Carbonic acid, $H_2CO_3$, dissociates to form hydrogen ions and hydrogencarbonate ions. This is also a reversible reaction and undissociated carbonic acid, hydrogen ions and hydrogencarbonate ions exist in dynamic equilibrium with one another

$$H_2CO_3 \rightleftharpoons H^+ + HCO_3^-$$

- Inside the erythrocytes negatively charged $HCO_3^-$ ions diffuse from the cytoplasm to the plasma.
- *This is balanced by diffusion of chloride ions, Cl⁻, in the opposite direction, maintaining the balance of negative and positive ions either side. This is called the* **'chloride shift'.**
- The dissociation of carbonic acid increases the acidity of the blood (decreases its pH). Hydrogen ions, $H^+$, then react with oxyhaemoglobin to release bound oxygen and reduce the acidity of the blood.
- This buffering action allows large quantities of carbonic acid to be carried in the blood without major changes in blood pH.

$$Hb.4O_2 + H^+ \rightleftharpoons HHb+ + 4O_2$$

- It is this reversible reaction that accounts for the Bohr Effect. Carbon dioxide is a waste product of respiration and its concentration is high in the respiring cell and so it is here that haemoglobin releases oxygen.
- Carbon dioxide is removed to reduce its concentration in the cell and is transported to the lungs were its concentration is lower.
- This process is continuous since the oxygen concentration is always higher than the carbon dioxide concentration in the lungs.
- The opposite is true in respiring cells.

# VII. VENTILATION- PERFUSION RELATIONSHIP

- *In the typical adult, 1 litre of blood can hold about 200 mL of oxygen;*
- *1 litre of dry air has about 210 mL of oxygen.*
- On the other side Ventilation-perfusion mismatch is the term used when the ventilation and the perfusion of a gas exchanging unit are not matched.
- The actual values in the lung vary depending on the position within the lung. If taken as a whole, the typical value is approximately 0.8.
- Because the lung is centered vertically around the heart, part of the lung is superior to the heart, and part is inferior.
- This has a major impact on the V/Q ratio:
  - Apex of lung – higher
  - Base of lung – lower

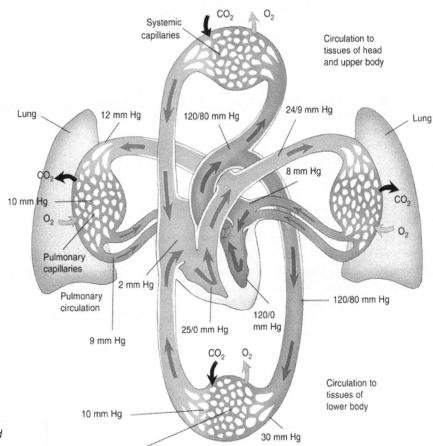

Fig. 2.2.8. Comparison of pulmonary and systemic blood flows and pressures.

## A. GRAVITY AND PULMONARY PERFUSION

- **Hydrostatic pressure**
  - o Pulmonary blood pressures (both arterial and venous) are low: mean pulmonary blood pressure = **15mmHg.**
  - o In an erect person, there is about 30cmH20 (23mmHg) difference between apex and base due to hydrostatic pressure.
  - o Both pulmonary arterial and venous pressure increases from apex to base.
  - o Blood flows at different levels change as per West's zone.

### WEST'S ZONES

- o **Zone 1** - PA>Pa>Pv (PA - pressure in alveoli)
- o **Zone 2** - Pa>PA>Pv (Pa - pressure in pulmonary artery)
- o **Zone 3** - Pa>Pv>PA (Pv - pressure in pulmonary vein)
- o **Zone 4** - very low volume

- **Zone 1 - PA>Pa>Pv**
  - o Pressure in alveoli is > than pulmonary arterial pressure.
    - capillary is squashed flat
    - no perfusion
    - "alveolar dead space"
  - o Zone 1 doesn't happen in normal person but happens when
    - PA increased - e.g. positive pressure ventilation
    - Pa decreased - e.g. massive haemorrhage

- **Zone 2 - Pa>PA>Pv**
  - o Moving down from zone 1, hydrostatic pressure raises both Pa and Pv so that PA is less than Pa but greater than Pv.
  - o Blood flow is present but dependent on the pressure difference between Pa and PA.
  - o Recruitment effect dominates here.
  - o Pv has no effect on blood flow
  - o Capillaries collapse at downstream end and pressure at the point of collapse (PA) limits flow: => **"Starling resistor" or "waterfall effect"**

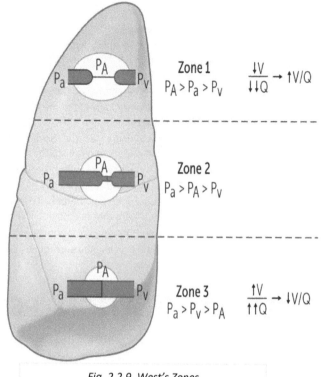

*Fig. 2.2.9. West's Zones*

- **Zone 3 - Pa>Pv>PA**
  - o Moving down from zone 2, hydrostatic pressure increases both Pa and Pv further and now PA is less than Pv.
  - o Blood flow is dependent on the pressure difference between Pa and Pv. Distension effect dominates here.

- **Zone 4 - very low volume**
  - o At very low volume:
    - Reduction in radial traction
    - Extra-alveolar vessels narrow
    - Pulmonary vascular resistance increase
    - Decrease in blood flow

## B. PATHOLOGY (V/Q MISMATCH)

- *Shunt*: an area with perfusion but no ventilation and thus a V/Q of zero.
- *Dead space*: an area with ventilation but no perfusion and thus a V/Q undefined though approaching infinity.
- Of note, few conditions constitute "pure" shunt or dead space as they would be incompatible with life, and thus the term V/Q mismatch is more appropriate for conditions in between these two extremes.
  - o P-V = S >>> perfusion without ventilation =Shunt= 0
  - o V-P = D >>> ventilation without perfusion = Dead Space= ∞
- The ventilation/perfusion (V/Q) ratio is the major determinant of PACO2 and PAO2:
  - o *A higher V/Q ratio (more ventilation relative to perfusion) decreases PACO2 but increases PAO2.*
  - o *A lower V/Q ratio (more perfusion relative to ventilation) raises PACO2 is high and lowers PAO2.*
- **Increased V/Q ration in:**
  - o Pulmonary embolism (normal ventilation, reduced perfusion)
  - o COPD (some areas have increased ventilation)
- **Decreased V/Q ratio occurs in:**
  - o Inhaled foreign body/ aspiration (reduced ventilation, normal perfusion)
  - o COPD (some areas have decreased ventilation)

o   Respiratory depression e.g. coma, sedative poisoning (reduced ventilation, normal perfusion)

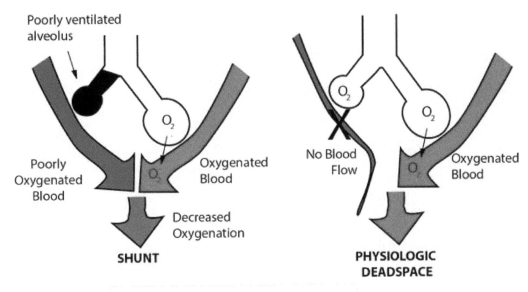

Fig. 2.2.10. Shunt and Dead space

## C. DEAD SPACE

o   The volume occupied by gas which does not participate in gas exchange in lung.
o   A few different types, including:
- Anatomical dead space
- Physiological dead space
- Alveolar dead space
- Apparatus dead space (Anesthetic equipment)

### 1. ANATOMICAL DEAD SPACE
- Anatomical dead space is the volume of the conducting airways from the nose or mouth down to the level of the terminal bronchioles.
- It is about 150mL in an average adult or 2.2mLs/kg
- Anatomical dead space is constant regardless of circulation.
- It is measured using **Fowler's method**: Based on rapid dilution of gas already in lung (N2 or CO2) by inspired gas (100% O2).

### 2. PHYSIOLOGICAL DEAD SPACE
- Physiological dead space is the part of the tidal volume which does not participate in gas exchange.
  *Physiological dead space includes all the non-respiratory parts of the bronchial tree included in anatomic dead space, but also factors in alveoli which are well-ventilated but poorly perfused and are therefore less efficient at exchanging gas with the blood.*
  o   The difference between anatomical dead space and physiological dead space is **alveolar dead space.**
  o   With increased cardiac output (during exercise), physiological dead space is reduced (due to reduction in alveolar dead space).
- It is measured using **Bohr's equation and Bohr's method**: Based on "all expired CO2 comes from alveolar gas", and dead space doesn't eliminate CO2.
- **Enghoff modification**: using measured arterial PaCO2 as an estimate of the ideal alveolar PACO2

#### FACTORS INFLUENCING ANATOMICAL DEAD SPACE
- **Size of subject**: increases with body size
- **Age**: at infancy, anatomical dead space is higher for body weight (3.3mL/kg)
- **Posture**: sitting 147mL, supine 101mL
- **Position of neck and jaw**
- **Lung volume at the end of inspiration**: anatomical dead space increases by 20mL for each Liter of lung volume
- **Drugs**: bronchodilator will increase dead space

#### FACTORS INFLUENCING ALVEOLAR DEAD SPACE
- Low cardiac output can increase alveolar dead space (increasing West's zone 1)
- Pulmonary embolism

# VIII. ALTITUDE AND HUMAN BODY

## 1. ACCLIMATIZATION TO ALTITUDE

- The human body can adapt to high altitude through both immediate and long-term acclimatization.
- In the short term:
  - Increase in the breathing rate (hyperventilation).
  - Respiratory alkalosis,
  - Tachycardia;
  - The stroke volume is slightly decreased
- Full acclimatization, however, requires days or even weeks:
  - Gradually, the body compensates for the respiratory alkalosis by renal excretion of bicarbonate, allowing adequate respiration to provide oxygen without risking alkalosis.
  - It takes about four days at any given altitude and can be enhanced by drugs such as acetazolamide.
  - Eventually, the body has lower lactate production (because reduced glucose breakdown decreases the amount of lactate formed),
  - Decreased plasma volume, Increased haematocrit (polycythaemia),
  - Increased RBC mass, Increased myoglobin,
  - Increased mitochondria, Increased aerobic enzyme concentration,
  - Increase in 2,3-DPG,
  - Hypoxic pulmonary vasoconstriction, and right ventricular hypertrophy.
  - Pulmonary artery pressure increases in an effort to oxygenate more blood.

| LEVEL OF ALTITUDE (FEET) | COMMON EFFECTS | TREATMENT | |
|---|---|---|---|
| 5,000 | • No effect | **Mild Acute Mountain Sickness (AMS)** | • Supportive, wait until acclimatization<br>• Acetazolamide 125-250mg 12 hly<br>• Dexamethasone 2-4mg 6hly |
| 10,000 | • No hypoxia up to pO2 60mmHg<br>• Rapid ascent up to 10,000ft is **safe zone of ascent** | | |
| 15,000 | • Moderate hypoxia with CVS and respiratory symptoms | **Moderate to Severe AMS** | • Should be treated like Early cerebral Edema<br>• Dexamethasone and Acetazolamide |
| 18,000 | • Severe hypoxia with involvement of CNS | | |
| 20,000 | • Hypoxia aggravates. Unconsciousness when Hb saturation falls below 60%<br>• Critical survival altitude | **High Altitude Cerebral Edema (HACE)** | • **Immediate descent**: descending 500m can improve symptoms<br>• Supplemental O2<br>• Portable hyperbaric O2 chamber<br>• Dexamethasone<br>  ○ 8mg IV/IM/PO stat<br>  ○ then 4mg IV/IM/PO 6hly |
| 30,000 | • Severe hypoxia even with oxygen therapy | | |

- Above 10,000 ft, the arterial O2 saturation falls rapidly
- It is due to **increased 2,3 DPG concentration**
- It is slightly less than 70% at 20,000 ft and much less at higher altitudes.

## 2, 3-DPG (2, 3-DIPHOSPHOGLYCERATE)

- An inorganic phosphate produced in red cells by the Rapoport-Luebering shunt;
- 2,3 DPG binds to the betachain of reduced haemoglobin (Hb), lowering Hb's affinity for O2 and by extension, facilitating O2 release to tissues causing a "right shift" of the O2 dissociation curve.
- 2,3-DPG further shifts the curve to the right by lowering the red cells' pH,
- When transfused, red cells regain 50% of the 2,3-DPG within 3–8 hours and 100% within 24 hours.

| FACTORS AFFECTING 2,3- DPG | |
|---|---|
| **INCREASED 2,3-DPG** | **DECREASED 2,3-DPG** |
| ○ High altitude,<br>○ Anaemia,<br>○ Hyperthyroidism,<br>○ Chronic hypoxia,<br>○ Chronic alkalosis | ○ Storage of blood,<br>○ Hypothyroidism,<br>○ Hypophosphatemia,<br>○ Acidosis |

- Note that levels of 2,3-DPG transiently increase after exercise.

# IX. OXYGEN DELIVERY METHODS

| Device | Flow rate (L/min) | O2 (%) |
|---|---|---|
| Nasal cannula | 1-6 | 21-44 |
| Venturi mask | 4-12 | 24-50 |
| Partial rebreather mask (simple mask) | 6-10 | 36-60 |
| Nonrebreather O2 mask with reservoir | 6-15 | 60-100 |
| Bag-mask with nonrebreather "tail" | 15 | 95-100 |

- Oxygen delivery is function of cardiac output, Hb and Saturation. At rest, O2 consumption is approximately 250ml/min, with about 25% of the total O2 delivered. Approximately 1.5% of O2 is dissolved, most being delivered bound to Hb.
- When Hb levels fall, O2 delivery to tissues is maintained by a compensatory increase in cardiac output.
- The extraction ratio increases when consumption increases (exercises).
  - **97% SaO2= 13.3KPa (100mmHg)**
  - **90% SaO2= 8KPa (60mmHg)**
  - **75% SaO2= 5.3 Kpa (40mmHg)**
- Administer to all patients of ACS for the first 6hrs. Continue if pulmonary congestion, ongoing ischaemia, or Sat < 90%
- Also, indicated in patient with stroke and hypoxaemia and any suspect of cardiopulmonary emergency. *Supplementary oxygen does not benefit stroke patients with normal lung function.*
- Pulse oximetry may be inaccurate in low cardiac output states, with vasoconstriction, or with CO exposure.
- Observe closely when using with pulmonary patients known to be dependent on hypoxic respiratory drive.
- *In Patient with Opiates Overdose or Brain Injury, supplementary Oxygen corrects hypoxia but not Ventilation. Therefore, saturation is not a valuable technique to monitor ventilation.*
- *Supplemental oxygen does not correct hypoxia caused by shunt.*

# X. PULSE OXIMETER

## FACTORS AFFECTING READING

- **Carbon Monoxide:** Carbon monoxide molecules, even in a small amount, can attach to the patient's hemoglobin replacing oxygen molecules. A pulse oximeter cannot distinguish the differences and the reading will show the total saturation level of oxygen and carbon monoxide. If 15% of hemoglobin has carbon monoxide and 80% has oxygen, the reading would be 95%.
- *A pulse oximeter should not be used on people with smoke inhalation, CO poisoning, and heavy cigarette smoking.*
- **Hemoglobin Deficiency (Anaemia):** Low quantity of hemoglobin may affect the result.
- **Blood Volume Deficiency**
  - Conditions, such as hypovolemia, hypotension, and hypothermia, may have adequate oxygen saturation, but low oxygen carrying capacity.
  - Due to the reduction in blood flow, the sensor may not be able to pick up adequately the pulsatile waveform resulting in no signal or loss of accuracy. Taking measurement on sick patients with cold hands can be challenging.
- **Irregular Signals:** The irregular signals can be caused by irregular heartbeats or by patient's movements. If this is the problem, one can tell by looking at the SpO2 waveform which is available on some pulse oximeters.
- **External Interference**
  - Exposure to strong external light while taking measurement may result in inaccurate readings. Shield the sensors from bright lights.
  - Strong electromagnetic fields may also affect readings.
- **Fingernail Polish and Pressed on Nails:** Nail polish and pressed-on nails may interfere with readings.
- **Skin Pigmentation:** Dark skin pigmentation can give over-estimated SpO2 readings when it is below 80%. Find a place where the skin color is lighter.
- **Intravenous Dyes:** Intravenous dyes (such as methylene blue, indigo carmine, and indocyanine green) can cause inaccurate readings.
- **Methaemoglobin**
  - Methaemoglobin is a form of hemoglobin that does not carry O2.
  - It is normal to have 1-2% of haemoglobin in this form.
  - A high level of methaemoglobin would cause a pulse oximeter to have a reading of around 85% regardless of the actual oxygen saturation level.
  - The higher percentage of methaemoglobin can be genetic or caused by exposure to certain chemicals and medications.

# Past Asked Questions

**The following are true of Pulse oximetry:**

| | |
|---|---|
| Bilirubinaemia gives a falsely high saturation? | F |
| Carboxyhaemoglobin gives falsely low readings? | F |
| Readings of 90% roughly correspond to a PO2 of 8.0 kPa as measured by arterial blood gas analysis? | T |
| Peripheral vasodilatation due to CO2 retention causes unreliable readings? | F |

**The following are true of non-invasive ventilation in the emergency department:**

| | |
|---|---|
| Most devices use in ED are driven by air? | T |
| Should be avoided in acidotic COPD patients? | F |
| Increases tidal volume? | T |
| Has no effect on gas exchange? | F |

**Intubation and positive pressure ventilation:**

| | |
|---|---|
| Increases dead space? | T |
| Can cause Pneumothorax? | T |
| Can cause hypocapnia? | T |
| Reduces venous return to the right atrium? | T |

**Regarding the pulmonary circulation:**

| | |
|---|---|
| The mean pulmonary artery pressure is typically 15mmHg? | T |
| Pulmonary blood flow equals cardiac output? | T |
| The ventilation/perfusion ratio is highest in the mid zones of the lungs? | F |
| High right atrial pressures predispose to pulmonary oedema? | F |

**In unacclimatised persons ascending to high altitudes:**

| | |
|---|---|
| Respiratory acidosis occurs? | F |
| The oxyHb dissociation curve shifts to the left? | F |
| Pulmonary oedema may occur? | T |
| An increased in haematocrit may be seen after 3 days? | T |

**The respiratory system adapts to pregnancy in the following ways:**

| | |
|---|---|
| Tidal volume increases? | T |
| Progesterone stimulates ventilation? | T |
| Hb falls by term? | T |
| By term residual volume has decreased by 20% but total lung capacity remains the same? | T |

**Regarding ventilation/perfusion (V/Q) relationship in the lung of a healthy person in the upright position**

| | |
|---|---|
| In the upright position, ventilation is highest at the base of the lung | T |
| The V/Q ratio is lowest at the apex of the lung | F |
| An increased V/Q ratio will lower PACO2 and raise PAO2 | T |
| Pulmonary embolism lowers the V/Q ratio | F |

**Alveolar surfactant has the following properties**

| | |
|---|---|
| It is synthesized by type II pneumocytes | T |
| It is a mixture of glycoproteins | F |
| Surfactant increases alveolar surface tension | F |
| Surfactant is deficient in hyaline membrane disease | T |

**Lung compliance has the following features**

| | |
|---|---|
| Compliance is equivalent to the unit volume change of the lungs divided by unit pressure change ($\Delta V/\Delta P$) | T |
| Compliance is decreased in patients with emphysema | F |
| Compliance decreases with age | F |
| Surfactant increases compliance | T |

**Spirometry can be used to measure the following**

| | |
|---|---|
| Vital capacity (FVC) | T |
| Functional residual capacity (FRC) | F |
| Forced expiratory volume at 1 second (FEV1) | T |
| Total lung capacity (TLC) | F |

**Lung compliance**

| | |
|---|---|
| Is the measure of the ease of expansion of the lung | T |
| Is decreased by pulmonary surfactant | F |
| Is increased in chronic obstructive pulmonary disease | T |
| Dynamic compliance is greater than static compliance in asthmatics | F |

**Regarding lung volumes and capacities of an adult male weighing 70kg**

| | |
|---|---|
| The residual volume (RV) is around 1.3L | T |
| The functional residual capacity (FRC) is around 2.5L | T |
| The tidal volume (TV) is around 650ml | F |
| The vital capacity (VC) is over 6.0L | F |

| Right shift of the haemoglobin-oxygen dissociation curve is caused by: | |
|---|---|
| Carbon monoxide | F |
| Increased 2,3 diphosphoglycerate (2,3 DPG) | T |
| Increasing pH | F |
| Reduced affinity of haemoglobin for oxygen | T |

| Regarding the oxygen dissociation curve | |
|---|---|
| Left shift reduces the affinity of oxygen for haemoglobin | F |
| Increasing acidity (pH decreases) shifts the dissociation curve to the right | T |
| 2,3 diphosphoglyceric acid (2,3 DPG) increases the affinity of Hb for oxygen | F |
| Oxygen binding to the fetal Hb (HBF) has a dissociation curve to the right of the adult curve | F |

| The following are true of pulmonary function tests: | |
|---|---|
| The vital capacity includes the residual volume | F |
| The functional residual capacity can be measured by spirometry | F |
| The tidal volume is around 500ml | T |
| A normal FEV1/FVC ratio is around 0.85-0.95 | F |

| True or False | |
|---|---|
| The aortic chemoreceptors lose sensitivity in chronic hypoxia? | F |
| The hering_Breuer reflex is a spinal reflex? | F |
| FRC is measured by spirometry? | F |
| FRC corresponds to the volume at 50% of the inspiratory flow volume curve? | F |
| FVC equals the sum of IRV and ERV? | F |
| 15 liters/min (normal wall O2 on full) exceeds peaks inspiratory flow demand? | F |
| The Physiological Dead space equals the sum of Anatomical Dead space and Residual volume? | F |
| Helium dilution gives higher estimates of TLC than plethysmography? | F |
| Alveolar Oxygen tension is approximately 2/3 of atmospheric oxygen? | T |
| Physiological Dead space is reduced in COPD? | F |
| Alveolar ventilation is approximately 2/3 of Total Minute ventilation? | T |
| SPO2 is valuable technique for monitoring ventilation in head injury? | F |
| CO2 crosses the alveolar membrane readily? | T |
| Alveolar PO2 averages 1kPa greater than arterial PO2 in normal? | T |
| Supplemental oxygen corrects hypoxia caused by shunt? | F |
| Doubling arterial PO2 from 8 to 16kPa doubles tissue oxygen delivery? | F |
| Myoglobin contains 4 atoms of Iron? | F |
| Altitude acclimatisation moves the oxyhaemoglobin curve to the right? | T |
| CO2 returns to the lung bound to plasma proteins? | F |
| The oxyhaemoglobin curve of fetal Hb is to the right of adult? | F |
| Supplementary oxygen does not benefit stroke patients with normal lung function | T |
| As high a concentration of O2 as possible should be given to patients with CO poisoning? | T |
| The target O2 saturation for patients on O2 should be 100%? | F |
| A venturi mask provides a higher concentration of O2 than a non-rebreathing mask? | F |

# Section 3: Cardiovascular Physiology

## I. CARDIAC OUTPUT

### 1. DEFINITIONS

- **Cardiac Output** is the volume of blood pumped by the heart per minute (mL blood/min).
- Cardiac output is a function of heart rate and stroke volume.

  **Cardiac Output in mL/min = Heart Rate (beats/min) X Stroke Volume (mL/beat)**

$$CO = HR \times SV$$

- **The Heart Rate** is simply the number of heart beats per minute.
- **The Stroke Volume** is the volume of blood, in millilitres (mL), pumped out of the heart with each beat.

  **Stroke Volume = End-Diastolic volume – End-Systolic Volume**

$$SV = EDV - ESV$$

- Increasing either heart rate or stroke volume increases cardiac output.
- The total volume of blood in the circulatory system of an average person is about 5 liters (5000 mL).
- This entire volume of blood within the circulatory system is pumped by the heart each minute (at rest). During vigorous exercise, the cardiac output can increase up to 7-fold (35 liters/minute)

### 2. CONTROL OF CARDIAC OUTPUT

- Cardiac output depends on stroke volume and heart rate.
- Stroke volume is dependent on three important factors:
  - Preload,
  - Afterload and
  - Contractility.

### A. PRELOAD= END-DIASTOLIC PRESSURE

- Preload is the force distending the ventricles.
- It can be assessed by measuring end-diastolic pressure.
- Preload depends on **venous return.**
- An intrinsic property of myocardial cells, within normal limits, is that the force of their contraction depends on the length to which they are stretched.
- The greater the stretch (within certain limits), the greater the force of contraction.
- This property is known as the **Frank-Starling phenomenon.**
- It occurs because stretching of the myofibrils results in more efficient creation of cross-bridges between the contractile proteins.
- An increase in preload (End-Diastolic Volume) will result increase in Stroke Volume, therefore in a concomitant increase in cardiac output.

| Factors affecting Preload | Comment |
|---|---|
| **Venous Return /Blood volume/ Heart rate** | ○ Any increase will increase the SV |
| **Body position and Gravity** | ○ Standing up position >>> ↓Venous return |
| | ○ When a person initially stands and before the baroreceptor reflex is activated, CO and arterial pressure decrease because right atrial pressure and ventricular preload falls, which decreases stroke volume. |
| **Phase of respiration** | ○ Inspiration: ↓Rt Atrial Pressure >>> ↑ Venous return >>> ↑ SV |
| **Vena cava compression.** | ○ ↓ venous return (Valsalva maneuver or late pregnancy) |
| **Decreased venous compliance** | ○ ↑central venous pressure and promotes venous return |
| **Locomotion** | ○ ↑venous return by the muscle pump mechanism |

### FRANK-STARLING MECHANISM (STARLING'S LAW)

- Starling's Law describes the relationship between end-diastolic volume and stroke volume.
- If the end-diastolic volume doubles then stroke volume will double. Starling's law of the heart, states that the heart will eject a greater stroke volume if it is filled to a greater volume at the end of diastole.
- ***Thus, increasing left ventricular end diastolic volume or pressure (LVEDP) leads to increased stroke volume.***
- This is true for a healthy heart across the physiological range of end-diastolic volumes (typically 80 to 200ml).
- Cardiac filling outside this physiological range leads to decreased stroke volume; either decreased cardiac output of the under-filled heart or, at the opposite extreme, fluid overload cardiac failure.

## B. AFTERLOAD

- Afterload is the force against which the ventricles must act in order to eject blood (it is the resistance to ventricular ejection).
- This is largely dependent on **Aortic Blood Pressure**, which in turn depends on **Vascular Resistance**.
- Afterload is increased when aortic pressure and systemic vascular resistance are increased, by aortic valve stenosis, and by ventricular dilation.
- When afterload increases, there is an increase in end-systolic volume and a decrease in stroke volume
- *Increasing afterload increases myocardial oxygen consumption and may decrease stroke volume.*
- *As shown in the figure above, an increase in afterload shifts the Frank-Starling curve down and to the right, which decreases stroke volume (SV) and at the same time increases left ventricular end-diastolic pressure (LVEDP).*
- *However, reductions in afterload may also result in an increase in stroke volume and this will maintain blood pressure, within limits.*

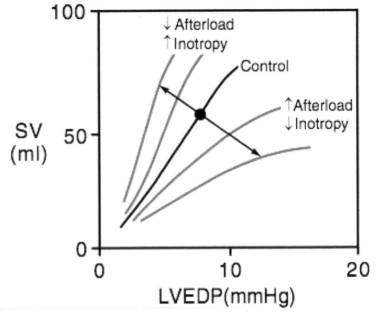

Fig. 2.3.1. Frank-Starling mechanism

## C. CONTRACTILITY

- The strength of the force of myocardial contraction is dependent on direct autonomic control affecting preload and afterload but also on the contractility of the myocardium.

| FACTORS AFFECTING AFTERLOAD | FACTORS AFFECTING CONTRACTILITY | |
|---|---|---|
| | **Increased by:** | **Decreased by:** |
| o Heart rate | • Sympathetic Nervous System | • Beta-blockade |
| o Vascular tone (and therefore blood pressure) | • Drugs: | • Cardiac failure |
| o Aortic stiffness |   o Adrenaline | • Acidosis |
| o Myocardial tension (affected by hypoxia, volume overload) |   o Dobutamine | • sepsis |
| |   o Levosimendan | • Hypoxia |
| o Metabolic rate |   o Ephedrine | • Hypercapnia. |
| o Preload |   o Digoxin | |
| o Valvular regurgitation |   o Calcium | |
| |   o Milrinone... | |

*Laplace's Law: a dilated heart needs more tension to generate a given pressure*

## DISTRIBUTION OF CARDIAC OUTPUT AT REST AND DURING EXERCISE

| | At Rest | | During exercise | |
|---|---|---|---|---|
| **ORGANS** | **CO= 5000mls** | | **CO= 25000mls** | |
| **Liver** | 27% | 1350 mls | 2% | 500 mls |
| **Muscles** | 20% | 1000 mls | 84% | 21000 mls |
| **Kidneys** | 20% | 1000 mls | 1% | 250 mls |
| **Brain** | 15% | 750 mls | 4% | 1000 mls |
| **Skin** | 6% | 300 mls | 2% | 500 mls |
| **Heart** | 4% | 200 mls | 4% | 1000 mls |
| **Other** | 8% | 400 mls | 3% | 750 mls |
| **Total** | 100% | 5000mls | 100% | 25000mls |

# II. ANATOMY OF THE HEART

## 1. CORONARY ANATOMY AND BLOOD FLOW

| RCA | LCA |
|---|---|
| • Arises from Anterior Aortic Sinus<br>• Supplies RV wall and parts of the posterior septum<br>• In 2/3 of patients, the RCA supplies the SA Node<br>• 85% RCA dominant | • Arise from the Posterior Aortic Sinus<br>• Supplies the anterior 2/3 of the septum<br>• LCX artery supplies the LV lateral<br>• 15% patient supplies the inferior wall (No PDA) |

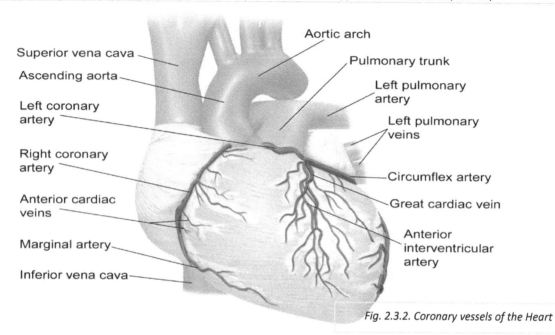

Fig. 2.3.2. Coronary vessels of the Heart

## A. LOCATION MI AND ECG CHANGES

| LOCATION OF MI | LEADS AFFECTED | VESSELS INVOLVED | ECG CHANGES |
|---|---|---|---|
| **Anterior wall** | V2-V4 | LAD (Diagonal branch) | Poor R progression, ST elevation T inversion |
| **Septal wall** | V1-V2 | LAD (septal branch) | R wave disappears, ST rises T inverts |
| **Lateral wall** | I, aVL, V5, V6 | LCX | ST elevation |
| **Inferior wall** | II, III, aVF | RCA (posterior descending branch) | T inversion ST elevation |
| **Posterior wall** | V1-V4 (V7-V9) | LCX RCA | Tall R waves, ST depression Upright T waves |
| *Rt Ventricle MI* | V1, V4R | RCA | |
| *Atrial MI* | PTa in I, V5, V6 | RCA | |

## 2. CARDIAC INNERVATION

○ **Right vagus nerve** supplies the SA Node

○ **Left vagus nerve** supplies the AV Node

○ **Sympathetic nerve** supply originates from **C2-T4**

○ **Phrenic nerve** innervates both layers of the pericardium

**Parasympathetic innervation**

Nucleus ambigus of Vagal Nerve
↓                    ↓
Rt vagus ↓          ↓ Lt Vagus
↓                    ↓
SA Node            AV Node
↓
Reduced gradient phase 4
hyperpolarization
↓
**Reduced Heart Rate**

**Sympathetic innervation**

Rostral ventrolateral Medulla
↓                    ↓
Rt sympathetics ↓   ↓ Lt sympathetics
↓                    ↓
SA Node            AV Node
↓                    ↓
Increased gradient phase 4
↓
**Increased Heart Rate**

# III. REGULATION OF BLOOD PRESSURE

## 1. MEAN ARTERIAL PRESSURE (MAP)

- Mean arterial pressure represents the average pressure in the arterial system.
- This value is important because it is the difference between MAP and the venous pressure that drives blood through the capillaries of the organs.
- A simple formula for calculation of MAP is:

$$MAP = \frac{SABP + 2DABP}{3} \qquad MAP = P_{diastolic} + \frac{1}{3}PP$$

MAP = Diastolic Pressure + 1/3 Pulse Pressure or (2/3DBP) + (1/3SBP)

Pulse pressure = Systolic Pressure - Diastolic Pressure

MAP = Cardiac Output X Total Peripheral Resistance

Ejection Fraction=SV/EDV, SV=EDV-ESV >>EF=EDV-ESV/EDV
Normal 0.5-0.75

### A. MAJOR FACTORS THAT EFFECT MAP

- The three most important variables effecting MAP are:
  - Total peripheral resistance (TPA)
  - cardiac output
  - Blood volume.

### B. CONTROLLING OF MEAN ARTERIAL PRESSURE

- **Increasing in TPR, SV or HR >>> increases of MAP**
- **Increasing arterial compliance >>> reduces MAP**
- **Baroreceptors:**
  - Aortic Arch & Carotid Sinus >>> detect changes in MAP
- **Peripheral Chemoreceptors:**
  - In Aorta and Carotid: PO2 detectors increase Blood Pressure in times of low PO2

### C. ACTION OF ANGIOTENSIN II

- Vasoconstriction >>> increase SVR
- Increase Na and Fluid retention
- Release of Aldosterone and ADH
- Its actions are opposed by ANP (Atrial Natriuretic Peptide)

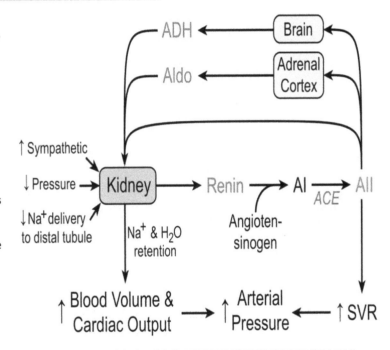

*Fig. 2.3.3. Action of Angiotensin II*

## 2. ORTHOSTASIS AND ORTHOSTATIC HYPOTENSION

- Standing up from a supine position (orthostasis) causes pooling of blood in the veins of the lower limbs under the influence of gravity. This in turn causes a sudden reduction in systemic arterial pressure which is sensed by the arterial baroreceptors of the carotid sinus and aortic arch.
- Reduced firing of the baroreceptors is fed via the glossopharyngeal (carotid sinus baroreceptors) and vagus (aortic arch baroreceptors) nerves to the cardiovascular control centres in the medulla which respond by increasing sympathetic activity to cause:
  - Increased heart rate via stimulation of the sinoatrial node
  - Constriction of venous capacitance vessels to push blood back into the active circulation
  - Systemic arterial vasoconstriction
- These events occur rapidly over seconds to one or two minutes after standing to stabilise arterial pressure and maintain cerebral perfusion.
- **Postural hypotension – and orthostatic syncope – occur due to failure of these compensatory mechanisms.**
- Changes in blood volume do occur over time but are too slow to be significant in the immediate response to orthostasis.

# V. CARDIAC CYCLE I

## A. CARDIAC ELECTRICAL CONDUCTION SYSTEM

### 1. CONTROL OF HEARTBEAT

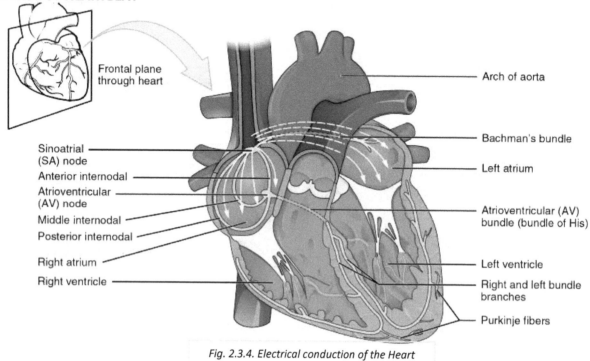

Fig. 2.3.4. Electrical conduction of the Heart

## A. SA NODE

- The sinoatrial node (SA node or SAN, also called the sinus node) is the impulse generating (pacemaker) tissue located on the wall of the right atrium, near the entrance of the superior vena cava. These cells are modified cardiac myocytes.
- They possess some contractile filaments, though they do not contract.
- Because the sinoatrial node is responsible for the rest of the heart's electrical activity, it is sometimes called the **primary pacemaker**.
- Cells in the SA node will naturally discharge (create action potentials) at about 70-80 times/minute.
- Although all of the heart's cells possess the ability to generate the electrical impulses (or action potentials) that trigger cardiac contraction, the sinoatrial node is what normally initiates it, simply because it generates impulses slightly faster than the other areas with pacemaker potential. Because cardiac myocytes, like all nerve cells, have refractory periods following contraction during which additional contractions cannot be triggered, their pacemaker potential is overridden by the sinoatrial node.
- The SA node emits a new impulse before either the AV or purkinje fibers reach threshold.
- If the SA node doesn't function, or the impulse generated in the SA node is blocked before it travels down the electrical conduction system, a group of cells further down the heart will become the heart's pacemaker.
- These cells form the atrioventricular node (AV node), which is an area between the right atrium and ventricle, within the atrial septum.
- The impulses from the AV node will maintain a slower heart rate (about 40-60 beats per a minute).
- When there is a pathology in the AV node or purkinje fibers, an ectopic pacemaker can occur in different parts of the heart.
- The ectopic pacemaker typically discharges faster than the SA node and causes an abnormal sequence of contraction.
- *The SA node is richly innervated by vagal and sympathetic fibers. This makes the SA node susceptible to autonomic influences.*
- ***Stimulation of the vagus nerve causes decrease in the SA node rate*** *(thereby causing decrease in the heart rate).*
- ***Stimulation via sympathetic fibers causes increase in the SA node rate*** *(thereby increasing the heart rate).*
- *Parasympathetic stimulation from the vagal nerves decreases the rate of the AV node* **by causing the release of acetylcholine at vagal endings** *which in turn increases the K+ permeability of the cardiac muscle fiber.*
- *Vagal stimulation can block transmission through AV junction or stop SA node contraction which is called* **"ventricular escape."**
- **When this happens, the purkinje fibers in the AV bundle develops a rhythm of their own.**
- The sympathetic nerves are distributed to all parts of the heart, especially in ventricular muscles. The parasympathetic nerves mainly control SA and AV nodes, some atrial muscle and ventricular muscle. In the majority of patients, the SA node receives blood from the right coronary artery, meaning that a myocardial infarction occluding it will cause ischemia in the SA node unless there is a sufficiently good anastomosis from the left coronary artery. If not, death of the affected cells will stop the SA node from triggering the heartbeat.

## B. AV NODE

- The atrioventricular node (AV node) is the tissue between the atria and the ventricles of the heart, which conducts the normal electrical impulse from the atria to the ventricles. The AV node receives two inputs from the atria: posteriorly via the *crista terminalis*, and anteriorly via the *interatrial septum*. An important property that is unique to the AV node is **decremental conduction:**
  - This is the property of the AV node that prevents rapid conduction to the ventricle in cases of rapid atrial rhythms, such as atrial fibrillation or atrial flutter.
  - The AV node delays impulses for 0.1 second before spreading to the ventricle walls.
  - The reason it is so important to delay the cardiac impulse is to ensure that the atria are empty completely before the ventricles contract.
- The blood supply of the AV node is from a branch of the right coronary artery in 85% to 90% of individuals, and from a branch of the left circumflex artery in 10% to 15% of individuals. In certain types of supraventricular tachycardia, a person could have two AV Nodes; this will cause a loop in electrical current and uncontrollably-rapid heartbeat.
- When this electricity catches up with itself, it will dissipate and return to normal heart-beat speed.

## C. AV BUNDLE OR BUNDLE OF HIS

- The bundle of HIS is a collection of heart muscle cells specialized for electrical conduction that transmits the electrical impulses from the AV node to the point of the apex of the fascicular branches. There are two branches of the bundle of His: the **left bundle branch** and the **right bundle branch**, both of which are located along the interventricular septum.
- The left bundle branch further divides into the **left anterior fascicles** and the **left posterior fascicles**.
- These structures lead to a network of thin filaments known as Purkinje fibers.

## D. PURKINJE FIBERS

- These fibers distribute the impulse to the ventricular muscle.
- Together, the bundle branches and purkinje network comprise the ventricular conduction system.
- It takes about 0.03-0.04s for the impulse to travel from the bundle of HIS to the ventricular muscle.
- During the ventricular contraction portion of the cardiac cycle, *the Purkinje fibers carry the contraction impulse from the left and right bundle branches to the myocardium of the ventricles.* This causes the muscle tissue of the ventricles to contract and force blood out of the heart — either to the pulmonary circulation (from the right ventricle) or to the systemic circulation (from the left ventricle).

## E. PACEMAKER

- The contractions of the heart are controlled by electrical impulses, these fire at a rate which controls the beat of the heart.
- The cells that create these rhythmical impulses are called pacemaker cells, and they directly control the heart rate.

# 2. ELECTROCARDIOGRAM (ECG)

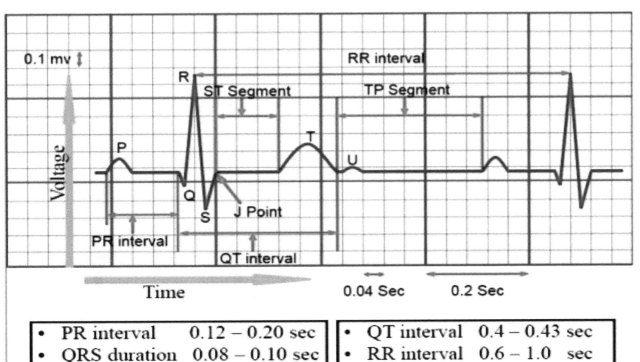

*Fig. 2.3.5. ECG*

| ECG AXIS | QRS COMPLEX |
|---|---|
| Normal | [-30° to +90°] |
| Left Axis Deviation | [-30° to -90°] (LVH, LBBB, Left ant. fascicular block) |
| Right Axis Deviation | > +90° (RVH, RBBB, Lt post fascicular block, COPD, PE...) |
| Extreme Axis Deviation | [-90° and +180°] |

## A. P WAVE

- The P wave represents the *atrial depolarization.*
- It takes usually *0.08 to 0.1 seconds* (80-100 ms) in duration.
- The brief isoelectric (zero voltage) period after the P wave represents the time in which the impulse is travelling within the AV node (where the conduction velocity is greatly retarded) and the bundle of His.

## P-R INTERVAL

- The PR interval is the time from the onset of the P wave to the start of the QRS complex. It reflects conduction through the AV node.
- The normal PR interval is between **0.12 – 0.2s** (120-200ms) duration (three to five small squares).
- If the PR interval is > 200 ms, **First Degree Heart Block** is said to be present.
- PR interval < 120 ms suggests **Pre-Excitation** (the presence of an accessory pathway between the atria and ventricles) or **AV nodal (junctional) rhythm**.

## PRE-EXCITATION SYNDROMES

- Wolff-Parkinson-White (WPW) & Lown-Ganong-Levine (LGL) syndromes.
- These involve the presence of an accessory pathway connecting the atria and ventricles.
- The accessory pathway conducts impulses faster than normal, producing a short PR interval.
- The accessory pathway also acts as an anatomical re-entry circuit, making patients susceptible to re-entry tachyarrhythmias.

## PR SEGMENT

- The PR segment is the flat, usually isoelectric segment between the end of the P wave and the start of the QRS complex.
- It represents the duration of the conduction from the atrioventricular node, down the bundle of His and through the bundle branches to the muscle.

### PR SEGMENT ABNORMALITIES OCCUR IN TWO MAIN CONDITIONS

- Atrial Ischemia
- Pericarditis:
  - ✓ PR segment depression.
  - ✓ Widespread concave ('saddle-shaped') ST elevation.
  - ✓ Reciprocal ST depression and PR elevation in aVR and V1
  - ✓ Absence of reciprocal ST depression elsewhere.

## B. Q WAVE

- The Q wave represents the normal left-to-right depolarisation of the interventricular septum.
- Small 'septal' Q waves are typically seen in the left-sided leads (I, aVL, V5 &V6)

### PATHOLOGICAL Q WAVE

- Q waves are considered pathological if:
  - ✓ > 40 ms (1 mm) wide
  - ✓ > 2 mm deep
  - ✓ > 25% of depth of QRS complex
  - ✓ Seen in leads V1-3

### DIFFERENTIAL DIAGNOSIS OF ABNORMAL Q WAVE

- Myocardial infarction
- Cardiomyopathies: Hypertrophic (HOCM), infiltrative myocardial disease
- Rotation of the heart: Extreme clockwise or counter-clockwise rotation
- Lead placement errors: e.g. upper limb leads placed on lower limbs

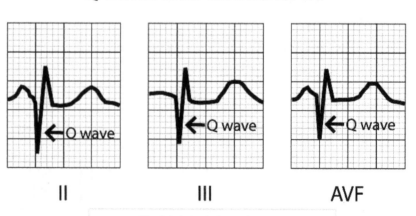

Fig. 2.3.6. Pathological Q wave

## C. QRS COMPLEX
- The QRS complex represents *ventricular depolarization.*
- *It takes* normally **0.08 to 0.1 seconds**.

### NARROW OR SUPRAVENTRICULAR COMPLEXES
- o **Arise from three main places**
- o Narrow complex tachycardias are **Supraventricular tachycardias**, meaning only that they originate above the ventricles.

### BROAD QRS COMPLEXES
- A QRS duration > 100 ms is abnormal
- A QRS duration > 120 ms is required for the diagnosis of bundle branch block or ventricular rhythm.
- Broad complexes may be ventricular in origin or due to aberrant conduction secondary to:
  - o Bundle branch block
  - o Hyperkalaemia
  - o Poisoning with sodium-channel blocking agents (e.g. TCAs)
  - o Pre-excitation (i.e. Wolff-Parkinson-White syndrome)
  - o Ventricular pacing
  - o Hypothermia
  - o Intermittent aberrancy (e.g. rate-related aberrancy)

## D. ST SEGMENT
- It is the time at which the entire ventricle is depolarized and roughly *corresponds to the plateau phase of the ventricular action potential*.
- The ST segment is important in the diagnosis of ventricular ischemia or hypoxia.

## E. J POINT
- The J point is the junction between the termination of the QRS complex and the beginning of the ST segment.
- Elevation or depression of the J point is seen with the various causes of ST segment abnormality.
- Notching of the J point occurs with benign early repolarization.
- *A positive deflection at the J point is termed a J wave **(Osborn wave) and** is characteristically seen with **hypothermia**.*

50 mm/s

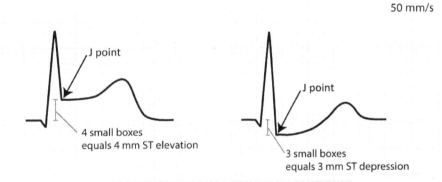

Fig. 2.3.7. J Point

## F. T WAVE
- The T wave represents *ventricular repolarization*
- Is longer in duration than depolarization (i.e., conduction of the repolarization wave is slower than the wave of depolarization).
- Sometimes a small positive U wave may be seen following the T wave: This wave represents the last *remnants of ventricular repolarization*. Inverted or prominent U waves indicate underlying pathology or conditions affecting repolarization.

## Q-T INTERVAL
- The QT interval is defined from the beginning of the QRS complex to the end of the T wave.
- The Q-T interval represents *the time for both ventricular depolarization and repolarization to occur.* This interval can range *from 0.2 to 0.4 seconds* depending upon heart rate.

  - *The QT interval is inversely proportional to heart rate:*
    - o *The QT shortens at faster heart rates*
    - o *The QT lengthens at slower heart rates*
  - *An abnormally prolonged QT is associated with an increased risk of ventricular arrhythmias, especially Torsade's de Pointes.*
- The recently described congenital short QT syndrome has been found to be associated with an increased risk of paroxysmal atrial and ventricular fibrillation and sudden cardiac death.

## CORRECTED Q-T (QTC)

- In practice, the Q-T interval is expressed as a "corrected Q-T (QTc)" *by taking **the Q-T interval and dividing it by the square root of the R-R interval** (interval between ventricular depolarizations).*
- This allows an assessment of the Q-T interval that is independent of HR.
  - **Bazett's formula**         : $QT_C = QT / \sqrt{RR}$
  - **Fredericia's formula**     : $QT_C = QT / RR^{1/3}$
  - **Framingham formula**       : $QT_C = QT + 0.154 (1 - RR)$
  - **Hodges formula**           : $QT_C = QT + 1.75 (HR - 60)$
- *Normal corrected Q-Tc intervals are less than **0.44 sec.***

### CAUSES OF A PROLONGED QTC (>440MS):

**4H** Must **Raise C**ardiac **P**ressure with **Drugs**
  - **H**ypokalaemia
  - **H**ypomagnesaemia
  - **H**ypocalcaemia
  - **H**ypothermia
  - **M**yocardial ischemia
  - **Raised** intracranial pressure
  - **C**ongenital long QT syndrome
  - **P**ost-cardiac arrest
- **DRUGS:        Triple AAA T**ears        First Endothelium
  - ✓ **A**ntihistaminics
  - ✓ **A**nticholinergics
  - ✓ **A**ntiarrythmics (specially Quinidine and Sotalol)
  - ✓ **T**CAS
  - ✓ **F**luoroquinolones
  - ✓ **E**rythromycin

**Other drugs are:** Chloroquine, Mefloquine, Haloperidol, Risperidone, Methadone, and HIV protease Inhibitors.

NORMAL EKG

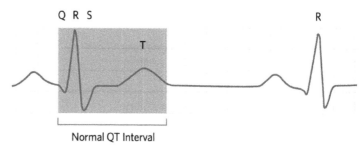

Normal QT Interval

EKG WITH LQTS

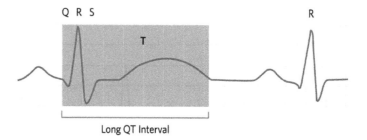

Long QT Interval

Fig. 2.3.8. Prolonged QTc

## 3. ECG DIFFERENTIAL DIAGNOSIS

### HYPERKALAEMIA
- Tall, tented narrow T waves
- Decreased P wave amplitude
- Widened QRS complexes
- AV Block
- Absent P waves very broad, bizarre QRS
- VT/VF or ventricular asystole

### HYPOKALAEMIA
- Widened T waves
- Prolonged PR
- ST depression
- U waves
- Ventricular ectopic
- Ultimately ST/VT

### HYPERCALCAEMIA
- Shortened QT

### HYPOCALCAEMIA
- Prolonged QT

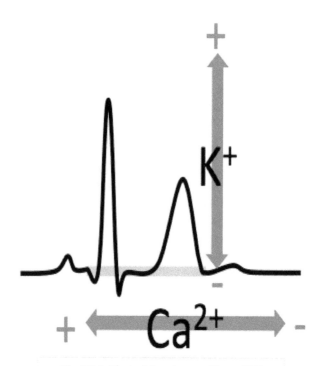

Fig. 2.3.9. Electrolytes abnormality on ECG

# LEFT BUNDLE BRANCH BLOCK

- **DIAGNOSTIC CRITERIA OF LBBB:**
  - ✓ QRS duration of > 120 ms
  - ✓ Dominant S wave in V1
  - ✓ Broad monophasic R wave in lateral leads (I, aVL, V5-V6)
  - ✓ Absence of Q waves in lateral leads (I, V5-V6; small Q waves are still allowed in aVL)
  - ✓ Prolonged R wave peak time >60ms in left precordial leads (V5-6)
- **ASSOCIATED FEATURES:**
  - ✓ Appropriate discordance: the ST segments and T waves always go in the opposite direction to the main vector of the QRS complex.
  - ✓ Poor R wave progression in the chest leads.
  - ✓ Left axis deviation

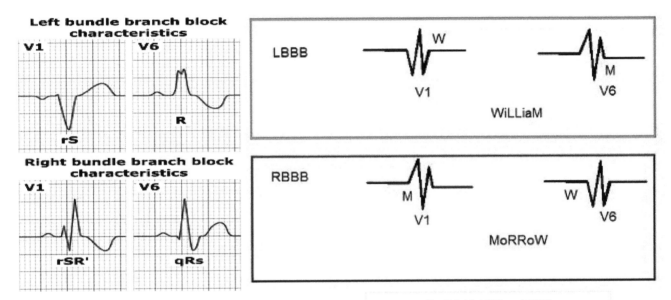

# RIGHT BUNDLE BRANCH BLOCK

- **DIAGNOSTIC CRITERIA:**
  - ✓ Broad QRS > 120 ms
  - ✓ RSR' pattern in V1-3 ('M-shaped' QRS complex).
  - ✓ Wide, slurred S wave in the lateral leads (I, aVL, V5-6).
- **ASSOCIATED FEATURES:**
  - ✓ ST depression and T wave inversion in the Rt precordial leads (V1-V3).

*Fig. 2.3.10. LBBB and RBBB*

# ECG CHANGES IN PULMONARY EMBOLISM

- RBBB
- Sinus Tachycardia
- Extreme right axis deviation (+180 degrees)
- S1 Q3 T3
- P Pulmonale
- T-wave inversions in V1-4 and lead III
- Clockwise rotation with persistent S wave in V6

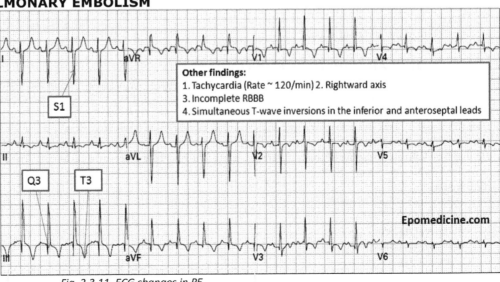

Other findings:
1. Tachycardia (Rate ~ 120/min) 2. Rightward axis
3. Incomplete RBBB
4. Simultaneous T-wave inversions in the inferior and anteroseptal leads

Epomedicine.com

*Fig. 2.3.11. ECG changes in PE*

## CAUSES OF ST-SEGMENT ELEVATION

- Acute MI (myocardial infarction)
- Coronary vasospasm (Printzmetal's angina)
- Pericarditis and myocarditis
- Benign early repolarisation
- LBBB: Left bundle branch block
- LVH: Left ventricular hypertrophy
- Ventricular aneurysm
- Brugada syndrome
- Ventricular paced rhythm
- Raised ICP

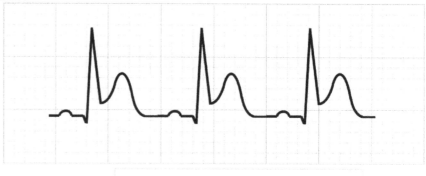

Fig. 2.3.12. STEMI

## ECG CHANGES IN POSTERIOR MI  :
- Tall, broad R waves in leads V1-V3
- ST depression in leads V1-V3
- Dominant R wave in lead V2
- Upright T waves in leads V1-V3

## SGARBOSSA CRITERIA (NEW)

- A new LBBB is always pathological and can be a sign of myocardial infarction. The most important change is the modification of the rule for **excessive discordance**.
- The use of a 5 mm cut off for excessive discordance was arbitrary and non-specific — for example, patients with LBBB and large voltages will commonly have ST deviations > 5 mm in the absence of ischaemia.
- The modified rule is positive for STEMI if there is discordant ST elevation with amplitude > 25% of the depth of the preceding S-wave.
- **MODIFIED SGARBOSSA CRITERIA:**
  - ≥ 1 lead with ≥1 mm of concordant ST elevation
  - ≥ 1 lead of V1-V3 with ≥ 1 mm of concordant ST depression
  - ≥ 1 lead anywhere with ≥ 1 mm STE and proportionally excessive discordant STE, as defined by ≥ 25% of the depth of the preceding S-wave

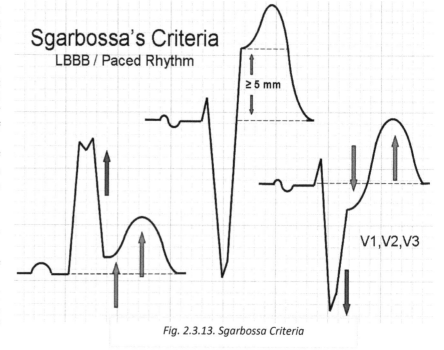

Fig. 2.3.13. Sgarbossa Criteria

## LEFT VENTRICULAR HYPERTROPHY (LVH)
- The left ventricle hypertrophies in response to pressure overload secondary to conditions such as **Aortic Stenosis** and **Hypertension**.
- This results in increased R wave amplitude in the left-sided ECG leads (I, aVL and V4-6) and increased S wave depth in the right-sided leads (III, aVR, V1-3).
- The thickened LV wall leads to prolonged depolarization (increased R wave peak time) and delayed repolarization (ST and T-wave abnormalities) in the lateral leads.
- To diagnose left ventricular hypertrophy on the ECG one of the following criteria should be met: **The Sokolow-Lyon criterion:** R in V5 or V6 + S in V1 >35 mm. (S wave depth in V1 + tallest R wave height in V5-V6 > 35 mm). This criterion is not reliable **below age 40 years.**
- **CAUSES OF LVH**
  - ✓ Hypertension (most common)
  - ✓ Aortic stenosis
  - ✓ Aortic regurgitation
  - ✓ Mitral regurgitation
  - ✓ Coarctation of the aorta
  - ✓ Hypertrophic cardiomyopathy

## RIGHT VENTRICULAR HYPERTROPHY (RVH)

- Right axis deviation of +110° or more.
- Dominant R wave in V1 (> 7mm tall or R/S ratio > 1).
- Dominant S wave in V5 or V6 (>7mm deep or R/S ratio <1).
- *QRS duration < 120ms (i.e. changes not due to RBBB).*
- **CAUSES OF RVH**
  - ✓ Pulmonary hypertension
  - ✓ Mitral stenosis
  - ✓ Pulmonary embolism
  - ✓ Chronic lung disease (cor pulmonale)
  - ✓ Congenital heart disease (e.g. Tetralogy of Fallot, pulmonary stenosis)
  - ✓ Arrhythmogenic right ventricular cardiomyopathy

## WOLFF-PARKINSON-WHITE SYNDROME

- A shortened PR interval (often < 120 ms). A slurring and slow rise of the initial upstroke of the QRS complex (Delta Wave).
- A widened QRS complex (total duration >0.12 seconds)
- ST segment–T wave changes, generally directed opposite the major delta wave and QRS complex

## WELLENS' SYNDROME

- **DIAGNOSTIC CRITERIA:**
  - ✓ Deeply-inverted or biphasic T waves in V2-3 (may extend to V1-6)
  - ✓ Isoelectric or minimally-elevated ST segment (< 1mm)
  - ✓ No precordial Q waves
  - ✓ Preserved precordial R wave progression
  - ✓ Recent history of angina
  - ✓ ECG pattern present in pain-free state
  - ✓ Normal or slightly elevated serum cardiac markers
- There are 2 patterns of T-wave abnormality in Wellens' syndrome:
  - ○ **Type A** = Biphasic, with initial positivity & terminal negativity (25% of cases)
  - ○ **Type B** = deeply and symmetrically inverted (75%)

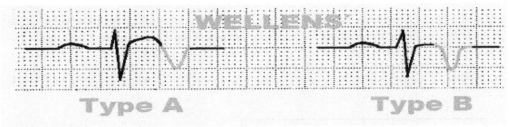

*Fig. 2.3.14. Wellen's syndrome*

## 4. ATRIOVENTRICULAR BLOCK

- AV block occurs when atrial depolarisation fails to reach the ventricles because of a block involving the AV node or the His-Purkinje system. If block is at the AV nodal level complexes will be narrow.
- If block is lower down in the His-Purkinje system complexes will be wide.
- The higher the block the more likely it will respond to increases in sympathetic tone or the use of atropine.
- Three degrees of block are recognised and described below:

### 1. FIRST DEGREE AV BLOCK

- PR interval > 0.20 sec; *all* P waves conduct to the ventricles.

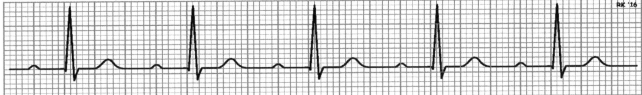

- This may be a sign of **early fibrosis or ischaemia** in the AV node but is most commonly a normal variant and is asymptomatic.
- In the context of an acute coronary syndrome it requires monitoring in case of progression to other forms of heart block.
- ***It does not require treatment.***

## 2. SECOND DEGREE AV BLOCK

- The QRS remains narrow but atrial impulses fail to conduct normally to the ventricles in one of the following ways:

### A. MOBITZ TYPE I (WENCKEBACH)

- o The PR interval lengthens progressively after each successive P wave until a P wave is not conducted.
- o This is common following **inferior acute myocardial infarction** (AMI) when it may progress to complete heart block.
- o Mobitz type 1 heart block (Wenckebach) is normally asymptomatic and resolves without the need for urgent intervention

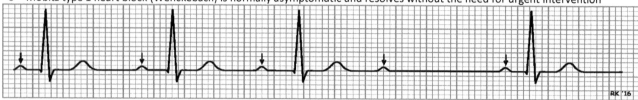

### B. MOBITZ TYPE II

- o There is a constant PR interval but some P waves fail to conduct to the ventricles
- o The ratio of conducted and non-conducted beats may be fixed (e.g. 2:1 or 3:1).
- o This is less common than Mobitz type I, often symptomatic and of more concern.
- o It signifies **septal involvement** in the setting of **AMI** and commonly progresses to complete heart block.
- o Patients who have this diagnosed on pre-operative assessment are fitted with pacemakers before undergoing anaesthesia.
- o *Mobitz type 2 heart block commonly progresses to complete heart block which may require urgent intervention.*
- o In Type II block several consecutive P waves may be blocked as illustrated below:

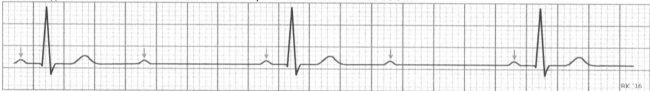

## 3. THIRD DEGREE AV BLOCK (COMPLETE HEART BLOCK)

- All P waves fail to conduct to the ventricles resulting in a broad complex ventricular escape rhythm.

- A rhythm originating in the high septal region will have a rate of 40-50 beats per minute. If originating from a lower ventricular site, the rate will be lower at 30-40 beats per minute. Although this may be a coincidental finding it usually presents with lethargy and syncope.

- It signifies **significant fibrosis or ischaemia** in the AV node and **requires a permanent pacemaker.** Following an **anterior AMI,** it indicates extensive damage to the septal region and indicates a worse prognosis. *Complete heart block in the setting of acute anterior MI indicates extensive septal damage and is a poor prognostic sign.*

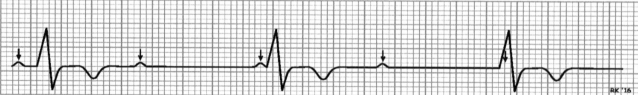

## 4. TRIFASCICULAR BLOCK

- A trifascicular block is the combination of:
  - o *A right bundle branch block,*
  - o *Left anterior or posterior fascicular block and*
  - o *A first-degree AV block (prolonged PR interval).*

- A trifascicular block is a precursor to complete heart block. Trifascicular block is usually present in various heart diseases (it is definitely not a normal finding) and sometimes can progress into the **third-degree AV block**. While a trifascicular block itself does not require any treatment, high doses of AV blocking agents likely should be avoided.

- Some series report a 50% lifetime need for a **permanent pacemaker** in the setting of a trifascicular block.

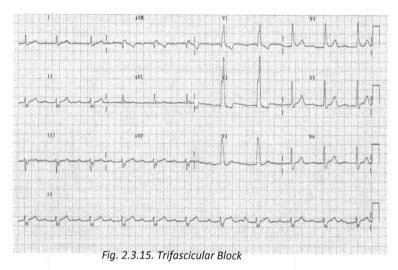

*Fig. 2.3.15. Trifascicular Block*

# V. CARDIAC CYCLE II

## A. THE CYCLE & ECG

- The cardiac cycle describes the electromechanical events occurring in the heart during a single beat.
- These events can be related to the heart sounds on auscultation, the features of the ECG and the visible waves of the jugular venous pulse. Traditionally the cardiac cycle is divided into 5 phases:

### 1. PHASE I - ATRIAL CONTRACTION
- o At the end of diastole, the atria contract pushing blood through the open atrioventricular valves into the relaxed ventricles.
- o This completes ventricular filling in preparation for systole.

### 2. PHASE 2 – ISOVOLUMETRIC CONTRACTION
- o At the onset of systole, the atrioventricular valves snap shut (1st heart sound) and isometric contraction of ventricles causes sharp increase in intraventricular pressure.
- o This phase ends when ventricular pressures exceed aortic and pulmonary artery pressures and the aortic and pulmonary valves open.

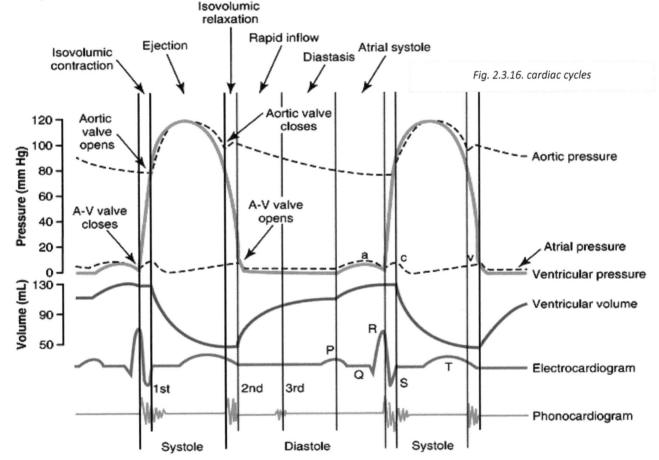

Fig. 2.3.16. cardiac cycles

### 3. PHASE 3 – VENTRICULAR EJECTION
- o During the ventricular ejection phase blood is pumped out of the ventricles into the aorta and pulmonary arteries.
- o When ventricular contraction is complete, ventricular pressure wanes and falls below aortic and pulmonary pressures causing the aortic and pulmonary valves to close (2nd heart sound).
- o The end of this phase marks the onset of diastole.

### 4. PHASE 4- ISOVOLUMETRIC RELAXATION
- o During this phase, all four heart valves are closed and there is a sharp decrease of intraventricular pressure.
- o At the end of this phase, the atrioventricular valves opens.

### 5. PHASE 5 – VENTRICULAR FILLING
- o Blood returning via the venae cava flows through the atria and open atrioventricular valves to fill the ventricles.
- o Ventricular pressures remain low during diastole.

## CARDIAC CYCLE AND CORRESPONDING ECG SEGMENTS AND HEART SOUNDS

| STAGE | VALVES | ECG | HEART SOUNDS |
|---|---|---|---|
| *Early (ventricular) Diastole* | VP drops<br>AV valves opened SL valves closed | Isoelectric line | **3rd Heart sound may be heard** |
| *Atrial systole/ contraction* | AV valves opened<br>SL valves closed | P wave<br>PR interval | **4th Heart sound may be heard** |
| *Isovolumetric ventricular contraction* | All 4 valves are closed | QRS complex | **1st Heart sound (S1)** |
| *Ventricular ejection* | VP > AP/PP<br>AV valves closed SL Valves opened | ST segment<br>T wave | **No Heart sound** |
| *Isovolumetric ventricular relaxation* | All 4 valves are closed | Isoelectric line | **2nd Heart sound (S2)** |

*VP: Ventricular Pressure, AV: AtrioVentricular, SL: Semilunar*      *AP: Aortic Pressure, PP: Pulmonary Pressure*

## B. AUSCULTATION OF THE HEART

- **S1: Mitral and Tricuspid closure (systolic):** Loudest in the left 5th intercostal space
- **S2: Aortic and Pulmonary closure (systolic):** Loudest right/left upper sternal border
- **S3: Increased filling pressure (early diastole):** Most common in hypertrophy (CCF, dilated cardiomyopathy…); Can be Normal (Pregnancy, children, Athletes…)
- **S4: Atrial kick (late diastole):** High atrial pressure; Ventricular hypertrophy

- **Aortic murmurs**
  - **Aortic murmurs** are best heard with the stethoscope placed to the right of the upper sternum.
  - **Pulmonary murmurs** are best heard just to the left of the upper sternum.
- **The Third Heart Sound (S3)**
  - Caused by the reverberation of blood during rapid ventricular filling in early diastole. It may be normal in the young and athletes but in older adults is associated with heart failure.
- **A Fourth Heart Sound (S4)**
  - **It is always abnormal** and is caused by atrial contraction against a non-compliant (hypertrophied) ventricle.
  - Since it coincides with the atrial kick an S4 occurs in late diastole.
- **The Early Diastolic Murmur** of aortic regurgitation
  - Is best heard with the patient sitting forwards in full expiration.
- **Physiological splitting the second heart sound (S2)**
  - Occurs because the aortic valve tends to close slightly before the pulmonary valve.
  - However, in conditions causing significantly delay in left ventricular ejection such as aortic stenosis or LBBB, the pulmonary valve may close before the aortic, giving a **Paradoxically** or **Reverse Split S2.**
- **Some specific splits:**
  - **Wide splitting**
    - Pulmonary stenosis or RBBB
  - **Fixed splitting**
    - ASD/ VSD
  - **Paradoxal splitting**
    - Aortic stenosis or LBBB

| SYSTOLIC MURMURS | |
|---|---|
| **Mitral Regurgitation** | **Aortic Stenosis** |
| - Blowing<br>- Loudest at Apex<br>- Radiates to Axilla<br>- Enhanced by:<br>  o  Increasing TPR: squatting<br>  o  Increasing LA return (expiration) | - Crescendo-decrescendo<br>- Ejection click<br>- Radiates to carotid/apex<br>- Slow rising pulse<br>- Syncope |
| **DIASTOLIC MURMURS** | |
| **Aortic Regurgitation** | **Mitral Stenosis** |
| - Early diastolic<br>- Blowing<br>- Wide pulse pressure<br>- Patient sitting forwards<br>- Full expiration<br>- Soft S1 | - Follows opening snap<br>- Late diastolic murmur<br>- Rheumatic Fever<br>- Loud S1 |

- A very widened pulse pressure suggests **Aortic Regurgitation** (as in diastole, the arterial pressure drops to fill the left ventricle though the regurgitating aortic valve)
- A very narrow pulse pressure suggests **Cardiac Tamponade**, or any other sort of low output state (e.g. severe cardiogenic shock, massive pulmonary embolism or tension pneumothorax).

## C. NORMAL CARDIAC PRESSURES

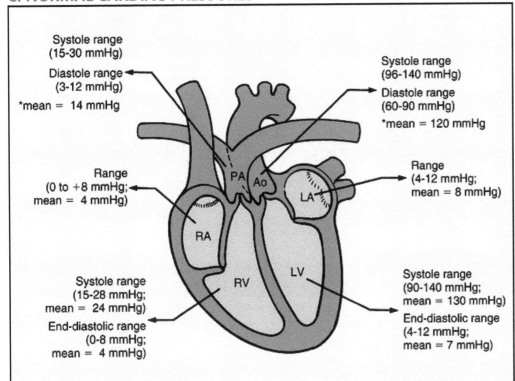

| Right Atrium | 5/3 mmHg |
|---|---|
| Left Atrium | 10/8 mmHg |
| Right Ventricle | 28/2 mmHg |
| Left Ventricle | 125/6 mmHg |
| Aorta | 120/70 mmHg |

*Fig. 2.3.17. Normal cardiac pressures*

## D. CENTRAL VENOUS PRESSURE

- Central venous access for CVP monitoring is obtained by inserting a catheter into a vein, typically the subclavian or jugular vein, and advancing it toward the heart until the catheter tip rests within the superior vena cava near its junction with the right atrium.
- CVP is a reflection of right atrial pressure, which is used as an estimate of left ventricular end-diastolic volume (preload).
- Normally, CVP ranges from **3 to 8 cm $H_2O$** or (2 to 6 mm Hg).

### FACTORS AFFECTING MEASURED CENTRAL VENOUS PRESSURE

- **Technical factors:**
  - Patient positioning
  - Level of transducer
  - Inconsistent measurement technique with water manometer
  - Inappropriate central venous catheter placement

- **PHYSIOLOGIC FACTORS AFFECTING CVP**
  - *Factors that increase CVP include*:
    - Pulmonary Hypertension
    - Pulmonary Embolism
    - Pleural effusion
    - Tension pneumothorax
    - Heart failure
    - Decreased cardiac output
    - Cardiac tamponade
    - Hypervolemia
    - Forced exhalation
    - Mechanical ventilation and the application of positive end-expiratory pressure (PEEP)

○   *Factors that decrease CVP include:*
   •   Hypovolemia
   •   Deep inhalation
   •   Distributive shock (vasodilation): Septic shock, Anaphylactic shock, neurogenic shock.

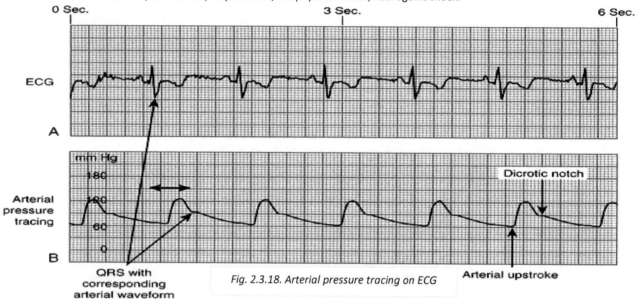

*Fig. 2.3.18. Arterial pressure tracing on ECG*

## CENTRAL VENOUS PRESSURE WAVEFORM COMPONENTS

| Waveform component | Phase of cardiac cycle | Mechanical Event | Comments |
|---|---|---|---|
| a wave | End diastole | Atrial contraction | Large in atrial enlargement and tricuspid stenosis<br>Canon waves |
| c wave | Early systole | Tricuspid bulging<br>Ventricular contraction (IVC) | Small canon waves |
| x descent | Mid systole | Tricuspid valve is closed<br>Atrium relaxation | Blood filling the atrium, draining the JVP |
| v wave | Late systole | Systolic filling of the atrium | Slow increase in JVP pressure<br>Elevated in tricuspid incompetence |
| y descent | Early diastole | Early ventricular filling | |

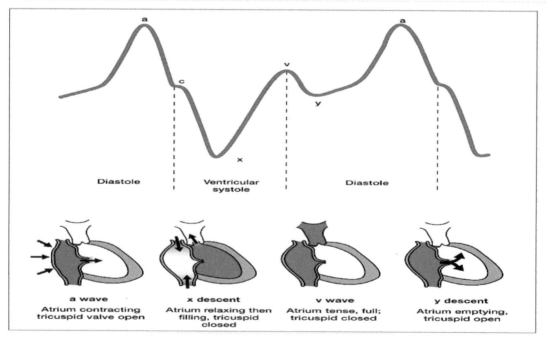

*Fig. 2.3.19. Central venous pressure waveform*

# VI. CARDIAC CYCLE III

## A. CARDIAC CONDUCTING SYSTEM

- Sinoatrial (SA) node normally generates the action potential, i.e. the electrical impulse that initiates contraction.
    - The SA node excites the right atrium (RA), travels through Bachmann's bundle to excite left atrium (LA).
    - The impulse travels through internodal pathways in RA to the atrioventricular (AV) node.
- From the AV node, the impulse then travels through the bundle of His and down the bundle branches, fibers specialized for rapid transmission of electrical impulses, on either side of the interventricular septum.
    - Right bundle branch (RBB) depolarizes the right ventricle (RV).
    - Left bundle branch (LBB) depolarizes the left ventricle (LV) and interventricular septum.
- Both bundle branches terminate in Purkinje fibers, millions of small fibers projecting throughout the myocardium.

## B. ELECTROPHYSIOLOGY

### A. ION CHANNELS

- Two main forces drive ions across cell membranes:
    - **Chemical potential**: an ion will move down its concentration gradient.
    - **Electrical potential**: an ion will move away from ions/molecules of like charge.
- The **Transmembrane Potential** (TMP) is the electrical potential difference (voltage) between the inside and the outside of a cell.
- When there is a net movement of positive ions into a cell, the TMP becomes more positive, and when there is a net movement of positive ions out of a cell, TMP becomes more negative.
- Ion channels help maintain ionic concentration gradients and charge differentials between the inside and outside of the cardiomyocytes.

### PROPERTIES OF CARDIAC ION CHANNELS

- **Selectivity:** they are only permeable to a single type of ion based on their physical configuration.
- **Voltage-sensitive gating:** a specific TMP range is required for a particular channel to be in open configuration; at all TMPs outside this range, the channel will be closed and impermeable to ions.
- Therefore, specific channels open and close as the TMP changes during cell depolarization and repolarization, allowing the passage of different ions at different times.
- **Time-dependence:** some ion channels (importantly, fast $Na^+$ channels) are configured to close a fraction of a second after opening; they cannot be opened again until the TMP is back to resting levels, thereby preventing further excessive influx.

### B. ACTION POTENTIAL AND IMPULSE CONDUCTION

- **Action potential:** electrical stimulation created by a sequence of ion fluxes through specialized channels in the membrane (sarcolemma) of cardiomyocytes that leads to cardiac contraction.

### 1. ACTION POTENTIAL IN CARDIOMYOCYTES

- The action potential in typical cardiomyocytes is composed of 5 phases (0-4), beginning and ending with phase 4.

### PHASE 4: THE RESTING PHASE

- The resting potential in a cardiomyocyte is –90 mV due to a constant outward leak of $K^+$ through inward rectifier channels.
- $Na^+$ and $Ca^{2+}$ channels are closed at resting TMP.

### PHASE 0: DEPOLARIZATION

- An action potential triggered in a neighbouring cardiomyocyte or pacemaker cell causes the TMP to rise above –90 mV.
- Fast $Na^+$ channels start to open one by one and $Na^+$ leaks into the cell, further raising the TMP.
- TMP approaches –70mV, the threshold potential in cardiomyocytes, i.e. the point at which enough fast $Na^+$ channels have opened to generate a self-sustaining inward $Na^+$ current.
- The large $Na^+$ current rapidly depolarizes the TMP to 0 mV and slightly above 0 mV for a transient period of time called the overshoot; fast $Na^+$ channels close (recall that fast $Na^+$ channels are time-dependent).
- L-type ("long-opening") $Ca^{2+}$ channels open when the TMP is greater than –40 mV and cause a small but steady influx of $Ca^{2+}$ down its concentration gradient.

### PHASE 1: EARLY REPOLARIZATION

- TMP is now slightly positive.
- Some $K^+$ channels open briefly and an outward flow of $K^+$ returns the TMP to approximately 0 mV.

### PHASE 2: THE PLATEAU PHASE

- L-type $Ca^{2+}$ channels are still open and there is a small, constant inward current of $Ca^{2+}$.
- This becomes significant in the excitation-contraction coupling process described below.

○ K⁺ leaks out down its concentration gradient through delayed rectifier K⁺channels.
○ These two countercurrents are electrically balanced, and the TMP is maintained at a plateau just below 0 mV throughout phase 2.

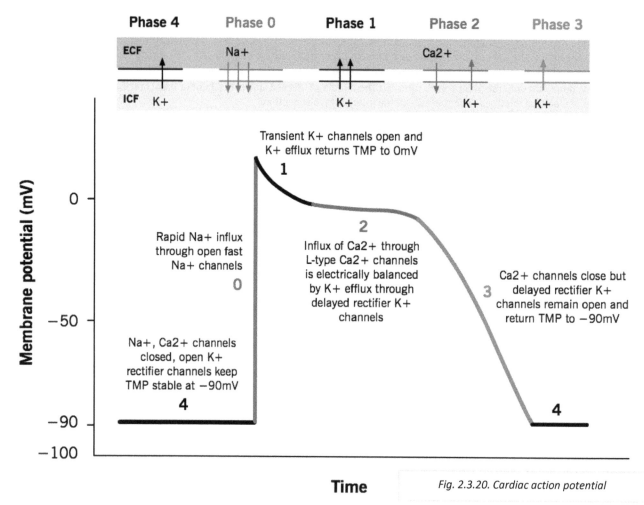

Fig. 2.3.20. Cardiac action potential

## PHASE 3: REPOLARIZATION

○ $Ca^{2+}$ channels are gradually inactivated.
○ Persistent outflow of K⁺, now exceeding $Ca^{2+}$ inflow, brings TMP back towards resting potential of –90 mV to prepare the cell for a new cycle of depolarization.
○ Normal transmembrane ionic concentration gradients are restored by returning Na⁺ and $Ca^{2+}$ ions to the extracellular environment, and K⁺ ions to the cell interior.
○ The pumps involved include the sarcolemmal **Na⁺-Ca²⁺ exchanger, Ca²⁺-ATPase and Na⁺-K⁺-ATPase**.

## 2. ACTION POTENTIAL IN CARDIAC PACEMAKER CELLS

○ **Automaticity:** unlike other cardiomyocytes, pacemaker cells do not require external stimulation to initiate their action potential; they are capable of self-initiated depolarization in a rhythmic fashion.
○ This property is known as automaticity, whereby the cells undergo spontaneous depolarization and an action potential is triggered when threshold voltage is reached.
○ **Unstable membrane potential**: Pacemaker cells have an unstable membrane potential and their action potential is not usually divided into defined phases.
○ **No rapid depolarization phase:** Pacemaker cells have fewer inward rectifier K⁺channels than do other cardiomyocytes, so their TMP is never lower than –60 mV.
○ As fast Na⁺ channels need a TMP of –90 mV to reconfigure into an active state, they are permanently inactivated in pacemaker cells so there is no rapid depolarization phase.

## 3. IMPLICATIONS OF PACEMAKER ACTIVITY ON GLOBAL CARDIAC DEPOLARIZATION

○ **Synchronous contraction:** all cardiomyocytes (including pacemaker cells) are electrically coupled through gap junctions. An action potential in one cell will cause all neighbouring cells to depolarize, allowing the heart chambers to act as a unit.
○ **Dominance:** the cell with the highest inherent rate of pacemaker activity will therefore also set the heart rate, as all other pacemaker cells will be depolarized and rendered inactive by this stimulus.

## 4. REFRACTORY PERIOD
- Defined as the time from phase 0 until the next possible depolarization of a myocyte, i.e. once enough fast $Na^+$ channels have recovered (as TMP decreases below −50 mV).
- Cardiomyocytes have a longer refractory period than other muscle cells given the long plateau from slow $Ca^{2+}$ channels (phase 2).
- This is a physiological mechanism allowing sufficient time for the ventricles to empty and refill prior to the next contraction.
- Different degrees of refractoriness are encountered during an action potential, reflecting the number of fast $Na^+$ channels that have recovered from their inactive state and are capable of reopening.
- **Absolute refractory period (ARP):** the cell is completely unexcitable to a new stimulus.
- **Effective refractory period (ERP):** ARP + short segment of phase 3 during which a stimulus may cause the cell to depolarize minimally but will not result in a propagated action potential (i.e. neighbouring cells will not depolarize).
- **Relative refractory period (RRP):** a greater than normal stimulus will depolarize the cell and cause an action potential.
- **Supranormal period:** a hyperexcitable period during which a weaker than normal stimulus will depolarize the cells and cause an action potential. Cells in this phase are particularly susceptible to arrhythmias when exposed to an inappropriately timed stimulus, which is why one must synchronize the electrical stimulus during cardioversion to prevent inducing ventricular fibrillation.

## C. EXCITATION-CONTRACTION COUPLING
- Excitation-contraction coupling represents the process by which an electrical action potential leads to contraction of cardiac muscle cells.
- This is achieved by converting a chemical signal into mechanical energy via the action of contractile proteins.
- Calcium is the crucial mediator that couples electrical excitation to physical contraction by cycling in and out of the myocyte's cytosol during each action potential.

## 1. CONTRACTILE PROTEINS
- Main contractile elements:
  - **Myosin:** thick filaments with globular heads evenly spaced along their length; contains myosin ATPase.
  - **Actin:** smaller molecule (thin filaments) consisting of two strands arranged as an alpha-helix, woven between myosin filaments.

**REGULATORY ELEMENTS:**
- **Tropomyosin:** double helix that lies in the groove between actin filaments. It prevents contraction in the resting state by inhibiting the interaction between myosin heads and actin.
- **Troponin:** complex with three subunits that sits at regular intervals along the actin strands.
  - **Troponin T (TnT):** Ties troponin complex to actin and tropomyosin molecules.
  - **Troponin I (TnI):** Inhibits activity of ATPase in actin-myosin interaction.
  - **Troponin C (TnC):** binds Calcium ions that regulate contractile process.

## 2. CALCIUM-INDUCED CALCIUM RELEASE (CICR)
- The initial influx of $Ca^{2+}$ into myocytes through L-type $Ca^{2+}$ channels during phase 2 of the action potential is insufficient to trigger contraction of myofibrils.
- This signal is amplified by the CICR mechanism, which triggers much greater release of $Ca^{2+}$ from the sarcoplasmic reticulum.
- The cell membrane of cardiomyocytes, called sarcolemma, contains invaginations (T-tubules) that bring L-type $Ca^{2+}$ channels into close contact with **Ryanodine Receptors**, specialized $Ca^{2+}$ release receptors in the sarcoplasmic reticulum (SR).
- When $Ca^{2+}$ enters the cells through L-type channels, ryanodine receptors change conformation and induce a larger release of $Ca^{2+}$ from abundant SR stores.
- Large levels of intracellular $Ca^{2+}$ act on tropomyosin complexes to induce myocyte contraction.

## 3. CONTRACTILE CYCLE
- $Ca^{2+}$ binds to TnC → TnI is inhibited → conformational change in tropomyosin that exposes active site between actin and myosin.
- Myosin heads interact with active sites on actin filaments and "flex," like oars on a boat, to "row" myosin along actin in an ATP-dependent reaction:
  - Hydrolysis of ATP by ATPase on myosin (no longer inhibited by TnI) induces crossbridge formation between myosin head and active site on actin. The strength of cardiac contraction is proportional to the number of crossbridges formed.
  - Interaction between myosin head and actin trigger "firing" of myosin head, causing it to pull itself along the actin filament in a process known as the **power stroke.**
  - ADP is released from the myosin head, which then binds a new ATP, releasing the actin filament.
  - The cycle can then repeat itself, allowing myosin to travel further along the actin molecules and progressively shorten the muscle fibers, as long as (i) the cytosolic $Ca^{2+}$ concentration remains sufficiently high to inhibit the action of TnI and (ii) there is enough ATP to drive crossbridge formation.

## 4. MYOCYTE RELAXATION
- As with myocyte contraction, this process is synchronized with the electrical activity of the cell.
- L-type $Ca^{2+}$ channels inactivate toward the end of phase 2 → $Ca^{2+}$ influx arrests → CICR trigger is abolished.
- At the same time, $Ca^{2+}$ is sequestered back into the SR by sarcoplasmic reticulum $Ca^{2+}$ ATPase (SERCA) and pumped out of the cell to a lesser extent by specialized $Ca^{2+}$ pumps.

○   $Ca^{2+}$ ions dissociate from TnC as their intracellular concentration falls, and tropomyosin inhibition of actin-myosin interaction is restored.

## D. NEURONAL MODULATION CONTRACTILITY

○   Heart is innervated by both parasympathetic and sympathetic afferent and efferent neurons.

○   Sympathetic: postganglionic sympathetic fibers from paravertebral sympathetic ganglia associated with T1-T5 innervate the atria, ventricles, and conduction system.

○   Parasympathetic: parasympathetic innervation is limited to vagal efferent fibers which innervate the SA node and the AV node; parasympathetic innervation to the ventricles is minimal.

○   Both sympathetic and parasympathetic tone is exerted on the heart at rest, but parasympathetic tone predominates.

○   **Sympathetic neurons:**

    ●   Release norepinephrine, a catecholamine, which activates β1 receptors on cardiac myocytes, leading to the following effects:

       ✓   **Chronotropic**: increased heart rate
       ✓   **Dromotropic**: faster conduction through AV node
       ✓   **Inotropic**: increased contractility
       ✓   **Lusitropic**: faster relaxation after contraction

    ●   Note: epinephrine, also a catecholamine, can be made by the adrenal glands and released into the circulation, and has the same effect on β1 receptors.

○   **Parasympathetic neurons**

    ➤   Release acetylcholine, a cholinergic hormone, which activates muscarinic $M_2$-receptors on cardiac myocytes, leading to just one main effect:

       ✓   **Negative chronotropic**: decreased heart rate.

# VII. PERIPHERAL VASCULAR PHYSIOLOGY

## STARLING'S FORCES

●   **Starling's hypothesis** states that the fluid movement due to filtration across the wall of a capillary is dependent on the balance between the hydrostatic pressure gradient and the oncotic pressure gradient across the capillary.

●   The four Starling's forces are:
    ○   Hydrostatic pressure in the capillary (Pc)
    ○   Hydrostatic pressure in the interstitium (Pi)
    ○   Oncotic pressure in the capillary (pc)
    ○   Oncotic pressure in the interstitium (pi)

●   *Oncotic pressure pulls fluid into the capillary with **Albumin** as the main determinant.*

**Starling's Equation**

**Net Flow/filtration pressure = (Pc-Pif) − (πp- πif)**

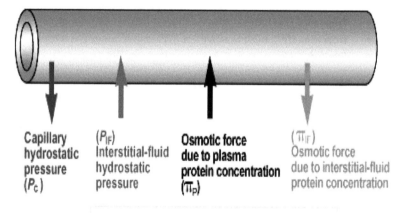

| Capillary hydrostatic pressure $(P_c)$ | $(P_{IF})$ Interstitial-fluid hydrostatic pressure | Osmotic force due to plasma protein concentration $(\pi_p)$ | $(\pi_{IF})$ Osmotic force due to interstitial-fluid protein concentration |

*Fig. 2.3.21. Starling Forces*

## Factors Precipitating Edema

●   **Increased capillary hydrostatic pressure**
    ○   Occurs when venous pressures become elevated by gravitational forces, in heart failure or with venous obstruction.

●   **Decreased plasma oncotic pressure**
    ○   Occurs with hypoproteinaemia during malnutrition.

●   **Increased capillary permeability**
    ○   Caused by proinflammatory mediators (e.g., histamine, bradykinin) or by damage to the structural integrity of capillaries so that they become more "leaky" (as occurs in tissue trauma, burns, and severe inflammation).

●   **Lymphatic obstruction**
    ○   Occurs in filariasis or with tissue injury.

# VIII. BRAIN CIRCULATION

## 1. CEREBRAL BLOOD FLOW (CBF)

- It is the blood supply to the brain in a given period of time.
- *In an adult, CBF is typically 750 millilitres per minute or 15% of the cardiac output. This equates to an average perfusion of 50 to 54 millilitres of blood per 100 grams of brain tissue per minute.*
- Cerebral blood flow is determined by a number of factors, such as viscosity of blood, how dilated blood vessels are, and the net pressure of the flow of blood into the brain, known as *cerebral perfusion pressure (CPP),* which is determined by the body's blood pressure.
- Cerebral blood vessels are able to change the flow of blood through them by altering their diameters in a process called autoregulation:
  - *They constrict:  if ↑BP or ↓PCO2*
  - *They dilate: if ↓BP or ↑PCO2*
- CBF is sensitive to changes in PCO2 and PO2

$$CBF = CPP / CVR$$

- CBF is directly proportional to PCO2
- Hypoventilation >>> ↑PCO2 >>> ↑CBF
- Hyperventilation >>> ↓PCO2 >>> ↓CBF
- Arterial Hypoxaemia >>> cerebral vasodilatation >>> ↓PO2 >>> ↑PCO2 >>> ↑CBF
- *CBF remains constant if MAP stays between 50-150mmHg*
- CBF is equal to the cerebral perfusion pressure (CPP) divided by the cerebrovascular resistance (CVR):

## 2. CEREBRAL PERFUSION PRESSURE (CPP)

- It is defined as the difference between the Mean Arterial Pressure (MAP) and the Intracranial Pressure (ICP).
- **Elevation head to 30° significantly reduced ICP without reducing CPP or CBF.**

$$CPP = MAP - ICP$$

>70mmHg    80mmHg    <10mmHg

## 3. INTRACRANIAL PRESSURE (ICP)

- Increased intracranial pressure (**normal 5-15mmHg**) causes decreased blood perfusion of brain cells by mainly two mechanisms:
  - Increased ICP constitutes an increased interstitial hydrostatic pressure that, in turn, causes a decreased driving force for capillary filtration from intracerebral blood vessels.
  - Increased ICP compresses cerebral arteries, causing increased cerebrovascular resistance (CVR).

| PHYSIOLOGICAL CHANGES IN PREGNANCY | CHILDREN vs ADULTS |
|---|---|
| ➢ **Cardiovascular system**<br>　○ 50% increase Plasma Volume<br>　○ Increased Cardiac Output<br>　○ Increased Blood flow to uteroplacental unit<br>　○ Red cell mass increases 20-30%<br>　○ Blood pressure dips slightly<br>　○ Increased hepatic blood flow<br>　○ ECG changes (LAD, ST sagging)<br>　○ Mild Anaemia develops<br><br>➢ **Respiratory system**<br>　○ Respiratory alkalosis<br>　○ Tidal volume increases 40%<br>　○ RR increases<br><br>➢ **Metabolism**<br>　○ Changes in activity of enzyme systems involved in drug metabolism<br>　○ Decreased serum Albumin<br><br>➢ **Renal system**<br>　○ Increased Glomerular filtration rate up to 50%<br><br>➢ **Gastrointestinal system**<br>　○ Delayed gastric emptying<br>　○ Increased transit time<br>　○ Decreased stomach acidity | ○ Large body surface area (BSA) volume ratio<br>○ Higher (age related) heart rate and respiratory rate<br>○ Higher oxygen metabolism<br>○ Immature blood brain barrier<br>○ Underdeveloped hypothalamus<br>○ Larger tongue relative to size oral cavity<br>○ Prominent occiput<br>○ Shorter narrower funnel shaped trachea |

# IX. THE BLOOD–BRAIN BARRIER

## A. OVERVIEW

- A mechanism that controls the passage of substances from the blood into the CSF and thus into the brain and spinal cord.
- The blood-brain barrier (BBB) lets essential metabolites, such as **oxygen** and **glucose**, pass from the blood to the brain and central nervous system (CNS) but blocks most molecules that are more massive than about 500 Daltons.
- This is a low mass in biomolecular terms and means that everything from hormones and neurotransmitters to viruses and bacteria are refused access to the brain by the BBB.
- It also means that many drugs, which would otherwise be capable of treating disorders of the CNS, are denied access to the very regions where they would be affective.
- **Key functions of the BBB are:**
  - ○ Protecting the brain from "foreign substances" (such as viruses and bacteria) in the blood that could injure the brain,
  - ○ Shielding the brain from hormones and neurotransmitters in the rest of the body,
  - ○ Maintaining a constant environment (homeostasis) for the brain.

## B. ANATOMY OF THE BBB

- A key aspect of the blood-brain barrier is the thin, flat cells known as **endothelial cells** which form the walls of capillaries.
- In most parts of the body, the endothelial cells in the capillaries overlap at what are called **junctions.**
- These junctions are leaky enough to let a lot of different materials move through the wall of the blood vessel into the tissue and back again.
- Substances can get into the surrounding tissues either by leaking out of the junctions or passing straight through the endothelial cells. However, in the brain there's a different arrangement where the endothelial cells join up.
- The endothelial cells meet each other at what are called **tight junctions.**
- These junctions block the passage of most things except for small molecules and are a crucial component of the blood-brain barrier. In order to traverse the walls of brain capillaries, substances must move through the endothelial cell membranes.
- Because the main constituent of cell membranes is lipid, it would seem that a molecule could only get into the brain if it were lipid-soluble.
- However, many ions and small molecules that aren't readily soluble in lipids do move quite readily from brain capillaries into brain tissue. In addition to tight junctions, the **"end feet" of astrocytes** (the terminal regions of astrocytic processes) surround the outside of capillary endothelial cells.
- The reason for this endothelial-glial allegiance is unclear, but may have reflected an influence of astrocytes on the formation and maintenance of the blood-brain barrier.

## C. CIRCUMVENTRICULAR ORGANS

- The circumventricular organs are regions of the brain where the blood-barrier barrier is weak or absent.
- These regions allow substances to cross into brain tissue more freely and thereby allow the brain to monitor the makeup of the blood.
- Hormones produced in the posterior pituitary gland such as **vasopressin and oxytocin** can pass directly into the blood stream because the BBB is absent there.
- Areas of brain without a BBB: MAPPPPE
  - ✓ **M**edian eminence
  - ✓ **A**rea postrema
  - ✓ **P**ituitary gland
  - ✓ **P**reoptic recess
  - ✓ **P**araphysis
  - ✓ **P**ineal gland
  - ✓ **E**ndothelium of choroid plexus

## D. FACTORS THAT CAN LOWER THE BBB:

- ✓ Hypertension,
- ✓ hyperosmolality
- ✓ Microwaves
- ✓ Radiation
- ✓ Infection
- ✓ Injury to the brain due to trauma, ischemia, inflammation, or pressure.

# Past Asked Questions

| **True or False:** | |
|---|---|
| Aortic murmurs are best heard at the left upper sternal border | F |
| A third heart sound (S3) may be heard in late diastole | F |
| The murmur of aortic regurgitation is exaggerated with the patient sitting forwards | T |
| Reverse splitting of the second heart sound (S2) occurs with left bundle branch block | T |
| Isovolumetric contraction follows closure of the tricuspid and mitral valves | T |

| **True or False:** | |
|---|---|
| The P wave of the ECG marks the onset of atrial systole | T |
| The a-wave of the jugular venous pulse corresponds to ventricular systole | F |
| Right ventricular pressure during systole is around 20-30 mmHg | T |
| The circumflex artery is a branch of RCA | F |
| The IV septum is supplied by branches of LAD | T |
| The carotid sinus baroreceptor firing decreases with falling blood pressure | T |
| The inotropic effects of digoxin are mediated by beta-receptors | F |
| The atrial Natriuretic peptide promotes water retention | F |
| Renin secretion from JGA increases with Hypotension | T |
| Pain of pericardial inflammation is transmitted via vagus nerve | F |
| Nitrates reduce both preload and afterload | T |
| LVEDP is inversely proportional to stroke volume | F |
| Positive inotropy shift the Frank-Starling curve to the left | T |

| **True or False:** | |
|---|---|
| At no single point are all 4 heart valves closed | F |
| Spontaneous depolarization is a feature of the SA node myocytes only | F |
| The Aortic valve always closes before the Pulmonary valve | F |
| A 4th heart sound should always be considered abnormal | T |
| A soft S1 is associated with Mitral stenosis | F |

| **True or False:** | |
|---|---|
| Normal Axis is between 0-90 degrees | F |
| The ECG changes in hyperkalaemia include T-wave inversion | F |
| In AV block, there is no atrial activity in complete Heart block | F |
| Regarding Starling's forces, hypoalbuminaemia reduces plasma oncotic pressure | T |
| The P-wave of the ECG occurs during diastole | T |
| ECG changes in hyperkalaemia include J waves | F |
| The normal PR interval is less than 0.12 sec | F |

| **The following cardiovascular changes occur in pregnancy** | |
|---|---|
| Blood volume increases by 45% | T |
| Circulating oestrogen and progesterone cause vasodilatation and reduce peripheral vascular resistance | T |
| Red cell mass declines causing the physiological anaemia of pregnancy | F |
| Pregnancy has no effect on the ECG | F |

| **The following occur as part of the cardiovascular response to orthostasis** | |
|---|---|
| Carotid and aortic arch baroreceptor firing increases | F |
| Heart rate | T |
| Venous capacitance vessels constrict | T |
| Blood volume increases | F |

| **True or False:** | |
|---|---|
| A wide QRS with Mobitz II AV block shows worsening AV block | T |
| Capillary fluid exchange is increased with histamine | T |
| Stroke volume is the amount of blood expelled from the ventricle in 1min | F |
| Cardiac output is proportional to stroke volume | T |
| Decreasing pH (acidaemia) reduces stroke volume | T |
| In the healthy heart, decreasing left ventricular end diastolic pressure (LVEDP) increases stroke volume | F |
| Atrial contraction coincides with isometric relaxation of the ventricles | F |
| The second heart sound is produced by opening of the aortic and pulmonary valves | F |
| All four heart valves are closed during isovolumetric relaxation of the ventricles | T |
| Ventricular pressure rises sharply during ventricular filling | F |

# Section 4: Gastrointestinal Physiology

## I. SALIVA

### 1. FUNCTIONS

1. Cleanses the mouth
2. Helps moisten and compact food into a round mass called a bolus
3. Contains enzymes that begin the chemical breakdown of starch
4. Dissolves food chemicals so they can be "tasted"

### 2. PRODUCTION

- Most saliva is produced by major or extrinsic salivary glands that lie outside the oral cavity and empty their secretions into it.
- Minor or intrinsic salivary glands within the oral cavity alter the output slightly (note: extrinsic glands lie outside of oral cavity; intrinsic glands lie within oral cavity).
- The major salivary glands are paired and develop from the oral mucosa and stay connected to it by small ducts.
- The large, triangle shaped parotid gland lies anterior to the ear between the skin and masseter muscle.
- Its main duct opens into the vestibule next to the second upper molar.
- Facial nerves run through the parotid gland to muscles in the face used for facial expression.
- The salivary glands are composed of two types of secretory cells, serous and mucous.
- Serous cells produce a watery secretion containing ions, enzymes, and a small amount of mucin.
- Mucous cells produce mucus.
- *The submandibular and parotid glands contain a large percentage of serous cells.*
- *The sublingual glands contain mostly mucous cells.*

### 3. COMPOSITION OF SALIVA

- Saliva is mainly water.
- It is 97-99.5% water which makes it hypoosmotic.
- Its osmolarity depends on the glands that are active and the amount and type of stimulus for salivation.
- Generally, saliva is a bit acidic (6.75-7.00), but the pH can vary.
- Its solutes include electrolytes (mainly sodium, potassium, chloride, and bicarbonate); the digestive enzymes salivary amylase and lingual lipase; the proteins mucin, IgA, and lysozyme; metabolic wastes (uric acid, urea).
- When dissolved in water, the glycoprotein mucin forms thick mucus that lubricates the oral cavity and hydrates foodstuffs.
- Saliva protects against microorganisms because it has:
  1. *IgA antibodies*
  2. *Lysozyme*
  3. *Defensins*: defensins function as cytokines and call defensive cells (lymphocytes) into the mouth.

### 4. CONTROL OF SALIVATION

- The minor salivary glands secrete saliva continuously, keeping the mouth optimally moist.
- When food enters, the major glands activate and large amounts of saliva pour out.
- The average human being produces around 1500ml of saliva per day, but it can be a great deal higher if the glands are stimulated properly. For the most part, salivation is controlled by the parasympathetic division of the autonomic nervous system.
- When food is ingested, chemoreceptors and mechanoreceptors in the mouth send signals to the salivatory nuclei in the brain stem to the pons and medulla.
- As a result, parasympathetic nervous system activity increases.
- Impulses sent by motor fibers in the facial (VII) and glossopharyngeal (IX) nerves dramatically increase the output of watery saliva.
- The chemoreceptors are activated the most by acidic foods and liquids.
- The mechanoreceptors are activated by almost any type of mechanical stimulus in the mouth (chewing).
- Even the sight and smell of food can get saliva flowing.
- Irritation of the lower gastrointestinal tract can also increase salivation (spicy food, toxins).
- In contrast to parasympathetic controls, the sympathetic division causes the release of thick, mucin-rich saliva.
- Heavy activation of the sympathetic division constricts blood vessels serving the salivary glands and inhibits the release of saliva, causing dry mouth.
- Dehydration also inhibits salivation.

# II. SWALLOWING

## A. PHASES

### 1. ORAL PREPARATORY PHASE
- Movement patterns depend on consistency of material swallowed
- Liquid Bolus has a certain degree of cohesiveness that may be maintained as bolus is held between tongue and anterior hard palate.
- Lip Closure
- Facial tone helps with labial seal.
- Rotary, lateral jaw movement
- Rotary, lateral tongue movement
- Anterior pulling of soft palate and rests against the back of the tongue, which is elevated serving to keep material in the oral cavity.

### 2. ORAL PHASE (1 sec)
- Intact labial seal
- Anterior to posterior tongue movement

### 3. PHARYNGEAL PHASE-PHARYNGEAL RESPONSE (1 sec)
- Triggering of the swallowing response occurs at the anterior faucial arch.
- Elevation and retraction of the velum and complete closure of velopharyngeal port to prevent material from entering the nasal cavity.
- Initiation of pharyngeal peristalsis to pick up the bolus as it passes the anterior faucial arch and carry it by sequential peristaltic (squeezing) action of the pharyngeal constrictors into and through the pharynx to the cricopharyngeal sphincter at the top of the oesophagus.
- Elevation and closure of the larynx at all three sphincters (epiglottis/aryepiglottic folds, false vocal folds, and true vocal folds) to prevent material from entering the airway.
- Relaxation of the cricopharyngeal sphincter to allow material to pass from pharynx into the oesophagus.
- laryngeal elevation and cricopharyngeus relaxation

### 4. ESOPHAGEAL PHASE (8-20 sec)
- Transit times can be measured from the point where the bolus enters the oesophagus at the cricoesophageal juncture until it passes into the stomach at the gastro-oesophageal juncture.

## B. NEURAL REGULATION OF SWALLOWING
- Swallowing is initiated by sensory impulses transmitted as a result of stimulation of receptors on the fauces, tonsils, soft palate, base of the tongue, and posterior pharyngeal wall.
- *Sensory impulses reach the brainstem primarily through the 7th, 9th, and 10 cranial nerves, while the efferent (motor) function is mediated through the 9th, 10th, 12th cranial nerves.*
- Cricopharyngeal sphincter opening is reflexive, relaxation occurring at the time when the bolus reaches the posterior pharyngeal wall prior to reaching this sphincter.
- **CRANIAL NERVES**
  - **CN V: Trigeminal**
    - Contains both sensory and motor fibers that innervate the face
    - Important in chewing
  - **CN VII: Facial**
    - Contains both sensory and motor fibers
    - Important for sensation of oropharynx & taste to anterior 2/3 of tongue.
  - **CN IX: Glossopharyngeal**
    - Contains both sensory and motor fibers
    - Important for taste to posterior tongue, sensory and motor functions of the pharynx.
  - **CN X: Vagus**
    - Contains both sensory and motor fibers
    - Important for taste to oropharynx, and sensation and motor function to larynx and laryngopharynx.
    - Important for airway protection.
  - **CN XII: Hypoglossal**
    - Contains motor fibers that primarily innervate the tongue

# III. THE STOMACH

## 1. OVERVIEW

- The wall of the stomach contains four layers.
- The inner layer, the mucosa, is modified for the specialized functions of the stomach.
- The innermost layer of the mucosa (facing the lumen) *contains a layer of simple columnar epithelium consisting of goblet cells.*
- Gastric pits on the surface penetrate deep into the layer, forming ducts whose walls are lined with various gastric glands.
- A summary of the glands in the mucosa follows:
  - *Mucous surface cells* are the goblet cells that make up the surface layer of the simple columnar epithelium. These cells *secrete mucus*, which protects the mucosa from the action of acid and digestive enzymes.
  - *Parietal (oxyntic) cells* are scattered along the neck and lower walls of the ducts. *They secrete hydrochloric acid (HCl) and intrinsic factor.* Intrinsic factor is necessary for the absorption of vitamin B $_{12}$ in the small intestine.
  - *Chief (zymogenic) cells* also line the lower walls of the ducts. *They secrete pepsinogen*, the inactive form of pepsin. Pepsin is a protease, an enzyme that breaks down proteins.
  - *Enteroendocrine cells* secrete various hormones that diffuse into nearby blood vessels. One important hormone, *gastrin*, stimulates other glands in the stomach to increase their output.

## 2. FUNCTIONS

- *Storage*
  - The stomach can expand to store two to four liters of material.
- *Mixing*
  - The stomach mixes the food with water and gastric juice to produce a creamy medium called *chyme*.
- *Physical breakdown*
- *Chemical breakdown*
  - Proteins are chemically broken down by the enzyme pepsin.
  - Chief cells are protected from self-digestion because chief cells produce and secrete an inactive form of pepsin, pepsinogen.
  - Pepsinogen is converted to pepsin by the HCl produced by the parietal cells.
  - Only after pepsinogen is secreted into the stomach cavity can protein digestion begin.
  - Once protein digestion begins, the stomach is protected by the layer of mucus secreted by the mucous cells.
- *Controlled release*
  - Movement of chyme into the small intestine is regulated by a sphincter at the end of the stomach, the pyloric sphincter.

### A. ROLE OF THE CHIEF AND PARIETAL CELLS

- Parietal cells are the epithelial cells that secrete hydrochloric acid (HCl) and intrinsic factor.
- These cells are located in the gastric glands found in the lining of the fundus and in the body of the stomach.
- They contain an extensive secretory network (called canaliculi) from which the HCl is secreted by active transport into the stomach.
- The enzyme hydrogen potassium ATPase ($H^+/K^+$ ATPase) is unique to the parietal cells and transports the $H^+$ against a concentration gradient of about 3 million to 1, which is the steepest ion gradient formed in the human body.
- *Parietal cells are primarily regulated via histamine, acetylcholine and gastrin signalling from both central and local modulators.*

## 3. SECRETION OF HYDROCHLORIC ACID

- **Parietal cells** in the stomach secrete roughly two liters of acid a day in the form of **hydrochloric acid**.
- The acid is important to establish the optimal pH (**1.8-3.5**) for the function of the digestive enzyme **pepsin**.
- A key protein for acid secretion is the **$H^+/K^+$-ATPase** (or **proton pump**).
- This protein, which is expressed on the apical membrane of parietal cells, uses the energy derived from ATP hydrolysis to pump hydrogen ions into the lumen in exchange for potassium ions.
- Stimulation of acid secretion involves the translocation of $H^+/K^+$-ATPases to the apical membrane of the parietal cell.
- When the cell is resting (not stimulated), $H^+/K^+$-ATPases are located in vesicles inside the cell.
- When the cell is stimulated, these vesicles fuse with the plasma membrane, thereby increasing the surface area of the plasma membrane and the number of proton pumps in the membrane.
- There are three regulatory molecules that stimulate acid secretion (**Acetylcholine**, **Histamine, and Gastrin**) and one regulatory molecule that inhibits acid secretion (**Somatostatin**).
- **Acetylcholine** is a **neurotransmitter** that is released by **enteric neurons**.
- **Histamine** is a **paracrine** that is released from **enterochromaffin-like (ECL) cells**.
- **Gastrin** is a **hormone** that is released by **G cells**, endocrine cells that are located in the gastric epithelium.
- **Somatostatin** is also secreted by endocrine cells (**Antral D cells**) of the gastric epithelium; it can act as either a paracrine or a hormone.

- Above figure shows how the positive and negative regulators interact to stimulate acid secretion.
- Acetylcholine and histamine directly stimulate parietal cells to increase acid secretion.
- Gastrin stimulates acid secretion by stimulating histamine release from ECL cells. (Gastrin also has a direct effect on parietal cells, which is to stimulate their proliferation).
- When the pH of the stomach gets too low, somatostatin secretion is stimulated.
- Somatostatin inhibits acid secretion by direct effects on parietal cells, and also by inhibiting release of the positive regulators histamine and gastrin.
- The balance of activity of the different regulators changes as food is consumed and passes through different segments of the upper GI tract.

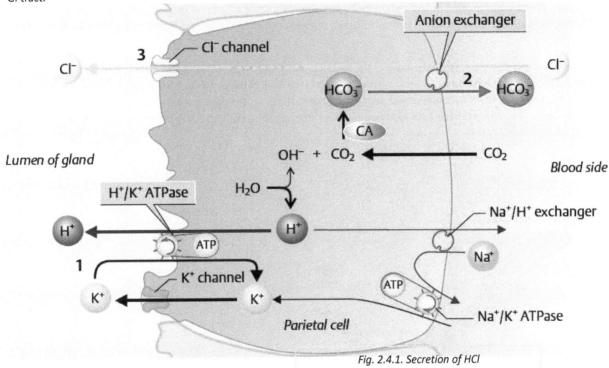

Fig. 2.4.1. Secretion of HCl

## A. CEPHALIC PHASE

- Cephalic phase stimuli are things like the sight, smell, taste or thought of food.
- These stimuli, processed by the brain, activate enteric neurons via parasympathetic preganglionic neurons traveling in **the vagus nerve.**

## B. GASTRIC PHASE

- The primary factor during the gastric phase is that there is food in the stomach, which stimulates acid secretion.
- There are three different ways that this occurs.
- Food will **stretch** the walls of the stomach; this is sensed by mechanoreceptors, activating a neural reflex to stimulate acid secretion.
- Peptides and amino acids in food **stimulate G cells** to release gastrin.
- Food also acts as a buffer, **raising the pH** and thus removing the stimulus for somatostatin secretion.

## C. INTESTINAL PHASE

- Once chyme enters the duodenum, intestinal phase stimuli activate negative feedback mechanisms to reduce acid secretion and prevent the chyme from becoming too acidic.
- This occurs by neural reflexes and hormonal reflexes.
- **Enterogastrones** are hormones that inhibit stomach processes (in this case, acid secretion).
- In addition to their other actions, **CCK, secretin, GLP-1,** and **GIP** act as enterogastrones.

## 4. DUODENAL STIMULATION OF GASTRIC SECRETION

- Presence of partially digested proteins and amino acids in the duodenum acid secretion in the stomach is stimulated by three methods.
  - *Peptones* stimulate duodenal G Cells to secrete gastrin.
  - Peptones stimulate an unknown endocrine cell to release an additional humoral signal, "*enterooxytonin*".
  - Amino Acids absorbed by the duodenum stimulate acid secretion by unknown mechanisms.

# 5. DUODENAL INHIBITION OF GASTRIC SECRETION

- The acid and semi-digested fats in the duodenum trigger the enterogastric reflex – the duodenum sends inhibitory signals to the stomach by way of the enteric nervous system, and sends signals to the medulla that (1) inhibit the vagal nuclei, thus reducing vagal stimulation of the stomach, and (2) stimulate sympathetic neurons, which send inhibitory signals to the stomach. Chyme also stimulates duodenal enteroendocrine cells to release **secretin** and **cholecystokinin**.
- *They primarily stimulate the pancreas and gall bladder, but also suppress gastric secretion and motility.*

## A. SECRETIN

- Produced by the Cells in the lining of the duodenum in response *to **acidic chyme*** emerging from the stomach.
- Stimulates the pancreas to produce and secrete pancreatic juice containing a high concentration of bicarbonate ions.
- Bicarbonate reacts with and neutralizes hydrochloric acid present in chyme to return the chyme to a neutral pH of around 7.

## B. CCK

- It is a hormone produced by cells in the lining of the duodenum in response to the presence of ***proteins and fats in chyme***.
- Travels through the bloodstream and binds to receptor cells in the acini of the pancreas.
- Stimulates these cells to produce and secrete pancreatic juice that has a high concentration of digestive enzymes.
- The high levels of enzymes in pancreatic juice help to digest large protein and lipid molecules that are more difficult to break down.

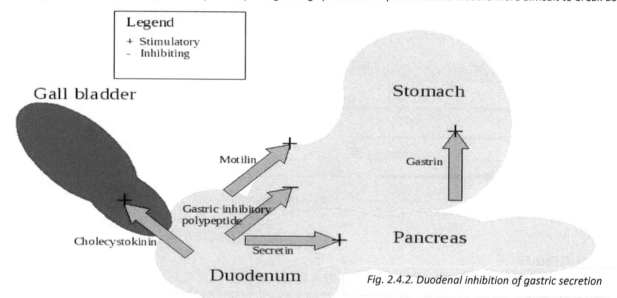

Fig. 2.4.2. Duodenal inhibition of gastric secretion

## GASTROINTESTINAL HORMONES

| Hormone | Source | Target | Triggers | Effects |
|---|---|---|---|---|
| Gastrin | Gastric mucosa | Stomach | Food in stomach, psychic factors | Increased HCl secretion & gastric emptying |
| Cholecystokinin (CCK) | Duodenal mucosa | Gallbladder & pancreas | Amino acids, peptides, fatty acids in duodenum | Contraction of gallbladder & secretion of pancreatic juice |
| Secretin | Duodenal mucosa | Pancreas | Acid in duodenum | Increased bicarbonate secretion |
| Enterogastrone: Gastric inhibitory peptide | Duodenal mucosa | Stomach | Fat digestion products in duodenum | Decreases gastric emptying |

| | |
|---|---|
| • HCL secretion from parietal cells occurs in the cardia | F |
| • Acid secretion is increased by Histamine | T |
| • Intrinsic factors from chief cells is vital for Vit B12 absorption | F |
| • NSAIDS predispose to Peptic Ulcer Disease by increasing acid secretion | F |

# IV. SMALL INTESTINE

## 1. FUNCTIONS

- Peristalsis moves the chyme through the small intestine.
- Chemical digestion.
  - Enzymes from the small intestine and pancreas break down all four groups of molecules found in food (polysaccharides, proteins, fats, and nucleic acids) into their component molecules.
- **Absorption:** The small intestine is the primary location in the GI tract for absorption of nutrients.
- The components of carbohydrates, proteins, nucleic acids, and water-soluble vitamins are absorbed by facilitated diffusion or active transport. They are then passed to blood capillaries.
- *Vitamin B $_{12}$:* Vitamin B $_{12}$ combines with intrinsic factor (produced in the stomach) and is absorbed by receptor-mediated endocytosis. It is then passed to the blood capillaries.
- *Lipids and fat-soluble vitamins:* Because fat-soluble vitamins and the components of lipids are insoluble in water, they are packaged and delivered to cells within water-soluble clusters of bile salts called micelles.
  - They are then absorbed by simple diffusion and, once inside the cells, mix with cholesterol and protein to form *chylomicrons*.
  - The chylomicrons are then passed to the lymphatic capillaries.
  - When the lymph eventually empties into the blood, the chylomicrons are broken down by lipoprotein lipase, and the breakdown products, fatty acids and glycerol, pass through blood capillary walls to be absorbed by various cells.
- *Water and electrolytes:* About 90 percent of the water in chyme is absorbed, as well as various electrolytes (ions), including $Na^+$, $K^+$, $Cl^-$, nitrates, calcium, and iron.

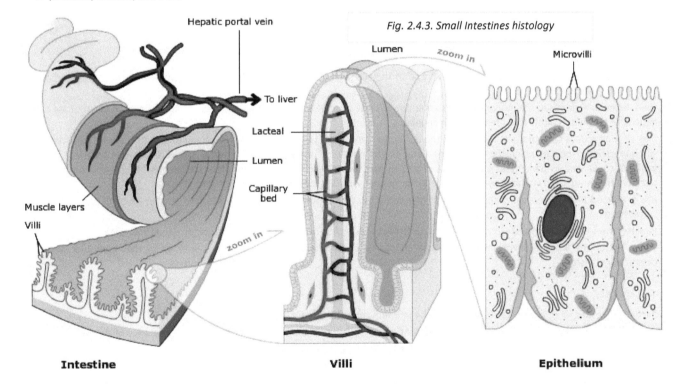

Fig. 2.4.3. Small Intestines histology

**Intestine**            **Villi**            **Epithelium**

a. **Modifications of the mucosa for its various specialized functions in the small intestine include the following:**
   - *The plicae circulares (circular folds)* are permanent ridges in the mucosa that encircle the inside of the small intestine. The ridges force the food to spiral forward. The spiral motion helps mix the chyme with the digestive juices.
   - *Villi (singular, villus)* are fingerlike projections that cover the surface of the mucosa, giving it a velvety appearance. They increase the surface area over which absorption and digestion occur.
   - The spaces between adjacent villi lead to deep cavities at the bases of the villi called intestinal crypts *(crypts of Lieberkühn)*. Glands that empty into the cavities are called intestinal glands, and the secretions are collectively called intestinal juice.
   - *Microvilli* are microscopic extensions of the outer surface of the absorptive cells that line each villus. Because of their brushlike appearance (microscopically), the microvilli facing the lumen form the brush border of the small intestine. Like the villi; the microvilli increase the surface area over which digestion and absorption take place.
   - The villi of the mucosa have the following characteristics: An outer epithelial layer (facing the lumen) consists of the following cell types:

- o **Absorptive cells**, the primary cell type of the epithelial layer, synthesize digestive enzymes called brush border enzymes that become embedded in the plasma membranes around the microvilli. Various nutrients in the chyme that move over the microvilli are broken down by these brush border enzymes and subsequently absorbed.
  - o **Goblet cells**, located throughout the epithelial layer, secrete mucus that helps protect the epithelial layer from digestion.
  - o **Enteroendocrine cells** secrete hormones into blood vessels that penetrate each villus.
  - o **Paneth cells**, located in the epithelial layer facing the intestinal crypts, secrete lysozyme, an enzyme that destroys bacteria.
  - o An inner core of lamina propria (connective tissues) contains blood capillaries and small lymphatic capillaries called lacteals.
- b. **The submucosa that underlies the mucosa of the small intestine bears the following modifications:**
  - o **Brunner's (duodenal) glands**, found only in the submucosa of the duodenum, secrete an alkaline mucus that neutralizes the gastric acid in the incoming chyme.
  - o **Peyer's patches** (aggregated lymphatic nodules), found mostly in the submucosa of the ileum, are clusters of lymphatic nodules that provide a defensive barrier against bacteria.
- In the duodenum, segmentations help to mix chyme with bile and pancreatic juice to complete the chemical digestion of the chyme into its component nutrients.
- Villi and microvilli throughout the intestines sway back and forth during the segmentations to increase their contact with chyme and efficiently absorb nutrients.
- Once nutrients have been absorbed by the mucosa, they are passed on into tiny blood vessels and lymphatic vessels in the middle of the villi to exit through the mesentery. Fatty acids enter small lymphatic vessels called *lacteals* that carry them back to the blood supply.
- All other nutrients are carried through veins to the liver, where many nutrients are stored and converted into useful energy sources.
- Chyme is slowly passed through the small intestine by waves of smooth muscle contraction known as peristalsis.
- Each wave moves the chyme a short distance, so it takes many waves of peristalsis over several hours to move chyme to the end of the ileum.

## 2. DUODENUM

- After being stored and mixed with hydrochloric acid in the stomach for about 30 to 60 minutes, chyme slowly enters the duodenum through the pyloric sphincter.
- Next, Brunner's glands in the mucosa of the duodenum secrete alkaline mucus containing a high concentration of bicarbonate ions to neutralize the hydrochloric acid present in the chyme.
- This alkaline mucus both protects the walls of the duodenum and helps the chyme to reach a pH conducive to chemical digestion in the small intestine. Upon reaching the ampulla of Vater in the middle of the duodenum, chyme is mixed with bile from the liver and gallbladder, as well as pancreatic juice produced by the pancreas. These secretions complete the process of chemical digestion that began in the mouth and stomach by breaking complex macromolecules into their basic units.
- Bile produced in the liver and stored in the gallbladder acts as an emulsifier, breaking lipids into smaller globules to increase their surface area.
- Pancreatic juice contains many enzymes to break carbohydrates, lipids, proteins and nucleic acids into their monomer subunits.
- These secretions are thoroughly mixed with the chyme by contractions of the duodenum until all of the digestible material is chemically digested.

## 3. JEJUNUM

- Partially digested food, known as chyme, enters the jejunum from the duodenum.
- As chyme enters the jejunum, it is mixed by segmentations, or localized smooth muscle contractions in the walls of the jejunum.
- These segmentations help to circulate chyme and increase its contact with the walls of the jejunum.
- The walls of the jejunum are folded many times over to increase its surface area and allow it to absorb nutrients.
- Each epithelial cell on the surface of the jejunum contains microscopic folds of cell membrane called microvilli that create tiny pockets and increase the contact between the cells and chyme.
- The entire wall of the jejunum is also folded into microscopic finger-like ridges known as villi that form larger pockets and further increase the surface area of the jejunum. The entire structure of the jejunum is optimized for the absorption of nutrients from chyme.
- By the time chyme has passed through the jejunum and enters the ileum, around 90% of all available nutrients have been absorbed into the body.

## 4. TERMINAL ILEUM

- Chyme is thoroughly processed by the duodenum, jejunum, and ileum before it enters the terminal ileum. It is then stored in the hollow lumen of the terminal ileum as it awaits the opening of the ileocecal sphincter. Small masses of chyme are pushed into the cecum by waves of peristaltic contraction of the walls of the terminal ileum coordinated with the opening of the ileocecal sphincter.
- While the chyme is stored, Peyer's patches lining the walls of the terminal ileum examine the contents of the chyme for any potentially dangerous pathogens.

# V. PANCREAS

## 1. DIGESTION

- The exocrine portion of the pancreas plays a major role in the digestion of food.
- It releases the following enzymes:
- **Today All Live To See (2C) 3P**: *Chymotrypsinogen, Trypsinogen, Proelastase, Procarboxypeptidase, Amylase, Lipase, Phospholipase A2 and Cholesteroesterase.*
- The stomach slowly releases partially digested food into the duodenum as a thick, acidic liquid called chyme.
- The acini of the pancreas secrete pancreatic juice to complete the digestion of chyme in the duodenum.
- Pancreatic juice is a mixture of water, salts, bicarbonate, and many different digestive enzymes.
- The bicarbonate ions present in pancreatic juice neutralize the acid in chyme to protect the intestinal wall and to create the proper environment for the functioning of pancreatic enzymes.
- The pancreatic enzymes each specialize in digesting specific compounds found in chyme.

### A. PANCREATIC AMYLASE

- Breaks large polysaccharides like starches and glycogen into smaller sugars such as maltose, maltotriose, and glucose.
- Maltase secreted by the small intestine then breaks maltose into the monosaccharide glucose, which the intestines can directly absorb.

### B. TRYPSIN, CHYMOTRYPSIN AND CARBOXYPEPTIDASE

- Are protein-digesting enzymes that break proteins down into their amino acid subunits.
- These amino acids can then be absorbed by the intestines.

### C. PANCREATIC LIPASE

- Lipid-digesting enzyme that breaks large triglyceride molecules into fatty acids and monoglycerides.
- Bile released by the gallbladder emulsifies fats to increase the surface area of triglycerides that pancreatic lipase can react with.
- The fatty acids and monoglycerides produced by pancreatic lipase can be absorbed by the intestines.

### D. RIBONUCLEASE AND DEOXYRIBONUCLEASE

- Are nucleases, or enzymes that digest nucleic acids.
- Ribonuclease breaks down molecules of RNA into the sugar ribose and the nitrogenous bases adenine, cytosine, guanine and uracil.
- Deoxyribonuclease digests DNA molecules into the sugar deoxyribose and the nitrogenous bases adenine, cytosine, guanine, and thymine.

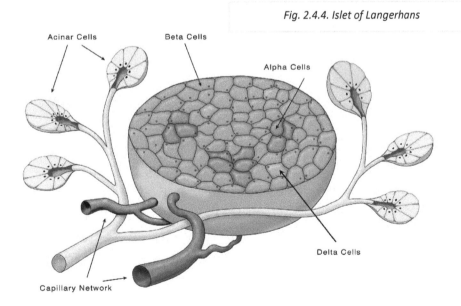

*Fig. 2.4.4. Islet of Langerhans*

## 2. BLOOD GLUCOSE HOMEOSTASIS

- The pancreas produces 2 antagonistic hormones to control blood sugar: glucagon and insulin. *The alpha cells of the pancreas produce* glucagon. Glucagon raises blood glucose levels by stimulating the liver to metabolize glycogen into glucose molecules and to release glucose into the blood.
- Glucagon also stimulates adipose tissue to metabolize triglycerides into glucose and to release glucose into the blood.

- *Insulin* is produced by **the beta cells of the pancreas**. This hormone lowers blood glucose levels after a meal by stimulating the absorption of glucose by liver, muscle, and adipose tissues. Insulin triggers the formation of glycogen in the muscles and liver and triglycerides in adipose to store the absorbed glucose.

## 3. REGULATION OF PANCREATIC FUNCTION

- The pancreas is controlled by both the autonomic nervous system (ANS) and the endocrine system.
- The ANS has 2 divisions: the sympathetic and the parasympathetic.

### A. NERVES OF THE SYMPATHETIC DIVISION

- o Become active during stressful situations, emergencies, and exercise.
- o Sympathetic neurons stimulate the alpha cells of the pancreas to release the hormone glucagon into the bloodstream.
- o Glucagon stimulates the liver to begin the breakdown of the energy storage molecule glycogen into smaller glucose molecules.
- o Glucose is then released into the bloodstream for the organs, especially the heart and skeletal muscles, to use as energy.
- o The sympathetic nerves also inhibit the function of beta cells and acini to reduce or prevent the secretion of insulin and pancreatic juice. The inhibition of these functions provides more energy for other parts of the body that are active in dealing with the stressful situation.

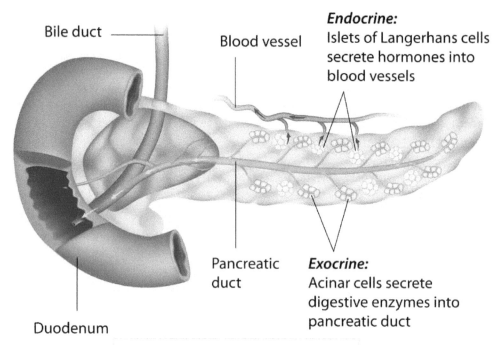

*Fig. 2.4.5. Endocrine and Exocrine pancreas*

### B. NERVES OF THE PARASYMPATHETIC DIVISION

- o Become active during restful times and during the digestion of a meal.
- o Parasympathetic nerves stimulate the release of insulin and pancreatic juice by the pancreas.
- o Pancreatic juice helps with the digestion of food while insulin stores the glucose released from the digested food in the body's cells.
- The endocrine system uses 2 hormones to regulate the digestive function of the pancreas: *secretin* and *cholecystokinin (CCK)*.

### a. SECRETIN

- Produced by the Cells in the lining of the duodenum in response *to acidic chyme* emerging from the stomach.
- Stimulates the pancreas to produce and secrete pancreatic juice containing a high concentration of bicarbonate ions.
- Bicarbonate reacts with and neutralizes hydrochloric acid present in chyme to return the chyme to a neutral pH of around 7.

### b. CCK

- It is a hormone produced by cells in the lining of the duodenum in response to the presence of *proteins and fats in chyme*.
- Travels through the bloodstream and binds to receptor cells in the acini of the pancreas.
- Stimulates these cells to produce and secrete pancreatic juice that has a high concentration of digestive enzymes.
- The high levels of enzymes in pancreatic juice help to digest large protein and lipid molecules that are more difficult to break down.

# VI. LIVER

## A. CONSTITUENTS OF A PORTAL TRIAD

- It is a component of the hepatic lobule.
  It consists of the following five structures: **PHC Like Bachelor**
  - ✓ *Portal Vein*
  - ✓ *Hepatic artery proper*
  - ✓ *Common bile duct*
  - ✓ *Lymphatic vessels*
  - ✓ *Branch of the vagus nerve*

## B. FUNCTIONS

### 1. DIGESTION

- The liver plays an active role in the process of digestion through the production of bile.
- Bile is a mixture of water, bile salts, cholesterol, and the pigment bilirubin.
- Hepatocytes in the liver produce bile, which then passes through the bile ducts to be stored in the gallbladder.
- When food containing fats reaches the duodenum, the cells of the duodenum release the hormone cholecystokinin to stimulate the gallbladder to release bile.
- Bile travels through the bile ducts and is released into the duodenum where it emulsifies large masses of fat.
- The emulsification of fats by bile turns the large clumps of fat into smaller pieces that have more surface area and are therefore easier for the body to digest.
- Bilirubin present in bile is a product of the liver's digestion of worn out red blood cells.
- Kupffer cells in the liver catch and destroy old, worn out red blood cells and pass their components on to hepatocytes.
- Hepatocytes metabolize hemoglobin, the red oxygen-carrying pigment of red blood cells, into the components heme and globin.
- Globin protein is further broken down and used as an energy source for the body.
- The iron-containing heme group cannot be recycled by the body and is converted into the pigment bilirubin and added to bile to be excreted from the body.
- Bilirubin gives bile its distinctive greenish color.
- Intestinal bacteria further convert bilirubin into the brown pigment stercobilin, which gives feces their brown color.

### 2. METABOLISM

- Because all of the blood leaving the digestive system passes through the hepatic portal vein, the liver is responsible for metabolizing carbohydrate, lipids, and proteins into biologically useful materials.
- The digestive system breaks down *carbohydrates* into the monosaccharide glucose, which cells use as a primary energy source.
- Blood entering the liver through the hepatic portal vein is extremely rich in glucose from digested food.
- Hepatocytes absorb much of this glucose and store it as the macromolecule glycogen, a branched polysaccharide that allows the hepatocytes to pack away large amounts of glucose and quickly release glucose between meals.
- The absorption and release of glucose by the hepatocytes helps to maintain homeostasis and protects the rest of the body from dangerous spikes and drops in the blood glucose level.
- *Fatty acids* in the blood passing through the liver are absorbed by hepatocytes and metabolized to produce energy in the form of ATP.
- *Glycerol*, another lipid component, is converted into glucose by hepatocytes through the process of *gluconeogenesis*.
- Hepatocytes can also produce lipids like cholesterol, phospholipids, and lipoproteins that are used by other cells throughout the body.
- Much of the cholesterol produced by hepatocytes gets excreted from the body as a component of bile.
- *Dietary proteins* are broken down into their component amino acids by the digestive system before being passed on to the hepatic portal vein. Amino acids entering the liver require metabolic processing before they can be used as an energy source.
- Hepatocytes first remove the amine groups of the amino acids and convert them into ammonia and eventually urea.
- Urea is less toxic than ammonia and can be excreted in urine as a waste product of digestion.
- The remaining parts of the amino acids can be broken down into ATP or converted into new glucose molecules through the process of gluconeogenesis.

### 3. DETOXIFICATION

- As blood from the digestive organs passes through the hepatic portal circulation, the hepatocytes of the liver monitor the contents of the blood and remove many potentially toxic substances before they can reach the rest of the body.
- Enzymes in hepatocytes metabolize many of these toxins such as alcohol and drugs into their inactive metabolites.
- And in order to keep hormone levels within homeostatic limits, the liver also metabolizes and removes from circulation hormones produced by the body's own glands.

## 4. STORAGE

- The liver provides storage of many essential nutrients, vitamins, and minerals obtained from blood passing through the hepatic portal system.
- Glucose is transported into hepatocytes under the influence of the hormone insulin and stored as the polysaccharide glycogen.
- Hepatocytes also absorb and store fatty acids from digested triglycerides.
- The storage of these nutrients allows the liver to maintain the homeostasis of blood glucose.
- The liver also stores vitamins and minerals - such as *vitamins A, D, E, K, and B12 and the minerals iron and copper* in order to provide a constant supply of these essential substances to the tissues of the body.

## 5. PRODUCTION OF PROTEINS

- The liver is responsible for the production of several vital protein components of blood plasma: prothrombin, fibrinogen, and albumins.
- Prothrombin and fibrinogen proteins are coagulation factors involved in the formation of blood clots.
- Albumins are proteins that maintain the isotonic environment of the blood so that cells of the body do not gain or lose water in the presence of body fluids.

## 6. IMMUNITY

- The liver functions as an organ of the immune system through the function of the *Kupffer cells* that line the sinusoids.
- Kupffer cells are a type of fixed macrophage that form part of the mononuclear phagocyte system along with macrophages in the spleen and lymph nodes.
- Kupffer cells play an important role by capturing and digesting bacteria, fungi, parasites, worn-out blood cells, and cellular debris.
- The large volume of blood passing through the hepatic portal system and the liver allows Kupffer cells to clean large volumes of blood very quickly.

# C. ORIGIN AND CONSTITUENTS OF HEPATIC BILE

- There are two fundamentally important functions of bile in all species:
  - Bile contains bile acids, which are critical for digestion and absorption of fats and fat-soluble vitamins in the small intestine.
  - Many waste products, including bilirubin, are eliminated from the body by secretion into bile and elimination in feces.
- Adult humans produce 400 to 800 ml of bile daily.
- The secretion of bile can be considered to occur in two stages:
  - Initially, hepatocytes secrete bile into canaliculi, from which it flows into bile ducts. This hepatic bile contains large quantities of bile acids, cholesterol and other organic molecules.
  - As bile flows through the bile ducts it is modified by addition of a watery, bicarbonate-rich secretion from ductal epithelial cells.
- Typically, bile is concentrated five-fold in the gallbladder by absorption of water and small electrolytes. Virtually all of the organic molecules are retained.
- Secretion into bile is a major route for eliminating cholesterol.
- Free cholesterol is virtually insoluble in aqueous solutions, but in bile, it is made soluble by bile acids and lipids like lecithin.
- Gallstones, most of which are composed predominantly of cholesterol, result from processes that allow cholesterol to precipitate from solution in bile.

# D. ROLE OF BILE ACIDS IN FAT DIGESTION & ABSORPTION

- In humans, roughly 500 mg of cholesterol are converted to bile acids and eliminated in bile every day.
- Bile acids are derivatives of cholesterol synthesized in the hepatocyte.
- Cholesterol, ingested as part of the diet or derived from hepatic synthesis is converted into the bile acids cholic and chenodeoxycholic acids, which are then conjugated to an amino acid (glycine or taurine) to yield the conjugated form that is actively secreted into canaliculi.
- Bile acids are facial amphipathic, that is, they contain both hydrophobic (lipid soluble) and polar (hydrophilic) faces.
- The cholesterol-derived portion of a bile acid has one face that is hydrophobic (that with methyl groups) and one that is hydrophilic (that with the hydroxyl groups); the amino acid conjugate is polar and hydrophilic.
- Their amphipathic nature enables bile acids to carry out two important functions:
  - *Emulsification of lipid aggregates*: Bile acids have detergent action on particles of dietary fat which causes fat globules to break down or be emulsified into minute, microscopic droplets.
    Emulsification is not digestion per se, but is of importance because it greatly increases the surface area of fat, making it available for digestion by lipases, which cannot access the inside of lipid droplets.
  - *Solubilization and transport of lipids in an aqueous environment*: Bile acids are lipid carriers and are able to solubilize many lipids by forming micelles - aggregates of lipids such as fatty acids, cholesterol and monoglycerides - that remain suspended in water.
- Bile acids are also critical for transport and absorption of the fat-soluble vitamins.

## E. ENTEROHEPATIC RECIRCULATION

- Large amounts of bile acids are secreted into the intestine every day, but only relatively small quantities are lost from the body.
- This is because approximately 95% of the bile acids delivered to the duodenum are absorbed back into blood within the ileum.
- Venous blood from the ileum goes straight into the portal vein, and hence through the sinusoids of the liver.
- Hepatocytes extract bile acids very efficiently from sinusoidal blood, and little escapes the healthy liver into systemic circulation.
- Bile acids are then transported across the hepatocytes to be resecreted into canaliculi. The net effect of this enterohepatic recirculation is that each bile salt molecule is reused about 20 times, often two or three times during a single digestive phase.

## F. PATTERN AND CONTROL OF BILE SECRETION

- The flow of bile is lowest during fasting, and a majority of that is diverted into the gallbladder for concentration.
- When chyme from an ingested meal enters the small intestine, acid and partially digested fats and proteins stimulate secretion of secretin and cholecystokinin.
- These enteric hormones have important effects on pancreatic exocrine secretion.
- They are both also important for secretion and flow of bile:
  - *Cholecystokinin*: The most potent stimulus for release of cholecystokinin is the presence of fat in the duodenum. Once released, it stimulates contractions of the gallbladder and common bile duct, resulting in delivery of bile into the gut.
  - *Secretin*: This hormone is secreted in response to acid in the duodenum. Its effect on the biliary system is very similar to what was seen in the pancreas - it simulates biliary duct cells to secrete bicarbonate and water, which expands the volume of bile and increases its flow out into the intestine.

## G. BILIRUBIN

- Bilirubin is conjugated with *glucuronic acid* in the liver by the enzyme *glucuronyltransferase*, making it soluble in water.
- Much of it goes into the bile and thus out into the small intestine.
- However, 95% of the secreted bile is reabsorbed by the small intestine.
- This bile is then resecreted by the liver into the small intestine.
- About half of the conjugated bilirubin remaining in the large intestine (about 5% of what was originally secreted) is metabolised by colonic bacteria to *urobilinogen*, which is then further oxidized to *urobilin and stercobilin*. Urobilin, stercobilin and their degradation products give feces its brown color. Just like bile, some of the urobilinogen is reabsorbed, and 95% of what is reabsorbed is resecreted in the bile which is also part of enterohepatic circulation. A small amount of the reabsorbed urobilinogen (about 5%) is excreted in the urine where it is converted to an oxidized form, urobilin, which gives urine its characteristic yellow color.
- This whole process results in only 1-20% of secreted bile being lost in the feces. The amount lost depends on the secretion rate of bile.

# VII. GALLBLADDER

## 1. STORAGE

- The gallbladder acts as a storage vessel for bile produced by the liver.
- Bile is produced by hepatocytes cells in the liver and passes through the bile ducts to the cystic duct.
- From the cystic duct, bile is pushed into the gallbladder by peristalsis then slowly concentrated by absorption of water through the walls of the gallbladder. The gallbladder stores this concentrated bile until it is needed to digest the next meal.

## 2. STIMULATION

- Foods rich in proteins or fats are more difficult for the body to digest when compared to carbohydrate-rich foods.
- The walls of the duodenum contain sensory receptors that monitor the chemical makeup of chyme that passes through the pyloric sphincter into the duodenum. When these cells detect proteins or fats, they respond by producing the hormone cholecystokinin (CCK).
- CCK enters the bloodstream and travels to the gallbladder where it stimulates the smooth muscle tissue in the walls of the gallbladder.

## 3. SECRETION

- When CCK reaches the gallbladder, it triggers the smooth muscle tissue in the muscularis layer of the gallbladder to contract.
- The contraction of smooth muscle forces bile out of the gallbladder and into the cystic duct.
- From the cystic duct, bile enters the common bile duct and flows into the ampulla of Vater, where the bile ducts merge with the pancreatic duct. Bile then flows from the ampulla of Vater into the duodenum where it breaks the fats into smaller masses for easier digestion by the enzyme pancreatic lipase.

## 4. GALLSTONES

- Gallstones are hard masses of bile salts, pigments, and cholesterol that develop within the gallbladder.
- These solid masses form when the components of bile crystallize.

# VIII. LARGE INTESTINE

- A slurry of digested food, known as chyme, enters the large intestine from the small intestine via the ileocecal sphincter.
- Chyme passes through the cecum where it is mixed with beneficial bacteria that have colonized the large intestine throughout a person's lifetime. The chyme is then slowly moved from one haustra to the next through the four regions of the colon.
- Most of the movement of chyme is achieved by slow waves of peristalsis over a period of several hours, but the colon can also be emptied quickly by stronger waves of mass peristalsis following a large meal.
- While chyme moves through the large intestine, bacteria digest substances in the chyme that are not digestible by the human digestive system. Bacterial fermentation converts the chyme into feces and releases vitamins including vitamins *K, B1, B2, B6, B12, and biotin*.
- *Vitamin K is almost exclusively produced by the gut* bacteria and is essential in the proper clotting of blood.
- Gases such as carbon dioxide and methane are also produced as a by-product of bacterial fermentation and lead to flatulence, or gas passed through the anus. The absorption of water by the large intestine not only helps to condense and solidify feces, but also allows the body to retain water to be used in other metabolic processes. Ions and nutrients released by gut bacteria and dissolved in water are also absorbed in the large intestine and used by the body for metabolism.
- The dried, condensed fecal matter is finally stored in the rectum and sigmoid colon until it can be eliminated from the body through the process of defecation.

## 1. THE CECUM

- Plays an important role in the digestive system by assisting in the formation of feces. Partially digested food, known as chyme, passes through the small intestine where it is digested and most of its nutrients are absorbed.
- The ileocecal sphincter at the end of the small intestine opens and closes to allow small amounts of chyme to enter the cecum at the beginning of the large intestine. Chyme is next mixed with bacteria by contractions in the walls of the cecum.

## 2. ASCENDING COLON

- About 90% of the nutrients present in digested food have been absorbed by the time it reaches the large intestine.
- This food is mixed with bacteria in the cecum to form feces. Waves of peristalsis move the feces slowly up the length of the ascending colon. As the feces pass through the ascending colon, bacteria digest the waste material that the human body cannot digest and liberate *vitamins K, B1, B2, and B12*.
- The walls of the colon absorb these vitamins along with most of the water present in the feces.
- Under normal conditions fecal matter enters the colon as chunky liquid waste and exits the colon as a condensed solid waste.
- The absorption of water by the colon helps to maintain water homeostasis in the body and prevent dehydration.

## 3. THE TRANSVERSE COLON

- Mixes feces by contracting small regions of the intestinal wall in a process known as segmentation.
- As the feces are mixed, bacteria ferment the waste material to release vitamins and a few trace nutrients remaining in the waste.
- Water, nutrients, and vitamins are absorbed through the walls of the colon to be used by the tissues of the body.
- The colon then uses slow longitudinal waves of muscle contraction known as peristalsis to push the feces along its length.

## 4. DESCENDING COLON

- By the time feces reach the descending colon, the vast majority of nutrients, vitamins and water have been extracted by the ascending and transverse colon, leaving mostly waste products.
- Still, some absorption of water and vitamins produced by bacterial fermentation of feces, including vitamins K, B1, B2 and B12, does occur in the descending colon.
- Its primary function, however, is the storage and accumulation of feces prior to defecation.
- During defecation, the descending colon helps to propel feces toward the sigmoid colon and rectum and eventually out of the body by contraction of its smooth muscle tissue.

## 5. THE SIGMOID COLON AND RECTUM

- Feces enter the rectum from the sigmoid colon, where they are stored until they can be eliminated through defecation.
- While feces are stored in the rectum, the walls of the rectum absorb some water and return it to the blood supply.
- Bacteria continue the fermentation of organic fecal matter that began in the colon and liberate some remaining nutrients that are absorbed by the rectal walls. As feces accumulate and fill the rectum, they exert increasing pressure on the rectal walls.
- The distention of the rectum stimulates stretch receptors in the rectal walls to send nerve impulses to the brain.
- These impulses are integrated in the brain and result in feelings of discomfort and mounting pressure to empty the rectum through defecation.
- *They also cause relaxation of the smooth muscle of the internal anal sphincter to allow defecation to proceed.*

# Section 5: Renal Physiology

## I. BASIC ANATOMY OF THE KIDNEYS

### 1. OVERVIEW

- The urinary system helps maintain homeostasis by regulating water balance and by removing harmful substances from the blood.
- The kidneys are surrounded by three layers of tissue:
  - **The renal fascia** is a thin, outer layer of fibrous connective tissue that surrounds each kidney (and the attached adrenal gland) and fastens it to surrounding structures.
  - **The adipose capsule** is a middle layer of adipose (fat) tissue that cushions the kidneys.
  - **The renal capsule** is an inner fibrous membrane that prevents the entrance of infections.
- Inside the kidney, three major regions are distinguished:
  - **The renal cortex** borders the convex side.
  - **The renal medulla** lies adjacent to the renal cortex.
    It consists of striated, cone-shaped regions called **renal pyramids** (medullary pyramids), whose peaks, called **renal papillae**, face inward.
    The unstriated regions between the renal pyramids are called **renal columns**.
  - **The renal sinus** is a cavity that lies adjacent to the renal medulla.
- The other side of the renal sinus, bordering the concave surface of the kidney, opens to the outside through the **renal hilus**.
- The ureter, nerves, and blood and lymphatic vessels enter the kidney on the concave surface through the renal hilus.
- The renal sinus houses the renal pelvis, a funnel-shaped structure that merges with the ureter.

### 2. BLOOD AND NERVE SUPPLY

#### ARTERIAL SUPPLY:

- Blood supply is delivered by the large renal arteries.
- The renal artery for each kidney enters the renal hilus and successively branches into segmental arteries and then into *interlobar arteries*.
- The interlobar arteries then branch into *the arcuate arteries*, which curve as they pass along the junction of the renal medulla and cortex.
- Branches of the arcuate arteries, called *interlobular arteries*, penetrate the renal cortex, where they again branch into afferent arterioles, which enter the filtering mechanisms, or glomeruli, of the nephrons.

#### VENOUS DRAINAGE:

- Blood leaving the nephrons exits the kidney through veins that trace the same path, in reverse, as the arteries that delivered the blood. Interlobular, arcuate, interlobar, and segmental veins successively merge and exit as a single renal vein.

#### INNERVATION

- Autonomic nerves from the renal plexus follow the renal artery into the kidney through the renal hilus.
- The nerve fibers follow the branching pattern of the renal artery and serve as vasomotor fibers that regulate blood volume.
- *Sympathetic fibers constrict arterioles (decreasing urine output); while less numerous parasympathetic fibers dilate arterioles (increasing urine output).*

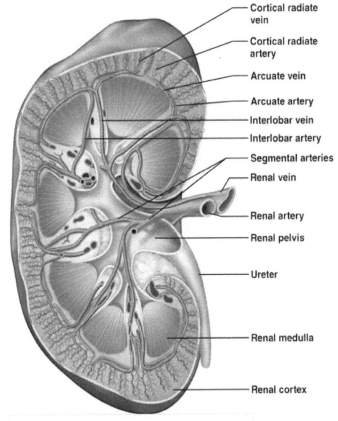

- Cortical radiate vein
- Cortical radiate artery
- Arcuate vein
- Arcuate artery
- Interlobar vein
- Interlobar artery
- Segmental arteries
- Renal vein
- Renal artery
- Renal pelvis
- Ureter
- Renal medulla
- Renal cortex

*Fig. 2.5.1. Renal blood supply*

### 3. NEPHRONS

- The kidney consists of over a million individual filtering units called *nephrons* (800,000 to 1,5 million nephrons)
- Each nephron consists of a filtering body, the renal corpuscle, and a urine-collecting and concentrating tube, the renal tubule.

# II. THE RENAL CORPUSCLE

- It is an assemblage of two structures, the glomerular capillaries and the glomerular capsule.

## 1. THE GLOMERULUS

- It is a dense ball of capillaries (glomerular capillaries) that branches from the afferent arteriole that enters the nephron.
- Because blood in the glomerular capillaries is under high pressure, substances in the blood that are small enough to pass through the pores (fenestrae, or endothelial fenestrations) in the capillary walls are forced out and into the encircling glomerular capsule.
- The glomerular capillaries merge, and the remaining blood exits the glomerular capsule through the efferent arteriole.
- **The Glomerular Capsule (Bowman's Capsule):**
  - Bowman's capsules are located in the renal cortex. It is a cup-shaped body that encircles the glomerular capillaries and collects the material (filtrate) that is forced out of the glomerular capillaries.

## 2. GLOMERULAR FILTRATION

- **20%** of glomerular plasma flow passes through the filter (filtration fraction)
- When blood enters the glomerular capillaries, water and solutes are forced into the glomerular capsule.
- Passage of cells and certain molecules are restricted as follows:
  - **The Fenestrae (pores)** of the capillary endothelium are large, permitting all components of blood plasma to pass except blood cells.
  - **A Basement Membrane** (consisting of extracellular material) that lies between the capillary endothelium and the visceral layer of the glomerular capsule blocks the entrance of large proteins into the glomerular capsule.
  - **The Filtration** slits between the pedicels of the podocytes prevent the passage of medium-sized proteins into the glomerular capsule.

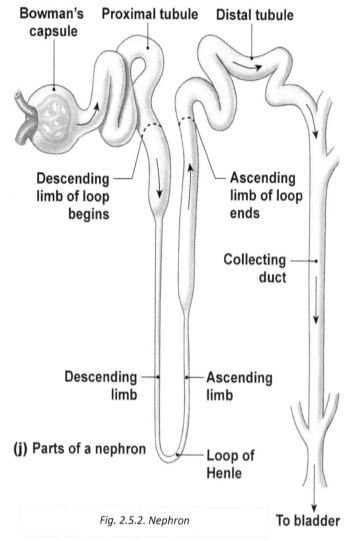

**(j) Parts of a nephron**

*Fig. 2.5.2. Nephron*

- The net filtration pressure (NFP) determines the quantity of filtrate that is forced into the glomerular capsule.
- The NFP, estimated at about *10 mmHg*, is the sum of pressures that promote filtration less the sum of those that oppose filtration.
- The glomerular filtration rate (GFR) is the rate at which filtrate collectively accumulates in the glomerulus of each nephron.
- The GFR, about 125 mL/min (180 liters/day), is regulated by the following:
  - Renal autoregulation
  - Neural regulation
  - Hormonal control of GFR is accomplished by the renin/angiotensinogen mechanism.
- When cells of the juxtaglomerular apparatus detect a decrease in blood pressure in the afferent arteriole or a decrease in solute ($Na^+$ and $Cl^-$) concentrations in the distal tubule, they secrete the enzyme renin.
- Renin converts angiotensinogen (a plasma protein produced by the liver) to angiotensin I.
- Angiotensin I in turn is converted to angiotensin II by the angiotensin-converting enzyme (ACE), *an enzyme produced principally by capillary endothelium in the lungs.* Angiotensin II circulates in the blood and increases GFR by doing the following:
  - Constricting blood vessels throughout the body, causing the blood pressure to rise
  - Stimulating the adrenal cortex to secrete aldosterone, a hormone that increases blood pressure by decreasing water output by the kidneys.

# III. THE RENAL TUBULE

o Consists of four sections:

## 1. THE PROXIMAL CONVOLUTED TUBULE (PCT)

o Exits the glomerular capsule as a winding tube in the renal cortex.
o The wall of the PCT consists of cuboidal cells containing numerous mitochondria and bearing a brush border of dense microvilli that face the lumen (interior cavity).
o The high-energy yield and large surface area of these cells support their functions of reabsorption and secretion.
o The initial glomerular filtrate has an osmolarity equivalent to that of the ECF; that is **300mOsm/L.**
o In the proximal tubule, two thirds of the primary urine volume with electrolytes are reabsorbed.
o *The net osmolarity of the tubular fluid does not change significantly in the proximal tubule or the thin Henle.*

### REABSORBTION WITHIN THE PCT

o *The PCT reabsorbs approximately*:
  - **100% of filtered Glucose (**pathway saturable only up to 10mmol/l...above that glucose is picked up in urine)
  - **100% of filtered Aminoacid**
  - **90% of filtered Bicarbonate**
  - **80% of filtered Phosphate**
  - **65% of filtered Potassium**
  - **65% of filtered Sodium**
  - **50% of filtered Urea (saturable pathway)**

- Electrolyte reabsorption leads to the water reabsorption with help of the leaky intercellular spaces of the proximal tubule epithelium.
- The solvent drug enables the paracellular absorption of water and chloride due to electrolyte concentrations between the tubule lumen and the renal interstitium.
- The drive of the sodium transport is accomplished through the basolateral sodium-potassium-pump.
- On the luminal side of the proximal tubule epithelium, sodium enters the cell via **symporter membrane proteins** (Co-transport with glucose, galactose, phosphate, sulfate or amino acids) or **antiporter membrane proteins** (Co-transport with protons).
- *The reabsorption of $HCO_3^-$ is linked to the sodium reabsorption and proton secretion with help of a luminal and intracellular carbonic anhydrase.*
- *The chloride reabsorption is not so clearly identified.* Beside the solvent drag, there are additional minor transcellular transport pathways for chloride in the luminal and basolateral membrane.

## 2. THE NEPHRON LOOP (LOOP OF HENLE)

- Is shaped like a hairpin and consists of a descending limb that drops into the renal medulla and an ascending limb that rises back into the renal cortex.
- As the loop descends, the tubule suddenly narrows, forming the thin segment of the loop.
- The loop subsequently widens in the ascending limb, forming the thick segment of the loop.
- Cells of the nephron loop vary from simple squamous epithelium (descending limb and thin segment of ascending limb) to cuboidal and low columnar epithelium (thick segment of ascending limb) and almost entirely lack microvilli.
- Around 85% of nephrons are cortical nephrons and possess only a short loop of Henle.
- The remaining 15% of nephrons are juxta-medullary nephrons which have long loop of Henle extending up to the tip of medullary pyramids.
- The medullary concentration gradient is produced and maintained by the juxtaglomerular nephrons with a long loop of Henle.
- *The thin descending limb contains water channels (aquaporins) and is highly permeable to water.*
- *Ascending limb of loop of Henle is almost completely impermeable to water.*

### ASCENDING PART OF THE HENLE LOOP

o *The thick ascending loop (TAL)* of Henle is impermeable to water and transports electrolytes into the interstitium of the kidney, producing a high osmotic pressure of the interstitium.
o *30% of the filtered sodium is reabsorbed using a luminal **Na-K-2Cl-cotransport*** mechanism.
o The effective prevention of a passive water flow with watertight tight junctions leads to a high osmotic pressure in the renal medulla.
o The urine at the end of the TAL is hypotonic.
o *Furosemide* inhibits the Na-K-2Cl cotransporter and leads to a massive natriuresis and loss of potassium, calcium and magnesium.

## 3. THE DISTAL CONVOLUTED TUBULE (DCT)

- Coils within the renal cortex and empties into the collecting duct. Cells here are cuboidal with few microvilli. Renal tubules of neighbouring nephrons empty urine into a single collecting duct.
- Here and in the final portions of the DCT, there are cells that respond to the hormones aldosterone and antidiuretic hormone (ADH), and there are cells that secrete H $^+$ in an effort to maintain proper pH.

- Various collecting ducts within the medullary pyramids merge to form papillary ducts, which drain eventually into the renal pelvis through the medullary papillae. Urine collects in the renal pelvis and drains out of the kidney through the ureter.
- The efferent arteriole carries blood away from the glomerular capillaries to form peritubular capillaries. These capillaries weave around the portions of the renal tubule that lie in the renal cortex.
- In portions of the nephron loop that descend deep into the renal medulla, the capillaries form loops, called **vasa recta**, that cross between the ascending and descending limbs. The peritubular capillaries collect water and nutrients from the filtrate in the tubule.
- They also release substances that are secreted into the tubule to combine with the filtrate in the formation of urine.
- The capillaries ultimately merge into an interlobular vein, which transports blood away from the nephron region.
- There are two kinds of nephrons:
  - **Cortical nephrons**, representing 85 percent of the nephrons in the kidney, have nephron loops that descend only slightly into the renal medulla.
  - **Juxtamedullary nephrons** have long nephron loops that descend deep into the renal medulla. *Only juxtamedullary nephrons have vasa recta that traverse their nephron loops.*
- *The juxtaglomerular apparatus (JGA) is an area of the nephron where the afferent arteriole and the initial portion of the distal convoluted tubule are in close contact.*
- *Here, specialized smooth muscle cells of the afferent arteriole, called granular juxtaglomerular (JG) cells, act as mechanoreceptors that monitor blood pressure in the afferent arteriole. In the adjacent distal convoluted tubule, specialized cells, called **macula densa**, act as chemoreceptors that monitor the concentration of $Na^+$ and $Cl^-$ in the urine inside the tubule.*
- *Together, these cells help regulate blood pressure and the production of urine in the nephron.*
- *Active sodium transport via **thiazide-sensitive Na-Cl-co-transporter;** about 10% of the filtered sodium is reabsorbed in the distal tubule. **Thiazides** inhibit the sodium reabsorption in the distal tubule and lead to a mild diuresis without loss of calcium (calcium-sparing diuretic).*

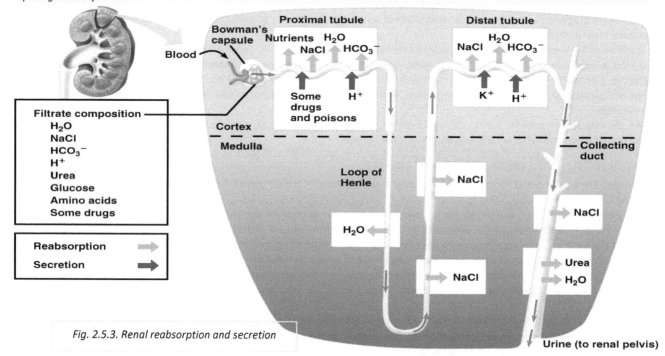

Fig. 2.5.3. Renal reabsorption and secretion

## 4. COLLECTING DUCTS

- The permeability of the collecting ducts for water lead to a concentration of the urine up to the fivefold osmolarity of the plasma.
- *The permeability of the collecting ducts is regulated with ADH (antidiuretic hormone, Vasopressin).*
- **ADH** causes the incorporation of additional water channels (aquaporins) into the luminal membrane.
- The high osmotic pressure of the renal medulla is the responsible force for the urine concentration.
- *ADH can control 10% of the primary urine volume, thus can regulate the diuresis between **1–20 L/d.***
- *In the absence of ADH, the permeability of the collecting ducts for water is low; the urine will not be concentrated.*
- *A deficiency of ADH secretion leads to diabetes insipidus, a disorder with massive diuresis and excessive thirst.*
- *Additional sodium reabsorption takes place in the collecting ducts via luminal sodium channels.*
- ***Aldosterone** regulates the sodium and water reabsorption and potassium secretion via expression of the sodium channels and the basolateral Na/K- pump.*
- *The luminal sodium channels can be inhibited by **Amiloride,** a potassium-sparing diuretic.*

# TUBULAR REABSORPTION

- The following mechanisms direct tubular reabsorption in the indicated regions:

**1. Active transport of Na $^+$**: PCT, DCT, and collecting duct.

- Because Na $^+$concentration is low inside tubular cells, Na $^+$ enters the tubular cells (across the luminal membrane) by passive diffusion.
- At the other side of the tubule cells, the basolateral membrane bears proteins that function as sodium-potassium (Na $^+$-K $^+$) pumps.
- These pumps use ATP to simultaneously export Na $^+$ while importing K $^+$.
- Thus, Na $^+$in the tubule cells is transported out of the cells and into the interstitial fluid by active transport.
- The Na $^+$in the interstitial fluid then enters the capillaries by passive diffusion.
- The K $^+$that is transported into the cell leaks back passively into the interstitial fluid.

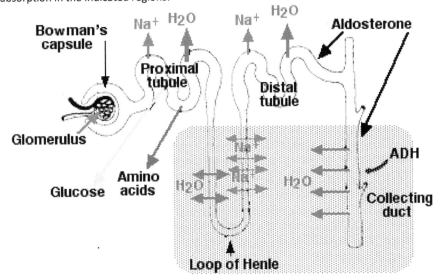

*Fig. 2.5.4. Renal reabsorption and secretion*

**2. Symporter transport (secondary active transport) of nutrients and ions**: PCT and Nephron Loop.

- Various nutrients, such as glucose and amino acids, and certain ions (K $^+$ and Cl $^-$) in the thick ascending limb of the nephron loop are transported into the tubule cells by the action of Na $^+$ symporters.
- A Na $^+$symporter is a transport protein that carries both Na $^+$ and another molecule, such as glucose, across a membrane in the same direction. Movement of glucose and other nutrients from the tubular lumen into the tubule cells occurs in this fashion.
- The process requires a low concentration of Na $^+$ inside the cells, a condition maintained by the Na $^+$-K $^+$ pump operating on the basolateral membranes of the tubule cells.
- The movement of nutrients into cells by this mechanism is referred to as secondary active transport, because the ATP-requiring mechanism is the Na $^+$-K $^+$ pump and not the symporter itself. Once inside the tubular cells, nutrients move into the interstitial fluid and into the capillaries by passive processes.

## RENAL REABSORBTION OF GLUCOSE

- ○ **Glucose** *is freely filtered at the glomerulus at a rate of **100mg/min**. Glucose is then almost completely **(nearly 100%)** reabsorbed from the proximal tubule by Na+ dependent secondary active transport processes.*
- ○ **At no point in the nephron is glucose secreted.**
- ○ **The renal threshold for glucose** *is the point where glucose reabsorption processes become saturated and glucose begins to appear in the urine. This occurs when the filtered glucose load exceeds around **250mg/min**, which corresponds to a venous blood glucose of around **11-12mmol/L (200 – 220 mg/dl)***

**3. Passive transport of H $_2$ O by osmosis**: PCT and DCT.

- The buildup of Na $^+$ in the peritubular capillaries creates a concentration gradient across which water passively moves, from tubule to capillaries, by osmosis. *Thus, the reabsorption of Na $^+$ by active transport generates the subsequent reabsorption of H $_2$O by passive transport, a process called obligatory H $_2$O reabsorption.*

**4. Passive transport of various solutes by diffusion**: PCT, DCT, and CD

- As H $_2$O moves from the tubule to the capillaries, various solutes such as K $^+$, Cl $^-$, HCO $_3$ $^-$, and urea become more concentrated in the tubule. As a result, these solutes follow the water, moving by diffusion out of the tubule and into capillaries where their concentrations are lower, a process called **solvent drag.**
- Also, the accumulation of the positively charged Na $^+$ in the capillaries creates an electrical gradient that attracts (by diffusion) negatively charged ions (Cl $^-$, HCO $_3$ $^-$).

**5. H $_2$ O and solute transport regulated by hormones**: DCT and CD

- The permeability of the DCT and Collecting Duct and the resultant reabsorption of H $_2$O and Na $^+$ are controlled by two hormones:
- **Aldosterone** *increases the reabsorption of Na $^+$ and H $_2$O by stimulating an increase in the number of Na $^+$-K $^+$ pump proteins in the principal cells that line the DCT and collecting duct.*
- **Antidiuretic hormone (ADH)** *increases H $_2$O reabsorption by stimulating an increase in the number of H $_2$O-channel proteins in the principal cells of the collecting duct.*

# TUBULAR SECRETION

- In contrast to tubular reabsorption, which returns substances to the blood, tubular secretion removes substances from the blood and secretes them into the filtrate.
- Secreted substances include $H^+$, $K^+$, $NH_4^+$ (ammonium ion), creatinine (a waste product of muscle contraction), and various other substances (including penicillin and other drugs).
- Secretion occurs in portions of the PCT, DCT, and Collecting Duct.

## A. SECRETION OF $H^+$

- Because a decrease in $H^+$ causes a rise in pH (a decrease in acidity), $H^+$ secretion into the renal tubule is a mechanism for raising blood pH.
- Various acids produced by cellular metabolism accumulate in the blood and require that their presence be neutralized by removing $H^+$.
- In addition, $CO_2$, also a metabolic by-product, combines with water (catalysed by the enzyme carbonic anhydrase) to produce carbonic acid ($H_2CO_3$), which dissociates to produce $H^+$, as follows:

$$CO_2 + H_2O \leftrightarrow H_2CO_3 \leftrightarrow H^+ + HCO_3^-$$

- This chemical reaction occurs in either direction (it is reversible) depending on the concentration of the various reactants.
- As a result, if $HCO_3^-$ increases in the blood, it acts as a buffer of $H^+$, combining with it (and effectively removing it) to produce $CO_2$ and $H_2O$. $CO_2$ in tubular cells of the collecting duct combines with $H_2O$ to form $H^+$ and $HCO_3^-$.
- The $CO_2$ may originate in the tubular cells or it may enter these cells by diffusion from the renal tubule, interstitial fluids, or peritubular capillaries.
- In the tubule cell, $Na^+/H^+$ antiporters, enzymes that move transported substances in opposite directions, transport $H^+$ across the luminal membrane into the tubule while importing $Na^+$.
- Inside the tubule, $H^+$ may combine with any of several buffers that entered the tubule as filtrate ($HCO_3^-$, $NH_3$, or $HPO_4^{2-}$).
- If $HCO_3^-$ is the buffer, then $H_2CO_3$ is formed, producing $H_2O$ and $CO_2$. The $CO_2$ then enters the tubular cell, where it can combine with $H_2O$ again. If $H^+$ combines with another buffer, it is excreted in the urine.
- Regardless of the fate of the H+ in the tubule, the $HCO_3^-$ produced in the first step is transported across the basolateral membrane by an $HCO_3^-/Cl^-$ antiporter. The $HCO_3^-$ enters the peritubular capillaries, where it combines with the $H^+$ in the blood and increases the blood pH. Note that the blood pH is increased by adding $HCO_3^-$ to the blood, not by removing $H^+$.

## B. SECRETION OF $NH_3$

- When amino acids are broken down, they produce toxic $NH_3$ (Ammonia).
- The liver converts most $NH_3$ to urea, a less toxic substance.
- Both enter the filtrate during glomerular filtration and are excreted in the urine.
- However, when the blood is very acidic, the tubule cells break down the amino acid glutamate, producing $NH_3$ and $HCO_3^-$.
- The $NH_3$ combines with $H^+$, forming $NH_4^+$, which is transported across the luminal membrane by a $Na^+$ antiporter and excreted in the urine. The $HCO_3^-$ moves to the blood (as discussed earlier for $H^+$ secretion) and increases blood pH.

## C. SECRETION OF $K^+$

- Nearly all of the $K^+$ in filtrate is reabsorbed during tubular reabsorption.
- When reabsorbed, quantities exceed body requirements, excess $K^+$ is secreted back into the filtrate in the collecting duct and final regions of the DCT.
- Because aldosterone stimulates an increase in $Na^+/K^+$ pumps, $K^+$ secretion (as well as $Na^+$ reabsorption) increases with aldosterone.

# RENAL CLEARANCE

- **Renal clearance** is the volume of plasma from which a substance is completely removed by the kidney in a given amount of time (usually a minute).
- Tests of renal clearance can detect glomerular damage or judge the progress of renal disease.

## 1. THE INULIN CLEARANCE TEST

- Uses inulin (not to be confused with insulin), a complex polysaccharide found in certain plant roots.
- In the test, a known amount of inulin is infused into the blood at a constant rate.
- The inulin passes freely through the glomerular membranes, so that its concentration in the glomerular filtrate equals that of the plasma.
- In the renal tubule, inulin is not reabsorbed to any significant degree, nor is it secreted.
- Consequently, the rate at which it appears in the urine can be used to calculate the rate of glomerular filtration.
- Similarly, the kidneys remove creatinine, which is produced at a constant rate as a result of muscle metabolism, from the blood. Like inulin, creatinine is filtered, but neither reabsorbed nor secreted by the kidneys.
- Thus, **the creatinine clearance test**, which compares a patient's blood and urine creatinine concentrations, can also be used to calculate the GFR.

- A significant advantage is that the bloodstream normally has a constant level of creatinine.
- Therefore, a single measurement of plasma creatinine levels provides a rough index of kidney function.
- For example, significantly elevated plasma creatinine levels suggest that GFR is greatly reduced.
- Because nearly all of the creatinine the kidneys filter normally appears in the urine, a change in the rate of creatinine excretion may reflect a renal disorder.

## 2. PARA-AMINOHIPPURIC ACID (PAH)

- A substance that filters freely through the glomerular membranes.
- However, unlike inulin, any PAH remaining in the peritubular capillary plasma after filtration is secreted into the proximal convoluted tubules.
- Therefore, essentially all PAH passing through the kidneys appears in the urine. For this reason, the rate of PAH clearance can be used to calculate the rate of plasma flow through the kidneys.
- Then, if the haematocrit is known, the rate of total blood flow through the kidneys can be calculated.

## MECHANISM OF ACTION OF DIURETICS

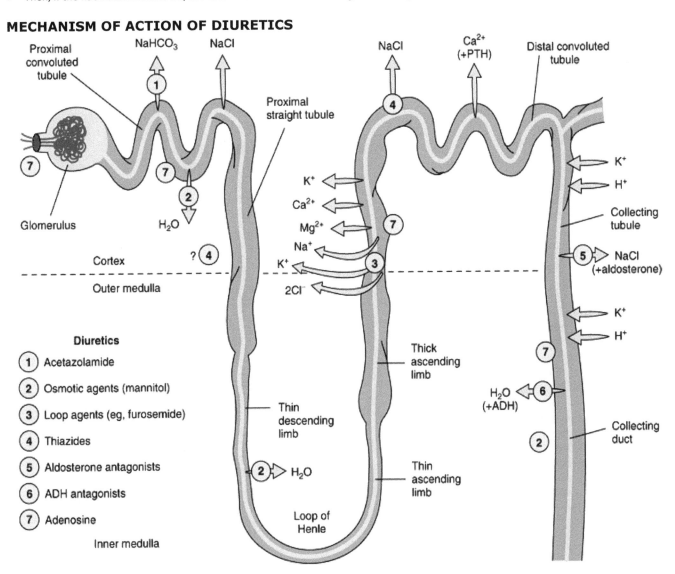

*Fig. 2.5.5. Mechanism of action of Diuretics*

# IV. REGULATION OF PLASMA OSMOLALITY

## A. WATER BALANCE (ADH)

- The consumption side is regulated by behavioural mechanisms, including **thirst** and **salt cravings**.
- One way the kidneys can directly control the volume of bodily fluids is by the amount of water excreted in the urine. Direct control of water excretion in the kidneys is exercised by vasopressin, or anti-diuretic hormone (ADH), a peptide hormone secreted by the hypothalamus. ADH causes the insertion of water channels into the membranes of cells lining the collecting ducts, allowing water reabsorption to occur.
- Without ADH, little water is reabsorbed in the collecting ducts and dilute urine is excreted.
- ADH secretion is influenced by several factors:

### FACTORS STIMULATING ADH RELEASE
- ○ Angiotensin II
- ○ Increase plasma osmolality (Hyperosmolality)
- ○ Increased sympathetic stimulation
- ○ Decreased blood volume and blood pressure

## CONTROL OF WATER/OSMOLARITY:

- Regulated by Thirst and ADH
- Body osmolality increases (285mosm+)
  \>>> osmoreceptors (hypothalamus)
  \>>> thirst and release of ADH
  \>>> increase permeability of CD to water
  \>>> water reabsorption from tubules
  \>>> concentrated urine + decreased osmolarity.

Osmolality= 2(Na+K) + urea + Glucose

## B. SODIUM BALANCE (ALDOSTERONE)

- Regulation of osmolarity is achieved by balancing the intake and excretion of sodium with that of water.
- As noted above, ADH plays a role in lowering osmolarity (reducing sodium concentration) by increasing water reabsorption in the kidneys, thus helping to dilute bodily fluids.
- To prevent osmolarity from decreasing below normal, the kidneys also have a regulated mechanism for reabsorbing sodium in the distal nephron.
- This mechanism is controlled by *aldosterone*, a steroid hormone produced by the adrenal cortex.

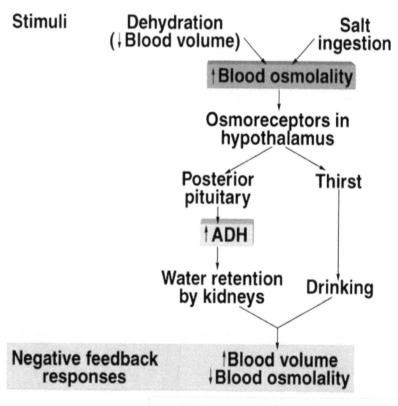

*Fig. 2.5.6. Control of Water/Osmolarity*

### FACTORS STIMULATING ALDOSTERONE RELEASE
- ✓ ACTH (transient effect only)
- ✓ Angiotensin II
- ✓ Hypoosmolarity and Low Blood volume
- ✓ Increased in plasma [K+] (Hyperkalaemia)
- ✓ **Standing:** Aldosterone release is increased in standing position because of:
  - ▪ Decreased hepatic clearance
  - ▪ Increase in renin and hence angiotensin II

# C. ELECTROLYTE REGULATION (RAAS)

## 1. RENIN-ANGIOTENSIN-ALDOSTERONE SYSTEM

### FACTORS STIMULATING RENIN RELEASE

- Sympathetic Nerve Activation (SNA; acting through $\beta_1$-adrenoceptors)
- Renal artery hypotension (caused by systemic hypotension or renal artery stenosis)
- Decreased Sodium delivery to the distal tubules of the kidney.

- Renin, which is primarily released by the kidneys, stimulates the formation of *angiotensin in blood and tissues*, which in turn stimulates the *release of aldosterone from the adrenal cortex.*

- Renin is a proteolytic enzyme that is released into the circulation primarily by the kidneys.
  - *A reduction in afferent arteriole pressure causes the release of renin from the JG cells, whereas increased pressure inhibits renin release.*
  - *Beta$_1$-adrenoceptors located on the JG cells respond to sympathetic nerve stimulation by releasing renin.*
  - *The macula densa senses the concentration of sodium and chloride ions in the tubular fluid.*
  - *When NaCl is elevated in the tubular fluid, renin release is inhibited.*
  - *In contrast, a reduction in tubular NaCl stimulates renin release by the JG cells.*
  - There is evidence that prostaglandins ($PGE_2$ and $PGI_2$) stimulate renin release in response to reduced NaCl transport across the macula densa.

Fig. 2.5.7. RAAS

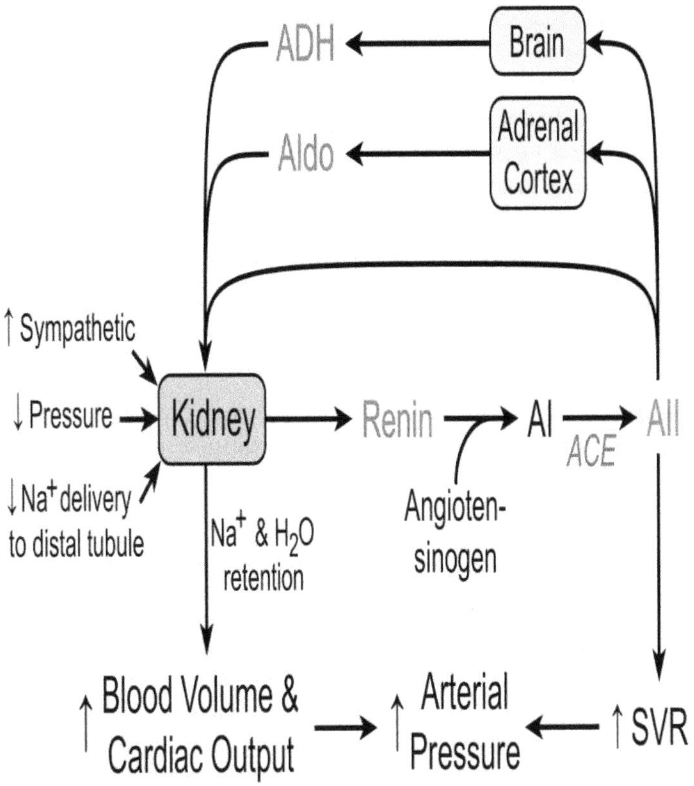

  - *When afferent arteriole pressure is reduced, glomerular filtration decreases, and this reduces NaCl in the distal tubule.*
  - This serves as an important mechanism contributing to the release of renin when there is afferent arteriole hypotension, which can be caused by systemic hypotension or narrowing (stenosis) of the renal artery that supplies blood flow to the kidney.
  - The renin-angiotensin-aldosterone pathway is not only regulated by the mechanisms that stimulate renin release, but it is also modulated by natriuretic peptides (ANP and BNP) released by the heart. These natriuretic peptides act as an important counter-regulatory system. Therapeutic manipulation of this pathway is very important in treating hypertension and heart failure.
  - ACE inhibitors, AII receptor blockers and aldosterone receptor blockers, for example, are used to decrease arterial pressure, ventricular afterload, blood volume and hence ventricular preload, as well as inhibit and reverse cardiac and vascular hypertrophy.
  - The renin-angiotensin-aldosterone system is one of the most complex and important systems in controlling the blood pressure in the body.

## CONTROL OF THE GLOMERULAR FILTRATION RATE (GFR) BY THE RAAS

- To maintain pressure in the glomerulus and therefore keep the glomerular filtration rate steady, angiotensin II constricts both the efferent and afferent arteriole, but with a much greater effect on the efferent arteriole. (*The effect of angiotensin II is greater on the efferent arteriole*). This means that the blood entering the glomerulus has a much harder time leaving it because the exit is far smaller than the entrance. This causes a backup of blood in the glomerulus, increases the pressure within it and, therefore, keeps the GFR at an appropriate rate. In addition, angiotensin II increases the absorption of sodium in the renal tubule.
- Since water follows sodium, it increases the amount of fluid in the blood vessels, further causing an increase in blood pressure in addition to the vasoconstriction that already occurred.

## 2. ALDOSTERONE

- Angiotensin causes the release of aldosterone from the adrenal glands. Aldosterone is a hormone that increases:
  - The absorption of water from the distal convoluted tubule and collecting duct of the kidney's nephrons.
  - The secretion of K into urine.
  - Aldosterone causes the absorption of sodium out of the renal tubule's filtrate and into the blood.
- Since water follows sodium, more water is reabsorbed back into the blood in order to increase the blood pressure.

## 3. ANTI-DIURETIC HORMONE (ADH)

- As if constricting blood vessels and releasing aldosterone to retain water and sodium weren't enough, angiotensin II also causes the release of a hormone called anti-diuretic hormone.
- ADH is a hormone released from the posterior pituitary gland that causes an increase in blood pressure by vasoconstriction of blood vessels and increasing water absorption from the distal tubule and collecting ducts.

# V. ACID – BASE BALANCE

## A. BLOOD GAS

**Normal values**

- pH = 7.35-7.45
- PaO2 = >10.6 kPa (70-100 mmHg)
- PaCO2 = 4.7-6 kPa (35-45 mmHg)
- HCO3 = 24-30 kPa (22-26 mEq/L)
- Base excess = 0(-2 to +2 mmol/l)

**COMMON CAUSES OF ABNORMAL BLOOD GAS**

| GAS DEVIATION | CHARACTERISTICS | COMMON CAUSES |
|---|---|---|
| Respiratory Acidosis | Acidosis with increased PaCO2 | Type II respiratory failure: Asthma/COPD<br>Muscle weakness (e.g. Guillain Barre syndrome),<br>Respiratory depression (e.g. sedatives) |
| Respiratory Alkalosis | Alkalosis with low PaCO2 | Commonly hyperventilation |
| Metabolic Acidosis | Acidosis with low HCO3 | **Normal anion gap:** HCO3 loss (e.g. diarrhoea), H retention (e.g. renal tubular acidosis)<br>**High anion gap:** Lactic acidosis (often post-MI), DKA, salicylate overdose |
| Metabolic Alkalosis | Alkalosis with high HCO3 | Potassium depletion, vomiting |

## B. CALCULATION OF ANION GAP

- The concentrations are expressed in units of milliequivalents/liter (mEq/L) or in millimoles/litre (mmol/L).
- **With potassium**
  - The anion gap is calculated by subtracting the serum concentrations of chloride and bicarbonate (anions) from the concentrations of sodium and potassium (cations):

$$\text{Anion Gap} = ([Na^+] + [K^+]) - ([Cl^-] + [HCO_3^-])$$

- **Without potassium (daily practice)**
  - Omission of potassium has become widely accepted, as potassium concentrations, being very low, usually have little effect on the calculated gap. This leaves the following equation:

$$\text{Anion Gap} = [Na^+] - ([Cl^-] + [HCO_3^-])$$

- The Anion Gap (AG) is a derived variable primarily used for the evaluation of metabolic acidosis to determine the presence of unmeasured anions. The normal anion gap depends on serum phosphate and serum albumin concentrations
- An elevated anion gap strongly suggests the presence of a metabolic acidosis
- The normal anion gap varies with different assays, but is typically **4 to 12mmol/L** (if measured by ion selective electrode) or **8 to 16mmol/L** (if measured by older technique of flame photometry).
  - *If AG > 30 mmol/L then metabolic acidosis invariably present*
  - *If AG 20-29mmol/L then 1/3 will not have a metabolic acidosis*

### 1. HIGH ANION GAP METABOLIC ACIDOSIS (HAGMA)

- HAGMA results from accumulation of organic acids or impaired H+ excretion
- **CAT MUD PILES**
  - ✓ CO, CN
  - ✓ Alcoholic ketoacidosis and starvation ketoacidosis
  - ✓ Toluene
  - ✓ Metformin, Methanol
  - ✓ Uremia
  - ✓ DKA
  - ✓ Pyroglutamic acidosis, paracetamol, phenformin, propylene glycol, paraldehyde
  - ✓ Iron, Isoniazid
  - ✓ Lactic acidosis
  - ✓ Ethylene glycol
  - ✓ Salicylates

### 2. NORMAL ANION GAP METABOLIC ACIDOSIS (NAGMA)

- NAGMA results from loss of HCO3- from ECF

**Causes:**
- **ABCD**
  - ✓ Addison's (adrenal insufficiency)
  - ✓ Bicarbonate loss (GI or Renal)
  - ✓ Chloride excess
  - ✓ Diuretics (Acetazolamide)

## C. HENDERSON-HASSELBACH EQUATION FOR BICARBONATE AND CO2 EQUILIBRIUM

o Bicarbonate as a buffer, tends to maintain a relatively constant plasma pH and counteract any force that would alter.

o In this system, carbon dioxide ($CO_2$) combines with water ($H_2O$) to form carbonic acid ($H_2CO_3$), which in turn rapidly dissociates to form hydrogen ions ($H^+$) and bicarbonate ($HCO_3^-$) as shown in the reactions below.

$$H2O + CO2 \rightleftharpoons H2CO3 \rightleftharpoons H+ + HCO3$$

o A modified version of the Henderson–Hasselbach equation can be used to relate the pH of blood to constituents of the bicarbonate buffering system:

$$pH= pK_{aH2CO3} + log\ ([HCO_3^-] / [H2CO3])$$

**Where:**

o $pK_{aH2CO3}$ is the negative logarithm (base 10) of the acid dissociation constant of carbonic acid. It is equal to 6.1.

o $[HCO_3^-]$ is the concentration of bicarbonate in the blood

o $[H_2CO_3]$ is the concentration of carbonic acid in the blood

- This is useful in arterial blood gas, but these usually state $pCO_2$, that is, the partial pressure of carbon dioxide, rather than $H_2CO_3$.
- However, these are related by the equation:

$$[H2CO3] = k_{H\ CO2}\ x\ pCO_2$$

**Where:**

o $[H_2CO_3]$ is the concentration of carbonic acid in the blood

o $k_{H\ CO2}$ is a constant including the solubility of carbon dioxide in blood. $k_{H\ CO2}$ is approximately 0.03 (mmol/L)/mmHg

o $pCO_2$ is the partial pressure of carbon dioxide in the blood

- Taken together, the following equation can be used to relate the pH of blood to the concentration of bicarbonate and the partial pressure of carbon dioxide:

$$pH= 6.1+ log\ ([HCO_3^-]/ 0.03x\ pCO_2)$$

**Where:**

o pH is the acidity in the blood

o $[HCO_3^-]$ is the concentration of bicarbonate in the blood, in mmol/L

o $pCO_2$ is the partial pressure of carbon dioxide in the blood, in mmHg

## D. RENAL REGULATION OF ACID – BASE BALANCE

### 1. BICARBONATE REABSORPTION

- The kidney filters approximately 4320 meq/day of HCO3- (24 meq/L ×180L/day).
- Under normal circumstances, the kidney is able to completely reabsorb all the filtered bicarbonate. This is vitally important, since any loss of bicarbonate in the urine would disturb acid base balance.
- *The process of bicarbonate reabsorption occurs predominantly in the proximal tubule (about 90%).*
- *The rest occur in the thick ascending limb and in the collecting tubule.*
- To completely reabsorb bicarbonate, the kidney must secrete 4320 meq/day of hydrogen ions in addition to the amount required to excrete the daily acid load. The primary step in proximal hydrogen secretion is the secretion of H+ by the Na+/H+ antiporter in the luminal membrane. Hydrogen ions are generated by the intracellular breakdown of $H_2O$ to OH- and H+. Hydrogen ions secreted combine with filtered HCO3- ions to form carbonic acid and then CO2 + H2O, which are then passively reabsorbed.
- HCO3- ions reabsorbed in this process are not the same as the ones filtered.
- Note that a new HCO3- ion is generated from the intracellular breakdown of $H_2O$ to OH- and H+ and subsequent reaction of OH- with CO2 to form HCO3- . This new bicarbonate then crosses the basolateral membrane via a Na+ - 3HCO3- cotransporter.
- The net effect is one mol of bicarbonate ion returned to systemic circulation for every H+ ion that is secreted and reabsorption of virtually all filtered bicarbonate. Similar processes occur in the thick ascending loop of Henle and intercalating cells of the collecting duct.
- In contrast to the proximal tubule, hydrogen ion secretion in the collecting tubule is mediated by an H+ ATPase pump in the luminal membrane and a Cl-HCO3- exchanger in the basolateral membrane.
- The H+ ATPase pump is influenced by aldosterone, which stimulates increased H+ secretion.
- Hydrogen ion secretion in the collecting tubule is the process primarily responsible for acidification of the urine, particularly during states of acidosis. The urine pH may fall as low as 4.0. Proximal reabsorption of bicarbonate can be affected by many factors, in particular, potassium balance, volume status and renin/angiotensin levels.
- Therefore, these factors can have very significant effects on acid base balance.

### 2. URINARY BUFFERING

- The role of urinary buffering serves two purposes; to excrete the daily acid load and regenerate bicarbonate lost during extracellular buffering.
- It is a process whereby secreted hydrogen ions are buffered in the urine by combining with weak acids (titratable acidity) or with NH3 (ammonia) to be excreted. It is a necessary process because the kidney cannot easily excrete free hydrogen ions.

## 3. TITRATABLE ACIDITY

- The major titratable acid buffer is $HPO_4^{2-}$. Other less important buffers are creatinine and uric acid.
- Excretion of titratable acids is dependent on the quantity of phosphate filtered and excreted by the kidneys, which is dependent on one's diet, and also PTH levels. As such, the excretion of titratable acids is not regulated by acid base balance and cannot be easily increased to excrete the daily acid load.
- Ammonium production can however be regulated to respond to acid base status.

## 4. AMMONIUM EXCRETION

- With increased acid load, there is increased hydrogen ion secretion, causing the urine pH to fall below 5.5.
- At this point, virtually all the urinary phosphate exist as H2PO4- and further buffering cannot occur unless there is an increase in urinary phosphate excretion.
- Phosphate excretion is mainly dependent on dietary phosphate intake and PTH levels and is not regulated in response to the need to maintain acid base balance. Without further urinary buffering, adequate acid excretion cannot take place.
- The major adaptation to an increased acid load is increased ammonium production and excretion. The role of ammonium production in the further generation of bicarbonate ions.
- The process of ammonium excretion takes place in 3 steps:
  - Ammonium Formation (ammoniagenesis) (proximal tubule)
  - Ammonium Reabsorption (Medullary Recycling) (thick ascending loop)
  - Ammonium Trapping (collecting tubule)

## 5. REGULATION OF BODY POTASSIUM

- $K^+$ is the major intracellular ion.
- Only 2% is in the ECF at a concentration of only 4 mEq/L.
- K is taken up by all cells via the Na-K ATPase pump.
- It is one of the most permeable ion across cell membranes and exits the cells mostly via K channels (and in some cells via K-H exchange or via K-Cl cotransport).

## A. ROLES OF K

- K is the major ion determining the resting membrane electrical potential, which in turn, limits and opposes K efflux.
- Thus, changes in K concentrations (particularly in the ECF) have marked effects on cell excitability (heart, brain, nerve, muscle).
- K is the mayor intracellular osmotically active cation and participates in cell (intracellular) volume regulation (exits with Cl when cells swell).
- A constant cell K concentration is critical for enzyme activities and for cell division and growth.
- Intracellular K participates in acid base regulation through exchange for extracellular H and by influencing the rate of renal ammonium production.
- Regulation of extracellular K is by tissue buffering (uptake of K excess) and by slower renal excretion.

## B. CELLULAR K BUFFERING

- When K is added to the ECF, most of the added K is taken up by the cells, reducing the ECF $K^+$ increase.
- Similarly, if K is lost from the ECF, some $K^+$ leaves the cells, reducing the ECF K decline.
- Buffering of ECF K through cell K uptake is impaired in the absence of aldosterone or of insulin or of catecholamines.
- Cell K exit to the ECF increases when osmolarity increases (as in diabetes mellitus) and in metabolic acidosis, when it is exchanged for ECF protons ($H^+$). When cells die, they release their very high K content to the ECF.

## C. RENAL REGULATION OF POTASSIUM

- In normal function, renal K excretion balances most of the K intake (about 1.5 mEq/Kg per day).
- The kidneys excrete about 15 % of the filtered K load of 10 mEq/Kg per day.
- Along the proximal tubule the K concentration remains nearly equal to that in plasma.
- Since the PCT reabsorbs about 2/3 of the filtrate water, it also reabsorbs about 2/3 (66%) of the filtered K.
- Along the descending limb of the loop of Henle, K is secreted into the tubule lumen from the interstitium.
- Along the thick ascending limb, K is reabsorbed via Na-K-2 Cl cotransport.
- In the loop, there is net K reabsorption of 25% of the filtered K.
- Along the distal tubule and collecting ducts (CD), there is net secretion of K which is stimulated by aldosterone and when there is dietary K excess.
- Regulation of renal K excretion is in the CD and is mostly by changes in the rate of K secretion.
- In the CD, K secretion is by the principal cells (via luminal K channels and basolateral Na-K ATPase) and K reabsorption is by the alpha intercalated cells via a luminal H-K ATPase.

# VI. LACTATE AND LACTIC ACIDOSIS

- Lactic acid exists in 2 optical isomeric forms, L-lactate and D-lactate.
- **L-lactate** is the most commonly measured level, as it is the only form produced in human metabolism. Its excess represents increased anaerobic metabolism due to tissue hypoperfusion.
- **D-lactate** is a by-product of bacterial metabolism and may accumulate in patients with short-gut syndrome or in those with a history of gastric bypass or small-bowel resection.
- A lactate level of > 4 mmol/l is associated with increased ICU admission and mortality in normotensive patients with sepsis.
- **Cryptic shock** is defined as a serum lactate greater than 4 mmol/l with a SBP of at least 90mmHg. Severe sepsis with cryptic shock has a mortality rate similar to that of patients with overt septic shock.

## COHEN & WOODS CLASSIFICATION OF LACTIC ACIDOSIS

- **Type A: Inadequate Oxygen Delivery**
  - **Anaerobic muscular activity:**
    - Sprinting, Generalised convulsions.

  - **Tissue hypoperfusion**
    - Shock, cardiac arrest/ cardiac failure
    - Regional hypoperfusion -> mesenteric ischemia.

  - **Reduced tissue oxygen delivery**
    - Hypoxaemia, anaemia, CO poisoning.

- **Type B: No Evidence of Inadequate Tissue Oxygen Delivery**
  - **B1: associated with underlying diseases**
    - **LUKE**: leukaemia, lymphoma.
    - **TIPS**: Thiamine Deficiency, Infection, Pancreatitis, Short Bowel Syndrome.
    - **FAILURES**: hepatic, renal, diabetic failures

  - **B2: associated with drugs & toxins**
    - Phenformin, Cyanide, Beta-agonists, Methanol
    - Adrenaline, Salicylates, Nitroprusside infusion
    - Ethanol intoxication in chronic alcoholics
    - Anti-retroviral drugs, Paracetamol, Salbutamol
    - Biguanides, Fructose, Sorbitol, Xylitol, Isoniazid

  - **B3: associated with inborn errors of metabolism**
    - ✓ Pyruvate carboxylase deficiency, G6PD and Fructose-1,6-bisphosphatase deficiencies.
    - ✓ Oxidative phosphorylation enzyme defects.

# HORMONES AND STRESS

➤ **HORMONES LEVELS FALL DURING ILLNESS OR STRESS: I TOT IT**
  - **I**nsulin
  - **T**estosterone
  - **O**estrogen
  - **T**SH
  - **I**GF-1
  - **T**hyroxine

➤ **HORMONES THAT RISE DURING ILLNESS AND STRESS: GAG GAP**
  - **G**rowth hormone
  - **A**CTH
  - **G**lucocorticoids
  - **G**lucagon
  - **A**drenaline
  - **P**rolactin

➤ **HORMONES ACT VIA A RISE IN INTRACELLULAR CALCIUM LEVELS: GTA**
  - **G**nRH
  - **T**RH
  - **A**drenaline (alpha receptors)

# VII. RENAL TUBULAR ACIDOSIS & URAEMIC ACIDOSIS

| RENAL TUBULAR ACIDOSIS | | | |
|---|---|---|---|
| | **Type 1 Distal** | **Type 2 Proximal** | **Type 4** |
| **Defect** | Reduced H+ excretion in distal tubule | Impaired HCO3 reabsorption in proximal tubule | Impaired cation exchange in distal tubule |
| **Hyperchloremic NAGMA** | Yes | Yes | Yes |
| **Minimum urine pH** | >5.5 | <5.5 (but usually >5.5 before acidosis becomes established) | <5.5 |
| **Plasma HCO3** | <15 | Usually >15 | Usually >15 |
| **Plasma K** | Low-normal | Low-normal | **High** |
| **Renal stones** | Yes | No | No |

## 1. URAEMIC ACIDOSIS

- Caused by failure to excrete acid anions (PO4 and SO4) due to decreased number of functional nephrons.
- GFR < 20ml/min.
- Low plasma HCO3.
- Patients often survive a long time and get chronic complications such as bone demineralization.

## 2. TYPE 1 RTA (Classic RTA, Distal)

- Reduced secretion of H+ in distal tubule >>> inability to maximally acidify the urine.
- **Causes:** HANDO
  - **H**ereditary
  - **A**utoimmune (Sjogren's, SLE, thyroiditis)
  - **N**ephrocalcinosis (e.g. primary hyperparathyroidism, vitamin D intoxification)
  - **D**rugs/toxins (e.g. amphotericin B, toluene inhalation)
  - **O**bstructive nephropathy
- **Investigation:**
  - Urine pH remains >5.5 despite severe acidaemia (HCO3 < 15mmol/L).
  - May require an acid load test to see whether urinary pH remains > 5.5.
  - *Hyperchloraemic acidosis + alkaline urine + renal stone formation.*
  - **Secondary hyperaldosteronism** >>> increased K+ loss in urine.

## 3. TYPE II RTA (Proximal)

- Termed proximal because the main problem is impaired reabsorption of bicarbonate in the proximal tubule.
- At normal plasma HCO3, 15% of filtered HCO3 is excreted in the urine >>> in acidosis when HCO3 levels are low the urine can become HCO3 free. Symptoms take place when there is an increase in plasma HCO3 >>> proximal tubule cannot reabsorb the increased filtered load >>> delivered to distal tubule and is unable to be reabsorbed >>> urinary loss of HCO3.
- Results = **metabolic acidosis with an inappropriately high urinary pH + hyperchloraemia** (Cl- replaces HCO3 in circulation).
- With increased distal tubular Na+ delivery >>> **hyperaldosteronism** >>> K+ wasting.
- **Causes:** CV PHLAM
  - **C**ystinosis
  - **V**itamin D deficiency
  - **P**roximal tubular defects: affects reabsorption of glucose, phosphate and amino acids.
  - **H**ereditary
  - **L**ead nephropathy
  - **A**myloidosis
  - **M**edullary cystic disease
- **Investigations:**
  - Metabolic acidosis (usually not as severe as distal RTA)
  - Plasma HCO3 usually > 15mmol/L
  - High urinary HCO3 (inappropriate)
  - Hypokalaemia
  - During the NH4Cl loading test urinary pH drops < 5.5

# 4. TYPE IV RTA

- Defect in cation-exchange in the distal tubule with reduced secretion of both H+ and K+. Associated with renal failure caused by disorders affecting the renal interstitium and tubules.
- GFR >20mL/min (unlike uraemic acidosis).
- **Always associated with hyperkalaemia** (unlike others).
- Associated with: **Addison's disease** or **post bilateral adrenalectomy.**
- Acidosis not common unless there is associated renal damage affect the distal tubule.
- The H+ pump in the tubule is not abnormal so that patients with this disorder are able to decrease their urinary pH to <5.5 in response to the acidosis.

## OSMOLAR GAP

- The osmolar gap is the difference between the measured serum osmolality and the calculated serum osmolarity.
- Calculating the osmolar gap can be helpful in determining the presence of toxic alcohols in cases of poisoning by an unknown agent.
- A normal osmolar gap is less than **10mosm/kg.**
- A raised osmolar gap indicates the presence of an unmeasured solute in the blood; usually either an:
  - alcohol (e.g. ethanol, methanol, ethylene glycol or acetone)
  - sugar (mannitol, maltose or sorbitol)
  - Protein (paraproteinaemia or hypergammaglobulinaemia)
  - Lipid (hypertriglyceridaemia)

| SERUM vs URINE OSMOLALITY | | |
|---|---|---|
| **SERUM OSMOLALITY** | **URINE OSMOLALITY** | **CAUSES** |
| Normal/ increased | Increased | Dehydration<br>Renal failure<br>CCF<br>Hyperglycaemia<br>Hypernatraemia<br>Hypercalcaemia<br>Addison's disease |
| Normal/ increased | Decreased | Diabetes insipidus |
| Decreased | Increased | SIADH |
| Decreased | Decreased (with no increase in fluid intake) | Overhydration<br>Hyponatraemia<br>Adrenocortical insufficiency<br>Sodium loss |

| Biochemistry | Prerenal Failure | Intrinsic Renal Failure |
|---|---|---|
| Urine specific gravity: | >1 | <1 |
| Urinary Na: | <20mmol/l | >40mmol/l |
| Urinary urea: | >250mmol/l | <185mmol/l |
| Osmolarity: | >500mosm/kg | 300-350mosm/kg |

| Regarding the pituitary gland | |
|---|---|
| It occupies the sella turcica of the sphenoid bone | T |
| The adenohypophysis constitutes the anterior 80% of the pituitary gland | T |
| ADH and oxytocin are released from the neurohypophysis | T |
| Dopamine stimulates prolactin release from the anterior pituitary | F |
| **Which statements regarding the hormone glucagon are true?** | |
| It is a steroid hormone | F |
| It stimulates gluconeogenesis in the liver and muscle | T |
| It inhibits glycogenesis in liver | T |
| It has a ketogenic function | T |
| **Regarding Thyroid function test** | |
| TSH levels are raised in hyperthyroidism | F |
| Aspirin dislodges T4 from its binding protein thyroid binding globulin | T |
| Both T4 and TSH may be low in the sick euthyroid state | T |
| Hashimoto's disease is the most common cause of hypothyroidism | T |

# Past Asked Questions

**Regarding Glomerular Filtration:**

| | |
|---|---|
| Around 5% cardiac output passes through the Kidney each minute? | F |
| In healthy adult GFR is dependent upon Blood pressure? | F |
| GFR can be calculated clinically by the rate at which a physiologically inert substance injected into the circulation is excreted in the urine? | T |
| Creatinine clearance increases with age? | F |

**When considering the control of glucose and electrolytes by the kidney:**

| | |
|---|---|
| The Proximal tubules reabsorbs 50% of glucose | F |
| 50% of Na in the glomerular filtrate is reabsorbed in the PCT? | F |
| Loop diuretics act on the Na/K/2Cl co-transporter in the ascending loop of Henle? | T |
| Net tubular excretion of K occurs in K excess? | T |

**Regarding the role of hormones in renal function:**

| | |
|---|---|
| Aldosterone stimulates salt and K retention? | F |
| Without ADH the collecting ducts are largely impermeable to water? | T |
| Spironolactone conserves K by inhibiting aldosterone? | T |
| SIADH is established cause of hypernatraemia? | F |

**When considering the handling of glucose by the kidney**

| | |
|---|---|
| It is reabsorbed by primary active transport? | ? |
| It is reabsorbed only in the proximal tubule? | T |
| Glucose appears in the urine once venous glucose concentration exceeds 20mmol/l? | F |
| The difference between the observed and predicted renal threshold for glucose is called splay? | T |

**The following are indications for dialysis in acute renal failure:**

| | |
|---|---|
| Pulmonary oedema with oliguria | T |
| Cardiac tamponade | T |
| Serum creatinine >600 | F |
| Uncontrolled HTN | F |

**The following statement are true of the renin-angiotensin system:**

| | |
|---|---|
| Renin is secreted by the juxtaglomerular cells in response to reduced renal perfusion | T |
| Angiotensin II inhibits aldosterone release? | T |
| Losartan (Ag. II receptor antagonist) stimulates angiotensin II receptors? | F |
| Angiotensin converting enzyme is primarily located in the liver? | F |

**The following are of importance in the regulation of plasma osmolality:**

| | |
|---|---|
| Angiotensin II promotes thirst? | T |
| Hypothalamic osmoreceptors influence ADH release from the juxtaglomerular apparatus of the kidney? | F |
| ADH promotes water re-absorption in the ascending Loop of Henle? | F |
| A fall in the plasma osmolality triggers ADH release? | F |

**The following occur in the PCT of the nephron:**

| | |
|---|---|
| Carbonic anhydrase catalyses the breakdown of carbonic acid into CO2 and water? | T |
| PTH reduces phosphate resorption?  (In the DCT, Not in the PCT) | F |
| Excess K is eliminated | F |
| Penicillin is secreted into tubular fluid? | T |

**Causes of a raised osmolar gap include**

| | |
|---|---|
| Methanol | T |
| Salicylates | F |
| Diarrhoea and vomiting | F |
| Liver cirrhosis | F |

**The following are true of the loop of Henle of the nephron**

| | |
|---|---|
| Most nephrons have only a short Loop of Henle | T |
| It is lined throughout by simple squamous epithelium | F |
| The thick segment of ascending limb of loop of Henle is impermeable to water | T |
| Tubular fluid becomes steadily more concentrated as it passes through the Loop of Henle. | F |

**Which statement regarding glucose reabsorption from nephrons is true/ false?**

| | |
|---|---|
| Glucose is reabsorbed by Na+ dependent secondary active transport processes | T |
| In the healthy adult, around 75% of glucose is reabsorbed from nephrons | F |
| Renal threshold values for glucose is exceeded at blood glucose concentrations of around 11-12 mmol/L | T |
| Excess glucose is secreted in the distal convoluted tubules of nephrons | F |

# SECTION 6: ENDOCRINE PHYSIOLOGY
## I. PITUITARY FUNCTION

## 1. OVERVIEW
- Pituitary gland is located **in the sella turcica** of the body of sphenoid bone.
- Pituitary gland has 2 distinct parts:
  - **Adenohypophysis:** Anterior 80%. Contains endocrine cells which secrete the following hormones-
    - **Acidophilic cells:** Growth hormone, Prolactin
    - **Basophilic cells:** TSH, ACTH, LH, FSH.
  - **Neurohypophysis:** Posterior 20%. It contains nerve ending of neurones who originate in hypothalamus. **ADH and oxytocin** are synthesized in hypothalamus and are secreted from nerve endings at neurohypophysis.
- As a general scheme, hormone secretion from the anterior pituitary is stimulated by upstream hypothalamic releasing hormones and inhibited by negative feedback from downstream hormones and neural responses.
- The exception is prolactin which is secreted in response to suckling and inhibited by hypothalamic dopamine.

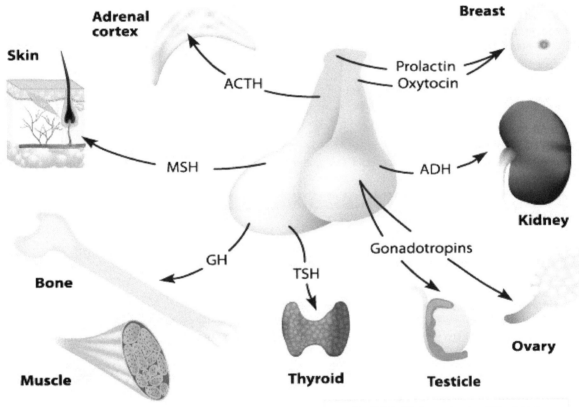

*Fig. 2.6.1. Pituitary gland and Hormones*

## A. ANTERIOR
- All releasing hormones (-RH) referred to, can also be referred to as releasing factors (-RF).

## 1. SOMATOTROPHINS:
- Human growth hormone (HGH), also referred to as 'growth hormone' (GH), and also as somatotropin, is released under the influence of hypothalamic growth hormone-releasing hormone (GHRH), and is inhibited by hypothalamic *somatostatin*.

## 2. THYROTROPHINS:
- Thyroid-stimulating hormone (TSH) is released under the influence of hypothalamic thyrotropin-releasing hormone (TRH) and is inhibited by *somatostatin*.

## 3. CORTICOTROPINS:
- Adrenocorticotropic hormone (ACTH), and Beta-endorphin are released under the influence of hypothalamic corticotropin-releasing hormone (CRH).

## 4. LACTOTROPHINS:

- Prolactin (PRL), also known as 'Luteotropic' hormone (LTH), whose release is inconsistently stimulated by hypothalamic TRH, oxytocin, vasopressin, vasoactive intestinal peptide, angiotensin II, neuropeptide Y, galanin, substance P, bombesin-like peptides (gastrin-releasing peptide, neuromedin B and C), and neurotensin, and inhibited by hypothalamic dopamine.

## 5. GONADOTROPINS:

- Luteinizing hormone (also referred to as 'Lutropin' or 'LH').
- Follicle-stimulating hormone (FSH), both released under influence of Gonadotropin-Releasing Hormone (GnRH)

## B. INTERMEDIATE

- The intermediate lobe synthesizes and secretes the following important endocrine hormone:

## 1. MELANOCYTE–STIMULATING HORMONE (MSH).

- This is also produced in the anterior lobe.
- When produced in the intermediate lobe, *MSHs are sometimes called "intermedins".*

## C. POSTERIOR

- The posterior pituitary stores and secretes (but does not synthesize) the following important endocrine hormones:

## MAGNOCELLULAR NEURONS:

## 1. ANTIDIURETIC HORMONE (ADH)

- Also known as vasopressin and arginine vasopressin (AVP), the majority of which is released from the supraoptic nucleus in the hypothalamus.

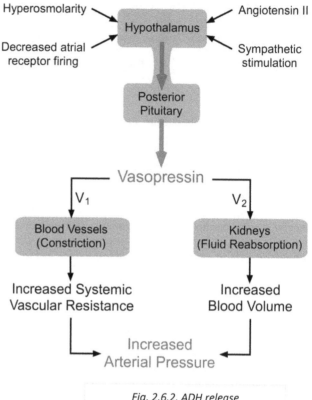

*Fig. 2.6.2. ADH release*

| FACTORS STIMULATING ADH RELEASE |
| --- |
| ○ Angiotensin II |
| ○ Increase plasma osmolality (Hyperosmolality) |
| ○ Increased sympathetic stimulation |
| ○ Decreased blood volume and blood pressure |

## 2. OXYTOCIN

- Most of which is released from the paraventricular nucleus in the hypothalamus.
- Oxytocin is one of the few hormones to create a positive feedback loop. For example, uterine contractions stimulate the release of oxytocin from the posterior pituitary, which, in turn, increases uterine contractions. This positive feedback loop continues throughout labour.

## 2. DISORDERS OF THE ANTERIOR PITUITARY GLAND

### 1. GROWTH HORMONE

### A. GH DEFICIENCY:

- ○ In children, this causes growth failure, and in adults features including decreased energy and quality of life, and increase in fat mass/decrease in muscle mass.
- ○ **The insulin tolerance test** is considered the 'gold standard' for diagnosis.

### B. GH EXCESS: ACROMEGALY

- Acromegaly can be an insidious disease.
- Symptoms, which may precede diagnosis by several years, can be divided into the following groups:
  - ○ Symptoms due to local mass effects of an intracranial tumor
  - ○ Symptoms due to excess of GH/IGF-I
- *Symptoms due to local mass effects of tumor*
  - ○ Headaches and visual field defects are the most common symptoms.
  - ○ Visual field defects depend on which part of the optic nerve pathway is compressed. The most common manifestation is a **bitemporal hemianopsia** caused by pressure on the optic chiasm.
  - ○ Hyperprolactinemia due to loss of inhibitory regulation of prolactin secretion by the hypothalamus.
  - ○ Deficiencies of glucocorticoids, sex steroids, and thyroid hormone.

- *Symptoms due to excess of GH/IGF-I*
  - o Soft tissue swelling and enlargement of extremities
  - o Increase in ring and/or shoe size
  - o Hyperhidrosis
  - o Coarsening of facial features
  - o Prognathism
  - o Macroglossia
  - o Arthritis
  - o Increased incidence of obstructive sleep apnea
  - o Increased incidence of glucose intolerance or frank diabetes mellitus, hypertension, and cardiovascular disease
  - o Hyperphosphatemia, hypercalcuria, and hypertriglyceridemia possible
  - o Increased incidence of congestive heart failure, which may be due to uncontrolled hypertension or to an intrinsic form of cardiomyopathy attributable to excess GH/IGF-I
  - o Increased incidence of colonic polyps and adenocarcinoma of the colon.

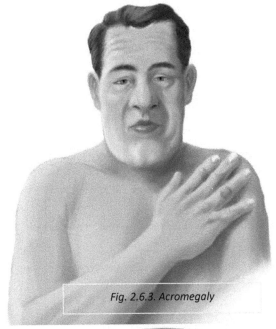

*Fig. 2.6.3. Acromegaly*

## 2. FSH and LH
### A. GONADOTROPIN DEFICIENCY:
  - o Women: oligo/amenorrhea, loss of libido, dyspareunia, hot flushes, and infertility.
  - o Men: loss of libido; impaired sexual function; mood impairment; loss of facial, scrotal and trunk hair; decreased muscle bulk and energy.
  - o Treatment comprises appropriate replacement therapy.

## 3. PROLACTIN
### A. PROLACTINOMAS:
  - o Most common pituitary adenomas and typically present with galactorrhoea and hypogonadism, manifesting in men as impotence, infertility, decreased libido and in women as oligo/amenorrhea and infertility.
  - o Secondary causes of hyperprolactinaemia must be excluded in any patient with an elevated serum prolactin and serum prolactin levels usually parallel tumour size in those with prolactinomas.
  - o **Dopaminergic agonists** like cabergoline, bromocriptine, pergolide, quinagolide are the primary therapy.

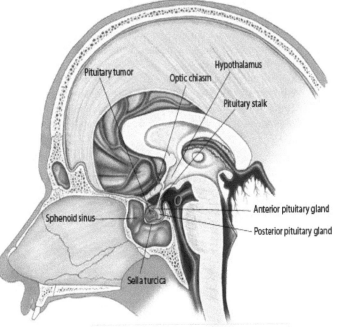

*Fig. 2.6.4. Pituitary Adenoma*

## 4. ACTH
### A. CHRONIC ACTH DEFICIENCY
  - o Associated with fatigue, pallor, anorexia, weight loss, hypotension, hyponatraemia, hypoglycaemia, and eosinophilia.
  - o **The insulin tolerance test** is considered the 'gold standard' for diagnosis.
  - o Replacement with hydrocortisone (or other steroid) in a dose and timing to mimic the normal pattern of cortisol secretion should begin as soon as the diagnosis is confirmed.

### B. CUSHING'S DISEASE
  - o Caused by chronic exposure to endogenous glucocorticoids (Cushing's syndrome) produced by the adrenal cortex in response to excess ACTH production by a pituitary corticotrophin adenoma.

## 5. TSH
### A. CENTRAL HYPOTHYROIDISM
  - o Diagnosed when the concentration of thyroxine is decreased and the level of TSH levels is usually normal or low.
  - o Clinical presentation is as for primary hypothyroidism.
  - o Treatment is with thyroxine.

# 6. OTHER DISEASES:

## 1. HYPOPITUITARISM:

○ Can be caused by a range of conditions including pituitary and nonpituitary tumours, hypophysitis, pituitary apoplexy, Sheehan's syndrome (postpartum), brain injury (traumatic, surgical, irradiation, post infective), and granulomatous diseases.
○ Clinical manifestations depend mainly on the underlying disease, as well as the type and the degree of the hormonal deficits.

## 2. PITUITARY ADENOMAS:

○ The most common cause of pituitary disease; may be functioning (resulting in syndromes of hormonal excess) or nonfunctioning (presenting with mass effects).

## 3. PITUITARY APOPLEXY:

○ Occurs primarily in patients with pre-existing pituitary adenomas; results from acute haemorrhage or infarction of the pituitary gland and is characterized by sudden onset of headache, vomiting, visual disturbance, ophthalmoplegia, and altered consciousness.

## 4. CRANIOPHARYNGIOMAS:

○ These epithelial tumours can present with pressure effects and/or compromised hypothalamo-pituitary function.

## 5. HYPOPHYSITIS:

• May be primary (granulomatous, xanthomatous or lymphocytic) or caused by a known agent or systemic disease.

# CLINICAL RELEVANCE:

## PHEOCHROMOCYTOMA

• **INTRODUCTION**
   ○ Pheochromocytomas are rare neuroendocrine tumours that arise from either adrenal medulla or extra adrenal chromaffin tissue.
   ○ They can produce a variety of nonspecific symptoms, which include headaches, sweating, anxiety and palpitations.
   ○ Pheochromocytoma is associated with Von Hippel Landau disease, Multiple Endocrine Neoplasia (MEN) type 2 syndromes and Neurofibromatosis type 1.
   ○ 80% are unilateral and solitary, 10% are bilateral and 10% are extra-adrenal.
   ○ Approximately 90% are benign and 10% are malignant.
   ○ Common signs include hypertension and tachycardia.
   ○ Surgery, especially adrenal laparoscopy, is the most common treatment for small pheochromocytomas.

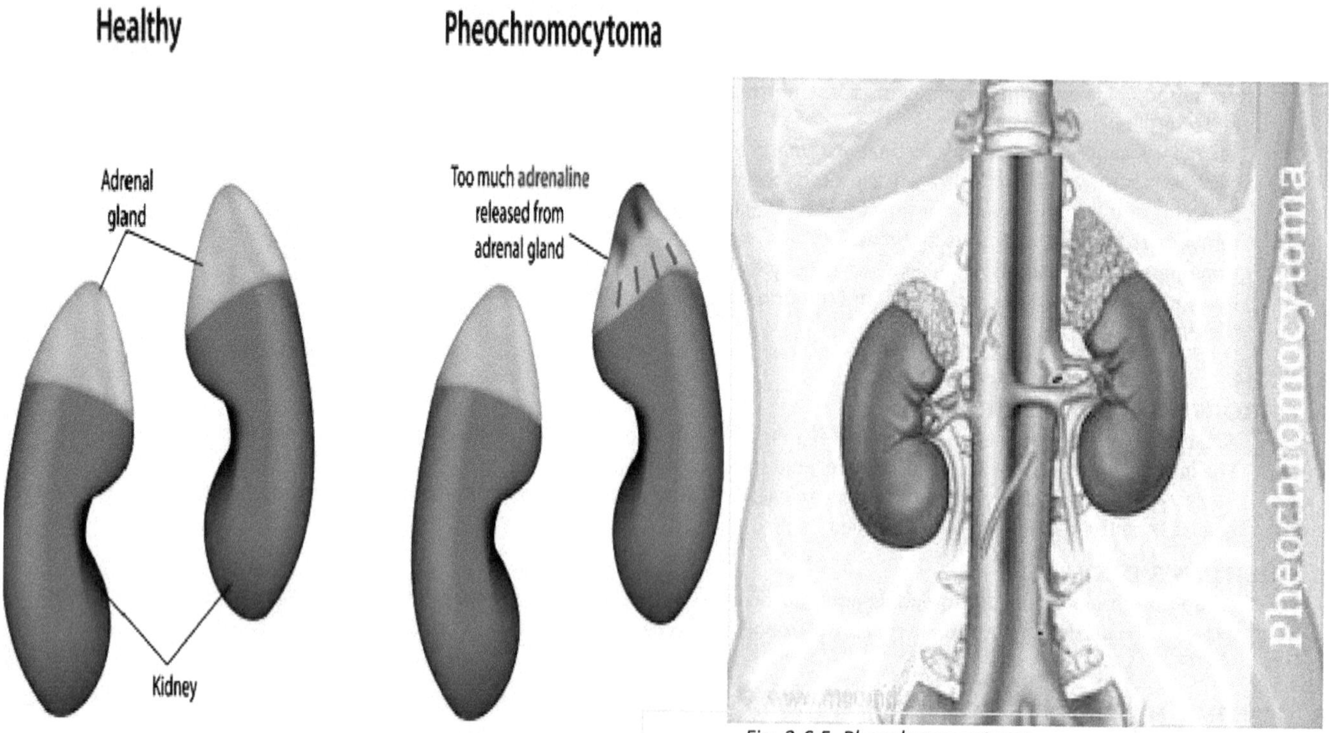

*Fig. 2.6.5. Pheochromocytoma*

- **PATHOPHYSIOLOGY**
  - The manifestations of pheochromocytoma are due mostly to the increased abnormal secretion of catecholamines, principally epinephrine, but also norepinephrine and dopamine.
  - The relative amounts of catecholamines secreted can differ between tumours and this determines the clinical picture.
  - The catecholamines can also be released episodically.
  - The effects of epinephrine and norepinephrine are caused by agonist activity at alpha and beta adrenoceptors and are detailed in the Pharmacology Section.

- **CLINICAL ASSESSMENT**
  - The presenting features of phaeochromocytoma are very wide and varied.
  - For this reason, it is referred to as the "great mimic".
  - Hypertension is a common presenting feature with SBP>220 mmHg or DBP<120 mmHg being generally accepted limiting values.
  - Hypertension is frequently associated with profound tachycardia, pallor and a feeling of anxiety or impending doom.
  - These symptoms are often paroxysmal and can occur many times a month or just once with a single fatal presentation.
  - The diagnosis should be considered in any patient presenting with acute hypertension or with a hypertensive crisis but be aware that hypertension can be episodic or absent and consider the diagnosis if there is a syndrome of appropriate clinical features compatible with the diagnosis.
  - Precipitants can include abdominal compression, anaesthesia, opiates, dopamine antagonists, cold medications, radiographic contrast media, catecholamine reuptake inhibitors and childbirth.

## DIFFERENTIAL DIAGNOSIS OF PHAEOCHROMOCYTOMA

| Endocrine | Cardiovascular | Neurological | Miscellaneous |
|---|---|---|---|
| Hyperthyroidism | Heart failure | Migraine | Essential hypertension |
| Carcinoid | Arrythmias | Stroke | Alcohol withdrawal |
| Hypoglycaemia | IHD | Diencephalic epilepsia | Pre-eclampsia |
| Medullary thyroid carcinoma | Baroreflex failure | Meningioma | Porphyria |
| Mastocytosis | Renovascular | Postural orthostatic tachycardia | Panic Disorder or Anxiety |
| Menopausal syndrome | hypertension | syndrome | Factitious Disorders |
| | | | Drug treatment |
| | | | Illegal Drug Use |

- **INVESTIGATION STRATEGIES**
  - ECG, Capillary Blood Glucose and FBC.
  - CT scan of the abdomen & MRI: Sensitivity 93-100%
  - Specific investigation for phaeochromocytoma is not usually instigated in the ED; appropriate subsequent tests include assay of plasma and urine metanephrines, catecholamines and urine vanillylmandelic acid (VMA).
  - The most sensitive test is Plasma Metanephrine Assay (99% sensitivity with a specificity of 89%)

- **MANAGEMENT OF PHEOCHROMOCYTOMA**
  - Definitive treatment is by **surgical resection of the tumour**, normally using a laparoscopic approach.
  - Prior to surgery the acute crisis is treated medically to control the effects of excess catecholamines.
  - This is normally achieved by alpha adrenoceptor blockade.
  - **Phenoxybenzamine** is advocated as it blocks adrenoceptors irreversibly and therefore its effect cannot be overcome by increasing catecholamine concentrations.
  - **Phentolamine and Doxazosin** are alternative alpha antagonists.
  - **Phenoxybenzamine IV 10-40 mg over one hour.**
  - It acts within one hour and its effects last for up to four days. It can be given orally in a dose of 10-60 mg/day in divided doses.
  - Side effects include hypotension, dizziness, sedation, dry mouth, paralytic ileus and impotence.
  - **Phentolamine 5-10 mg:** used in the diagnosis and perioperative management of pheochromocytoma. It causes vasodilatation, but also has positive inotropic and chronotropic effects.
  - It exerts its effect predominantly by competitive alpha adrenoceptor blockade.
  - **Side effects** include orthostatic hypotension, dizziness, abdominal discomfort and diarrhoea.
  - Cardiovascular collapse has occurred following treatment of pheochromocytoma.
  - Beta adrenoceptor blockade can be instituted to control tachycardia, but this should only be done after adequate alpha blockade, otherwise unopposed alpha activity can lead to worsening hypertension.
  - Treat arrhythmias if indicated.
  - IV fluid if fluid depleted.

# II. ADRENAL FUNCTION

## A. STRUCTURE

- The adrenal glands are located bilaterally in the retroperitoneum superior and slightly medial to the kidneys.
- In humans, the right adrenal gland is pyramidal in shape, whereas the left adrenal gland is semilunar in shape.
- The combined weight of the adrenal glands in an adult human range from 7 to 10 grams.
- The adrenal glands are surrounded by an adipose capsule and are enclosed within the renal fascia, a fibrous structure that also surrounds the kidney.
- A weak septum of connective tissue separates the glands from the kidneys and facilitates surgical removal of the kidneys without damage to the glands.
- The adrenal glands are in close relationship with the diaphragm, and are attached to the crura of the diaphragm by means of the renal fascia.
- Each adrenal gland has two anatomically and functionally distinct parts, the outer adrenal cortex and the inner medulla, both of which produce hormones.
- ***The cortex mainly produces aldosterone, cortisol and androgen.***
- ***While the medulla produces adrenaline and noradrenaline.***
- Each gland has an outer cortex made of steroid-producing cells surrounding a core of medulla, formed by chromaffin cells in direct relationship with the sympathetic nervous system.

## 1. THE ADRENAL CORTEX

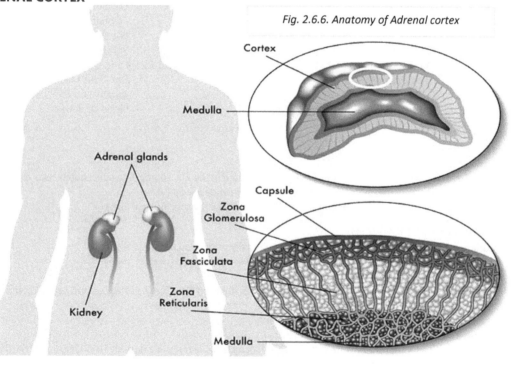

Fig. 2.6.6. Anatomy of Adrenal cortex

- o Divided into three zones according to their functions and microscopic appearance.
- o The adrenal cortex produces a class of steroid hormones, the corticosteroids, which are classified according to their effects:

## A. MINERALOCORTICOIDS (ALDOSTERONE)
- o Produced in the zona glomerulosa, help in the regulation of blood pressure and electrolyte balance.
- o The most important of which is aldosterone.

### FACTORS STIMULATING ALDOSTERONE RELEASE
- ✓ ACTH (transient effect only)
- ✓ Angiotensin II
- ✓ Hypoosmolarity and Low Blood volume
- ✓ Increased in plasma [K+] (Hyperkalaemia)
- ✓ **Standing:** Aldosterone release is increased in standing position because of:
  - ▪ Decreased hepatic clearance
  - ▪ Increase in renin and hence angiotensin II

## B. GLUCOCORTICOIDS (CORTISOL)

o   Synthesized in the zona fasciculata and their functions include regulation of glycogen and lipid metabolism and immune system suppression. This hormone is involved in the stress response and also helps to regulate body metabolism.
o   Cortisol stimulates glucose production by mobilising amino-acids and free fatty acids.
o   Cortisol also has significant anti-inflammatory effects.

## C. ANDROGENS (STEROID HORMONES)

o   Produced by the innermost layer of the cortex, the zona reticularis.
o   Androgens are converted to fully functional sex hormones in the gonads and other target organs. The production of steroid hormones is named steroidogenesis, and involves a number of reactions and processes that take place in cortical cells.
o   Adrenal androgens:
  ▪   Mainly dehydroepiandrosterone (DHEA) and testosterone.
  ▪   All have weak effects, but play a role in early development of the male sex organs in childhood, and in women during puberty.
  ▪   These are involved in creating and maintaining the differences between men and women.
• Regulation of synthesis and secretion of adrenal hormones is equally varied.
  o   **Mineralocorticoid production** is mainly under influence of the renin–angiotensin–aldosterone system (RAAS), in which specialized juxtaglomerular cells of the kidneys monitor blood volume and start a cascade of reactions that leads to the stimulation of aldosterone synthesis in the zona glomerulosa.
  o   **Cortisol and Androgen synthesis** are under control of the hypothalamic-pituitary-adrenal (HPA) axis in a classic example of a negative feedback loop, in which the hypothalamus and pituitary gland release stimulating hormones whenever cortisol levels are low.

## 2. THE MEDULLA

• Produces the catecholamines: epinephrine and norepinephrine.
• The release of medullary catecholamines is regulated by direct innervation from the sympathetic nervous system.

## B. BLOOD SUPPLY
## 1. ARTERIAL SUPPLY:

o   There are usually three arteries that supply each adrenal gland:
  ▪   **The superior suprarenal artery** (supplied by the inferior phrenic artery)
  ▪   **The middle suprarenal artery** (supplied by the abdominal aorta)
  ▪   **The inferior suprarenal artery** (supplied by the renal artery)

## 2. VENOUS DRAINAGE

o   Venous drainage of the adrenal glands is achieved via the suprarenal veins.
o   The right suprarenal vein drains into the inferior vena cava.
o   The left suprarenal vein drains into the left renal vein or the left inferior phrenic vein.
▪   The central adrenomedullary vein is a particular type of blood vessel in the adrenal medulla.
▪   The suprarenal vein exits the adrenal gland through a depression on its anterior surface known as the hilum.
▪   Note that the arteries supplying the suprarenal gland do not pass through the hilum.

## C. EFFECTS OF ADRENAL HORMONES
## 1. ADRENAL GLAND DISORDER
## 1.1. ADRENAL OVERPRODUCTION
## A. CUSHING'S SYNDROME: Secondary/Tertiary Hypercorticism

• **Cushing Syndrome** refers to the signs and symptoms associated with excess cortisol in the body, regardless of the cause.
• **Cushing Disease** is the hypercorticism caused by the pituitary adenoma oversecreting ACTH.
• The commonest cause of Cushing's syndrome is **iatrogenic administration of glucocorticoids.**
• It's can also be caused by an underlying disease which produces alterations in the Hypothalamo-Pituitary-Adrenal (HPA) axis or the production of cortisol. The most common cause of endogenous Cushing's syndrome is a pituitary adenoma (Secondary) which causes an excessive production of ACTH.
• Can also be due to excess production of hypothalamus CRH (tertiary hypercortisolism/hypercorticism) that stimulates the synthesis of cortisol by the adrenal glands. In the presence of Cushing's syndrome there is loss of the normal diurnal variation in cortisol levels. Under normal circumstances the midnight cortisol should be lower than the morning cortisol levels.
• *Patients with Cushing's syndrome are generally hypertensive due to cortisol enhancing the vasoconstrictive effect of endogenous adrenaline.*the following tests are recommended as screening tests for Cushing syndrome:
  o   **Midnight Serum or Salivary Cortisol**
  o   **24-hour Urine Free Cortisol**
  o   **Low dose Dexamethasone Suppression Test**
• Differentiation of Cushing syndrome from pseudo–Cushing syndrome can sometimes be a challenge.

## B. CONN'S SYNDROME: Primary Hyperaldosteronism

- When the zona glomerulosa produces excess aldosterone, the result is *primary aldosteronism*.
- Causes for this condition are bilateral hyperplasia of the glands and aldosterone-producing adenomas, which is called **Conn's syndrome.**
- Primary aldosteronism produces hypertension and electrolyte imbalance, increasing potassium depletion and sodium retention.
- **Biochemical markers:**          (MRCEM Part A question)
  - **Serum Potassium and Bicarbonate levels**
    - **Hypokalemia and Metabolic alkalosis**
    - Hypokalemia (K < 3.6 mEq/L) has a sensitivity of 75-80% while the patient is on a normal Na diet.
    - Typically, it is associated with mild metabolic alkalosis (serum bicarbonate level >31 mEq/L) and inappropriate kaliuresis (urinary potassium excretion >30 mmol/day).
  - **Low Renin level**
  - **Sodium and Magnesium levels**
    - **Mild serum hypernatremia** in the 143-147 mEq/L range and **Mild Hypomagnesemia** from renal magnesium wasting are other associated biochemical findings in established primary aldosteronism.
  - **Plasma aldosterone/plasma renin activity ratio**
    - Normal values are less than 270pmol/L, or are less than 10ng/dL.
    - A Plasma aldosterone/PRA ratio **> 20-25 ng/dL or 900 pmol/L** has 95% sensitivity and 75% specificity for primary aldosteronism.

# I.2. ADRENAL INSUFFICENCY (ADDISON'S DISEASE)

## A. PRIMARY ADRENAL INSUFFICIENCY

- Primary adrenal insufficiency, also known as **Addison's disease**, occurs when the adrenal glands cannot produce an adequate amount of hormones despite a normal or increased corticotropin (ACTH) level.
- This is a rare disease, occurring in approximately 35 to 120 people in every one million people.
- Most patients with Addison's disease experience fatigue, generalized weakness, loss of appetite, and weight loss.
- The type and severity of symptoms depends upon the speed with which the condition develops, the severity of the hormone deficiency, the underlying cause of the condition, and other stresses on the body.
- **Other common symptoms include:**
  - Darkening of the skin, especially on the face, neck, and back of hands
  - Gastrointestinal symptoms such as nausea and vomiting (vomiting and abdominal pain may be a sign of an **adrenal crisis)**
  - Low blood pressure with lightheadedness after standing or sitting up
  - Muscle and joint pain
  - Salt craving
  - In women, decreased hair in the armpits and pubic area and decreased sexual desire

## B. SECONDARY AND TERTIARY ADRENAL INSUFFICIENCY

- In **secondary adrenal insufficiency**, an insufficient amount of corticotropin (ACTH) is produced by the pituitary gland.
- In **tertiary adrenal insufficiency**, an insufficient amount of corticotropin-releasing hormone (CRH) is produced by the hypothalamus.
- **Symptoms**: The symptoms of secondary and tertiary adrenal insufficiency are similar to those of primary insufficiency, with a few exceptions:
  - Darkening of the skin and dehydration do not occur
  - Gastrointestinal symptoms are less common
  - Symptoms of **hypoglycemia** are more common, including sweating, anxiety, shaking, nausea, or heart palpitations
  - A tumor or other growth in the pituitary or hypothalamus can cause other symptoms, including headaches and difficulty seeing objects in the periphery of vision (to the far left and right).
  - Also, low levels of pituitary hormones can develop and may cause infertility, erectile dysfunction (impotence), fatigue, hoarseness, constipation, a delay in beginning puberty, or short stature in children.

| CAUSES OF ADRENAL INSUFFICIENCY ||
|---|---|
| **Primary causes** | **Secondary causes** |
| <ul><li>Idiopathic/Autoimmune</li><li>Infective: TB, AIDS, Fungal infection.</li><li>Haemorrhage: anticoagulant therapy, Waterhouse–Friderichsen syndrome (haemorrhage into the adrenal gland secondary to fulminant meningococcal septicaemia).</li><li>Infiltration: carcinoma, lymphoma, sarcoidosis, amyloidosis.</li><li>Drugs: ketoconazole, Etomidate</li></ul> | <ul><li>Abrupt withdrawal of long term steroids</li><li>Trauma to infundibular stalk</li><li>Necrosis (Sheehan's syndrome)</li><li>Neoplasms and granulomatous disease of pituitary</li><li>Radiation to pituitary</li></ul> |

## INVESTIGATION OF ADRENOCORTICAL INSUFFICIENCY

- U&E, Serum Cortisol & Plasma ACTH
- Infective Screen
- ECG
- **Adrenocortical deficiency results in:**
  - Hyponatraemia.
  - Hyperkalaemia.
  - Hypoglycaemia.
  - Elevated urea and creatinine.
  - Metabolic acidosis.
  - Serum cortisol and plasma ACTH levels should be sent, but should not delay treatment with hydrocortisone.

**Interpretation of the cortisol and ACTH results:**
- *Low serum cortisol (<200nmol/L): indicates adrenal insufficiency.*
- *A raised ACTH in this context suggests primary adrenal insufficiency and a low ACTH suggests secondary.*
- *High serum cortisol (>550nmol/L): excludes adrenal insufficiency.*
- *Intermediate serum cortisol (200–550 nmol/L): requires further investigation with a Synacthen (tetracosactrin) test.*

# ADRENAL CRISIS or ADDISONIAN CRISIS

## 1. OVERVIEW

- Do not confuse acute **adrenal crisis** with **Addison disease**.
- Adrenal crisis is a life-threatening condition that requires emergency medical treatment.
- The patient or a family member or friend should immediately give an emergency injection of a glucocorticoid at the first signs of adrenal crisis.
- Addison described a syndrome of long-term adrenal insufficiency that develops over months to years, with weakness, fatigue, anorexia, weight loss, and hyperpigmentation as the primary symptoms.
- In contrast, an acute adrenal crisis can manifest with vomiting, abdominal pain, and hypovolemic shock.
- Usually caused by concurrent illness, surgery, failure to take medications

## 2. CLINICAL:

- GI: abdominal pain, vomiting and diarrhoea
- CVS: dehydration, hypotension, refractory shock, poor response to inotropes/pressors
- Fever
- Confusion

## 3. INVESTIGATIONS

- **Diagnosis:**
  - Plasma cortisol level < 80mmol/L
  - Short synacthen test: 250mcg (normal response = cortisol > 525mmol/L
  - Other Low glucose
  - Low Na+
  - Hypo-osmolar
  - Raised K+
  - Raised Urea and Creatinine
  - Raised Ca2+ (primary only)
  - Eosinophilia

## 4. MANAGEMENT OF ACUTE ADRENOCORTICAL INSUFFICIENCY

- Treatment of a suspected adrenal crisis should not be delayed pending the results of cortisol and ACTH.
- ABCD Approach
- Hydrocortisone 100 mg IV should be given as soon as an adrenal crisis is suspected.
- Fludrocortisone is only required in primary adrenocortical insufficiency and is not commonly given in the ED.
- Fluid resuscitation should be directed by cardiovascular status.
- Patients should be monitored for hypoglycaemia and treated with 10% glucose IV if it develops.
- Any underlying infection should be treated with appropriate antibiotics.

# III. ENDOCRINE PANCREAS

## 1. INSULIN

- Insulin is synthesized in β cells
- Kallikrein, an enzyme present in the islets, aids in the conversion of proinsulin to insulin.
- In this conversion, a C peptide chain is removed from the proinsulin molecule producing the disulfide-connected α and β chains that are insulin.
- The major actions of insulin are:
  - facilitation of glucose transport through certain membranes (adipose and muscle cells),
  - Stimulation of the enzyme system for conversion of glucose to glycogen (liver and muscle cells);
  - slow-down of gluconeogenesis (liver and muscle cells);
  - Regulation of lipogenesis (liver and adipose cells);
  - Promotion of protein synthesis and growth (general effect).

Fig. 2.6.7. Endocrine pancreas

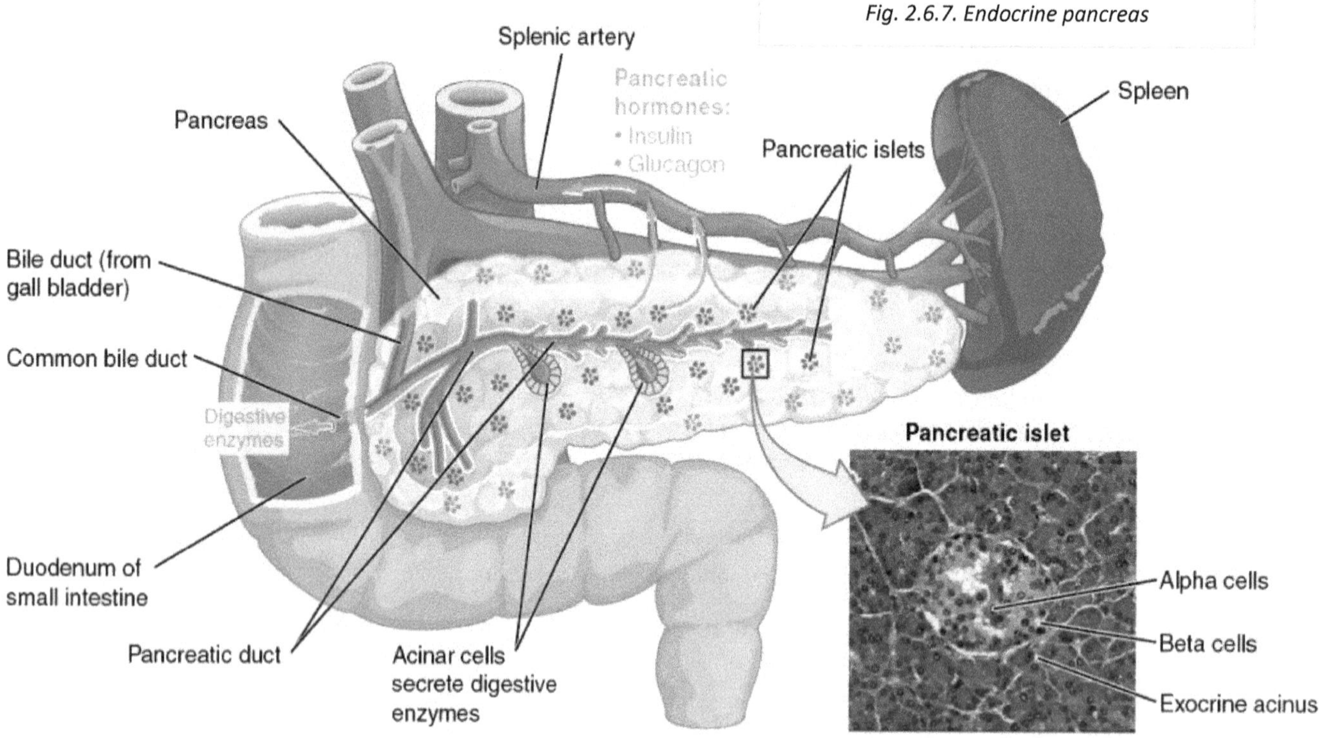

## 2. GLUCAGON

- Glucagon is the polypeptide hormone released from alpha cells of pancreatic islets.
- It is, like insulin, synthesised as a prohormone – proglucagon, and cleaved to the active form inside secretory granules.
- **Function:**
  - Stimulation of hepatic **glycogenolysis** (breakdown of glycogen stores to release glucose) and **gluconeogenesis** (synthesis of glucose from metabolic substrates such as pyruvate, glycerol and lactate).
  - Inhibit liver **glycogenesis**
  - High levels of glucagon will cause **lipolysis** and **production of keto-acids** (ketogenesis) as substrates for glucose synthesis.

| FACTORS AFFECTING GLUCAGON SECRETION ||
|---|---|
| **INCREASED GLUCAGON SECRETION** | **DECREASED GLUCAGON SECRETION** |
| o  Amino acids | o  Hyperglycaemia |
| o  CCK, gastrin | o  Following meals |
| o  Cortisol | o  Insulin |
| o  Exercise, Infection | o  Somatostatin |
| o  Beta adrenergic stimulants | o  Secretin |
| o  Theophylline | o  Free fatty acids |
| o  Acetylcholine | o  Blood ketones |
| o  Hypoglycaemia | |
| o  Fasting | |

# IV. THYROID PHYSIOLOGY

## SYNTHESIS AND RELEASE OF THYROID HORMONES

- Hormones are produced in the colloid when atoms of the mineral iodine attach to a glycoprotein, called **thyroglobulin**, that is secreted into the colloid by the follicle cells. The following steps outline the hormones' assembly:

  o Binding of TSH to its receptors in the follicle cells of the thyroid gland causes the cells to actively transport iodide ions ($I^-$) across their cell membrane, from the bloodstream into the cytosol. As a result, the concentration of iodide ions "trapped" in the follicular cells is many times higher than the concentration in the bloodstream.

  o Iodide ions then move to the lumen of the follicle cells that border the colloid. There, the ions undergo oxidation (their negatively charged electrons are removed).

  o The oxidation of two iodide ions ($2\ I^-$) results in iodine ($I_2$), which passes through the follicle cell membrane into the colloid.

  o In the colloid, peroxidase enzymes link the iodine to the tyrosine amino acids in thyroglobulin to produce two intermediaries: a tyrosine attached to one iodine and a tyrosine attached to two iodines. When one of each of these intermediaries is linked by covalent bonds, the resulting compound is **triiodothyronine** ($T_3$), a thyroid hormone with three iodines. Much more commonly, two copies of the second intermediary bond, forming tetraiodothyronine, also known as **thyroxine** ($T_4$), a thyroid hormone with four iodines.

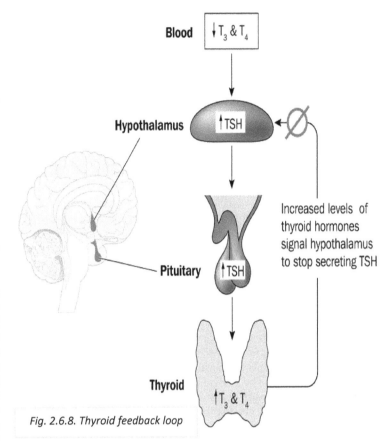

**Blood** $\downarrow T_3\ \&\ T_4$

**Hypothalamus** $\uparrow$TSH

**Pituitary** $\uparrow$TSH

Increased levels of thyroid hormones signal hypothalamus to stop secreting TSH

**Thyroid** $\uparrow T_3\ \&\ T_4$

*Fig. 2.6.8. Thyroid feedback loop*

  o These hormones remain in the colloid center of the thyroid follicles until TSH stimulates endocytosis of colloid back into the follicle cells. There, lysosomal enzymes break apart the thyroglobulin colloid, releasing free $T_3$ and $T_4$, which diffuse across the follicle cell membrane and enter the bloodstream.

  o In the bloodstream, less than one percent of the circulating $T_3$ and $T_4$ remains unbound. This free $T_3$ and $T_4$ can cross the lipid bilayer of cell membranes and be taken up by cells. The remaining 99 percent of circulating $T_3$ and $T_4$ is bound to specialized transport proteins called thyroxine-binding globulins (TBGs), to albumin, or to other plasma proteins. This "packaging" prevents their free diffusion into body cells.

  o When blood levels of $T_3$ and $T_4$ begin to decline, bound $T_3$ and $T_4$ are released from these plasma proteins and readily cross the membrane of target cells. $T_3$ is more potent than $T_4$, and many cells convert $T_4$ to $T_3$ through the removal of an iodine atom.

## REGULATION OF THYROID HORMONES SYNTHESIS

- The release of $T_3$ and $T_4$ from the thyroid gland is regulated by thyroid-stimulating hormone (TSH).
- Low blood levels of $T_3$ and $T_4$ stimulate the release of thyrotropin-releasing hormone (TRH) from the hypothalamus, which triggers secretion of TSH from the anterior pituitary.
- In turn, TSH stimulates the thyroid gland to secrete $T_3$ and $T_4$. The levels of TRH, TSH, $T_3$, and $T_4$ are regulated by a negative feedback system in which increasing levels of $T_3$ and $T_4$ decrease the production and secretion of TSH.

## FUNCTIONS OF THYROID HORMONES

- The thyroid hormones, $T_3$ and $T_4$, are often referred to as metabolic hormones because their levels influence the body's basal metabolic rate, the amount of energy used by the body at rest. When $T_3$ and $T_4$ bind to intracellular receptors located on the mitochondria, they cause an increase in nutrient breakdown and the use of oxygen to produce ATP.
- In addition, $T_3$ and $T_4$ initiate the transcription of genes involved in glucose oxidation. Although these mechanisms prompt cells to produce more ATP, the process is inefficient, and an abnormally increased level of heat is released as a byproduct of these reactions. This so-called calorigenic effect (calor- = "heat") raises body temperature.
- Adequate levels of thyroid hormones are also required for protein synthesis and for fetal and childhood tissue development and growth. They are especially critical for normal development of the nervous system both in utero and in early childhood, and they continue to support neurological function in adults.

- As noted earlier, these thyroid hormones have a complex interrelationship with reproductive hormones, and deficiencies can influence libido, fertility, and other aspects of reproductive function. Finally, thyroid hormones increase the body's sensitivity to catecholamines (epinephrine and norepinephrine) from the adrenal medulla by upregulation of receptors in the blood vessels.
- When levels of $T_3$ and $T_4$ hormones are excessive, this effect accelerates the heart rate, strengthens the heartbeat, and increases blood pressure. Because thyroid hormones regulate metabolism, heat production, protein synthesis, and many other body functions, thyroid disorders can have severe and widespread consequences.

## DISORDERS OF THE THYROID GLAND
### ENDOCRINE SYSTEM: IODINE DEFICIENCY, HYPOTHYROIDISM, AND HYPERTHYROIDISM

- Dietary iodine is required for the synthesis of $T_3$ and $T_4$. But for much of the world's population, foods do not provide adequate levels of this mineral, because the amount varies according to the level in the soil in which the food was grown, as well as the irrigation and fertilizers used.
- Marine fish and shrimp tend to have high levels because they concentrate iodine from seawater, but many people in landlocked regions lack access to seafood. Thus, the primary source of dietary iodine in many countries is iodized salt. Fortification of salt with iodine began in the United States in 1924, and international efforts to iodize salt in the world's poorest nations continue today.
- Dietary iodine deficiency can result in the impaired ability to synthesize $T_3$ and $T_4$, leading to a variety of severe disorders.
- When $T_3$ and $T_4$ cannot be produced, TSH is secreted in increasing amounts.
- As a result of this hyperstimulation, thyroglobulin accumulates in the thyroid gland follicles, increasing their deposits of colloid.
- The accumulation of colloid increases the overall size of the thyroid gland, a condition called a **goiter**. A goiter is only a visible indication of the deficiency. Other iodine deficiency disorders include impaired growth and development, decreased fertility, and prenatal and infant death. Moreover, iodine deficiency is the primary cause of preventable mental retardation worldwide.
- **Neonatal hypothyroidism** (cretinism) is characterized by cognitive deficits, short stature, and sometimes deafness and muteness in children and adults born to mothers who were iodine-deficient during pregnancy
- In areas of the world with access to iodized salt, dietary deficiency is rare. Instead, inflammation of the thyroid gland is the more common cause of low blood levels of thyroid hormones.
- Called **hypothyroidism**, the condition is characterized by a low metabolic rate, weight gain, cold extremities, constipation, reduced libido, menstrual irregularities, and reduced mental activity.
- In contrast, **hyperthyroidism**—an abnormally elevated blood level of thyroid hormones—is often caused by a pituitary or thyroid tumor. In Graves' disease, the hyperthyroid state results from an autoimmune reaction in which antibodies overstimulate the follicle cells of the thyroid gland. Hyperthyroidism can lead to an increased metabolic rate, excessive body heat and sweating, diarrhoea, weight loss, tremors, and increased heart rate. The person's eyes may bulge (**called exophthalmos**) as antibodies produce inflammation in the soft tissues of the orbits. The person may also develop a goiter.

## CALCITONIN

- The thyroid gland also secretes a hormone called **calcitonin** that is produced by the parafollicular cells (also called C cells) that stud the tissue between distinct follicles.
- Calcitonin is released in response to a rise in blood calcium levels. It appears to have a function in decreasing blood calcium concentrations by:
  - Inhibiting the activity of osteoclasts, bone cells that release calcium into the circulation by degrading bone matrix
  - Increasing osteoblastic activity
  - Decreasing calcium absorption in the intestines
  - Increasing calcium loss in the urine
- However, these functions are usually not significant in maintaining calcium homeostasis, so the importance of calcitonin is not entirely understood. Pharmaceutical preparations of calcitonin are sometimes prescribed to reduce osteoclast activity in people with osteoporosis and to reduce the degradation of cartilage in people with osteoarthritis. The hormones secreted by thyroid are summarized in table below.
- Of course, calcium is critical for many other biological processes. It is a second messenger in many signaling pathways, and is essential for muscle contraction, nerve impulse transmission, and blood clotting. Given these roles, it is not surprising that blood calcium levels are tightly regulated by the endocrine system. The organs involved in the regulation are the parathyroid glands.

| Thyroid Hormones | | |
|---|---|---|
| **Associated hormones** | **Chemical class** | **Effect** |
| Thyroxine ($T_4$), triiodothyronine ($T_3$) | Amine | Stimulate basal metabolic rate |
| Calcitonin | Peptide | Reduces blood $Ca^{2+}$ levels |

# III. THYROID EMERGENCIES

## 1. THYROID STORM

### DESCRIPTION

- **Malignant or critical thyrotoxicosis**, **thyroid storm**, is a life-threatening medical emergency in which excessive concentrations of thyroid hormone produce organ dysfunction. It is an uncommon manifestation of hyperthyroidism, occurring in less than 10% of patients hospitalized for thyrotoxicosis.
- However, it may be the presenting symptom of the condition and, if untreated, is associated with 80% to 90% mortality.
- Even with treatment, mortality from thyroid storm exceeds 20%. Recognition and immediate management is important in preventing the high morbidity and mortality associated with this disease. A spectrum of thyroid dysfunction exists.
- **Hyperthyroidism, or thyrotoxicosis**, refers to disorders that result from overproduction and release of hormone from the thyroid gland. Thyrotoxicosis refers to any cause of excessive thyroid hormone concentration, whereas **malignant thyrotoxicosis, or thyroid storm**, represents an extreme manifestation of thyrotoxicosis with resultant end-organ dysfunction.
- Incidence Thyroid storm can occur in both men and women of any age. However, it is more common in teenaged or young adult women. Although a history of hyperthyroidism is common, thyroid storm may be the initial manifestation in a significant number of patients. Thyroid storm can be precipitated by a variety of factors, including severe infection, diabetic ketoacidosis, surgery, trauma, and pulmonary thromboembolism.
- Direct trauma or surgical manipulation of the thyroid gland can also precipitate thyroid storm. Iodine, either from excessive ingestion, intravenous administration, or radiotherapy, has been reported to precipitate thyroid storm.
- It has also been described following discontinuation of antithyroid medications. Of interest, salicylates have been implicated in triggering thyroid storm by increasing the concentration of circulating free thyroid hormones to critical levels.

### CLINICAL MANIFESTATION AND DIAGNOSIS

- The clinical manifestations of thyroid storm are consistent with marked hypermetabolism resulting in multiorgan system dysfunction.
- The differential diagnosis of thyroid storm includes **sepsis, central nervous system infection, anticholinergic or adrenergic intoxication, other endocrine dysfunction, and acute psychiatric illness**.
- Symptoms include:
  - **Thermoregulatory dysfunction** (high fever, warm moist skin, diaphoresis),
  - **Neurologic manifestations** (mental status changes, seizure, coma, psychosis, hyperreflexia, lid lag),
  - **Cardiovascular dysregulation** (atrial fibrillation, tachycardia, hypertension, congestive heart failure),
  - The hypometabolic state and mental status depression may result in centrally mediated hypoventilation and hypercapnic respiratory failure.
  - **Respiratory distress** (dyspnoea, tachypnoea), and
  - **Gastrointestinal dysfunction** (diarrhoea, abdominal pain, nausea, vomiting).
- The diagnosis of thyroid storm relies heavily on clinical suspicion.
- It is strongly suggested by the constellation of these symptoms and is confirmed by means of thyroid function tests (TFT).
- However, treatment should not be delayed for verification by laboratory tests.
- **Thyroid stimulating hormone** (TSH) levels are virtually undetectable (<0.01 micro international units [mcIU]/L) with a concomitant elevation of free T4 and T3. Because of increased conversion of T4 to T3, the elevation of T3 is typically more dramatic.
- For this reason, it is essential to measure both T3 and free T4 levels when thyroid storm is suspected.
- *There are no differences in the results of TFT in patients with thyroid storm when compared with patients who have symptomatic hyperthyroidism, and levels of thyroid hormone cannot predict which patients will undergo decompensation from thyrotoxicosis to thyroid storm. The distinction is made clinically by documentation of acute organ dysfunction.*

# Graves' Disease

*Graves' disease*, also known as **toxic diffuse goiter**, is *an autoimmune disease that affects the thyroid.*
*It frequently results in and is the most common cause of hyperthyroidism*

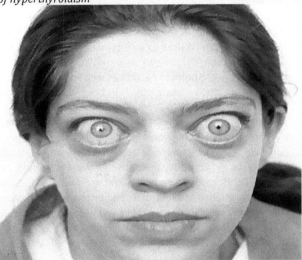

*Fig 2.6.9. The classic finding of exophthalmos and lid retraction in Graves' disease*

**Symptoms**
- Enlarged Thyroid, Irritability, Muscle weakness,
- Sleeping problems, **Fast heartbeat**,
- Poor tolerance of heat
- Complications: Graves' Ophthalmopathy

**Causes:** unknown
**Risk Factors:**
- Family history, Other autoimmune diseases
- Diagnostic Method
- Blood tests, Radioiodine uptake

**Treatment:**
- Radioiodine Therapy,
- Medications,
- Thyroid surgery

**Frequency:** 0.5% (males), 3% (females)

- Other laboratory abnormalities commonly seen are **hypercalcemia** from osteoclast-mediated bone resorption, **elevated alkaline phosphatase** caused by activated bone remodelling, and **hyperglycaemia** secondary to enhanced glycogenolysis and increased circulation of catecholamines.
- Adrenal insufficiency, especially among patients with **Graves' disease**, is common and should be evaluated prior to the initiation of treatment.

## EMERGENCY TREATMENT

- The treatment of thyroid storm involves 3 critical fundamentals:
  - ○ **First**, supportive care should be provided to minimize the secondary effects of organ failure. This should include respiratory and hemodynamic support and treatment of hyperthermia.
  - ○ **Second**, identification and treatment of the precipitating event is warranted to prevent further progression of disease.
  - ○ **Third**, and most critical, the release and effects of circulating thyroid hormone must be blocked. Inhibition of the peripheral conversion of T4 to T3 helps attenuate the effects of thyroid hormone.
- **Propylthiouracil (PTU)** blocks peripheral conversion of T4 to T3 and can be given as a 600- to 1000-mg loading dose, followed by 1200 mg/day divided into doses given every 4 to 6 hours.
- **Methimazole** can be used as an alternate agent but does not block peripheral T4 conversion. Both medications can be administered rectally if necessary.
- Peripheral thyroid hormone action as well as tachycardia and hypertension can be minimized by beta-blockers; typically, **Propranolol** administered intravenously initially in 1-mg increments every 10 to 15 minutes until symptoms are controlled or **Esmolol** administered as a loading dose of 250-500 mcg/kg followed by an infusion of 50-100 mcg/kg/minute.
- Thyroid hormone release can be reduced by the administration of **lithium, iodinated contrast, and corticosteroids**.
- **Hydrocortisone 100 mg** given intravenously every 8 hours has been shown to improve outcomes in patients. Steroid therapy is also beneficial, given the common association with adrenal insufficiency.
- Iodine acts by inhibiting hormone release but should not be given until 1 hour after PTU administration. In refractory cases, plasmapheresis, plasma exchange, and peritoneal hemodialysis can be used to remove circulating thyroid hormone.
- With appropriate treatment, clinic and biochemical improvement are typically seen within 24 hours.
- Full recovery usually occurs within a week of therapy. Thyroid storm poses diagnostic and therapeutic challenges.
- Treatment is aimed at halting the thyrotoxic process at all levels. Prompt recognition and treatment is essential for successful management and is paramount to decreasing the high mortality associated with this disease.

## 2. MYXEDEMA COMA

- **DESCRIPTION**
  - ○ Myxedema coma is an uncommon presentation of severe hypothyroidism that is potentially fatal. Published mortality rates exceed 60%, and even with early detection and appropriate treatment, death occurs in up to 30% of individuals.
  - ○ The term myxedema coma is a misnomer, as myxedema and coma are neither diagnostic criteria nor common presenting findings.
  - ○ A more proper description would be critical hypothyroidism.
  - ○ Because of its lethal nature and nonspecific features, the actual prevalence of myxedema coma is unknown.
  - ○ However, this syndrome is extensively cited in the literature and is not uncommon in clinical practice.

- **INCIDENCE**
  - ○ Myxedema coma, or **critical hypothyroidism**, occurs most often in patients with long-standing, preexisting hypothyroidism.
  - ○ Hypothyroidism is 4 times more common in women than in men, and 80% of cases of myxedema coma occur in females.
  - ○ It occurs almost exclusively in persons 60 years or older.
  - ○ There are approximately 300 cases of myxedema coma reported in the literature.
  - ○ Most cases occur during the winter, when thermoregulatory stressors are high.
  - ○ It can develop from all causes of hypothyroidism, including autoimmune thyroiditis, secondary hypothyroidism, and drug-induced hypothyroidism (e.g., caused by lithium or amiodarone).

- **CLINICAL MANIFESTATION AND DIAGNOSIS**
  - ○ Myxedema coma can be precipitated by several factors. **Infections,** especially pneumonia, are perhaps the most common precipitating factor.
  - ○ Even occult bacterial infections have been implicated and, as such, infections should be thoroughly evaluated for as a potential etiologic factor.
  - ○ Cardiac events (myocardial infarction, congestive heart failure), cerebral infarction, trauma, hemorrhage, hypothermia, hypoglycemia, and respiratory depression secondary to anesthetics or sedatives have also been implicated.
  - ○ Clinical findings in myxedema coma are similar to those encountered with hypothyroidism, but they are typically seen in greater magnitude. In short, it is a state of profound decreased metabolic activity.
  - ○ Cardinal features include:
    - ▪ **Impaired thermoregulation** (hypothermia),
    - ▪ **Hypotension,**
    - ▪ **Bradycardia, and**
    - ▪ **Mental status depression.**

- Mental status depression is a common clinical feature and may progress to stupor, obtundation, or frank coma.
- Concomitant endocrinopathies are commonly encountered, most notably adrenal insufficiency, which may contribute to the electrolyte, thermoregulatory, and cardiovascular derangements commonly seen.
- **Hyponatremia** resulting from an increased release of antidiuretic hormone and hypoglycemia caused by decreased gluconeogenesis, infection, or adrenal insufficiency are common features.
- Myxedema is characterized by generalized skin and soft tissue swelling, periorbital edema, ptosis, macroglossia, and the presence of cool, dry skin.
- Despite the name of the condition, clinically significant myxedema is infrequently identified and is not a diagnostic criteria.
- Unlike thyroid storm, most patients with myxedema coma have a prior diagnosis of hypothyroidism. Although it is necessary to confirm the diagnosis, thyroid function testing can be confusing.
- The diagnosis is suspected clinically and confirmed with TFT.
- Treatment should not be delayed for laboratory confirmation

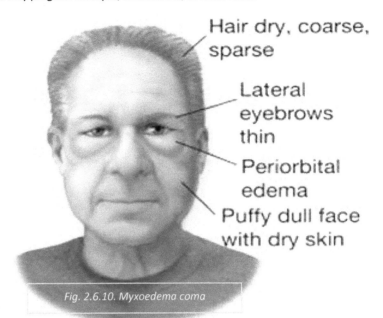

Fig. 2.6.10. Myxoedema coma

- *Hypothyroidism is diagnosed in individuals with elevated TSH levels and low levels of free T4 and T3.*
- *In myxedema coma, T3 and T4 levels may be profoundly diminished or even undetectable.*
- The degree of TFT abnormalities does not distinguish hypothyroidism from myxedema coma. Rather, the distinction is based on clinical findings. Abnormal TFT can be seen in other acute illnesses and does not necessarily reflect myxedema coma or even hypothyroidism.
- It is important for the clinician to be able to differentiate hypothyroidism from euthyroid sick syndrome, in which patients have a reduction in both TSH and thyroid hormone levels.
- Given the common association with adrenal insufficiency, a cosyntropin stimulation test should be considered, especially in those with hemodynamic instability.

- **EMERGENCY TREATMENT**
  - The treatment of myxedema coma involves rapid replacement of thyroid hormone, treatment of the precipitating cause, and general supportive measures. A stated, despite a prompt diagnosis and initiation of treatment, mortality from myxedema coma can still exceed 30%.
  - **Thyroid hormone replacement** should be given intravenously to ensure rapid restoration of bioactive thyroxine levels and resolution of symptoms. Both high-dose and low-dose strategies have been used. However, neither has been shown to be superior.
  - **High-dose intravenous thyroxine** is given as a bolus of 300-500 mcg, followed by 50-100 mcg daily depending on the patient's age, weight, and risk of complications.
  - This method provides a more rapid recovery of symptoms but carries the potential for unwanted cardiac events resulting from the rapid replacement of thyroxine.
  - In the low-dose method, thyroxine 25 mcg is given daily for 1 week followed by a gradually increased dose until the patient is able to resume normal thyroxine orally.
  - Alternatively, **5 mcg of triiodothyronine** can be given twice daily during the loading period.
  - **Intravenous triiodothyronine** can be used as well and may provide a more rapid resolution of symptoms and improved mental status, although high levels of triiodothyronine have been correlated with increased mortality.
  - Triiodothyronine is given as an initial bolus dose of 10-20 mcg, followed by 10 mcg every 4 to 24 hours, with taper to 10 mcg every 6 hours.
  - Regardless of the replacement method used, all patients should be continuously monitored for hypertension and cardiac ischemia, which portend the greatest risk of death among patients with myxedema coma.
  - Treatment should also be directed at identifying and reversing the underlying cause.
  - Supportive care should be provided while thyroid hormone levels are replaced.
  - Ventilatory support, passive external rewarming, and correction of underlying electrolyte abnormalities are commonly required.
  - **Glucose and steroid replacement** should also be considered until recovery. Given the strong association with infectious causes, antimicrobial therapy should be considered. Myxedema coma is a potentially fatal complication of a common disorder.
  - Prompt recognition based on clinical features and institution of aggressive comprehensive treatment can reduce mortality.

# V. CALCIUM, Vit D & PTH PHYSIOLOGY

## 1. VITAMIN D PHYSIOLOGY

- *Synthesis*
  - *7-Dehydrocholesterol*
    - Precursor to calcitriol is stored in the skin where UV exposure converts it to previtamin D3.
  - *cholecalciferol (Vitamin D3)*
    - Previtamin D3 is then bound to vitamin-D binding protein (DBP) where it is carried to the liver and metabolized to 25-hydroxyvitamin D3.
  - *25-hyrdoxyvitamin D3*
    - When calcium is low, parathyroid hormone (PTH) levels become elevated which activates 1-alpha-hydroxylase in the kidney.
    - 1-alpha-hydroxylase converts 25-hydroxyvitamin D to the active Vitamin D (calcitriol).
  - *1,25-dihydroxyvitamin D3 (Vitamin D, calcitriol)*
    - Active form that controls calcium homeostasis in body by targeting intestines and bones.
- *Function*
  - ↑ serum $Ca^{2+}$ and phosphate via
    - ↑ absorption of calcium and phosphate from the intestine
    - ↑ bone resorption of $Ca^{2+}$ and phosphate
  - recall PTH functions to ↑ serum $Ca^{2+}$ but ↓ serum phosphate
- *Regulation*
  - PTH stimulates 1,25-$(OH)_2$ vitamin D production.
  - Hypocalcaemia/hypophosphatemia stimulates 1,25-$(OH)_2$ vitamin D production.
  - 1,25-$(OH)_2$ vitamin D feedback negatively on itself.

## 2. PTH PHYSIOLOGY

- *Synthesis*
  - Secreted by the chief cells of parathyroid.
- *Function*
  - ↑ serum $Ca^{2+}$ and ↓ serum phosphate in response to hypocalcaemia/hypomagnesemia via:
    - ↑ Bone resorption of calcium and phosphate (bone is destroyed).
      - ✓ PTH receptor is on the osteoblasts which secretes IL-1 to activated osteoclasts
    - ↑ Kidney resorption of calcium in distal convoluted tubule.
    - ↓ Kidney resorption of phosphate.
    - ↑ 1,25-$(OH)_2$ vitamin D production.

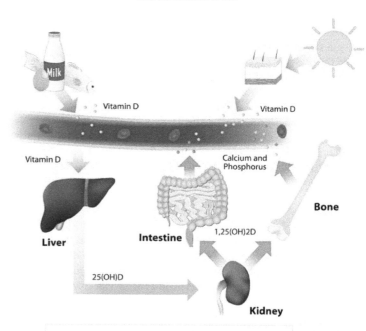

# VITAMIN D

*Fig. 2.6.11. Vit D Physiology*

## PARATHYROID GLANDS
(located on the back of the thyroid gland)

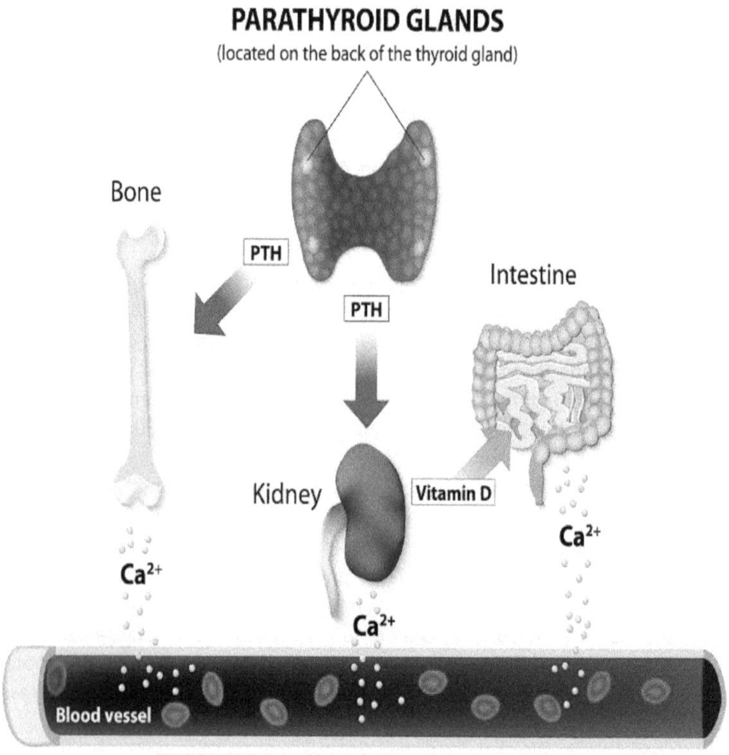

*Fig. 2.6.12. parathyroid physiology*

# 3. CALCIUM HOMEOSTASIS

- Calcium homeostasis regulates calcium flow to and from the bones.
- Inadequate calcium levels can result in osteoporosis.
- Calcium release from bone is regulated by parathyroid hormone.
- Vitamin D is converted to calcidiol (also called calcifediol) in the liver, which is then converted to calcitriol in the kidneys, the biologically active form of vitamin D.
- Calcitriol regulates the levels of calcium and phosphorus in the blood and helps maintain a healthy skeletal system.
- Bone resorption by osteoclasts releases calcium into the bloodstream, which helps regulate calcium homeostasis.
- **Calcitriol:** The active metabolite—1,25-dihydroxycholecalciferol—that is involved in the absorption of calcium.
- **Calcitonin:** Produced in humans by the thyroid gland, it acts to reduce blood calcium, opposing the effects of parathyroid hormone.
- **Calcium homeostasis:** Calcium homeostasis is the mechanism by which the body maintains adequate calcium levels in order to prevent hypercalcemia or hypocalcaemia, both of which can have important consequences for health.
- **Calcidiol:** A prehormone that is produced in the liver by the hydroxylation of vitamin D3 (cholecalciferol) by the enzyme cholecalciferol 25-hydroxylase.
- Calcium metabolism or calcium homeostasis is the mechanism by which the body maintains adequate calcium levels. Derangements of this mechanism lead to hypercalcemia or hypocalcaemia, both of which can have important consequences for health.

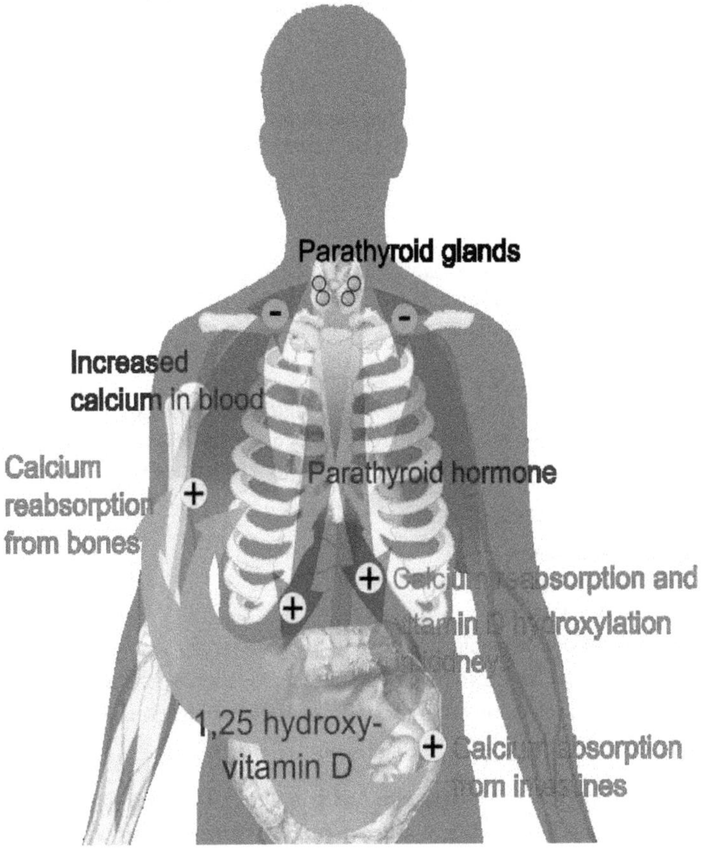

Fig. 2.6.13. Calcium regulation

- Although calcium flow to and from the bone is neutral, about five mmol is turned over a day. Bone serves as an important storage point for calcium, as it contains 99% of the total body calcium.
- Calcium release from bone is regulated by parathyroid hormone.
- Calcitonin stimulates incorporation of calcium in bone.
- Low calcium intake may be a risk factor in the development of osteoporosis.
- With a better bone balance, the risk of osteoporosis is lowered. Supplementation with vitamin D and calcium slightly improves bone mineral density.

## VITAMIN D AND CALCIUM HOMEOSTASIS

- Vitamin D is converted to calcidiol in the liver. Part of the calcidiol is converted by the kidneys to calcitriol, the biologically active form of vitamin D.
- It circulates as a hormone in the blood, regulating the concentration of calcium and phosphate in the bloodstream and promoting the healthy growth and remodeling of bone.

## RESPONSES TO BLOOD CALCIUM CHANGES

- The process of bone resorption by the osteoclasts releases stored calcium into systemic circulation and is an important process for regulating calcium balance.
- As bone formation actively fixes circulating calcium in its mineral form by removing it from the bloodstream, resorption actively unfixes it, thereby increasing circulating calcium levels.
- When blood calcium concentration rises, the parafollicular cells of the thyroid gland increase calcitonin secretion into the blood. At the same time, the parathyroid glands reduce parathyroid hormone secretion into the blood.
- The resulting high levels of calcitonin in the blood stimulate the bone to remove calcium from the blood plasma and deposit it as bone.
- Removal of calcium from the bone is also inhibited. When the blood calcium level is too low, calcitonin secretion is inhibited and PTH secretion is stimulated.
- This results in the removal of calcium from the bone to correct blood calcium levels.

# Section 7: Essential of Biochemistry

## I. CARBOHYDRATES

- **Starch** and **cellulose** are two common carbohydrates.
- Both are polymers (hence "**polysaccharides**"); that is, each is built from repeating units, monomers, much as a chain is built from its links. The monomers of both starch and cellulose are the same: units of the sugar **glucose**.

## 1. SUGARS

### A. MONOSACCHARIDES:
- ○ **Glucose**: "blood sugar", the immediate source of energy for cellular respiration.
- ○ **Galactose**: a sugar in milk (and yogurt)
- ○ **Fructose**: a sugar found in honey.

### B. DISACCHARIDES
- ○ **Sucrose**: common table sugar = **Glucose + Fructose**
- ○ **Lactose**: major sugar in milk = **Glucose + Galactose**
- ○ **Maltose**: product of starch digestion = **Glucose + Glucose**

### C. POLYSACCHARIDES
- • **Starches**
- ○ **Amylose**
- ○ **Amylopectin**
- Starches are insoluble in water and thus can serve as storage depots of glucose. Plants convert excess glucose into starch for storage.
- Rice, wheat, and corn (maize) are also major sources of starch in the human diet.
- Before starches can enter (or leave) cells, they must be digested. The hydrolysis of starch is done by **amylases**.

## 2. BIOSYNTHESIS OF GLYCOGEN AND GLUCOSE

- The goal of glycolysis, glycogenolysis, and the citric acid cycle is to conserve energy as ATP from the catabolism of carbohydrates.
- If the cells have sufficient supplies of ATP, then these pathways and cycles are inhibited.
- Under these conditions of excess ATP, the liver will attempt to convert a variety of excess molecules into glucose and/or glycogen.

### A. GLYCOGENESIS (INSULIN)
- Glycogenesis is the formation of **glycogen from glucose**.
- Glycogen is synthesized depending on the demand for glucose and ATP (energy). If both are present in relatively high amounts, then the excess of insulin promotes the glucose conversion into glycogen for storage **in liver and muscle cells.**
- In the synthesis of glycogen, one ATP is required per glucose incorporated into the polymeric branched structure of glycogen.
- **Glucose-6-phosphate** is synthesized directly from glucose or as the end product of gluconeogenesis.

### B. GLYCOGENOLYSIS (PEPTIDE, GLUCAGON & EPINEPHRINE)
- In glycogenolysis, glycogen stored in the liver and muscles, is converted first to **Glucose-1- Phosphate** and then into **Glucose-6-Phosphate**.
- Two hormones which control glycogenolysis are a **Peptide, Glucagon** from the pancreas and **Epinephrine** from the adrenal glands.
- Glucagon is released from the pancreas in response to low blood glucose and epinephrine is released in response to a threat or stress.
- Both hormones act upon enzymes to stimulate glycogen phosphorylase to begin glycogenolysis and inhibit glycogen synthetase (to stop glycogenesis).

### C. GLUCONEOGENESIS (GLUCAGON)
- The process of synthesizing glucose **from non-carbohydrate sources**. The starting point of gluconeogenesis is **Pyruvic Acid,** although oxaloacetic acid and dihydroxyacetone phosphate also provide entry points.
- **Lactic acid**, some amino acids from protein and glycerol from fat can be converted into glucose.
- *Gluconeogenesis is similar but not the exact reverse of glycolysis*, some of the steps are the identical in reverse direction and three of them are new ones.
- Gluconeogenesis occurs **mainly in the liver** with a small amount also occurring in **the cortex of the kidney.**
- **Very little** gluconeogenesis occurs in the **brain, skeletal muscles, heart muscles or other body tissue.**
- In fact, these organs have a high demand for glucose. Therefore, gluconeogenesis is constantly occurring in the liver to maintain the glucose level in the blood to meet these demands.

# Part Three:
## Pharmacology

Compiled and Edited by:
**Dr Moussa Issa**
MBChB MRCEM
Senior ED Registrar

# SECTION 1: BASIC PRINCIPLES OF PHARMACOLOGY

## I. PHARMACOKINETICS

What the body does to drug (**ADME**)
- Absorption
- Distribution
- Metabolism
- Excretion

## 1. BIOAVAILABILITY

- It is the amount of unchanged drug that reaches the systemic circulation, one of the principal pharmacokinetic properties of drugs.
- By definition, when a medication is administered intravenously, its **bioavailability** is "**1**" (100%).
- When the drug is administered orally the bioavailability depends on several factors.
- Physicochemical properties of the drug and its excipients that determine its dissolution in the intestinal lumen and its absorption across the intestinal wall.
  - Decomposition of the drug in the lumen.
  - pH and perfusion of the small intestine.
  - Surface and time available for absorption.
  - Competing reactions in the lumen (for example of the drug with food).
  - Hepatic first-pass effect

## 2. UNDERSTANDING FIRST PASS METABOLISM

- **First-pass effect** or also known as **first-pass metabolism** or **presystemic metabolism** is when an administered drug enters the liver and undergoes extensive biotransformation and thus decreasing the concentration rapidly before it reaches its target.
- It happens most commonly when the drug is administered orally.
- The drug then is absorbed in the GIT and enters the portal circulation before entering the systemic circulation.
- Via the portal circulation it enters the liver where some drugs undergo extensive biotransformation and the drug concentration is decreased. Lipid soluble drugs are better absorbed across the gut to enter the circulation. Clinically, first-pass metabolism is important when the fraction of the dose administered that escapes metabolism is small and variable.
- **The liver** is usually assumed to be the major site of first-pass metabolism of a drug administered orally, but other potential sites are: the gastrointestinal tract, blood, vascular endothelium, lungs, and the arm from which venous samples are taken.
- When several sites of first-pass metabolism are in series, the bioavailability is the product of the fractions of drug entering the tissue that escape loss at each site. The extent of first-pass metabolism in the liver and intestinal wall depends on a number of physiological factors. Many clinically important drugs undergo considerable first-pass metabolism after an oral dose.
- *Drugs in this category include: alprenolol, amitriptyline, dihydroergotamine, 5-fluorouracil, hydralazine, isoprenaline (isoproterenol), lignocaine (lidocaine), lorcainide, pethidine (meperidine), mercaptopurine, metoprolol, morphine, neostigmine, nifedipine, pentazocine and propranolol.*
- One major therapeutic implication of extensive first-pass metabolism is that much larger oral doses than intravenous doses are required to achieve equivalent plasma concentrations.
- For some drugs, extensive first-pass metabolism precludes their use as oral agents (e. g. Lignocaine, Naloxone and Glyceryl Trinitrate). Some drugs take benefit of the liver biotransformation. These drugs are administered as ***prodrugs*** and are converted from inactive to active form.
- E.g. Codeine is administered and demethylated (biotransformation in liver) into its active form Morphine proper.

## 3. VOLUME OF DISTRIBUTION

- The volume of distribution ($V_D$, also known as apparent volume of distribution) is the theoretical volume that would be necessary to contain the total amount of an administered drug at the same concentration that it is observed in the blood plasma.
- The volume of distribution is given by the following equation:

$$VD = \frac{\textbf{Amount Drug in the Body}}{\textbf{Concentration measured in plasma}}$$

  - **Low VD**:
    - Warfarin (binds to plasma),
    - Gentamycin (water soluble)

- o **Medium VD** : Diazepam
- o **High VD:**
    - Digoxin (bind to tissue)
    - Chloroquine (lipid soluble)
- **VD is related to:**
    - o Patient's weight and fat distribution
    - o Ratio of plasma to tissue binding
    - o Lipid or water solubility
    - o Can be used to calculate the Loading dose (LD)

    LD= [Drug] plasma x VD (*LD is given for drugs with long half-lives*)

# 4. METABOLISM

- is often divided into two phases:

➢ **PHASE I METABOLISM**

- 4 phases:
    - o **O**xidation (Cytochrome p450)
    - o **R**eduction
    - o **D**eamination
    - o **H**ydrolysis
- Makes the drug more water soluble or more reactive; Enzymes mostly produced and occurs in **the liver** (*not exclusively*)

➢ **PHASE II METABOLISM**

- Involves conjugation: addition of further molecules onto the drug to enhance metabolism:
    - o **A**cetylation
    - o **S**ulfation
    - o **G**lucuronidation
    - o **A**ddition of many other groups
- They make products less lipid-soluble, less likely to be reabsorbed in the urine.

## CYTOCHROME P450 (CYP)

- o *Part of phase I metabolism*
- o *CYP are responsible for 75% drug metabolism*
- o *Mostly found in the liver (not exclusively)*
- o *CYP3A4 metabolises most drugs*
- o *Drugs can be either inhibitors (AO DEVICES= slow metabolism of other drugs) or inducers (PC BRAS= increase metabolism of other drugs) of these enzymes.*
- o *AO DEVICES & PC BRAS: see Warfarin (**Section 2, Chap X, Part B**)*
- o *Pharmacogenetics: CYP2D6 polymorphic in 6% Caucasians.*

# 5. ELIMINATION

➢ **First order Kinetics**

- Elimination of the drug depends on plasma concentration; Fixed fraction of available drug is eliminated per unit time (Half-life)
- The Greater the concentration the greater the amount of drug eliminated.

➢ **Zero order kinetics**

- Enzymes are saturated
- Constant amount of drug is eliminated per unit time regardless of concentration.
- Drugs implicated are: **WATT Power**

| | | |
|---|---|---|
| o **W: Warfarin** | o **T: Tolbutamide** | o **T: Theophylline** |
| o **A: Alcohol & Aspirin** | o **P: Phenytoin** | |

# 6. HALF-LIFE

- It is the time required to reduce the plasma concentration to half its initial value in a study state.

$$t\tfrac{1}{2} = \frac{0.693 \; X \; VD}{clearance}$$

- o Increased VD >>> increases half-life
- o Reducing clearance >>>increases half-life

# II. PHARMACODYNAMIC

**What the drug does to the body**
- Drug-receptor interaction
- Dose-response
- Potency: amount of drug needed to produce a desired effect
- Therapeutic index

## 1. DOSE RESPONSE CURVE
- **$EC_{50}$** is the concentration at which 50% of the maximum effect occurs
- **$ED_{50}$** is the dose required for 50% of the population get the desired effect (Desired dose).
- **$TD_{50}$** is the dose required for 50% of the population get a Toxic effect (Toxic dose) **or $LD_{50}$** is the dose required for 50% of the population get a Lethal effect (Lethal dose).

## 2. THERAPEUTIC INDEX
- Also, referred to as therapeutic window or safety window (or sometimes as therapeutic ratio) is a comparison of the amount of a therapeutic agent that causes the therapeutic effect to the amount that causes toxicity.

$$TI = \frac{LD50}{ED50}$$

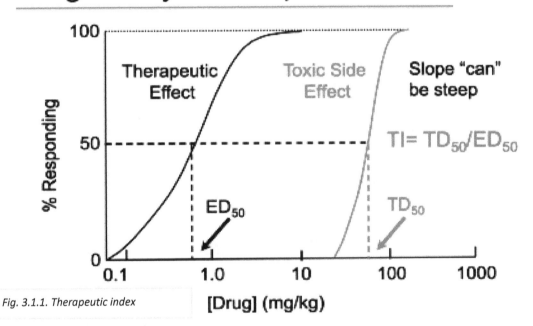

*Fig. 3.1.1. Therapeutic index*

### DRUGS WITH NARROW THERAPEUTIC RANGE

**RENALLY EXCRETED:**
- Digoxin
- Gentamycin
- Vancomycin
- Lithium
- (Metformin): in theory

**HEPATICALLY METABOLISED:**
- Phenytoin
- Ciclosporin

# Section 2: Gastrointestinal Pharmacology

## I. BULKING AGENTS, STOOL SOFTENERS, AND LAXATIVES

### 1. BULKING AGENTS
- o **Mechanism:** ease constipation by increasing the volume of stool and making it easier to pass.
- o **Example:** Bran or Psyllium

### 2. STOOL SOFTENERS
- o **Mechanism:** soften the stool, making it easier to pass. Stool softeners can be most effective by drinking plenty of water throughout the day.
- o **Example:** Colace and Docusate Calcium

### 3. OSMOTIC LAXATIVES
- o **Mechanism:**
  - ▪ Hold fluids in the intestine.
  - ▪ They also draw fluids into the intestine from other tissue and blood vessels.
  - ▪ This extra fluid in the intestines makes the stool softer and easier to pass.
- o **Example:**
  - ▪ Fleet Phospho-Soda,
  - ▪ Milk of Magnesia or Miralax
  - ▪ Nonabsorbable sugars (lactulose or sorbitol).

### 4. STIMULANT LAXATIVES
- o **Mechanism:**
  - ▪ Make stool move faster through the intestines by irritating the lining of the intestines.
  - ▪ Regular use of stimulant laxatives is not recommended.
  - ▪ Stimulant laxatives change the tone and feeling in the large intestine with risk of dependency on using laxatives all the time to have a bowel movement.
- o **Example:** Correctol, Ex-Lax, and Senokot.

## II. ANTIEMETIC AGENTS

### A. PHARMACOLOGY OF ANTIEMETIC DRUGS

| NEUROTRANSMITTERS | RECEPTORS OF EMESIS | DRUGS |
|---|---|---|
| Histamine | $H_1$ | • **Cyclizine**<br>• **Promethazine** |
| Acetylcholine | Muscarinic | • **Hyoscine** |
| Dopamine | $D_2$ | • **Prochlorperazine**<br>• **Metoclopramide**<br>• **Domperidone** |
| Serotonin | $5HT_3$ and $5HT_4$ | • **Granisetron**<br>• **Ondansetron** |
| Substance P | Neurokinin 1 ($NK_1$) | • **Aprepitant** |

### 1. ANTIHISTAMINES
- • **Mechanism of action:**
  - o **Cyclizine:** A piperazine derived drug that primarily acts antagonistically on $H_1$ receptors but also has notable antimuscarinic activity as well.
  - o **Promethazine:** Derived from the phenothiazine family. Similarly, with cyclizine, it has notable antimuscarinic activity as well as antagonism of several serotonergic receptors as well (5HT2A; 5HT-2C).
- • **Metabolism:**

- o **Routes:** orally and can also be given by IM or IV administration. Promethazine is vulnerable to a considerable first-pass effect.
- o **Half-life:** Promethazine: **10 hours**, Cyclizine: **20 hours**.
- o **Elimination:** Hepatic.
- **Indications:**
  - o Cyclizine is widely employed in drug-induced vomiting.
  - o Promethazine is free of teratogenic potential and hence can be given to treat vomiting in pregnancy.
- **Side effects:**
  - o The most common side-effect by far is the experience of drowsiness.
  - o Anticholinergic symptoms such as xerostomia (dry mouth), urinary retention and blurred vision are *quite common*.

## 2. ANTIMUSCARINIC DRUGS
- **Mechanism of action:**
  - o **Hyoscine:** It acts as a competitive inhibitor at $M_1$ receptors.
- **Metabolism:**
  - o **Routes:** Parenteral, Transdermal and Oral routes, where the latter has reasonably good absorption
  - o **Half-life:** approximately **8 hours**.
  - o **Elimination:** Hepatic.
- **Indications:**
  - o Treatment of motion sickness and postoperative vomiting.
- **Side effects:**
  - o As an antimuscarinic drug, it carries with it the typical side-effects of dry mouth, urinary retention and blurred vision.

## 3. DOPAMINE RECEPTOR ANTAGONISTS
- **Mechanism of action:**
  - o These drugs act as antagonists at $D_2$ receptors.
  - o Thus, they're involved in the inhibition of dopaminergic stimulation on the CTZ (chemoreceptor trigger zone).
  - o **Metoclopramide** acts as a dopamine receptor antagonist at regular doses but higher doses also have the effect of acting as a $5HT_3$ receptor antagonist. This double efficacy can come into play when trying to treat cytotoxic-induced vomiting such as that which occurs with anticancer agents.
  - o In addition to this, Metoclopramide also has significant *prokinetic effects* which increase the rate of gastric emptying while also increasing the tone of the gastroesophageal sphincter.
- **Metabolism:**
  - o *Metoclopramide and Domperidone undergo extensive first-pass metabolism* and thereby have very limited oral bioavailability.
  - o **Routes:** Metoclopramide can be given IV or IM while Domperidone can be administered rectally through the use of suppositories.
  - o **Half-life:** Metoclopramide: **4 hours**, Domperidone: **14 hours**.
  - o **Elimination:** Hepatic.
- **Indications:**
  - o *Dopamine receptor antagonists are chiefly used in vomiting that occurs due to drugs or operations*.
  - o **Domperidone** lack any antimuscarinic effect and thereby become ineffective when trying to treat motion sickness.
  - o **Prochlorperazine** can be used to treat various vestibular disorders and motion sickness primarily due to this additional antimuscarinic effect. It is also classified as an antipsychotic drug but the dose at which it's administered for its antiemetic effect is approximately a third of that than its dose for psychosis.
- **Side effects:**
  - o CNS effects are typical with Metoclopramide and Prochlorperazine due to the ability to cross the blood brain barrier to some extent - this crossing is much less appreciable with Domperidone.
  - o ***Due to the inhibition of dopamine receptors, dystonias, extrapyramidal effects and parkinsonian-like symptoms are potential.*** (MRCEM Part A Dec 2015)

## 4. 5HT₃ RECEPTOR ANTAGONISTS
- **Mechanism of action:**
  - o These drugs act as antagonists at $5HT_3$ receptors located at the level of the gut but also at the level of the CTZ.
- **Metabolism:**
  - o **Routes:** oral, IV and IM, or even via the rectal route.
  - o **Half-life: 3 hours**
  - o **Elimination:** It goes through a very partial first-pass effect and is also primarily eliminated by metabolism in the liver.
- **Indications:**
  - o Used in cancer treatment
  - o Have also proven useful in postoperative nausea and vomiting.
- **Side effects:**
  - o Commonly cause headache as well as constipation.

## 5. NEUROKININ RECEPTOR ANTAGONISTS

- **Mechanism of action:**
  - The mechanism of action of aprepitant involves blocking $NK_1$ receptors at the level of the CNS.
  - Aprepitant also enhances the effects of $5HT_3$ receptor antagonists as well as corticosteroid drugs in the prevention of acute or delayed emesis due to chemotherapeutic drugs.
- **Metabolism:**
  - Aprepitant is an inhibitor of the isoenzyme CYP 3A4 and an inducer of CYP 2C9. Due to these effects, it would decrease the effect of Warfarin should the two be taken together.
  - Aprepitant has very good absorption from the gut
  - **Routes:** Oral, IV and IM, or even via the Rectal route.
  - **Half-life: 10 hours**
  - **Elimination:** Extensively metabolised via CYP 3A4 in the liver
- **Side effects:**
  - CNS: Dizziness, headache and tiredness.
  - GI: abdominal pain and diarrhoea.

# III. PROTON-PUMP INHIBITORS

## 1. Mechanism of action

- Proton pump inhibitors act by irreversible inhibition of the H+/K+ ATPase, in the parietal cells of the stomach.
- It markedly inhibits gastric acid secretion and has a long duration of action.
- They are used for treatment of gastric and duodenal ulcers, gastroesophageal reflux disease and other excessive gastrointestinal acid secretory disorders.

## 2. Cautions

- PPI drugs may cause low serum magnesium levels (hypomagnesemia) if taken for prolonged periods of time (in most cases, longer than one year).
- Low serum magnesium levels can result in serious adverse events including muscle spasm (tetany), irregular heartbeat (arrhythmias), and convulsions (seizures); however, patients do not always have these symptoms.
- Treatment of hypomagnesemia generally requires magnesium supplements.
- In approximately one-quarter of the cases reviewed, magnesium supplementation alone did not improve low serum magnesium levels and the PPI had to be discontinued.

## 3. Side-effects

- Usually rare
- The most common side effects of proton pump inhibitors are:
  - Headache,
  - Diarrhoea,
  - Constipation,
  - Abdominal pain,
  - Flatulence
  - Nausea
  - Rash.
- Per a meta-analysis, the overall risk of pneumonia is about 25% higher among PPI users.

| True or False: | |
|---|---|
| Most drugs initially given with a loading dose have a short half-life | F |
| Cytochrome P450 is part of phase II metabolism | F |
| Half-life can only be calculated for first-order elimination drugs | T |
| Pharmacokinetics is the study of the drug effect upon the body | F |
| **True or False:** | |
| First pass metabolism reduces plasma half-life | F |
| Warfarin has a low therapeutic index | F |
| Loading dose must be proportionally reduced in renal failure | F |
| Volume of distribution is an important variable in calculating loading dose | T |
| **True or False:** | |
| Half life of a drug is a pharmacokinetic concept | T |
| Lithium has a narrow therapeutic range | T |
| Paracetamol has a narrow therapeutic index | F |

# Section 3: Cardiac & ACLS Core Drugs

## I. DIGOXIN

### 1. MECHANISM OF ACTION

- **Inhibits Na/K-ATPase pump** in myocardial cells, which subsequently promotes calcium influx via Na/Ca-exchange pump >>> increased contractile force (Positive Inotropy)
- **Parasympathetic activation:** increases vagal activity >>> suppresses AV node conduction >>> decreased ventricular rate.
- **Decreases Renin release**

### 2. INDICATIONS

- CCF: by increasing contractility
- AF: by decreasing AV node conduction

### 3. PRECAUTIONS

- Toxic effects are common and are frequently associated with serious arrhythmias.
- Avoid electrical cardioversion if patient is receiving digoxin unless condition is life-threatening, use lower dose (10 to 20 J).

### 4. SIDE EFFECTS

- Cholinergic effects; Nausea, Vomiting, Diarrhoea, blurry yellow-green visions/halos
- Atrial tachycardia and AV block
- Hyperkalaemia
- Toxic doses >>> arrhythmias

- **Digoxin is contraindicated in the following conditions: Sick Wolf Vows At Making Rats Cry**
  - Sick sinus syndrome
  - WPW syndrome
  - VF (Ventricular fibrillation)
  - AV block
  - MI (Myocardial infarction)
  - Restrictive cardiomyopathy
  - Cor pulmonale
- **Amiodarone interaction:** reduce digoxin dose by 50% when initiating amiodarone

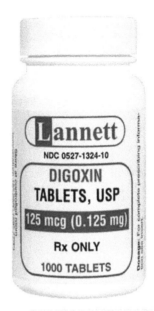
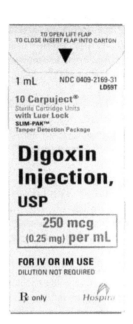

Fig. 3.3.1. Digoxin

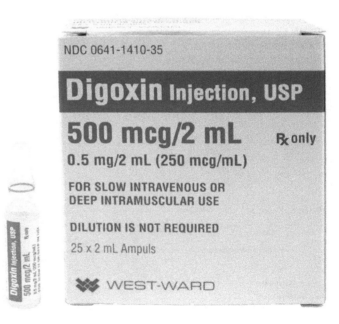

Fig. 3.3.2. Digoxin injection

# II. DIURETICS

## A. MECHANISM OF ACTION OF DIURETICS

- **Aquaretics:**
  - Increases blood flow in kidneys
- **Arginine vasopressin receptor 2 antagonists:**
  - Inhibits vasopressin's action
  - Example: Amphotericin B, Lithium citrate
- **Carbonic anhydrase inhibitors:**
  - Inhibits $H^+$ secretion, resultant promotion of $Na^+$ and $K^+$ excretion
  - Examples: Acetazolamide, Dorzolamide
- **Loop diuretics:**
  - Inhibits the Na-K-2Cl symporter
  - Example: Bumetanide, Ethacrynic acid, Furosemide, Torsemide
- **Na-H exchanger antagonists:**
  - Promotes $Na^+$ excretion. (e.g. Dopamine)
- **Osmotic diuretics:**
  - Promotes osmotic diuresis
  - Example: Glucose (especially in uncontrolled diabetes), Mannitol
- **Potassium-sparing diuretics:**
  - Inhibition of Na+/K+ exchanger:
  - Spironolactone inhibits aldosterone action,
  - Amiloride inhibits epithelial sodium channels

  Examples: Amiloride, Spironolactone, Eplerenone, Triamterene, Potassium Canrenoate
- **Thiazides:**
  - Inhibits reabsorption by $Na^+/Cl^-$ symporter

  Example: Bendroflumethiazide, Hydrochlorothiazide
- **Xanthines:**
  - Inhibits reabsorption of $Na^+$,
  - increase glomerular filtration rate
  - Examples: Caffeine, Theophylline, Theobromine

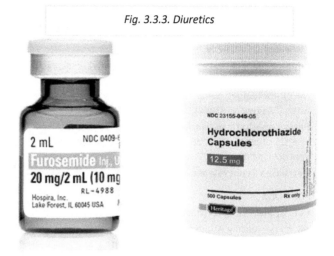

*Fig. 3.3.3. Diuretics*

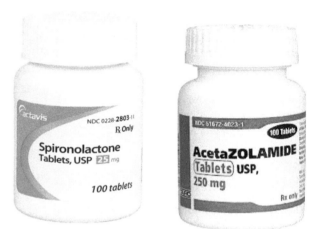

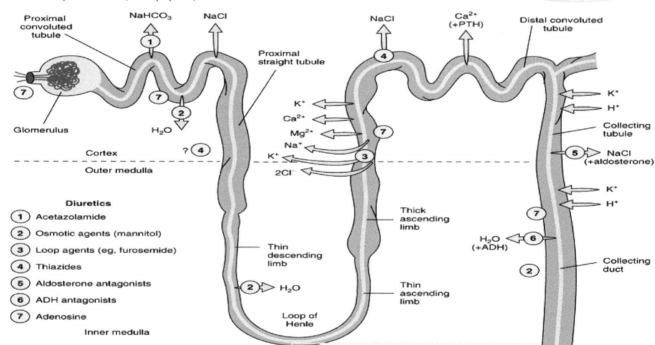

*Fig. 3.3.4. Mechanism of action of Diuretics*

## B. SIDE EFFECTS & CONTRAINDICATIONS

- The most important and frequent problem with thiazide and loop diuretics is hypokalemia.
- A potentially serious side effect of potassium-sparing diuretics is hyperkalemia.

- **Other side effects are list below:**

| CLASS | ADVERSE SIDE EFFECTS |
|---|---|
| **Thiazide** | Hypokalemia<br>Metabolic alkalosis<br>Dehydration (hypovolemia), leading to hypotension<br>Hyponatremia<br>Hyperglycemia in diabetics<br>Hypercholesterolemia; hypertriglyceridemia<br>Increased low-density lipoproteins<br>Hyperuricemia (at low doses)<br>Azotemia (in renal disease patients) |
| **Loop** | Hypokalemia<br>Metabolic alkalosis<br>Hypomagnesemia<br>Hyperuricemia<br>Dehydration (hypovolemia), leading to hypotension<br>Dose-related hearing loss (ototoxicity) |
| **K+-sparing** | Hyperkalemia<br>Metabolic acidosis<br>Gynecomastia (aldosterone antagonists)<br>Gastric problems including peptic ulcer |
| ***Carbonic anhydrase inhibitors*** | Hypokalemia and Metabolic acidosis |

## A. FUROSEMIDE

### 1. INDICATIONS
- For adjuvant therapy of acute pulmonary edema in patients with SBP>90 to 100mmHg (without signs and symptoms of shock).
- Hypertensive emergencies
- Increased ICP.

### 2. PRECAUTIONS
- Dehydration, hypovolemia, hypotension, hypokalaemia, or other electrolyte imbalance may occur.

### 3. DOSAGE
- 0.5 to 1mg/Kg over 1 to 2 minutes.
- If no response, double dose to 2mg/Kg, slowly over 1 to 2 minutes.
- For new onset, pulmonary edema with hypovolemia: < 0.5 mg/Kg.

## B. BENDROFLUMETHIAZIDE (BTZ)

- It is known to decreases pancreatic release of Insulin and peripheral utilization of glucose and care is required when BTZ is given to patients with both diabetes and impaired glucose tolerance. Hyponatraemia and hypokalaemia are common side effects of both the loop and thiazide diuretics. **Other toxicities of BTZ are:**
  - o Hyperuricaemia (beware in patients with gout)
  - o Pancreatitis
  - o Intrahepatic cholestasis
  - o Hyperlipidaemia
  - o Weakness and fatigability

## C. MANNITOL

- ➢ **INDICATIONS**
  - Increased ICP in management of neurologic Emergencies.
- ➢ **PRECAUTIONS**
  - Monitor fluid status and serum osmolarity (not to exceed 310 mOsm/kg)
  - Caution in renal failure because fluid overload may result.
- ➢ **DOSAGE**
  - **IV administration:**
    - o 0.5 to 1 g/kg over 5 to 10 minutes through in-line filter.
    - o Additional doses of 0.25 to 2g /kg can be given every 4 to 6 hours as needed.
    - o Use with support of oxygenation and ventilation.

# III. ANTI-ARRHYTHMICS

## VAUGHAN-WILLIAMS-SINGH CLASSIFICATION OF ANTIARRHYTHMIC DRUGS

| Class | | Basic Mechanism | Drugs | Comments |
|---|---|---|---|---|
| I | | Sodium-channel blockade | | Reduce phase 0 slope and peak of action potential. |
| | IA | - Moderate | Quinidine<br>Procainamide<br>Disopyramide | Moderate reduction in phase 0 slope;<br>Increase APD; increase ERP. |
| | IB | - Weak | Lidocaine<br>Phenytoin | Small reduction in phase 0 slope;<br>Reduce APD; decrease ERP. |
| | IC | - Strong | Flecainide<br>Propafenone | Pronounced reduction in phase 0<br>No effect on APD or ERP. |
| II | | Beta-blockade | Propranolol<br>Esmolol<br>Timolol<br>Metoprolol<br>Atenolol | Block sympathetic activity;<br>Reduce rate and conduction.<br>Decreases slope of phase 4 |
| III | | Potassium-channel blockade | Amiodarone<br>Sotalol<br>Ibutilide<br>Dofetilide | Delay repolarization (phase 3) and thereby increase APD and ERP.<br>Amiodarone also acts on phases 1, 2&4<br>Sotalol also decreases slope of phase 4 |
| IV | | Calcium-channel blockade | Verapamil<br>Diltiazem | Block L-type calcium-channels; most effective at SA and AV nodes; Reduce rate and conduction.<br>Prolongs phase 2 |
| V | | Variable mechanism | Adenosine<br>Digoxin<br>Magnesium sulfate | |

APD: action potential duration; ERP: effective refractory period;                    SA: sinoatrial node; AV: atrioventricular node.

## A. ADENOSINE

### 1. MECHANISM OF ACTION

- Adenosine is a **purine nucleoside** composed of a molecule of adenine attached to a ribose sugar molecule (ribofuranose) moiety via a β-N$_9$-glycosidic bond.
- **PSVT:** Slows conduction through AV node and interrupts AV reentry pathways, which restore normal sinus symptoms.
- **Stress testing:** A2A adenosine receptor agonist; activation of the A2A adenosine receptor produces coronary vasodilation and increases coronary blood flow.
- Adenosine should be administered by RAPID intravenous bolus so that a significant bolus of adenosine reaches the heart before it is metabolized.
- A change from the 2010 guidelines now has adenosine given up to two times rather than three.

### 2. PHARMACOKINETICS

- Half-Life: <10 sec
- Duration: <10 sec
- Onset: 20-30 sec

### 3. INDICATIONS

- PSVT
- Stress testing (Diagnostic)
- Sustained ventricular tachycardia (SVT)
- DOES NOT CONVERT ATRIAL FIBRILLATION, ATRIAL FLUTTER OR VT.

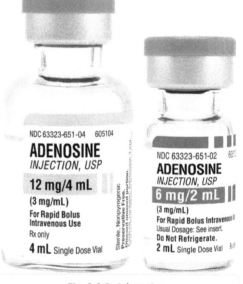

Fig. 3.3.5. Adenosine

### 4. DOSING

- The first dose of adenosine should be 6 mg administered rapidly over 1-3 seconds followed by a 20 ml NS bolus.
- If the patient's rhythm does not convert out of SVT within 1 to 2 minutes, a second 12 mg dose may be given in similar fashion.
- All efforts should be made to administer adenosine as quickly as possible.

### 5. INTERACTIONS

- *Prolonged asystole has been seen with the use of normal doses of adenosine in heart transplant patients and central line use.*
- *Therefore, the lower dose (3mg) may be considered for patients with a central venous line or a history of heart transplant.*

- *A lower initial dose of 3mg should be used for patients taking dipyridamole or carbamazepine as these two medications potentiate the effects of adenosine.*
- *Theophylline decreases effects of adenosine by pharmacodynamic antagonism. Larger doses may be required in patients taking Theophylline or caffeine.*

### 4. PRECAUTIONS/CONTRAINDICATIONS

- Some side effects of adenosine administration include flushing, chest pain/tightness, brief asystole or bradycardia.
- Make sure that adenosine is not used for irregular, polymorphic wide-complex tachycardia and unstable VT.
- Use in these cases may cause clinical deterioration.
- Transient periods of sinus bradycardia and ventricular ectopy are common after termination of SVT.
- Safe and effective in pregnancy.

## B. AMIODARONE

### 1. MECHANISM OF ACTION

- Amiodarone is considered a class III antiarrhythmic agent and is used for various type tachyarrhythmias.
- Because of its associated toxicity and serious side-effects, it should be used cautiously and care should be taken to ensure that cumulative doses are not exceeded.
- The mechanism of action of amiodarone remains unknown, but within the framework of ACLS, amiodarone is used primarily to treat VF & VT (ventricular fibrillation and ventricular tachycardia) that occurs during cardiac arrest and is unresponsive to shock delivery, CPR, and vasopressors.

### 2. INDICATIONS FOR ACLS

- **Pulseless Ventricular Fibrillation/Ventricular Tachycardia (VT/VF)**
- Amiodarone should not be used in individuals with polymorphic VT as it associated with a prolonged QT interval which is made worse with antiarrhythmic drugs.
  - *Amiodarone should only be used after defibrillation/cardioversion and first line drugs such as epinephrine and vasopressin have failed to convert VT/VF.*

### 3. ROUTE

- Amiodarone can be administered by intravenous or intraosseous route.

### 4. DOSING

- The maximum cumulative dose in a 24-hour period should not exceed 2.2 grams.
- Within the **VT/VF pulseless arrest algorithm**, the dosing is as follows: 300mg IV/IO push → (if no conversion) 150 mg IV/IO push → **(after conversion)** Infusion#1: 360 mg IV over 6 hours (1mg/min) → Infusion#2: 540 mg IV over 18 hours (0.5mg/min)

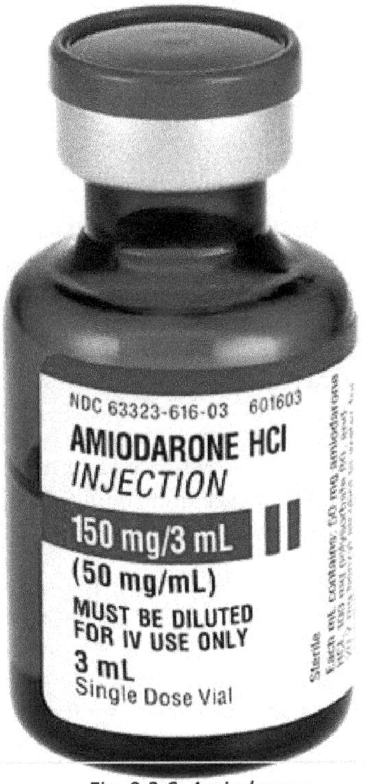

*Fig. 3.3.6. Amiodarone*

- For tachyarrhythmias other than life threatening, expert consultation should be considered before use.
- For **Tachycardia, other than pulseless VT/VF**, Amiodarone dosing is as follows: 150 mg over 10 minutes → repeat as needed if VT recurs → maintenance infusion of 1mg/min for 6 hours

- *Amiodarone should only be diluted with D5W and given with an in-line filter.*
- *Amiodarone and Erythromycin both increase QTc interval*
- *Infusions exceeding 2 hours must be administered in glass or polyolefin bottles containing D5W.*

## C. FLECAINIDE

### 1. MECHANISM OF ACTION

- ➤ *Class IC antidysrhythmic;*
- ➤ *slows conduction in cardiac tissue by altering transport of ion across membranes;*
- ➤ *causes slight prolongation of refractory periods,*
- ➤ *Decreases rate of rise of action potential without affecting its duration;*
- ➤ *Local anesthetic and moderate negative inotropic effects.*

### 2. COMMON ADVERSE EFFECTS

- Visual disturbances (5-16%)
- Dizziness (10-19%)

### 3. WARNING

- Reserve class IC antiarrhythmics use for life-threatening ventricular arrhythmias only.

- Ventricular proarrhythmic effects with AF/flutter
- Not recommended for chronic atrial fibrillation
- 10.5% incidence of ventricular tachycardia/fibrillation in patients treated for chronic atrial fibrillation
- Proarrhythmic effects with flecainide for atrial fibrillation/flutter: Increased risk of PVCs, ventricular tachycardia, ventricular fibrillation, and fatality
- *Flecainide use should be restricted to patients with life-threatening ventricular arrhythmias.*
- *As with other class I agents, use of flecainide for atrial flutter has been reported with 1:1 atrioventricular conduction due to atrial rate slowing.*

### 4. CONTRAINDICATIONS
- Hypersensitivity.
- 2nd or 3rd degree AV block
- RBBB when associated with left hemiblock (bifascicular block),
- Unless pacemaker is present to sustain cardiac rhythm; discontinue therapy immediately

### 5. CAUTIONS
- Atrial fibrillation, CHF, hypotension, HTN, post MI patients, geriatrics, proarrhythmia events, hepatic/renal impairment, and sick sinus syndrome.
- May slow cardiac conduction to produce dose-related increases in PR, QRS, and QT intervals; manage patient on lowest effective dose.
- Discontinuation should be done in hospital.
- Causes increased mortality in post-AMI period, also with chronic atrial fibrillation
- May affect endocardial pacemaker reversibly by increasing endocardial pacing thresholds or suppressing ventricular escape rhythms; do not administer to patients with existing poor thresholds or nonprogrammable pacemakers unless suitable pacing rescue is available
- Correct preexisting hypokalemia or hyperkalemia before initiating therapy

## D. LIDOCAINE
- Although lidocaine was removed from the 2010 Simplified Pulseless Arrest Diagram, it is still considered a suitable alternative if amiodarone is ineffective in cardiac arrest from VT/VF.
- Lidocaine was removed in the AHA Simplified Pulseless Arrest Diagram to help reduce emphasis on the use of medications and place more emphasis on **high quality CPR and early defibrillation.**

### 1. INDICATIONS FOR ACLS
- In ACLS, Lidocaine is used intravenously for the treatment of ventricular arrhythmias. (VT/VF)
- It is also useful for the treatment of **stable** monomorphic VT with preserved ventricular function and for **stable** polymorphic VT with preserved left ventricular function, normal QT interval, and correction of any electrolyte imbalances.
- The overall benefits of lidocaine for the treatment arrhythmias in cardiac arrest has come under scrutiny.
- It has been shown to have no short term or long term efficacy in cardiac arrest.
- Routine prophylactic use is contraindicated for acute myocardial infarction.

### 2. SIDE EFFECTS
- Lidocaine should be used with caution due to negative cardiovascular effects which include hypotension, bradycardia, arrhythmias, and/or cardiac arrest.
- Some of these side effects may be due to hypoxemia secondary to respiratory depression.

## E. PROCAINAMIDE
### 1. INDICATIONS
- Useful for treatment of a wide variety of arrhythmias, including stable monomorphic VT with normal QT interval and preserved LV function. May use for treatment of PSVT uncontrolled by adenosine and vagal manoeuvres if BP stable.
- Stable wide-complex tachycardia of unknown origin.
- A. fib with rapid rate in WPW syndrome.

### 2. PRECAUTIONS
- If cardiac or renal dysfunction is present, reduce maximum total dose to 12mg/kg and maintenance infusion to 1 to 2 mg/min.
- Proarrhythmic, especially in setting of AMI, hypokalaemia, or hypomagnesemia.
- May induce hypotension in patients with impaired LV function.
- Use with caution with other drugs that prolong QT interval.

### 3. DOSAGE
- **Recurrent VF/VT:**
  - 20mg/min IV infusion (maximum total dose 17mg/kg)
  - In urgent situations, up to 50mg/min may be administered to total dose of 17mg/kg.

- **Other indications:**
  - 20mg/min IV infusion until one of the following occurs:
    - Arrhythmia suppression
    - Hypotension
    - QRS widens by >50%
    - Total dose of 17mg/kg is given
  - Use in cardiac arrest limited by need for slow infusion & uncertain efficacy.
- **Maintenance infusion:**
  - 1 to 4mg/min (dilute in D5W or NS).
  - Reduce dose in presence of renal insufficiency.

## F. SODIUM BICARBONATE

### 1. INDICATIONS

- Known pre-existing hyperkalaemia.
- Known pre-existing bicarbonate-responsive acidosis; eg, DKA, TCA or aspirin overdose, cocaine, or diphenhydramine.
- Prolonged resuscitation with effective ventilation; upon return of spontaneous circulation after long arrest interval. Not useful or effective in hypercarbic acidosis (eg, cardiac arrest and CPR without intubation).

### 2. PRECAUTIONS

- Adequate ventilation and CPR, not bicarbonate, are the major "buffer agents" in cardiac arrest.
- Not recommended for routine use in cardiac arrest patients.

### 3. DOSAGE

**IV administration:**

- 1 mEq/kg IV bolus
- If rapidly available, use arterial blood gas analysis to guide bicarbonate therapy (calculated base deficits or bicarbonate concentration).
- ABG results not reliable indicators of acidosis during cardiac arrest.

**Exam Questions**

50 mL Single-dose

**8.4% Sodium Bicarbonate Inj., USP**  ℞ only

50 mEq (1 mEq/mL)
4.2 grams (84 mg/mL)

HOSPIRA, INC., LAKE FOREST, IL 60045 USA

NDC 0409-6625-02

Each mL contains sodium bicarbonate, 84 mg. 2 mOsmol/mL (calc.). pH 7.8 (7.0 to 8.5). Single-dose container. Contains no bacteriostat. Discard unused portion. Do not resterilize. For intravenous use. Usual dose: See insert. Sterile, nonpyrogenic. Use only if clear and seal is intact and undamaged. Do not use the injection if it contains precipitate.

RL-0059 (4/04)

Hospira

## G. MAGNESIUM SULFATE

### 1. INDICATIONS

- Recommended for use in cardiac arrest only if torsades de pointes or suspected hypomagnesemia is present.
- Life-threatening ventricular arrhythmias due to digitalis toxicity.
- Routine administration in hospitalized patients with AMI is not recommended.

### 2. PRECAUTIONS

- Occasional fall in blood pressure with rapid administration.
- Use with caution if renal failure is present.

### 3. DOSAGE

- **Cardiac arrest:** due to hypomagnesemia or torsades de pointes
  - 1- 2g (2-4ml of 50% slt) diluted in 10ml of D5W IV/IO over 5-20min

- **Torsades de Pointes with a pulse or AMI with Hypomagnesemia.**
  - Loading dose of 1 to 2 g mixed in 50 to 100 ml of D5W, over 5 to 60 min IV.
  - Follow with 0.5 to 1 g/hr IV (titrate to control torsades).

# IV. BETA-ADRENOCEPTOR BLOCKERS

## 1. INDICATIONS
- Administer to all patients with suspected Myocardial infarction and unstable angina in the absence of contraindication.
- These are effective antianginal agents and can reduce incidence of VF.
- Useful in adjunctive agent with fibrinolytic therapy.
- May reduce nonfatal reinfarction and recurrent ischemia.
- To convert to normal sinus rhythm or to slow ventricular response (or both) in SVT (PSVT, Afib or Atrial flutter).
- Beta-blockers are second line   agents (with Ca Channel Blockers) after adenosine.
- To reduce MI and damage in AMI patients with elevated heart rate, blood pressure or both.
- For emergency, antihypertensive therapy for hemorrhagic and acute ischemic stroke.

## 2. PRECAUTIONS/ CONTRAINDICATIONS
- *Concurrent IV administration   with IV Ca Channel Blocking agents like Verapamil or Diltiazem can cause severe hypotension.*
- *Avoid in bronchospastic diseases, cardiac failure, or severe abnormalities in cardiac conduction.*
- *Monitor cardiac and pulmonary status during administration.*
- *May cause myocardial depression. Contraindicated in presence of severe bradycardia, SBP <100mmHg, severe LV failure, hypoperfusion, or second-or third- degree AV Block. Propanolol is contraindicated in cocaine-induced ACS.*

## A. PROPANOLOL
- *Is a competitive, nonselective beta-adrenergic receptor antagonist.*
- *Propanolol inhibits sympathetic stimulation; this results in a reduction in resting heart rate, cardiac output, systolic and diastolic blood pressure, and reflex orthostatic hypotension.*
- Half life: **4 hours**
- Total dose: 0.1mg/Kg by slow IV push divided into 3 equal doses at 2-to 3-minute interval.
- Do not exceed 1mg/min
- Repeat in 2 min after total dose is given if necessary.

## B. ESMOLOL
- *Class II antiarrhythmic; selective beta1-blocker with little or no effect on beta-2 receptors except at high doses.*
- *Short acting and rapid onset.*
- *It does not have intrinsic sympathomimetic activity*
- *Esmolol has a short half-life: 2 to 9 minutes*

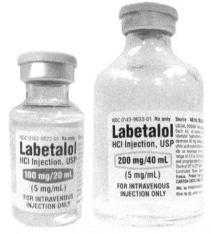

Fig. 3.3.7. Labetalol

**DOSAGE:**
- 0.5mg/Kg over 1 min, followed by 4-minute infusion at 50µg/Kg (0.05mg/Kg) per minute, maximum 0.3mg/Kg/min for a total of 200µg/Kg.
- If initial response inadequate, second 0.5mg/Kg bolus over one minute, then increase infusion to 100 µg/Kg/minute; max infusion rate 300 µg/Kg (0.3mg/Kg) per minute.

## C. LABETALOL
### 1. MECHANISM OF ACTION
- *Nonselective beta blocker with intrinsic sympathomimetic activity; also, alpha blocker. Has an arterial vasodilating action.*

### 2. DOSING FORMS
- 10mg labetalol IV push over 1 to 2 minutes
- May repeat or double Labetolol every 10minutes to a maximum dose of 150mg, or give initial as bolus, then start Labetolol infusion at 2 to 8mg/min.

## D. METOPROLOL
### 1. MECHANISM OF ACTION
- *Blocks response to beta-adrenergic stimulation;*
- *Cardioselective for beta1 receptors at low doses, with little or no effect on beta2 receptors.*

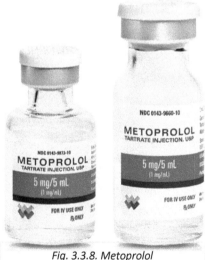

Fig. 3.3.8. Metoprolol

### 2. DOSAGE
- Initial IV dose: 5mg slow IV at 5-minute intervals to a total of 15mg.
- Oral regimen to follow IV dose: 50mg BD for 24hrs, then increase to 100mg BD.

## E. SOTALOL

### 1. MECHANISM OF ACTION
- *Antiarrhythmic: Class II (beta blockade) and class III (action potential prolongation) properties.*
- *Has adrenoceptor-blocking effect and markedly prolongs action potential and repolarization.*

### 2. INDICATIONS
- Ventricular & Supraventricular Arrhythmias in patients without structural heart disease.
- Refractory Life-Threatening Ventricular Arrhythmias

### 3. PRECAUTIONS
- Avoid in patients with poor perfusion because of significant negative inotropic effects.
- Must be infused slowly.
- Adverse effects include bradycardia, hypotension, and arrhythmias (torsades de pointes)
- Use with caution with other drugs that prolong QT interval (procainamide, amiodarone).

### 4. DOSAGE
- 1 to 1.5mg/Kg body weight, then infused at a rate of 10mg/min.
- Must be infused slowly.
- Reduce dose with renal impairement.

## F. CALCIUM CHLORIDE

➤ **INDICATIONS**
- Known or suspected hyperkalaemia (eg, renal failure).
- Ionized hypocalcaemia (eg, after multiple blood transfusions).
- As an antidote for toxic effects (hypotension and arrhythmias) from ca Channel Blocker overdose or beta-Blocker overdose.

➤ **PRECAUTIONS**
- Do not use routinely in cardiac arrest.
- Do not mix with Sodium Bicarbonate

➤ **DOSAGE**
- 500mg to 1000mg (5 to 10 ml of a 10% solution) IV for hyperkalaemia and Ca Channel Blocker overdose.
- May be repeated as needed.

# V. VASODILATORS (ANTI-ANGINAL AGENTS)

## 1. GLYCERYL TRINITRATE / NITROGLYCERIN

### 1. MECHANISM OF ACTION
- Organic nitrate which causes systemic venodilation, decreasing preload.
- Cellular mechanism: nitrate enters vascular smooth muscle and converted to nitric oxide (NO) leading to activation of cGMP & vasodilation.
- Relaxes smooth muscle via dose-dependent dilation of arterial and venous beds to reduce both preload and afterload, and myocardial O2 demand.
- Also improves coronary collateral circulation.
- Lower BP; increase HR, occasional paradoxical bradycardia.

### 2. INDICATIONS
- Initial antianginal for suspected ischemic pain.
- For initial 24 to 48 hrs in patients with AMI and CHF, large anterior wall infarction, persistent or recurrent ischemia, or hypertension.
- Continued use (beyond 48hrs) for patients with recurrent angina or persistent pulmonary congestion.
- Hypertensive urgency with ACS.

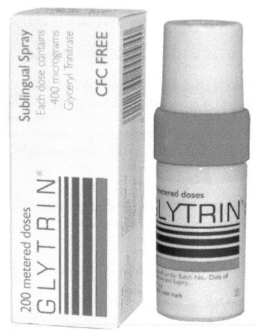

*Fig. 3.3.9. GTN spray*

### 3. PHARMACOLOGY

- Half-Life: 1-4 min
- Onset: 2 min
- Duration: Up to 1 hr
- Metabolism: Mainly in liver,
- Metabolites: 1,3-glyceryl dinitrate, 1,2-glyceryl dinitrate, & glyceryl mononitrate (inactive)
- Excretion: Urine

### 4. CONTRAINDICATIONS

- SBP < 90mmHg or more than 30mmHg below baseline.
- Severe bradycardia (<50bpm) or tachycardia (>100bpm).
- RV infarction
- Use of phosphodiesterase inhibitors for erectile dysfunction (eg sildenafil and vardenafil within 24hrs; tadalafil within 48hrs).

### 5. PRECAUTIONS

- With evidence of AMI, limit SBP drop to 10% if patient is normotensive; 30% drop if Hypertensive, and avoid drop below 90mmHg.
- Do not mix with other drugs.
- Patient should sit or lie down when receiving this medication.
- Do not shake aerosol spray because this affects metered dose.

### 6. DOSAGE

- IV Bolus: 12.5 to 25 µg (if no SL or spray given)
- Infusion: begin at 10 to 20µg/min. titrate to effect, increase by 5 to 10µg/min every 5 to 10 minutes until desired effect.
  - Route of choice for emergencies
  - Use appropriate IV sets provided by pharmaceutical companies.
  - Dilute in D5W or NS.
- Sublingual Route: 1 tab (0.3 to 0.4mg), repeated for total of 3 doses at 5-minutes intervals.
- Aerosol spray: 1 to 2 sprays for 0.5 to 1sec at 5-minute intervals (provides 0.4mg/dose). Maximum 3 sprays within 15minutes.

## 2. SODIUM NITROPRUSSIDE

### 1. INDICATIONS

- Hypertensive crisis
- To reduce afterload in heart failure and acute pulmonary edema.
- To reduce afterload in acute mitral or aortic valve regurgitation.

### 2. PRECAUTIONS

- May cause hypotension, thiocyanate toxicity, and $CO_2$ retention.
- May reverse hypoxic pulmonary vasoconstriction in patients with pulmonary disease, exacerbating intrapulmonary shunting, resulting in hypoxemia.
- Other side effects include: headaches, nausea, vomiting, and abdominal cramps.
- *Not suitable for direct injection; requires dilution prior to infusion*
- *Hypotension may occur, leading to irreversible ischemic injury or death; requires appropriate monitoring equipment and experienced personnel*
- *Cyanide toxicity may occur because of accumulation of cyanide ion.*
- *Caution with phosphodiesterase inhibitors (eg, sildenafil)*
- *Light-sensitive, cover drug reservoir and tubing with opaque material.*

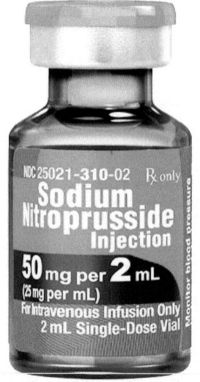

Fig. 3.3.10. Sodium Nitroprusside

### 3. DOSAGE

- IV administration: add 50 to 100 mg to 250 ml D5W.
- Begin at 0.1µg/kg/min and titrate upward every 3 to 5 minutes to desired effect (usually up to 5µg/kg/min but higher doses up to 10µg/kg may be needed).
- Use with an infusion pump; use hemodynamic monitoring for optimal safety.
- Action occurs within 1 to 2 minutes.

# VI. ALPHA-BLOCKERS

## A. DOXASOCIN (CARDURA)

### 1. MECHANISM OF ACTION

- Selective blockade of alpha-1 receptors results in vasodilation.
- These agents decrease blood pressure by decreasing total peripheral resistance and venous return.
- Hypertension: Blocks postsynaptic alpha1 receptors; alpha blockade causes arterial, arteriolar, and venous dilation; decreases total peripheral resistance and blood pressure
- Benign prostatic hyperplasia (BPH): Blocks alpha1 receptors in prostatic stromal and bladder tissues; reduces sympathetic tone-induced urethral stricture responsible for BPH symptoms

### 2. INDICATIONS

- Hypertension (Off-label)
- Immediate release: 1-4 mg PO once daily in AM or PM

### 3. ADVERSE EFFECTS

- Dizziness (5-19%), Fatigue (8-12%),
- Headache (6-10%), Vertigo (7%),
- Upper respiratory tract infection (URTI) (5%),
- Edema (3-4%), Rhinitis (3%)

### 4. CONTRAINDICATIONS

- Hypersensitivity to doxazosin or other quinazolines

### 5. CAUTIONS

- Use with caution in liver disease or recent cerebrovascular accident (CVA)
- Rule out prostate cancer before initiating therapy
- May cause first-dose syncope or sudden loss of consciousness
- Risk of orthostatic hypotension (dose dependent)
- Potential for hypotension, dry mouth, and urinary complications in elderly
- Priapism
- Extended-release form not indicated for hypertension

### 6. PREGNANCY & LACTATION

- Pregnancy category:

# VII. RENIN-ANGIOTENSIN SYSTEM DRUGS

## A. ACE INHIBITORS

### 1. INDICATIONS

- ACE inhibitors reduce mortality and improve LV dysfunction in post-AMI patients.
- They help prevent adverse LV remodeling, delay progression of heart failure, and decrease sudden death and recurrent MI.
- An ACE inhibitor should be administered orally within the first 24 hours of onset of symptoms and continued long term.
- Clinical heart failure without hypotension in patients not responding to digitalis or diuretics.
- Clinical signs of AMI with LV dysfunction
- LV ejection fraction < 40%.

### 2. APPROACH

- ACE Inhibitor therapy should start with low-dose oral administration (with possible IV doses for some preparations) and increase steadily to achieve a full dose within 24 to 48 hours.
- An Angiotensin receptor blocker (Losartan, Olmesartan...) should be administered to patients intolerant of ACE inhibitors.

### 3. PRECAUTIONS AND CONTRAINDICATIONS

- Contraindicated in:
  - Pregnancy (may cause fetal injury or death)
  - Angioedema
  - Hypersensitivity to ACE inhibitors
- *Reduce dose in Renal failure: Cr>2.5mg/dl in men and >2mg/dl in women.*

- *Avoid in bilateral renal artery stenosis*
- *Serum K >5mEq/l*
- *Do not give if patient is hypotensive (SBP <100mmHg or more than 30mmHg below baseline) or volume depleted.*
- *Generally, not started in ED; after reperfusion therapy has been completed and Blood pressure has stabilized, start within 24 hours.*
- *IV Enalapril is contraindicated in STEMI, risk of hypotension.*

## I. ENALAPRIL
- PO: start with single dose of 2.5mg. Titrate to 20mg PO BD
- IV: 1.25mg IV 6hourly

## II. CAPTOPRIL
- Start with a single dose of 6.25mg PO.
- Advanced to 25mg TDS and then 50mg TDS if tolerated.

## III. LISINOPRIL
- Start with 5mg within 24 hours of onset of symptoms, then
- 5mg given after 24 hours, then
- 10mg given after 48 hours, then
- 10mg once daily.

## IV. RAMIPRIL
- Start with a single dose of 2.5mg PO
- Titrate to 5mg Po BD as tolerated.

## CLINICAL: ACEI INDUCED ANGIOEDEMA
- The pathobiologic mechanism of angioedema with regard to ACE inhibitor therapy is believed to relate to the kallikrein-kinin plasma effector system.
- One hypothesis is that bradykinin, which is normally degraded by kininase II/ACE, accumulates in tissues.
- In this regard, plasma bradykinin has been shown to increase up to 12-fold during acute angioedema attacks in patients with hereditary or acquired forms of angioedema.

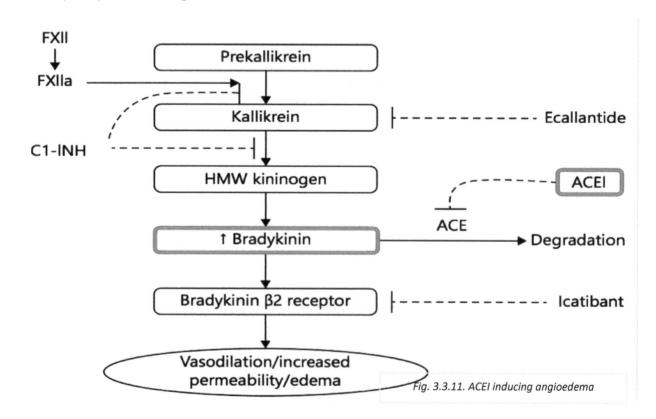

Fig. 3.3.11. ACEI inducing angioedema

# VIII. CALCIUM-CHANNEL BLOCKERS

## A. VERAPAMIL

### 1. MECHANISM OF ACTION
- Inhibition of the influx of calcium through slow channels in the vascular smooth muscles and myocardial tissue during depolarization.
- This results in systemic and coronary artery vasodilation, decreased myocardial contractility, and sinoatrial (SA) and atrioventricular (AV) nodal depression.

### 2. INDICATIONS
- Alternative drug (after adenosine) to terminate PSVT with narrow QRS complex and adequate BP and preserved LV function.
- May control ventricular response in patients with atrial fibrillation, flutter, or multifocal atrial tachycardia.

### 3. PRECAUTIONS
- Give only to patients with narrow-complex PSVT or known supraventricular arrhythmias.
- Do not use for wide-QRS tachycardias of uncertain origin, and avoid use for WPW syndrome and Afib, sick sinus syndrome, or second- or third-degree AV block without pacemaker.
- May decrease myocardial contractility and can produce peripheral vasodilation and hypotension.
- IV calcium may restore BP in toxic cases.
- Concurrent IV administration with IV beta-blockers may produce severe hypotension.
- **Use with extreme caution in patients receiving beta-blockers.**

### 4. DOSAGE
- **IV administration:**
  - o **First dose**: 2.5 to 5 mg IV bolus over 2 minutes (over 3 minutes in older patients)
  - o **Second dose**: 5 to 10 mg, if needed, every 15 to 30 minutes. Maximum dose 20mg.
  - o **Alternatives:** 5mg bolus every 15 minutes to a total dose of 30mg.

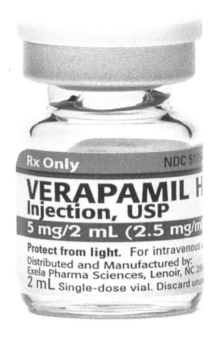

*Fig. 3.3.12. Verapamil*

## B. DILTIAZEM

### 1. INDICATIONS
- To control ventricular rate in atrial fibrillation and atrial flutter.
- May terminate reentrant arrhythmias that require AV nodal conduction for their continuation.
- Use after adenosine (second-line agent) to treat refractory reentry SVT in patients with narrow QRS complex and adequate blood pressure.

### 2. PRECAUTIONS
- See Verapamil

### 3. DOSAGE
- **Acute Rate Control**:
  - o 15 to 20 mg (0.25mg/Kg) IV over 2 minutes
  - o May give another IV dose in 15 minutes at 20 to 25mg (0.35 mg/Kg) over 2 minutes.
- **Maintenance Infusion:**
  - o 5 to 15 mg/h, titrated to physiologically appropriate heart rate (can dilute in D5W or NS).

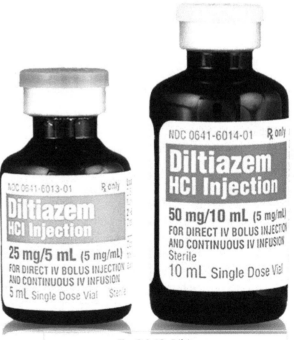

*Fig. 3.3.13. Diltiazem*

## C. NIFEDIPINE

### 1. MECHANISM OF ACTION

- See Verapamil

### 2. ADVERSE EFFECTS

- Adverse effects differ between short-acting (conventional) and extended-release formulations, with the conventional preparations having more serious adverse drug reactions in some cases
- Peripheral edema (10-30%), Dizziness (23-27%), Flushing (23-27%), Headache (10-23%), Heartburn (11%), Nausea (11%)

### 3. CONTRAINDICATIONS

- Hypersensitivity to nifedipine or other calcium-channel blockers
- Cardiogenic shockConcomitant administration with strong CYP3A4 inducers (e.g., rifampin, rifabutin, phenobarbital, phenytoin, carbamazepine, St John's wort) significantly reduces nifedipine efficacy
- Immediate release preparation (sublingually or orally) for urgent or emergent hypertension

### 4. CAUTIONS

- Use with caution in (≤4 weeks) myocardial infarction
- congestive heart failure,
- Advanced aortic stenosis, peripheral edema,
- Symptomatic hypotension, unstable angina,
- Concurrent use of beta blockers, hepatic or renal impairment, persistent progressive dermatologic reactions, exacerbation of angina (during initiation of treatment, after a dose increase, or after withdrawal of beta blocker)
- Short-acting nifedipine may be less safe than other calcium-channel blockers in management of angina, hypertension, or acute MI
- Use cautiously in combination with quinidine

### 5. PREGNANCY & LACTATION

- Pregnancy category: C
- Lactation: Drug is distributed into breast milk;

## D. NIMODIPINE

### 1. MECHANISM OF ACTION

- Ca channel blocker with minimal effects on conduction in heart; primary effect is upon cerebral arteries to prevent vasospasm.
- Highly lipophilic, allowing it to cross the blood-brain barrier.

### 2. ADVERSE EFFECTS

- Reduction in systemic blood pressure (1-8%), Diarrhea (2-4%), Headache (1-4%), Abdominal discomfort (2%), Rash (1-2%).

### 3. WARNING

- Do not administer contents of gel capsule or oral solution IV or by other parenteral routes
- Deaths and serious life-threatening adverse events (ie, significant hypotension requiring pressor support) have occurred when injected parenterally.

### 4. CONTRAINDICATIONS

- Hypersensitivity
- Parenteral administration; risk of death.

### 5. CAUTIONS

- Congestive heart failure
- Reflex tachycardia resulting in angina and/or MI in patients with obstructive coronary disease reported
- Metabolism decreased in patients with hepatic impairment
- Use caution in hepatic impairment or hypertrophic subaortic stenosis
- Peripheral edema may occur within 2-3 weeks of initiating therapy
- Hypotension with or without syncope is possible (particularly with severe aortic stenosis)
- Intestinal pseudo-obstruction and ileus have been reported rarely
- A decreased dose may be required with strong CYP3A4 inhibitors.

# IX. SYMPATHOMIMETICS

## A. VASOACTIVE AGENTS

- **INOTROPES:**
  - ○ Agents that increase myocardial contractility or inotropy (β1 effect)
  - ○ e.g. **Dobutamine**, Adrenaline, Isoprenaline, Ephedrine

- **VASOPRESSORS:**
  - ○ Agents that cause vasoconstriction leading to **increased** systemic and/or pulmonary vascular resistance (↑SVR, PVR/ α1 effect)
  - ○ e.g. **Noradrenaline**, Vasopressin, Metaraminol, methylene blue

- **INODILATORS:**
  - ○ Agents with inotropic effects that also cause vasodilation leading to **decreased** systemic and/or pulmonary vascular resistance (↓SVR, PVR)
  - ○ e.g. **Milrinone**, Levosimendan
- Some agents (Dopamine) don't fit any of these categories.

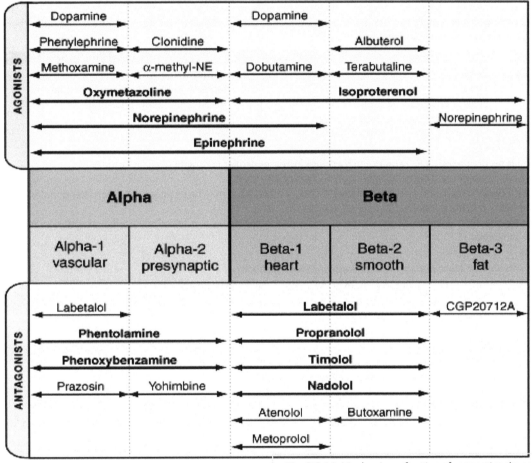

Fig. 3.3.14. Mechanism of action of vasoactive drugs

## 1. INOTROPES AND VASOPRESSORS

- ○ Inotropes are a group of drugs that alter the contractility of the heart.
  - ▪ **Positive inotropes** increase the force of contraction of the heart.
  - ▪ **Negative inotropes** weaken the force of contraction of the heart.

**INDICATIONS:**

- ○ Inotropes are indicated in acute conditions where there is low cardiac output (CO), such as cardiogenic shock following myocardial infarction, acute decompensated heart failure and low CO states after cardiac surgery.

- ○ *It is important to optimise preload by correcting fluid balance before starting inotropes, since there is little point in increasing the contractility of the heart if its chambers are not filled optimally.*

- ○ *Central venous pressure (CVP) can be used as a surrogate measure of preload.*

- ○ Inotropes increase CO, thereby increasing MAP and maintaining perfusion to vital organs and tissues.

o   Inotropes increase CO by increasing both SV and HR.
o   In the failing heart, SV can only increase to a certain level before the cardiac muscle fibres become overstretched and CO will start to drop. This phenomenon is known as Starling's law.

**MECHANISM OF ACTION**

o   The main mechanism of action for most inotropes involves increasing intracellular calcium, either by increasing influx to the cell during the action potential or increasing release from the sarcoplasmic reticulum.
o   Choice of inotrope will depend on factors such as the patient's underlying disease state and the clinician's preference.

## 1. CATECHOLAMINES

o   Most commonly used inotropes are the catecholamines; These can be:
  ▪   **Endogenous:** Adrenaline, Noradrenaline
  ▪   **Synthetic:** Dobutamine, Isoprenaline.
o   These medicines act on the sympathetic nervous system.
o   Most commonly their cardiac effects are attributed to stimulation of alpha and beta-adrenergic receptors (specifically $\alpha_1$, $\beta_1$, and $\beta_2$).
o   The main receptor in the cardiac muscle that affects the rate and force of contraction is the $\beta_1$ receptor.
o   Binding to $\beta_1$ receptors results in increased calcium entry into the cell via the opening of L-type calcium channels and release of intracellular calcium from the sarcoplasmic reticulum.
o   More calcium is available to bind with troponin-C, thereby enhancing myocardial contractility.
o   Most catecholamines have a **short half-life** (about 2 minutes) and steady-state blood concentrations are reached within 10 minutes.
o   They are therefore usually given by continuous infusion.

| Receptor | Location | Action |
|---|---|---|
| $\alpha_1$ | Peripheral, renal and coronary circulation | Vasoconstriction |
| $\beta_1$ | Heart | Increase in contractility and heart rate |
| $\beta_2$ | Lungs; peripheral and coronary circulation | Vasodilation, bronchodilation |
| **Dopaminergic** | Mesenteric, renal, coronary arteries | Vasodilation |

## A. DOBUTAMINE

o   Dobutamine **is predominantly a $\beta_1$ agonist** and therefore increases cardiac contractility and heart rate.
o   It also acts at $\beta_2$ receptors causing vasodilation and decreasing afterload.
o   Because of this vasodilation, and to ensure adequate MAP is achieved, it may be necessary to administer dobutamine in combination with a vasopressor (eg, noradrenaline).
o   **The main side effects** of dobutamine are increased heart rate, arrhythmias and raised myocardial oxygen demand. These can cause myocardial ischaemia.
o   **Precautions**
  ●   *Avoid with systolic blood pressure < 100 mmHg and signs of shock.*
  ●   *May cause tachyarrhythmias, fluctuations in blood pressure, headache, and nausea.*
  ●   *Elderly patients may have a significantly decreased response.*
  ●   *DO NOT MIX WITH SODIUM BICARBONATE.*

## B. ISOPRENALINE

o   Isoprenaline has a similar profile to dobutamine but tends to cause more tachycardia.
o   It is sometimes used for bradycardic patients requiring inotropic support.

## C. NORADRENALINE

o   Because noradrenaline **acts primarily via $\alpha_1$ receptors**, it is usually used as a **vasopressor** (increasing SVR to maintain MAP) rather than an inotrope.
o   It is often used with other inotropes, such as dobutamine, to maintain adequate perfusion, as discussed above.

## D. ADRENALINE

o   Adrenaline has activity at all adrenergic receptors (**predominantly acting as a $\beta$-agonist in low doses and an $\alpha$-agonist at higher doses**); other more specific inotropes are often preferred over adrenaline.
o   Adrenaline is used mainly during resuscitation after cardiac arrest (in this case it is given as a bolus).
o   **It is not recommended for use in cardiogenic shock** because of metabolic side effects, including **hyperlactataemia and hyperglycaemia.**

## E. DOPAMINE

o   Dopamine is a complicated inotrope because it has dose-dependent pharmacological effects:
  ▪   **Low-dose dopamine (2–5µg/kg/min):** Mainly Dopaminergic effects,
  ▪   **Medium doses (5–10µg/kg/min):** $\beta_1$ inotropic effects predominate
  ▪   **High doses (10–20µg/kg/min):** $\alpha_1$ vasoconstriction predominates.

**MECHANISM OF ACTION**

- Endogenous catecholamine, acting on both Dopaminergic and Adrenergic neurons:
  - **Low dose** stimulates mainly dopaminergic receptors, producing renal and mesenteric vasodilation;
    - 1-5 mcg/kg/min IV (low dose): May increase urine output and renal blood flow
  - Medium dose stimulates both beta1-adrenergic and dopaminergic receptors, producing cardiac stimulation and renal vasodilation;
    - 5-10 mcg/kg/min IV (medium dose): May increase renal blood flow, cardiac output, heart rate, and cardiac contractitlity
  - Large dose stimulates alpha-adrenergic receptors
    - 10-20 mcg/kg/min IV (high dose): May increase blood pressure and stimulate vasoconstriction; may not have a beneficial effect in blood pressure; may increase risk of tachyarrhythmias

## F. PHOSPHODIESTERASE-3 INHIBITORS (MILRINONE)

- Phosphodiesterase-3 (PDE3) is an enzyme found in cardiac and smooth muscle cells. Inhibition of PDE3 increases intracellular calcium causing vasodilation and increased myocardial contractility.
- The mechanism of action is independent of adrenergic receptors and therefore PDE3 inhibitors are particularly useful if these receptors have become down-regulated (eg, in patients with chronic heart failure).
- **Milrinone** is the most commonly used PDE3 inhibitor. It has a relatively long half-life (**two hours**) and can accumulate in patients with renal failure.

## G. LEVOSIMENDAN (unlicensed)

- Levosimendan is a novel inotrope that sensitises troponin-C to calcium, thereby increasing the force of contraction.
- It also acts on potassium channels in smooth muscle to cause vasodilation.
- Levosimendan increases CO without increasing myocardial oxygen consumption.
- Levosimendan is administered as a continuous infusion (with or without an initial bolus dose) over 24 hours.
- It has a half-life of about one hour, but active metabolites mean that the inotropic effect can continue for up to five days after the infusion has finished.

## B. DRUGS USED FOR BRADYCARDIA

## 1. ATROPINE

- Atropine is the first drug used to treat bradycardia in the bradycardia algorithm.
- May be beneficial in presence of AV nodal block or ventricular asystole.
- Second drug (after epinephrine and vasopressin) for asystole and bradycardic pulseless electrical activity.
- The dosing for Atropine is 0.5 mg IV every 3-5 minutes as needed, and the maximum total dosage that can be give is 3 mg.
- *It is classified as an Anticholinergic drug and increases firing of the SA Node by blocking the action of the Vagus Nerve on the Heart resulting in an increased Heart Rate.*
- *Atropine should be used cautiously in the presence of Myocardial Ischemia and Hypoxia since it increases oxygen demand of Heart and can worsen ischemia.*
- *Avoid in Hypothermic Bradycardia.*
- *Atropine will not be effective for Mobitz type II and complete Heart Block.*

---

*Atropine is not effective for 2nd degree block type II (Mobitz II) and 3rd degree block (Complete Heart Block):*

- Atropine may speed the firing rate of the SA node (atria), but the ventricles are not responding to anything the atria (SA node) puts out. Thus, the heart rates will not increase.
- There may be some action at the AV-node with atropine, but the effect will be negligible and typically not therapeutic.
- Atropine in most cases will not hurt the patient with 3rd degree block unless they are unstable and you delay pacing to give atropine.
- It is important to note that Mobitz II and Complete Heart Block may be associated with acute myocardial ischemia.
- In this case, if atropine is used and it increases the heart rate there is a high potential for worsening of the myocardial ischemia due to the increased oxygen consumption.
- The increased heart rate will also reduce diastolic filling time which may worsen coronary perfusion. Since new onset mobitz II and Complete Heart Block are commonly associated with myocardial infarction, it would be ideal to keep the HR slow (50-60) to increase diastolic filling time. Anytime you increase HR, the diastolic filling time is what takes the biggest hit.
- ***Transcutaneous Pacing should be the first line in symptomatic Mobitz II and Symptomatic Complete Heart Block.***

---

**DOSING:**

- *Asystole or PEA*
  - **1mg IV/IO push**
  - **May repeat every 3 to 5 min (if asystole persists) to a maximum of 3 doses (3mg).**

- *Bradycardia*
  - ○ *0.5mg IV every 3 to 5 min as needed, not to exceed total dose of 0.04mg/kg (total 3mg).*
- *Acs*
  - ○ *0.6 to 1mg IV repeated every 5min for acs patients (total 0.04mg/kg).*
- *Endotracheal administration*
  - ○ *2 to 3mg diluted in 10mls of ns.*
- *Organophosphate poisoning*
  - ○ *Extremely large doses: 2 to 4 mg or higher may be needed.*

## 2. EPINEPHRINE AND DOPAMINE

- Epinephrine and dopamine are second-line drugs for symptomatic bradycardia. They are both used as infusions in the bradycardia algorithm if atropine is ineffective.
- 2010 ACLS guidelines state that if bradycardia is unresponsive to atropine, an equally effective alternative to transcutaneous pacing is the use of an IV infusion of the beta-adrenergic agonists (dopamine or epinephrine).

### 1. DOSING:

- Begin the epinephrine infusion at **2 to 10 mcg/min** and titrate to patient's response.
- The goal of therapy is to improve the patient's clinical status rather than target an exact heart rate.
- Begin the dopamine infusion at **2 to 10 mcg/kg/min** and titrate to the patient's response.

### 2. PRECAUTIONS

- Prior to use of ACLS drugs in the treatment of symptomatic bradycardia, contributing factors of the bradycardia should be explored then ruled out or corrected.
- Moderate beta-1 & weak alpha effects resulting in alpha- and beta- adrenergic stimulation that increase CO & BP, decrease renal perfusion & variable peripheral vascular resistance (PVR).

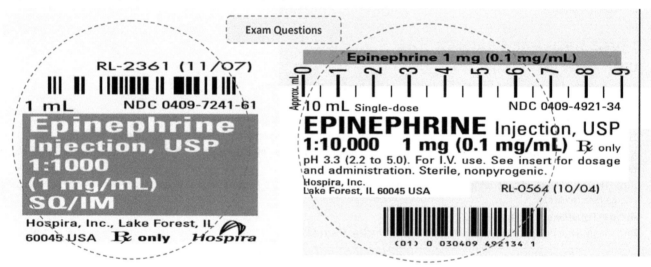

Exam Questions

## C. DRUGS USED IN RESUSCITATION

## 1. ADRENALINE/EPINEPHRINE

### 1. MECHANISM OF ACTION

- Epinephrine is the primary drug used in the pulseless arrest algorithm.
- It is used for its potent **vasoconstrictive effects** and also for its ability to **increase cardiac output**.
- Epinephrine is considered a vasopressor.
- **Vasoconstriction effects:** epinephrine binds directly to alpha-1 adrenergic receptors of the blood vessels (arteries and veins) causing direct vasoconstriction, thus, *improving perfusion pressure to the Brain and Heart.*
- **Cardiac Output:** Epinephrine also binds to beta-1-adrenergic receptors of the heart. This indirectly improves cardiac output by:
  - ○ Increasing Heart Rate
  - ○ Increasing Heart Muscle Contractility
  - ○ Increasing Conductivity through the AV Node

## 2. INDICATIONS FOR ACLS

- Epinephrine is used in the pulseless arrest algorithm as a direct IV push and also in the bradycardia algorithm as an infusion.

## 3. ROUTES

- During ACLS, epinephrine can be given 3 ways: intravenous; intraosseous, and endotracheal tube

## 4. DOSING

- **Intravenous Push/IO**: 1mg (10ml of 1:10 000 solution) epinephrine IV is given every 3-5 minutes. Follow each dose with 20ml flush, elevate arm for 10 to 20 seconds after dose.
- **Higher Dose:** up to 0.2mg/kg may be used for specific indications (beta-blocker or calcium channel blocker overdose).
- **Continuous Infusion:** Add 1mg epinephrine (1ml of 1:1000 solution) to 500ml NS or D5W. Initial infusion rate of 1μg/min titrated to effect (typical dose: 2 to 10μg/min).
- **Profound Bradycardia or Hypotension:** 2 to 10μg/min infusion; titrate to patient response.
- **IV infusion for post-cardiac arrest hypotension:** 0.1-0.5 mcg/kg/min (for example a 70kg adult: 7-35 mcg/min would be given).
- **Endotracheal Tube:** 2-2.5mg epinephrine is diluted in 10ml NS and given directly into the ET tube.
- *Epinephrine should be used with caution in patients suffering from Myocardial Infarction since Epinephrine increases Heart Rate and raises Blood Pressure. This increase in HR and BP can increase myocardial oxygen demand and worsen ischemia.*
- *There is no clinical evidence that the use of Epinephrine, when used during cardiac arrest, increases rates of survival to discharge from the hospital. However, studies have shown that epinephrine and vasopressin improve rates of ROSC (return of spontaneous circulation.*

# 2. NOREPINEPHRINE

## 1. INDICATIONS

- Severe cardiogenic shock and hemodynamically significant hypotension (SBP < 70mmHg) with low total Peripheral resistance.
- Agent of last resort for management of Ischemic heart disease and shock.

## 2. PRECAUTIONS

- *Increases myocardial oxygen requirements, raises blood pressure and heart rate. May induce arrhythmias.*
- *Use with caution in patients with acute ischaemia; monitor cardiac output.*
- *Extravasation causes tissue necrosis.*
- *If extravasation occurs, administer PHENTOLAMINE 5 to 10mg in 10 to 15ml saline solution, infiltrated into area.*

## 3. DOSAGE

- **IV administration (ONLY ROUTE):**
  - 0.5 to 1μg/min titrated to improve BP (up to 30μg/min)
  - Add 4mg of Norepinephrine or 8 mg of Norepinephrine bitartrate to 250ml of D5W or D5NS, but not NS alone.
  - Poison/drug-induced hypotension may require higher doses to achieve adequate perfusion.

# 3. VASOPRESSIN

## 1. MECHANISM OF ACTION

- Vasopressin is a primary drug used in the pulseless arrest algorithm. In high concentrations, it raises blood pressure by inducing moderate vasoconstriction, and it has been shown to be **more effective than epinephrine in asystolic cardiac arrest.**
- One major indication for vasopressin over epinephrine is its **lower risk for adverse side effects** when compared with epinephrine.
- With epinephrine, some studies have shown a risk of increased myocardial oxygen consumption and post arrest arrhythmias because of an increase in heart rate and contractility (beta 1 effects).
- Vasopressin also is thought to cause cerebral vessel dilation and theoretically increase cerebral perfusion.

## 2. INDICATIONS

- May be used as alternative pressor to epinephrine in the treatment of adult shock-refractory VF.
- May be useful alternative to epinephrine in asystole, PEA.

## 3. PRECAUTIONS

- Potent peripheral vasoconstrictor.
- Increased PVR may provoke cardiac ischemia and angina.
- Not recommended for responsive patients with coronary artery disease.

## 4. ROUTES

- Vasopressin may be given IV/IO or by endotracheal tube.

## 5. DOSING

- 40 units of vasopressin IV/IO push may be given to replace the first or second dose of epinephrine, and at this time, there is insufficient evidence for recommendation of a specific dose per the endotracheal tube.
- In the ACLS pulseless arrest algorithm, vasopressin may replace the first or second dose of epinephrine.

## 4. METARAMINOL

- **CLINICAL PHARMACOLOGY**
  - Metaraminol is a potent sympathomimetic amine that increases both systolic and diastolic blood pressure.
  - Acts mainly as an alpha 1 adrenergic receptor agonist (Vasopressor)
  - It also has some effect on beta adrenergic receptors
- **Administration Route:** IV
- **Alternative Names:** Aramine
- **Indications**
  - Hypotension (particularly during induction of anaesthesia)
- **PRESENTATION AND ADMINISTRATION**
  - *IV:*
    - 10mg in 1ml vial
    - Dilute 10mg in 20ml of compatible IV fluid (i.e. make up to a concentration of 0.5mg/ml)
  - Compatible with the following IV fluids: Sodium Chloride, 5% dextrose, Hartmanns
  - Store at room temperature
- **Dosage:** *IV:* 0.5-1mg PRN
- **Dosage in Paediatrics:** *IV:* 0.01mg/kg PRN
- **Contraindications:** hypersensitivity to metaraminol
- **WARNINGS**
  - Metaraminol contains sodium bisulfite, a sulfite that may cause allergic-type reactions including anaphylactic symptoms and life-threatening or less severe asthmatic episodes in certain susceptible people.
  - The overall prevalence of sulfite sensitivity in the general population is unknown and probably low.
  - Sulfite sensitivity is seen more frequently in asthmatic than in non-asthmatic people.
- **PRECAUTIONS**
  - *General:*
    - Avoid excessive blood pressure response.
    - Rapidly induced hypertensive responses have been reported to cause acute pulmonary oedema, arrhythmias, cerebral haemorrhage, or cardiac arrest.
    - Because of its vasoconstrictor effect metaraminol should be given with caution in heart or thyroid disease, hypertension, or diabetes.

## IMPORTANT DRUG INTERACTIONS FOR THE ICU

- ***Digoxin:*** *Metaraminol should be used with caution in digitalized patients, since the combination of digitalis and sympathomimetic amines may cause ectopic arrhythmias.*
- ***MAOI & TCAs (Monoamine oxidase inhibitors or tricyclic antidepressants):*** *may potentiate the action of sympathomimetic amines.*
- *Therefore, when initiating pressor therapy in patients receiving these drugs, the initial dose should be small and given with caution.*

- **Adverse Reactions**
  - Most adverse effects seen arise due to inadvertent excess dosing.
  - *Cardiovascular:*
    - Hypertension, tachycardia, bradycardia
    - Pulmonary oedema, atrial or ventricular arrhythmia.
  - *Central nervous system:*
    - Cerebral hemorrhage, convulsions.

## SYMPATHOMIMETIC, INOTROPIC & INODILATOR DRUGS

| DRUG | IV INFUSION | ADRENERGIC EFFECT | | ANTIARRHYTMOGENIC POTENTIAL |
|---|---|---|---|---|
| | | α | β | |
| Epinephrine | 2 to 10 μg/min | ++ | +++ | +++ |
| Norepinephrine | 0.5 to 12 μg/min | +++ | ++ | |
| Dopamine | 2 to 4 μg/kg/min | + | + | + |
| | 5 to 10 μg/kg/min | ++ | ++ | ++ |
| | 10 to 20 μg/kg/min | +++ | ++ | +++ |
| Dobutamine | 2 to 20 μg/kg/min | + | +++ | ++ |
| Isoproterenol | 2 to 10 μg/kg/min | 0 | +++ | +++ |
| Inamrinone (formerly Amnirinone) | 5 to 15 μg/kg/min (after loading dose of 0.75mg/Kg not to exceed 1mg/Kg, give over 2 to 3 minutes or longer) | 0 | 0 | ++ |

Source: American Heart Association /2006 ACLS core Drugs

# X. ANTICOAGULANTS

# A. PARENTERAL PREPARATIONS

## I. HEPARIN

### 1. MECHANISM OF ACTION
- **Mechanism for low dose:** Inactivates factor Xa and inhibits conversion of prothrombin to thrombin.
- **Mechanism for high dose:** Inactivates factors IX, X, XI, and XII and thrombin and inhibits conversion of fibrinogen to fibrin.
- Also inhibits activation of factor VIII

### 2. INDICATIONS
- Adjuvant therapy in AMI.
- Begin Heparin with fibrin-specific lytics (Alteplase, Reteplase, Tenecteplase).

### 3. PRECAUTIONS
- Same contraindications as for fibrinolytic therapy: active bleeding, recent intracranial, intraspinal, or eye surgery; severe hypertension; bleeding disorders; GIT bleeding.
- Doses and laboratory targets appropriate when used with fibrinolytic therapy. Do not use if platelet count is or falls below <100 000 or with history of heparin-induced thrombocytopaenia. For these patients consider direct antithrombins.

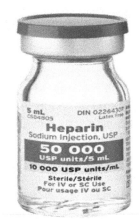

*Fig. 3.3.15. Heparin injection*

### 6. DOSAGE
- **UFH IV Infusion- STEMI:**
  - Initial bolus 60IU/Kg (max. bolus 4000IU)
  - Continue 12IU/kg/hr, round to the nearest 50IU (max. 1000IU/hr for patients > 70kg).
  - Adjust to maintain aPTT 1.5 to 2 times the control values (about 50 to 70 seconds) for 48hours or until angiography.
  - Check initial aPTT at 3 hours, then every 6 hours until stable, then daily.
  - Platelet count daily.

- **UFH IV Infusion- NSTEMI:**
  - Initial bolus 60 to 70IU/kg (max. 5000IU)
  - 12 to 15IU/Kg/hr (max. 1000IU/hr)
  - Check initial aPTT at 3 hours, then every 6 hours until stable, then daily.
  - Platelet count daily.

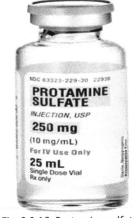

*Fig. 3.3.16. Protamine sulfate*

## II. ENOXAPARIN (CLEXANE)

### 1. MECHANISM OF ACTION
- LMWH; antithrombotic that inhibits factor Xa by increasing inhibition rate of clotting proteases that are activated by antithrombin III.
- Generally, does not increase PT or PTT. **Not neutralized by heparin-binding proteins.**

### 2. INDICATIONS
- For use in ACS, specifically patients with NSTEMI/unstable Angina.

### 3. PRECAUTIONS
- Hemorrhage may complicate any therapy with LMWH.
- Contraindicated in presence of hypersensitivity to heparin or pork products or history of sensitivity to drug.
- Use with extreme caution, in patients with type II heparin-induced thrombocytopaenia. Adjust dose for renal insufficiency.
- Contraindicated if platelet count < 100000. For these patients consider direct antithrombins.

### 4. DOSAGE
- **NSTEMI Enoxaparin protocol:** 1mg/Kg SQ BID; the first dose may be preceded by 30mg IV bolus.
- **STEMI Enoxaparin Protocol**: as ancillary therapy with fibrinolytic:
  - 30mg IV bolus, then 1mg/Kg SQ BID until hospital discharge.
  - For patients <75 years with no clinically significant renal insufficiency.
  - Contraindicated for creatinine > 2.5mg/dl in men or 2mg/dl in women (when administered with Tenecteplase).
- **Enoxaparin: Renal insufficiency:** For Cr clearance < 30ml/min, reduce dose to 1mg/kg SQ QID.
- **Heparin Reversal:** ICH or Life-threatening bleed: Administer protamine.

## DIFFERENCES BETWEEN UFH AND LMWH

|  | UFH | LMWH |
| --- | --- | --- |
| Bioavailability | Erratic SC absorption | Good SC absorption |
| Onset | Immediate IV | SC 3-4hrs |
| Duration | Appr. 4hrs | 12hrs |
| Monitoring | Required | Not required |
| Monitoring Test | aPTT | Antifactor Xa |
| Factor II: Factor Xa | Predominantly factor II | Predominantly factor Xa |
| Inpatient vs outpatient | Inpatient only | Inpatient and outpatient |

## III. PROTAMINE SULPHATE (ANTIDOTE)

### 1. MECHANISM OF ACTION

- Protamine that is strongly basic combines with acidic heparin forming a stable complex and neutralizes the anticoagulant activity of both drugs.

### 2. CONTRAINDICATIONS & CAUTIONS

- Protamine sulfate can cause severe hypotension, cardiovascular collapse, noncardiogenic pulmonary edema, catastrophic pulmonary vasoconstriction, and pulmonary hypertension.
- Allergy to fish, previous vasectomy, severe left ventricular dysfunction, and abnormal preoperative pulmonary hemodynamics also may be risk factors.
- In patients with any of these risk factors, the risk to benefit of administration of protamine sulfate should be carefully considered.
- Protamine should not be given when bleeding occurs without prior heparin use.

### 3. CAUTIONS

- Heparin rebound causing bleeding may occur 8-9 hr after protamine administration.
- May be ineffective in cardiac surgery patients despite adequate dose.
- Rapid infusion reactions can cause severe hypotensive reactions.

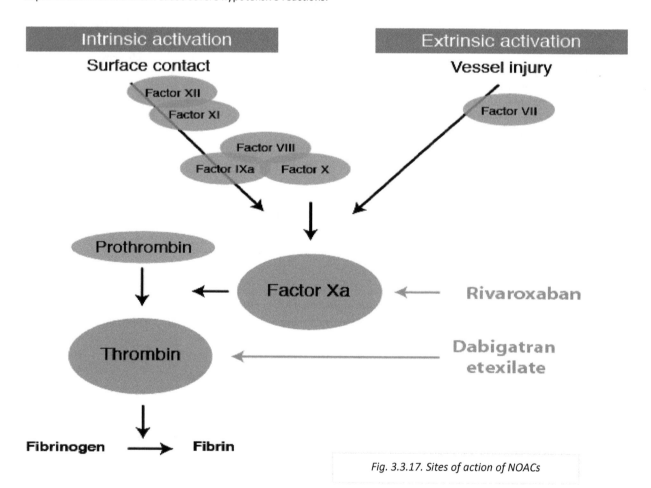

*Fig. 3.3.17. Sites of action of NOACs*

# B. ORAL PREPARATIONS

## 1. WARFARIN

### WARFARIN VS NEWER ANTICOAGULANT DRUGS

| Characteristic | Warfarin | Dabigatran | Rivaroxaban | Apixaban |
|---|---|---|---|---|
| Site of action | Vit K antagonist | Direct Thrombin inhibitor (IIa) | Factor Xa inhibitor | Factor Xa inhibitor |
| Maximum time to onset | 2-5 days | 2 hrs | 2.5-4hrs | 3 hrs |
| Half-life | 2-5 days | 14-17 days | 5-9 hrs in healthy patient<br>9-12 hrs in elderly patients | 8-15 hrs |
| Drug interactions | Acetaminophen<br>Aspirin<br>NSAIDS<br>SSRIs Phenytoin | P-gp inducers (Rifampicin)<br>Dronedarone<br>Ketoconazole<br>Aspirin<br>NSAIDS<br>Clopidogrel | Strong inhibitors and inducers of CYP3A4<br>Aspirin<br>NSAIDS<br>Clopidogrel | Aspirin<br>Clopidogrel<br>Potentially, strong inhibitors and inducers of CYP3A4 and P-gb |

### 1. MECHANISM OF ACTION
- Interferes with hepatic synthesis of vitamin K-dependent clotting factors II, VII, IX, and X, as well as proteins C and S (**910-27CS**).
- S-warfarin is 4 times more potent than R-warfarin.
- Warfarin depletes functional vitamin K reserves, which in turn reduces synthesis of active clotting factors, by competitively inhibiting subunit 1 of the multi-unit vitamin K epoxide reductase complex 1 (VKOR1).

### 2. DOSING FORMS
- **INR 2-2.5**
  - o  Prophylactic treatment for DVT (short-term).
- **INR 2-3**
  - o  Prophylactic treatment for hip surgery and surgery for femur fractures (short to medium term).
  - o  Treatment of venous thromboembolism - deep vein thrombosis (DVT) or pulmonary embolism (PE).
    - Anticoagulation for 1 month is inadequate treatment after an episode of VTE.
    - At least 6 weeks anticoagulation is recommended after calf vein thrombosis and at least 3 months after proximal DVT or PE.
    - For patients with temporary risk factors and a low risk of recurrence 3 months of treatment may be sufficient.
    - For patients with idiopathic VTE or permanent risk factors at least 6 months anticoagulation is recommended.
    - Target INR of 2·5 is recommended for long-term oral anticoagulant therapy for secondary prevention of VTE.
    - Target INR of 2·5 is recommended for patients with DVT or PE associated with antiphospholipid syndrome.
    - Target of 3·5 is also recommended for patients who suffer recurrence of VTE whilst on warfarin with an INR between 2·0 & 3·0.
  - o  **Cardioversion**
    - Target INR of 2·5 is recommended for 3 weeks before and 4 weeks after cardioversion.
    - To minimise cardioversion cancellations due to low INRs on the day of the procedure a higher target INR, e.g. 3·0, can be used prior to the procedure.
  - o  **Peripheral arterial thrombosis and grafts**
    - Antiplatelet drugs remain first line intervention for secondary antithrombotic prophylaxis.
    - If long-term anticoagulation is given to patients at high risk of femoral vein graft failure a target INR of 2·5 is recommended.
  - o  **Coronary artery thrombosis**
    - If oral anticoagulant therapy is prescribed a target INR of 2·5 is recommended.
  - o  **Systemic embolism after MI**
  - o  **Mitral stenosis with embolism (long term)**
  - o  **Atrial fibrillation (long-term)** - it may be safer to aim for an INR of 2 in those aged over 75 years.
    - Risk of stroke is 3 times greater in patients with atrial fibrillation with mitral stenosis than in those without valve disease.
    - Based on its apparent effectiveness in non-randomized studies and its effect in non-rheumatic atrial fibrillation, warfarin is usually given to maintain an INR of 2.5.
- **INR 3.0 or more**
  - o  **Treatment of recurrent DVT, PE (long term)**
    - Target of 3·5 is also recommended for patients who suffer recurrence of VTE whilst on warfarin with an INR between 2·0 & 3·0.

- ○ **Prosthetic Heart Valves (long-term)**
  - ▪ For patients in whom valve type and location are known, specific target INRs are recommended.
  - ▪ Bileaflet valve (aortic)                              2·5
  - ▪ Tilting disk valve (aortic)                           3·0
  - ▪ Bileaflet valve (mitral)                              3·0
  - ▪ Tilting disk (mitral)                                 3·0
  - ▪ Caged ball or caged disk (aortic or mitral)          3·5
  - ▪ Otherwise a target INR of 3·0 is recommended for valves in the aortic position and 3·5 in the mitral position.

**Notes:**

- • **Bioprosthetic valves:**
  - ○ Long-term warfarin not required in absence of atrial fibrillation.
  - ○ Oral anticoagulants are not required for valves in the aortic position in patients in sinus rhythm, although many centres anticoagulate patients for 3 or 6 months after any tissue valve implant.
  - ○ Patients with bioprostheses in the mitral position should receive oral anticoagulants to achieve an INR of 2.5 for the first 3 months. After 3 months, patients with atrial fibrillation should receive lifelong therapy to achieve an INR of 2.5.
  - ○ Patients with bioprosthetic valves with a history of systemic embolism and those with intracardiac thrombus should also be anticoagulated to achieve an INR of 2.5.
  - ○ Patients who do not require oral anticoagulants after the first 3 months may be considered for antiplatelet therapy, e.g. aspirin.
- • **INR values and risk of haemorrhage versus risk of thromboembolism in treatment of DVT/PE**
  - ○ Risks of haemorrhage and thromboemboli are minimized at international normalized ratios of 2-3.
  - ○ Ratios that are moderately higher than this therapeutic range appear safe and more effective than subtherapeutic ratios.

**Reference:** Baglin TP et al. British Committee for Standards in Haematology - Guidelines on oral anticoagulation (warfarin): third edition - 2005 update British Journal of Haematology 2006; 132 (3): 277-285.

## 5. CONTRAINDICATIONS

- • Pregnancy, except in women with mechanical heart valves.
- • Hemorrhagic tendencies or blood dyscrasias.
- • Recent or contemplated CNS or eye surgery or traumatic surgery resulting in large open surfaces.
- • Bleeding tendencies associated with CNS hemorrhage, cerebral aneurysms, dissecting aorta, pericarditis and pericardial effusions, bacterial endocarditis, and active ulceration or overt bleeding of the GI, GU, or respiratory tract.
- • Threatened abortion, eclampsia, and preeclampsia.
- • Unsupervised patients with conditions associated with potential high level of noncompliance (eg, dementia, alcoholism, psychosis).
- • Spinal puncture and other diagnostic or therapeutic procedures with potential for uncontrollable bleeding
- • Major regional or lumbar block anesthesia.
- • Known hypersensitivity.
- • Malignant hypertension.

| INTERACTIONS OF WARFARIN | |
|---|---|
| **Liver enzymes inducers (INR Reduction) = PC BRAS** | **LIVER ENZYME INHIBITORS (INR Elevation) = AO DEVICES** |
| Phenytoin | Amiodarone and Allopurinol |
| Carbamazepine | Omeprazole |
| Barbiturates | Disulfiram (Metronidazole) |
| Rifampicin | Erythromycin |
| Alcohol excess | Valproate |
| Sulphonurea | Isoniazid |
| | Cimetidine (and Ciprofloxacin) |
| | Acute Ethanol intoxication |
| | Sulphonamide |

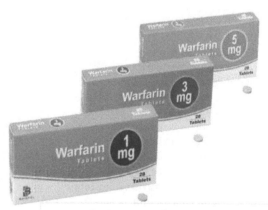

*Fig. 3.3.18. Warfarin interactions*

## 2. NOVEL ORAL ANTICOAGULANTS (NOACs)

| Anticoagulant | Mechanism of action |
|---|---|
| **Warfarin** | Reduce synthesis of factors II, VII, IX, X |
| **Novel Oral Anticoagulants (NOACs)** | |
| **Dabigatran** | Direct competitive reversible inhibition of thrombin |
| **Rivaroxaban** | Direct competitive reversible inhibition of Factor Xa |
| **Apixaban** | Direct competitive reversible inhibition of Factor Xa |
| **Edoxaban** | Direct competitive reversible inhibition of Factor Xa |

## SUMMARY OF BLOOD CLOTTING DISORDER DRUGS

| | | | |
|---|---|---|---|
| **Anticoagulants**<br>**Rx: arterial & venous Thrombosis** | Direct thrombin inhibitor | • Dabigatran<br>• Argatroban<br>• Lepuridin | |
| | Indirect thrombin inhibitor | • Heparin | • Enoxaparin<br>• UFH<br>• LMWH |
| | | • Fondaparinux | |
| | Vit K epoxide reductase inhibitor | • Warfarin | |
| | Direct Xa inhibitor | • Rivaroxaban<br>• Apixaban | |
| **Antiplatelet Drugs**<br>**Rx: arterial disease** | Cox-1 inhibitors | • Aspirin | |
| | Glycoprotein IIb/IIIa inhibitors | • Abciximab<br>• Eptifibatide<br>• Tirofiban | |
| | ADP inhibitors | • Clopidogrel<br>• Prasugrel | |
| | Phosphodiesterase inhibitor | • Dipyridamole<br>• Cilostazol | |
| **Thrombolytics**<br>**Rx: arterial & venous Thrombosis** | Plasminogen activators | • Streptokinase<br>• Reteplase<br>• Tenecteplase<br>• Alteplase | |

# XI. ANTIPLATELET DRUGS

## 1. PRECAUTIONS
- Active internal bleeding or bleeding disorder in past 30 days
- History of intracranial hemorrhage or other bleeding,
- Surgical procedure or trauma within 1 month
- Platelet count < 150 000/mm³,
- Hypersensitivity and concomitant use of another GP IIb/IIIa inhibitor.

## 2. ANTIPLATELET DRUGS AND MECHANISM OF ACTION

| DRUGS | MECHASNISM |
|---|---|
| Aspirin | Cyclooxygenase inhibitors |
| Clopidogrel, Prasugrel | ADP receptor inhibitor |
| Cilostazol | Phosphodiesterase inhibitor |
| Abciximab, Tirofiban, Eptifibatide | Glycoprotein IIb/IIIa inhibitors |
| Dipyridamole | Adenosine reuptake inhibitor |

## A. ABCIXIMAB AS A TYPE GIIB/IIIA INHIBITOR SUBSTANCE

### 1. MECHANISM OF ACTION
- Chimeric monoclonal antibody; prevents binding of fibrinogen, vWF to glycoprotein IIb/IIIa receptor sites on platelets.

### 2. INDICATIONS
- For patients with NSTEMI or unstable angina with planned PCI within 24 hours.

### 3. PRECAUTIONS
- Must use with Heparin
- Binds irreversibly platelets.
- Platelet function recovery requires 48 hours (regeneration)
- Readministration may cause hypersensitivity reaction.

### 4. DOSAGE
- **ACS with planned PCI within 24 hours**: 0.25mg/Kg IV bolus (10 to 60 minutes before procedure), then 0.125µg/Kg/min IV infusion for 12 to 24 hours.

**PCI only**: 0.25mg/Kg IV bolus, then 10µg/min IV infusion

## B. EPTIFIBATIDE

### 1. INDICATIONS
- Unstable angina/NSTEMI managed medically, and
- Unstable angina/NSTEMI patients undergoing PCI.

### 2. ACTIONS/PRECAUTIONS
- Platelet function recovers within 4 to 48 hours after discontinuation.

### 3. DOSAGE:
- **ACS**
  - 180µg/Kg IV bolus over 1-2 min, then 2µg/Kg/min IV infusion for 72 to 96hours.
- **PCI**
  - 180µg/Kg IV bolus over 1-2 min, then begin 2µg/Kg/min IV infusion, then repeat bolus in 10 minutes.
  - Maximum dose (121kg patient) for ACS/PCI: 22.6mg bolus; 15mg/h infusion.
  - Adjust dose if creatinine clearance < 50ml/min.

## C. TIROFIBAN

### 1. INDICATIONS AND PRECAUTIONS: see Eptifibatide
### 2. DOSAGE:
- **ACS or PCI:**
  - 0.4µg/Kg/min IV for 30minutes then 0.1µg/kg/min IV infusion for 48 to 96hours.
  - Adjust dose if creatinine clearance < 30ml/min.

# D. ASPIRIN

## 1. MECHANISM OF ACTION

- *Inhibits synthesis of prostaglandin by cyclooxygenase;*
- *Inhibits platelet aggregation; has antipyretic and analgesic activity.*
- *COX-1 is responsible for the formation of Prostaglandin H2 (PG H2), the precursor of Thromboxane $A_2$ ($TXA_2$).*
- *The non-linear relationship between inactivation of platelet COX-1 and inhibition of $TXA_2$-dependent platelet function by low-dose aspirin (Aspirin do not directly inhibit TXA2).*

## 2. ADVERSE EFFECTS

- Angioedema, Bronchospasm, CNS alteration, Hearing loss, Nausea
- Dermatologic problems, GI pain, ulceration, bleeding, Hepatotoxicity,
- Platelet aggregation inhibition, Premature hemolysis,
- Pulmonary edema (salicylate-induced, noncardiogenic),
- Renal damage.

## 3. CONTRAINDICATIONS

- Hypersensitivity to aspirin or NSAIDs.
- Aspirin-associated hypersensitivity reactions include aspirin-induced urticaria, aspirin-intolerant asthma.
- Allergy to tartrazine dye.

**Absolute**

- Bleeding GI ulcers, hemolytic anemia from pyruvate kinase (PK) and glucose-6-phosphate dehydrogenase (G6PD) deficiency, hemophilia,
- Hemorrhagic diathesis, hemorrhoids, lactating mother, nasal polyps associated with asthma, sarcoidosis, thrombocytopenia, ulcerative colitis.

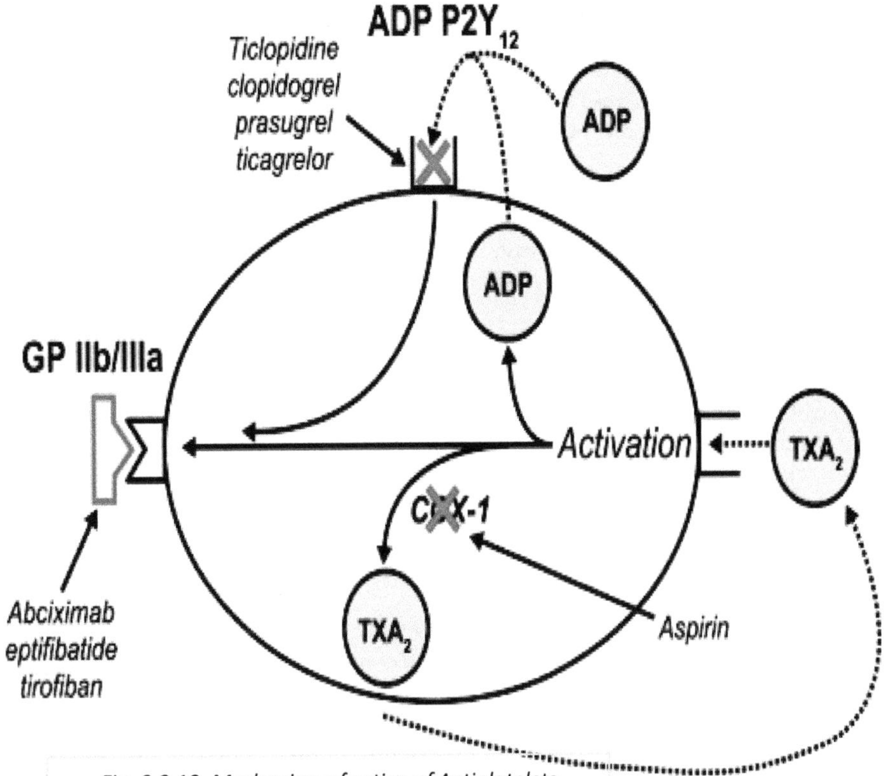

**Relative**

- Appendicitis, asthma (bronchial), chronic diarrhea,
- Bowel outlet obstruction (for enteric-coated formulations), dehydration, erosive gastritis, hypoparathyroidism

Fig. 3.3.19. Mechanism of action of Antiplatelets

## 4. CAUTIONS

- *Ethanol use may increase bleeding*
- *Discontinue therapy if tinnitus develops.*
- *Not indicated for children with viral illness: Use of salicylates in pediatric patients with varicella or influenzalike illness is associated with increased incidence of Reye syndrome.*

# E. CLOPIDOGREL (PLAVIX)

## 1. MECHANISM OF ACTION

- Inhibitor of adenosine diphosphate (ADP)-induced pathway for platelet aggregation.

## 2. PRECAUTIONS/ CONTRAINDICATIONS

- Do not administer to patients with active pathologic bleeding (eg, peptic ulcer).
- Use with caution in patients with risk of bleeding.
- Use with caution in the presence of hepatic impairement.
- DO NOT ADMINISTER IN ACS IF CABG PLANNED WITHIN 5 TO 7 DAYS.

## 3. DOSAGE

- Initial dose 300mg PO, followed by 75mg PO once daily for 1 to 9 months, full effects will not develop for several days.

# XII. MYOCARDIAL INFARCTION & FIBRINOLYSIS

## 1. INDICATIONS

- For cardiac Arrest: insufficient evidence to recommend routine use.
- For AMI in adults:
  - ST elevation (>1mm in ≥2 contiguous leads) or new or presumably new LBBB.
  - In context of signs and symptoms of AMI.
  - Time from onset of symptoms ≤ 12 hours.
- For Acute ischemic Stroke (AIS):
- Alteplase is the only fibrinolytic agent approved for acute Ischemic Stroke
  - Sudden onset of focal neurologic deficits or alterations in consciousness (eg, facial droop, arm drift, abnormal speech)
  - Absence of variable or rapidly improving neurologic deficits.
  - Alteplase can be started in <3 hours from symptom onset.

## 2. PRECAUTIONS

- Active internal bleeding (except menses) within 21days.
- History of cerebrovascular, intracranial, or intraspinal event within 3 months (stroke, arteriovenous malformation, neoplasm, aneurysm, recent trauma, recent surgery).
- Major surgery or serious trauma within 14 days.
- Aortic dissection, Severe, uncontrolled hypertension.
- Known bleeding disorders.
- Prolonged CPR with evidence of thoracic trauma.
- Lumbar puncture within 7 days.
- Recent arterial puncture at noncompressible site.
- During the first 24hours of fibrinolytic therapy for ischemic stroke, do not administer **aspirin or heparin.**

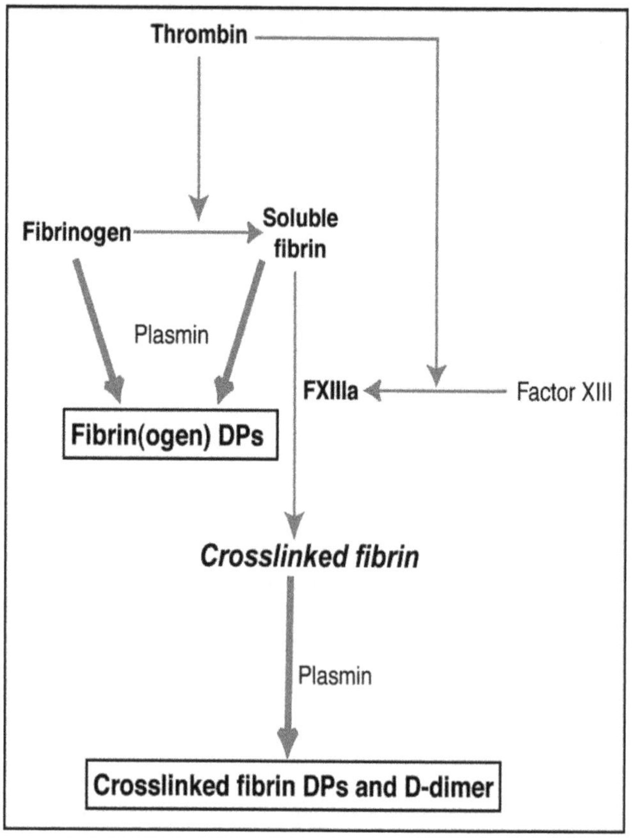

## 3. DOSAGE

- For all 4 agents, use 2 peripheral IV lines, one line exclusively for fibrinolytic administration.

Fig. 3.3.20. Fibrinolytic pathway

## A. ALTEPLASE, recombinant (tpa)

- Recommended total dose is based on patient's weight.
- For AMI the total dose should not exceed 100mg;
- For acute Ischemic stroke the total dose should not exceed 90mg.
- Note that there is a dose regimen for STEMI patients and different regimen for AIS.
- **For AMI:**
  - Accelerated infusion (1.5 hours)
  - Give 15mg IV bolus
  - Then 0.75mg/Kg over next 30 minutes (not to exceed 50mg).
  - Then 0.5mg/Kg over 60 minutes (not to exceed 35mg).
- **For AIS:**
  - Give 0.9 mg/kg (maximum 90mg) infused over 60minutes.
  - Give 10% of the total dose as an initial IV bolus over 1 minute.
  - Give the remaining 90% over the next 60 minutes.

## B. STREPTOKINASE

### 1. MECHANISM OF ACTION

- Streptokinase is a bacterial enzyme secreted by many species of beta-hemolytic Streptococcus bacteria. Streptokinase binds to the protein plasminogen to form an activator complex.
- This complex then cleaves other plasminogen molecules to the active proteolytic form, plasmin. The increased plasmin levels in the blood accelerate fibrinolysis and the dissolution of the blood clot, reducing vessel occlusion and improving blood flow.

### 2. ADMINISTRATION

- The normal intravenous infusion dose for a myocardial infarction patient is 1,500,000 IUs in 45 mL, administered intravenously over 1 hour with an infusion pump.

## C. TENECTEPLASE
### 1. MECHANISM OF ACTION
- Genetically engineered variant of alteplase with multiple point mutations of tPA (tissue plasminogen activator) molecule resulting in longer plasma half-life, enhanced fibrin specificity, & increased resistance to inactivation by plasminogen activator inhibitor 1 (PAI-1) compared to alteplase.
- Promotes thrombolysis by converting plasminogen to plasmin which degrades fibrin & fibrinogen.

### 2. DOSING FORMS
### a. Acute MI
○ Administer ASAP (within 30 minutes) after onset of acute MI
○ 30-50 mg IV bolus over 5 sec once (based on weight).
   - **<60 kg: 30 mg**
   - **60-70 kg: 35 mg**
   - **70-80 kg: 40 mg**
   - **80-90 kg: 45 mg**
   - **>90 kg: 50 mg**

## D. RETEPLASE
### 1. MECHANISM OF ACTION
- Reteplase is the r-PA (recombinant plasminogen activator) with nonglycosylated deletion mutant of wild-type tissue plasminogen activator (tPA); has less high-affinity fibrin binding, longer half-life, & greater thrombolytic potency than tPA.
- Promotes thrombolysis by converting plasminogen to plasmin which degrades fibrin & fibrinogen.

### 2. DOSAGE
- Give first 10U IV bolus over 2 minutes.
- 30 minutes later give second 10U IV bolus over 2 minutes. (Give NS flush before and after each bolus.)
- Give **heparin and aspirin conjunctively.**

| TRANEXAMIC ACID |
| --- |
| • Stops conversion of plasminogen to plasmin |
| • Stops plasmin activity |
| • Binds to both plasminogen and plasmin |

| FONDAPARINUX |
| --- |
| • Inactivates Factor Xa |
| • Works via anti-thrombin |
| • Selective for factor Xa |

# XIII. LIPID-REGULATING DRUGS

## I. STATINS
### GENERAL CONTRAINDICATIONS AND CAUTIONS
- Hypersensitivity to the individual statin or to any of the excipients.
- Active liver disease (AST or ALT level > 100iu/L) or unexplained persistent isolated elevations of serum transaminases.
- Statin use is contraindicated in both pregnancy and lactation.
- Consideration should be given to delaying statin therapy or addressing contraceptive needs in women of child-bearing age
- Concomitant use of fibrates and statins increases the risk of muscle toxicity.
- The co-administration of statins and nicotinic acid should be used with caution.
- Patients with excess alcohol intake (more than 50 units per week)

### SIDE -EFFECTS
○ Although side effects can vary between different statins, common side effects (which affect up to 1 in 10 people) include:
   - Nosebleeds, sore throat, a runny or blocked nose (non-allergic rhinitis)
   - Headache, nausea
   - Problems with the digestive system, such as constipation, diarrhoea, indigestion or flatulence.
   - Muscle and joint pain
   - Increased blood sugar level (hyperglycaemia)
   - An increased risk of diabetes

# Past Asked Questions

### True and False

| | |
|---|---|
| Flecanaide must be given by rapid infusion | F |
| Adenosine is contraindicated in patients using beta-blockades | F |
| Flecainide has a positive inotropic effect | F |
| Amiodarone decreases the QT interval | F |

### Digoxin is contraindicated in which of the following conditions?

| | |
|---|---|
| A stable patient with atrial fibrillation and a ventricular rate of 165/min | F |
| Congestive cardiac failure | F |
| Wolff-Parkinson-White syndrome | T |
| Myocardial infarction | T |

### The following are features of acute digoxin toxicity

| | |
|---|---|
| Hyperkalaemia | T |
| Nausea and vomiting | T |
| Atrial tachycardia | T |
| Maximal cardiotoxicity at 6hrs post ingestion | F |

### Furosemide has the following actions

| | |
|---|---|
| Increases glomerular filtration of sodium and water | T |
| Inhibition of Na+/K+/2Cl- co-transporters in the ascending limb of the loop of Henle | T |
| Stimulates the Na-CL co-transporter in the distal collecting duct | F |
| Venous vasodilatation | T |

### Side effects of bendroflumethiazide include

| | |
|---|---|
| Hyperglycaemia | T |
| Hyponatraemia | T |
| Ototoxicity | F |
| Pancreatitis | T |

### True and False

| | |
|---|---|
| Adrenaline has both alpha and beta-adrenergic effects | T |
| Dobutamine is used for its vasopressor effects | F |
| Ligands are receptor molecules expressed on cell walls | F |
| The effect of Atropine in the Heart is by stimulating vagus nerve | F |
| Noradrenaline has greater effect on alpha receptors | T |
| Tirofiban stops platelet activation by inhibiting GPIIa/IIIb | F |
| Rivaroxaban is a synthetic indirect inhibitor of factor Xa | F |

### A 60yr old man with hypertension takes captopril 5mg daily presents to the ED with angioedema of the lips and tongue. Which of the following occur in ACE inhibitor induced angioedema?

| | |
|---|---|
| Angiotensin I is converted to angiotensin II (patient is on ACE Inhibitor) | F |
| IgE mediated mast cell degranulation and histamine release occurs | F |
| Bradykinin metabolism is inhibited | T |
| Inflammatory mediators cause increased vascular permeability in mucosal tissues | T |

### The following commonly prescribed Drugs prolongs the INR in patients on warfarin

| | |
|---|---|
| Allopurinol | T |
| Phenytoin | F |
| Clarithromycin | T |
| Codeine phosphate | F |
| Amiodarone | T |
| Carbamazepine | F |

### The following commonly prescribed drugs prolong the INR in patients on warfarin

| | |
|---|---|
| Fluconazole | T |
| Phenytoin | F |
| Clarithromycin | T |
| Codeine phosphate | F |
| St John's wort | F |

### The following are true of platelet aggregation in thrombosis:

| | |
|---|---|
| TX A2 stimulates platelet activation? | T |
| Glucoprotein IIb/IIIa receptors bind activated platelet to the walls of damaged blood vessels? | F |
| Activated platelets express Von Willebrand's factor on their surface membrane | F |
| Clopidogrel and prasugrel inversibly block platelet ADP receptors | T |

# Section 4: Respiratory Pharmacology

## A.  SELECTIVE BETA-2 AGONISTS

### I.  SALBUTAMOL

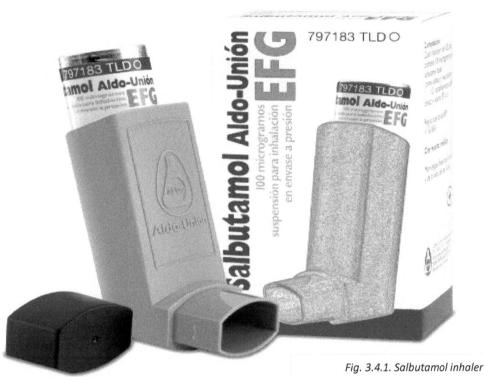

*Fig. 3.4.1. Salbutamol inhaler*

#### 1. MECHANISM OF ACTION
- Beta2 receptor agonist with some beta1 activity;
- Relaxes bronchial smooth muscle with little effect on heart rate.

#### 2. INDICATIONS
- Acute asthma attack where normal inhaler failed to relieve symptoms
- Expiratory wheezes associated with allergy, anaphylaxis, some inhalation...
- Exacerbation COPD
- Hyperkalaemia
- Shortness of breath in patients with severe breathing difficulty due to LV failure

#### 3. SIDE EFFECTS
- Tremor (20%), Nervousness in children aged 2-6 years (20%), Insomnia in children aged 6-12 years receiving 4-12 mg q12hr (11%).
- Tachycardia, Palpitations, Headache
- Peripheral vasodilatation

#### 4. CONTRAINDICATIONS
- None in the emergency situation

#### 5. CAUTIONS
- Risk of hypokalemia (usually transient). Late pregnancy (may relax uterus)
- Salbutamol should be administered cautiously to patients suffering from hyperthyroidism, cardiovascular disease and diabetes.
- Use face mask in children <4 years. Salbutamol will enhance the activity of other β2 sympathomimetics.
- Beta-receptor blocking agents such as propranolol inhibit the activity of salbutamol.
- Severe hypertension may occur in patients on beta-blockers and half dose should be used unless there is profound hypertension.
- The effects of salbutamol may be enhanced by concomitant administration of aminophylline or other xanthines.

# B. ANTIMUSCARINICS

## I. IPRATROPIUM

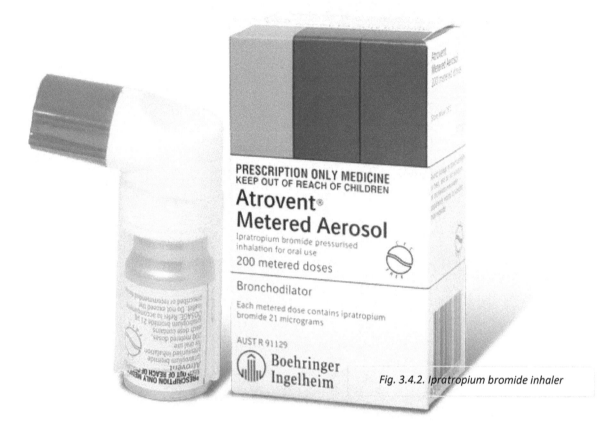

*Fig. 3.4.2. Ipratropium bromide inhaler*

### 1. MECHANISM OF ACTION

- Ipratropium bromide is an anticholinergic (parasympatholytic) agent.
- Anticholinergics prevent the increases in intracellular concentration of cyclic guanosine monophosphate (cyclic GMP) which are caused by interaction of acetylcholine with the muscarinic receptor on bronchial smooth muscle.

### 2. DOSING CONSIDERATIONS

- In treatment of acute asthma exacerbation with inhaler, short-acting beta agonist (SABA) must be coadministered.
- In treatment of allergic rhinitis, do not use for >3 weeks.
- Interaction of acetylcholine with muscarinic receptors on bronchial smooth muscle.

### 3. ADVERSE EFFECTS

- Bronchitis (10-23%), chronic obstructive pulmonary disease (COPD) exacerbation (8-23%), Sinusitis (1-14%)
- Cardiovascular: Hypotension, palpitations, tachycardia
- General: Dry throat, throat irritation.
- Gastrointestinal (GI): Constipation, stomatitis, mouth edema.
- Sensory: Narrow-angle glaucoma, glaucoma, halo vision, conjunctival hyperemia, corneal edema, mydriasis, acute eye pain, blurry vision.
- Respiratory: Bronchospasm, including paradoxical bronchospasm.
- Renal: Urinary retention

### 4. CONTRAINDICATIONS

- Documented hypersensitivity to ipratropium.
- Atropine or derivatives.

### 5. CAUTIONS

- Use for maintenance treatment only; should not be used as rescue therapy.
- May cause life-threatening paradoxical bronchospasm or hypersensitivity reactions (skin rash, pruritus, angioedema, urticaria/giant urticaria, laryngospasm); discontinue immediately, and use alternative treatment.
- May cause urinary retention; use with caution in patients with benign prostatic hyperplasia (BPH) or bladder-neck obstruction.
- May worsen narrow-angle glaucoma. Contact with eye can cause burning, stinging, mydriasis, visual halos.

# C. THEOPHYLLINE

## I. AMINOPHYLLINE

### 1. MECHANISM OF ACTION
- Methylxanthine; directly relaxes smooth muscles of respiratory tract

### 2. DOSING FORMS
- Acute Bronchospasm

### 3. CONTRAINDICATIONS
- Hypersensitivity,
- Active peptic ulcer disease,
- Underlying uncontrolled seizure disorder

### 4. SIDE EFFECTS
- Peak serum concentration <20 mcg/mL
- Central nervous system excitement, headache, insomnia, irritability, restlessness, seizure
- Diarrhea, nausea, vomiting
- Diuresis (transient), Exfoliative dermatitis, Skeletal muscle tremors
- Tachycardia, flutter
- Peak serum concentration >30 mcg/mL
- Acute myocardial infarction
- Seizures (resistant to anticonvulsants)
- Urinary retention

### 5. PREGNANCY CATEGORY: C
- Lactation: Theophylline is excreted into breast milk

# D. CORTICOSTEROIDS

## I. HYDROCORTISONE

### 1. MECHANISM OF ACTION
- Glucocorticoid; elicits mild mineralocorticoid activity and moderate anti-inflammatory effects;
- Controls or prevents inflammation by controlling rate of protein synthesis, suppressing migration of polymorphonuclear leukocytes (PMNs) and fibroblasts, and reversing capillary permeability.

### 2. ADVERSE EFFECTS
- Acne, Adrenal suppression, Arthralgia, Bladder dysfunction,
- Cardiomegaly, Cataract, Cushing syndrome, Delayed wound healing, Delirium,
- Depression, Diabetes mellitus, Epistaxis, Fat embolism,
- Hirsutism, Hyperglycemia, Hypokalemic alkalosis,
- Myopathy, Osteoporosis, Pseudotumor cerebri

### 3. CONTRAINDICATIONS
- Idiopathic thrombocytopenic purpura
- Intrathecal administration (injection)
- Documented hypersensitivity.
- Administration of live or live-attenuated vaccines is contraindicated in patients receiving immunosuppressive doses of corticosteroids.

### 4. CAUTIONS
- Patients receiving corticosteroids should avoid chickenpox or measles-infected persons if unvaccinated.
- Latent tuberculosis may be reactivated (patients with positive tuberculin test should be monitored).
- Prolonged corticosteroid use may result in elevated intraocular pressure, glaucoma, or cataracts.
- Killed or inactivated vaccines may be administered; however, the response to such vaccines cannot be predicted.
- Epidural injection.

### 5. PREGNANCY & LACTATION
- Pregnancy category: C
- Lactation: Drug enters breast milk; use with caution.

# II. BECLOMETHASONE

## 1. MECHANISM OF ACTION
- Potent anti-inflammatory glucocorticoid;
- Inhibits inflammatory cells and release of inflammatory mediators.

## 2. INDICATION
- Chronic Asthma

## 3. ADVERSE EFFECTS
- Pharyngitis (5-27%), Headache (8-25%), URI (5-11%)

## 4. CONTRAINDICATIONS
- Hypersensitivity.
- Primary treatment of status asthmaticus, acute bronchospasm.

## 5. CAUTIONS
- Respiratory tract TB; Untreated fungal or bacterial infections.
- Viral/parasitic infections, Ocular herpes simplex
- Nasal septum perforation, Wheezing, Cataracts, Glaucoma, Increased IOP.
- May decrease growth velocity in children. Risk of infections of nose and pharynx, including Candida albicans; must rinse mouth after inhalation to reduce risk. Risk of bronchospasm with immediate increase in wheezing after administration;
- Excessive use may suppress HPA function; monitor closely, especially postoperatively or during periods of stress.
- Switching from systemic steroids to therapy may unmask allergic conditions (eg, conjunctivitis, eczema, and rhinitis).
- Prolonged corticosteroid use may result in elevated IOP, glaucoma, and/or cataracts.
- Not a bronchodilator; should not be administered for rapid relief of acute bronchospasm.

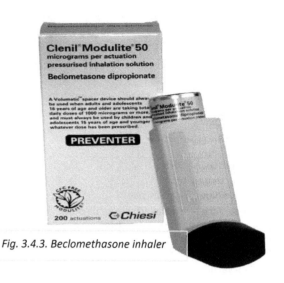

*Fig. 3.4.3. Beclomethasone inhaler*

# III. DEXAMETHASONE

## 1. CLINICAL PHARMACOLOGY
- Dexamethasone is a glucorticoid which is 25 times more potent than hydrocortisone with respect to its glucocorticoid activity;
- It has no mineralocorticoid effect.

## 2. INDICATIONS
- Cerebral oedema
- Upper airway oedema
- Nausea and vomiting
- Croup
- Other inflammatory conditions

## 3. DOSAGE:
- IV/PO:
  - *Cerebral oedema:* 8-16mg stat, then 4-8mg 4 hourly reducing over 3-5 days to 2mg 8 to 12 hourly
  - Nausea: 4-8mg IV stat
  - *Adult airway oedema:* 8-16mg 1hr pre extubation (may be repeated 8 hourly)
- **Dosage in paediatrics:**
- **IV / PO:**
  - *Cerebral oedema:* 0.25-1mg/kg stat then 0.1-0.2mg/kg 4 hourly reducing over 3-5 days to 0.05mg/kg 8-12 hourly
  - Severe croup or extubation stridor: 0.6mg/kg stat IV, then 1mg/kg prednisolone 8-12 hourly

## 4. CONTRAINDICATIONS
- Systemic fungal infections
- Hypersensitivity to dexamethasone or any component of the product

## 5. WARNINGS
- Anaphylaxis: Dexamethasone sodium phosphate injection contains sodium bisulfite.
- Exacerbation of fungal infections
- Relative steroid deficiency: Drug-induced secondary adrenocortical insufficiency may result from too rapid withdrawal of corticosteroids and may be minimized by gradual reduction of dosage.
- Masking of signs of infection

# SECTION 5: CENTRAL NERVOUS SYSTEM

## A. HYPNOTICS & ANXIOLYTICS

### I. DIAZEPAM

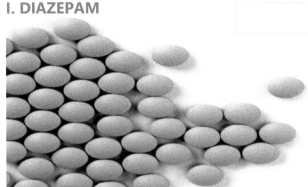

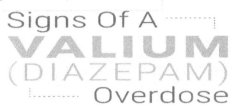

Fig. 3.5.1. Diazepam

Valium (diazepam), within the class of benzodiazepine drugs, is a central nervous system depressant that may cause addiction, overdose, and even death

#### 1. MECHANISM OF ACTION
- Modulates postsynaptic effects of GABA-A transmission, resulting in an increase in presynaptic inhibition.
- As with other benzodiazepines it has anticonvulsant, anxiolytic, sedative and muscle relaxant properties.

#### 2. PHARMACOLOGY
- Bioavailability: 90%
- Duration: Variable, dependent on dose and frequency (PO [hypnotic action]); 15-60 min (IV [sedative action])
- Peak plasma time: 30-90 min (PO), 5-90 min (PR)
- Metabolized by hepatic P450 enzymes
- Metabolites: N-desmethyldiazepam, 3-hydroxdiazepam, oxazepam
- Half-life: 20-70 hr (active metabolite)
- Excretion: Urine

#### 3. ADVERSE EFFECTS
- Ataxia (3%), Euphoria (3%, rectal gel), Incoordination (3%, rectal gel), Somnolence (>1%),
- Rash (3%, rectal gel), Diarrhea (4%, rectal gel).
**Common**
- Hypotension, Fatigue, Muscle weakness, Respiratory depression.
- Urinary retention, Depression, Incontinence, Blurred vision.
- Dysarthria, Headache, Skin rash, Changes in salivation.
**Serious**
- Neutropenia, Jaundice
- Local effects: Pain, swelling, thrombophlebitis, carpal tunnel syndrome, tissue necrosis.

#### 4. INDICATIONS
- Agitation
- Alcohol and benzodiazepine withdrawal
- Seizures

#### 5. CONTRAINDICATIONS
- Documented hypersensitivity
- Acute alcohol intoxication
- Myasthenia gravis, Narrow angle glaucoma (questionable)
- Severe respiratory depression, Depressed neuroses, psychotic reactions, Breastfeeding, Sleep apnea
- Children <6 months

#### 6. CAUTIONS
- Use caution in COPD, sleep apnea, renal/hepatic disease, open-angle glaucoma (questionable),
- Depression, suicide ideation, impaired gag reflex, history of drug abuse.
- Anterograde amnesia reported with benzodiazepine use. Avoid extravasation with IV dosing.
- Paradoxical reactions may occur including hallucinations, aggressive behavior, and psychoses; dinscontinue use if reactions occur.
- Abrupt withdrawal may result in temporary increase of seizures. Reduce opiate dose one-third when diazepam is added.

## II. CHLORDIAZEPOXIDE

### 1. MECHANISM OF ACTION

- Binds receptors at several sites within the CNS, including the limbic system and reticular formation.
- Effects may be mediated through the GABA receptor system.
- Increase in neuronal membrane permeability to chloride ions enhances the inhibitory effects of GABA; the shift in chloride ions causes hyperpolarization (less excitability) and stabilization of the neuronal membrane.

### 2. ADVERSE EFFECTS

- Ataxia, Drowsiness, Memory impairment, Sedation,
- Muscle weakness, Rash, Decreased libido, Menstrual disorders,
- Xerostomia, Salivation decreased, Increased/decreased appetite,
- Weight gain/loss, Micturition difficulties.

### 3. CONTRAINDICATIONS

- See Diazepam

### 4. CAUTIONS

- Patient should be observed for up to 3 hours following administration.
- Anterograde amnesia associated with treatment
- Use caution in renal and hepatic impairment.
- Use caution in respiratory disease (COPD), sleep apnea, porphyria, open-angle glaucoma (questionable), depression, suicidal ideation, impaired gag reflex.
- May impair ability to perform hazardous tasks.
- Paradoxical reactions, including hyperactive or aggressive behavior, reported.

## III. LORAZEPAM

### 1. MECHANISM OF ACTION

- Sedative hypnotic with short onset of effects and relatively long half-life;
- By increasing the action of gamma-aminobutyric acid (GABA), which is a major inhibitory neurotransmitter in the brain, lorazepam may depress all levels of the CNS, including limbic and reticular formation.

### 2. PHARMACOLOGY

- Onset: 1-3 min (IV in sedation); 15-30 min (IM in hypnosis)
- Duration: Up to 8 hr
- Peak plasma time: 2 hr (PO); <3 hr (IM)
- Metabolites: Inactive
- Undergoes glucuronic acid conjugation
- Half-life: 18 hr (children 2-12 years); 42 hr (neonates); 28 hr (adolescents); 18 hr (end stage renal disease); 14 hr (adults)
- Excretion: Urine (88% mainly as inactive metabolites); feces (7%)

### 3. CONTRAINDICATIONS

- Documented hypersensitivity
- Acute narrow angle glaucoma
- Intra-arterial administration
- Severe respiratory depression
- Sleep apnea

### 4. CAUTIONS

- Not recommended for use in patients with primary depressive disorder or psychosis.
- Risk of physical and psychological dependence (alcohol or drug abuse).
- Use caution in patients with history of suicide attempt or drug abuse.
- Do not withdraw abruptly after prolonged use; terminate dosage gradually.
- Use caution in patients with impaired gag reflex
- Anterograde amnesia reported with use. Use caution in patients with respiratory disease, including COPD or sleep apnea.

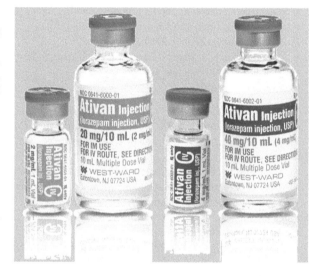

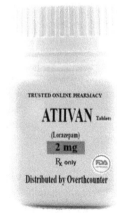

*Fig. 3.5.2. Lorazepam*

# B. ANTIPSYCHOTICS

## I. TYPICAL ANTIPSYCHOTICS

- First-generation antipsychotics are strong dopamine D2 antagonists.
- However, each drug in this class has various effects on other receptors, such as serotonin type 2 (5-HT2), alpha1, histaminic, and muscarinic receptors. First-generation antipsychotics have a high rate of extrapyramidal side effects, including rigidity, bradykinesia, dystonias, tremor, and akathisia.
- Neuroleptic malignant syndrome (NMS) can occur with these agents.
- Tardive dyskinesia (involuntary movements in the face and extremities) is another adverse effect that can occur with first-generation antipsychotics.

### 1. CHLORPROMAZINE

- Chlorpromazine is a phenothiazine antipsychotic that is a dopamine D2 receptor antagonist.
- It was the first conventional antipsychotic developed and is still in wide use for treatment of schizophrenia.
- Chlorpromazine is a low-potency medication and is associated with sedation and weight gain.

### 2. FLUPHENAZINE (Modecate, Moditen)

- Fluphenazine is a high-potency typical antipsychotic that blocks postsynaptic dopaminergic D1 and D2 receptors.
- It has some alpha-adrenergic and anticholinergic effects. Fluphenazine is clinically comparable to haloperidol, a first-generation antipsychotic with similar potency, route of administration, side effects, and efficacy.

### 3. HALOPERIDOL (Haldol, Haldol Decanoate)

- Haloperidol is a dopamine D2 antagonist noted for high potency and low potential for causing orthostasis.
- The drawback is the high potential for extrapyramidal symptoms or dystonia.
- Haloperidol can interact with CYP3A4 and CYP2D6 inhibitors and inducers.
- It also can interact with drugs that prolong QTc intervals.
- *Other drugs include*: Perphenazine, Thiothixene, Trifluoperazine

## II. ATYPICAL ANTIPSYCHOTICS

- Second-generation antipsychotics, with the exception of aripiprazole, are dopamine D2 antagonists, but are associated with lower rates of extrapyramidal adverse effects and tardive dyskinesia than the first-generation antipsychotics.
- However, they have higher rates of metabolic adverse effects and weight gain.

### 1. CLOZAPINE (Clozaril, FazaClo)

- Clozapine is the oldest atypical antipsychotic agent and probably the most effective.
- Because it is associated with about a **1% risk of agranulocytosis ($\downarrow$WCC):**
  - ✓ patients must undergo white blood cell (WBC) count monitoring every week for the first 6 months (the period of greatest risk),
  - ✓ Then every 2 weeks for 6 months, and finally every 4 weeks, as long as the absolute neutrophil count (ANC) is normal.
  - ✓ If the ANC drops, a strict protocol of monitoring and possibly medication cessation must then be followed.
- Clozapine is an antagonist at adrenergic, cholinergic, histaminergic, and serotonergic receptors.
- It has some dopamine D2 antagonism and high D4 affinity.
- **Side effects:**
  - o The anticholinergic adverse effects like:
    - ▪ Sedation, drooling, constipation.
  - o Possible cardiac effects.

### 2. OLANZAPINE

- Olanzapine is a selective monoaminergic antagonist at serotonin, dopamine D1-4, muscarinic, histamine H1, and alpha1-adrenergic receptors.
- The most common side effects of olanzapine include weight gain, sedation, akathisia, hypotension, dry mouth, and constipation.

### 3. QUETIAPINE (Seroquel)

- Quetiapine may act by antagonizing dopamine and serotonin receptors.
- It is used for treatment of schizophrenia.
- Major adverse effects include sedation, orthostatic hypotension, akathisia, dry mouth, and weight gain.

### 4. RISPERIDONE (Risperdal)

- Risperidone has both dopamine D2 and serotonin 5-HT2 antagonism.
- It has few anticholinergic effects.
- Primary adverse effects of risperidone include mild sedation, hypotension, akathisia, increase in prolactin, and weight gain.

- *Other drugs include*:
  - Iloperidone (Fanapt)
  - Asenapine (Saphris)
  - Lurasidone (Latuda)
  - Paliperidone (Invega)
  - Ziprasidone (Geodon)
  - Cariprazine (Vraylar)
  - Loxapine inhaled (Loxitane)

## NEUROLEPTIC MALIGNANT SYNDROME

- NMS is characterized by altered mental status, muscle rigidity, hyperthermia (T° > 38° C and often > 40° C) and autonomic hyperactivity that occur when certain neuroleptic drugs are used.
- Symptoms begin most often during the first 2 weeks of treatment but may occur earlier or after many years.
- **Malignant hyperthermia and withdrawal of intrathecal baclofen** can cause findings similar to those of neuroleptic malignant syndrome, but they are usually easily differentiated by history.
- **Serotonin Syndrome** can often be differentiated from NMS by use of an SSRI or other serotonergic drug (and often developing within 24 h of administration of its drug trigger) and hyperreflexia.
- Treatment is rapid cooling, control of agitation, and other aggressive supportive measures.
- Among patients taking neuroleptic drugs, about 0.02 to 3% develop neuroleptic malignant syndrome. Patients of all ages can be affected.

### DRUGS CAUSING NMS

| Atypical Antipsychotics | Typical Antipsychotics | Antiemetics |
|---|---|---|
| Chlorpromazine | Aripiprazole | Domperidone |
| Fluphenazine | Clozapine | Droperidol |
| Haloperidol | Olanzapine | Metoclopramide |
| Perphenazine | Paliperidone | Prochlorperazine |
| Thioridazine | Quetiapine | Promethazine |
| Thiothixene | Risperidone | |
| Trifluoperazine | Ziprasidone | |

# III. EXTRAPYRAMIDAL SIDE EFFECTS

## 1. AKATHISIA

- Akathisia is fundamentally a subjective disorder characterized by a desire to be in constant motion resulting in an inability to sit still and a compulsion to move.

**Treatment of Akathisia:**

- The treatment of choice for this poorly understood phenomenon is to lower the dosage of the antipsychotic. This strategy, however, is clinically unrealistic in many acutely ill psychiatric patients. This is a side effect that is not typically responsive to the addition of anticholinergic agents.
- The alpha-2 agonist **clonidine** has been consistently associated with efficacy.

## 2. ACUTE DYSTONIA

- A state of abnormal muscle tone resulting in muscular spasm and abnormal posture.
- The muscles of the trunk, shoulders, and neck go into spasm, so that the head and limbs are held in unnatural positions.

**Treatment of Dystonia:**

- Acute dystonias respond remarkably well to anti-Parkinsonian agents. Intramuscular **Benztropine or Diphenhydramine** will generally produce complete resolution in 20 to 30 minutes.
- The dose can be repeated after 30 minutes if complete recovery does not occur. Oral anticholinergics may be used in milder cases.

## 3. TARDIVE DYSTONIA

- Tardive dystonia is a more severely disabling condition, and symptoms are more sustained compared to the acute form, distinguishable only by the duration. The condition is apparently identical to idiopathic torsion dystonia associated with **Huntington's disease and Wilson's disease**, and there is some overlap with the features of Tardive Dyskinesia, with which it may coexist.

**Treatment of Tardive Dystonia:**

- There are no controlled studies regarding treatment for this condition. Some patients have responded to high doses of **Trihexyphenydyl 60 to 80mg/day**. Dopamine depleting agents, such as **Tetrabenazine or Reserpine**, have been used.
- **Procyclidine** is an anticholinergic drug principally used for the treatment of drug-induced Parkinsonism, akathisia and acute dystonia; Parkinson disease; and idiopathic or secondary dystonia.
- Large doses of **clonazepam, baclofen, or benzodiazepines** have given mixed results.
- Tardive dystonia responds to **Deep Brain Stimulation**. This is particularly useful for patients with focal dystonia. **The globus pallidus internus** has emerged as the most promising target for dystonia.

## 4. TARDIVE DYSKINESIA

- Tardive dyskinesia (TD) is the main late onset condition among the EPSEs.
- These are involuntary movements, mainly of the tongue and mouth with twisting of the tongue, chewing, and grimacing movements of the face.
- It develops after chronic exposure to antipsychotics for about six months.

**Treatment of TD:**

- When clinically appropriate, pharmacologic interventions may be considered for patients who are developing signs of TD. The two main strategies are:
  - o  Discontinuation of the offending drug
  - o  Switching from a first to a second generation antipsychotic drug
- For patients with a diagnosis of TD, additional pharmacologic interventions include the following:
- Use of **benzodiazepines, botulinum toxin injections, valbenazine, or tetrabenazine** to control symptoms of TD
- Paradoxically, resuming treatment with antipsychotic drugs in order to suppress TD
- *Procyclidine should never be used to treat tardive dyskinesia. Not only it is ineffective for this use, it can actually worsen Tardive Dyskinesia.*

## DRUGS CAUSING DYSKINESIA: (MRCEM Part A Dec 2015)

- TD can be caused by long-term treatment with dopamine antagonists.
- It can also be caused by both high-potency and low-potency traditional neuroleptics, including long-acting depot formulations (eg, **Decanoate and Enanthate**).
- **Amisulpride** has been associated with TD, but in general, newer atypical antipsychotic agents, including olanzapine and risperidone (and its metabolite Paliperidone), appear to carry less risk of TD.
- The antiemetic **Metoclopramide and Prochlorperazine**, potent $D_2$ dopamine receptor antagonists, may cause TD (in elderly patients).
- TDs have also been reported with the use of **Antihistamines**, **Fluoxetine**, **Amoxapine** (a tricyclic antidepressant) etc.
- **These drugs are:**

| | | | |
|---|---|---|---|
| *Chlorpromazine* | *Flunarizine* | *Phenytoin* | *TCAs* |
| *Fluphenazine* | *Fluoxetine* | *Procyclidine (worsen)* | *Alprazolam* |
| *Haloperidol* | *Sertraline* | *Metoclopramide* | *Bromocriptine* |
| *Perphenazine* | *Carbamazepine* | *Prochlorperazine* | *Levodopa* |
| *Trifluoperazine* | *Phenobarbital* | | |

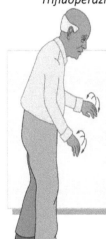

**Pseudoparkinsonism**
- ▲ Stooped posture
- ▲ Shuffling gait
- ▲ Rigidity
- ▲ Bradykinesia
- ▲ Tremors at rest
- ▲ Pill-rolling motion of the hand

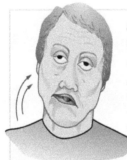

**Acute dystonia**
- ▲ Facial grimacing
- ▲ Involuntary upward eye movement
- ▲ Muscle spasms of the tongue, face, neck, and back (back muscle spasms cause trunk to arch forward)
- ▲ Laryngeal spasms

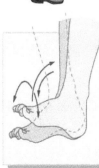

**Akathisia**
- ▲ Restless
- ▲ Trouble standing still
- ▲ Paces the floor
- ▲ Feet in constant motion, rocking back and forth

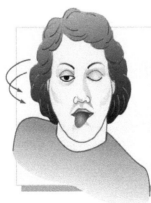

**Tardive dyskinesia**
- ▲ Protrusion and rolling of the tongue
- ▲ Sucking and smacking movements of the lips
- ▲ Chewing motion
- ▲ Facial dyskinesia
- ▲ Involuntary movements of the body and extremities

# C. ANTIMANIC DRUGS

## I. LITHIUM

### 1. MECHANISM OF ACTION

- Inhibits postsynaptic D2 receptor supersensitivity.
- Alters cation transport in nerve and muscle cells and influences reuptake of serotonin or norepinephrine.
- Inhibits phosphatidylinositol cycle second messenger systems.

### 2. INDICATION

- Bipolar Disorder.
- Huntington's disease.

### 3. ADVERSE EFFECTS

- **Leukocytosis (↑WCC** in most patients),
- Extrapyramidal symptoms,
- Electrocardiographic (ECG) changes (Risk of Brugada Syndrome)
- Neurology: Confusion, Coma, Hand tremor, Lethargy, Seizures,
- Renal toxicity
- Polyuria/polydypsia (30-50%), Dry mouth (20-50%), Nausea, vomiting, diarrhea (10-30% initially, 1-10% after 1-2 years of treatment).

### 4. CONTRAINDICATIONS

- Documented hypersensitivity.
- Severe cardiovascular disease.
- Pregnancy in 1st trimester.
- Unstable renal function, sodium depletion, severe dehydration.
- Debilitated patients.

### 5. CAUTIONS

- Cardiovascular disease; reports of possible association between lithium treatment and unmasking of Brugada syndrome.
- Use with caution in patients with thyroid disease.
- Maintain geriatric patients on dosages that produce serum lithium concentrations at lower end of desired range.
- May cause central nervous system (CNS) depression and impair ability to operate heavy machinery.
- Use with caution in patients at risk for suicide.
- Risk of nephrogenic diabetes insipidus.

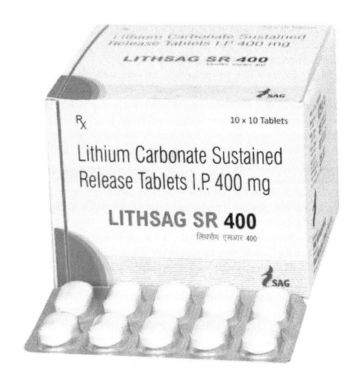

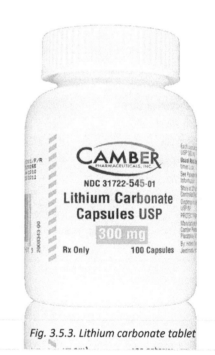

*Fig. 3.5.3. Lithium carbonate tablet*

*Lithium-sensitive patients may experience toxicity symptoms with serum lithium concentrations of 1-1.5 mEq/L. Lithium toxicity is closely related to serum levels and can occur at therapeutic dosages; if manifestations of toxicity occur, discontinue for 24-48 hours, then resume at lower dosage.*

# D. TRICYCLIC ANTIDEPRESSANTS

## TRICYCLIC ANTIDEPRESSANTS:

- Amitriptyline.
- Amoxapine.
- Desipramine (Norpramin)
- Doxepin.
- Imipramine (Tofranil)
- Nortriptyline (Pamelor)
- Protriptyline (Vivactil)
- Trimipramine (Surmontil)

## I. AMITRYPTILINE

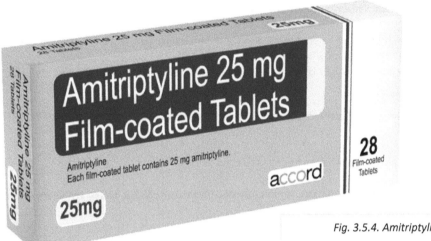

Fig. 3.5.4. Amitriptyline tablet

### 1. MECHANISM OF ACTION
- Neurotransmitter (especially norepinephrine and serotonin) reuptake inhibitor; anticholinergic.

### 2. PHARMACOLOGY
- Peak serum time: 4 hr
- Metabolized by hepatic CYP2C19, CYP3A4
- Metabolites: Nortriptyline
- Half-life: 9-27 hr
- Excretion: Urine (18%), small amounts in feces

### 3. CONTRAINDICATIONS
- Hypersensitivity.
- Acute recovery phase following MI.
- Concurrent use with cisapride.
- *Contraindicated within 14 days of MAOIs*
- *If linezolid or IV methylene blue (MAOIs) must be administered, discontinue serotonergic drug immediately and monitor for CNS toxicity; may resume 24 hr after last linezolid or methylene blue dose, or after 2 weeks of monitoring, whichever comes first.*

### 4. CAUTIONS
- Bone marrow suppression reported.
- Avoid use in narrow-angle glaucoma.
- May cause sedation and impair mental and physical abilities.
- Avoid use with any drugs or conditions that prolong QT interval
- May cause orthostatic hypotension.
- May worsen mania symptoms or precipitate mania in patients with bipolar disorder.
- Clinical worsening and suicidal ideation may occur despite medication in adolescents and young adults (18-24 years).
- Risk of anticholinergic side effects; may cause constipation, urinary retention, blurred vision, and xerostomia.
- Use caution in patients with urinary retention, open-angle glaucoma, BPH, decreased gastrointestinal motility, or paralytic ileus.
- Possibility of EPS and neuroleptic malignant syndrome.

# E. ANALGESICS

## I. OPIOIDS AND THEIR RECEPTORS

- Opioid receptors are members of the G protein-coupled receptors (GPCRs) that act to inhibit adenylate cyclase and thereby reduce intracellular levels of cyclic adenosine monophosphate (cAMP). Opioid receptors are found extensively in the brain and spinal cord, as well as in vascular, gut, lung airway, cardiac, and some immune system cells.
- There are three family members of opioid receptors, with similar protein sequences and structures (Kane et al., 2006): **Mu, Delta, and Kappa Receptors.**
- They are all transmembrane proteins of the rhodopsin family of GPCRs, embedded in the cell membrane and crossing it seven times.
- **The Mu opioid receptors (MOR)** give most of their analgesic effects in the central nervous system, as well as many side effects including sedation, respiratory depression, euphoria, and dependence. Most analgesic opioids are agonists on MOR.
- **The Delta opioid receptors (DOR)** are more prevalent for analgesia in the peripheral nervous system.
- **The Kappa opioid receptors (KOR)** contribute to analgesia in the spine and may exhibit dysphoria and sedation, but do not generally lead to dependence. Some drugs are relatively KOR-specific (Goodman & Gilman, 2011). At the cellular level, all three receptor types act similarly, though their distribution in the body and sensitivity to various opioid drugs leads to markedly different pharmacologic reactions. In addition, all three of these subtypes are present in some tissues at various levels, further modulating the responses.
- In the membrane, opiate receptors can form both homo- and heterodimers, altering the pharmacologic properties of the respective receptors. For example, DORs can form heterodimers with both KORs and MORs.
- Thus, MOR-DOR and DOR-KOR heterodimers show less affinity for highly selective agonists and reduced receptor recycling.

## II. AGONISTS AND ANTAGONISTS OPIOIDS

- Opioids can be classified as agonists (activators), antagonists (blockers), or partial agonist/ antagonists on their target receptors.
- **PURE AGONISTS:**
  - Most common morphine-like drugs.
  - They have high affinity for the Mu receptors and varying affinities for the kappa and delta receptors.
- **WEAK AGONISTS:**
  - Their maximal pain relief and side effects are much less than those of morphine and they usually do not lead to addiction.
  - E.g. methadone, codeine, dextropropoxyphene.
- **PARTIAL AGONISTS**
  - Have mixed agonist-antagonist character;
  - For example, Nalorphine and Pentazocine have a degree of agonism or antagonism on different receptors.
  - **Nalorphine** can be an agonist in some tissues, yet competitively block the otherwise stronger effects of morphine there.
  - **Pentazocine and Nalbuphine** are antagonists on Mu receptors but are partial agonists on KOR and DOR.
  - This class of drugs usually results in dysphoria (emotional state marked by anxiety, depression, and restlessness) rather than euphoria.
- **ANTAGONISTS**
  - Including **Naloxone** and **Naltrexone** they block the binding sites for agonists on the receptors.
- **NALOXONE**
  - Is a pure opioid antagonist at all three receptors and also blocks the endogenous neuropeptides such as endorphins and enkephalins.
  - It can rapidly reverse the effects of morphine and other related opiates, and causes hyperalgesia in stressful situations where natural endorphins would have normally reduced pain.
  - Given by IV, its action is almost immediate, but the short 1 to 2-hour time of action, due to rapid liver metabolism, may require repeat dosing.
  - Though it has no effects alone, it is effective in diagnosing addiction to opiates by rapidly inducing withdrawal.

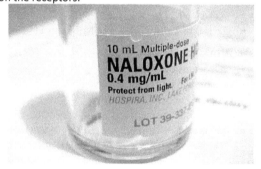

*Fig. 3.5.5. Naloxone*

## III. OPIOID ANALGESIA

### A. MORPHINE SALTS

#### 1. MECHANISM OF ACTION
- Narcotic agonist-analgesic of opiate receptor.
- Inhibits ascending pain pathways, thus altering response to pain; produces analgesia, respiratory depression, and sedation.
- Suppresses cough by acting centrally in medulla.

#### 2. INDICATIONS
- ACLS: Chest pain with ACS unresponsive to Nitrates
- Acute cardiogenic Pulmonary Edema (if BP is adequate).
- Pain control in ED

### 3. PRECAUTIONS
- Administer slowly and titrate to effect.
- May cause respiratory depression.
- Causes hypotension in volume-depleted patients.
- Use with caution in right ventricular infarction
- May reverse with naloxone 0.4 to 2 mg IV.

### 4. DOSAGE
- Initial dose: 2 to 4mg IV (over 1 to 5 minutes) every 5 to 30 minutes.
- Repeat dose: 2 to 8 mg at 5-to 15-minute interval.

## B. NALOXONE
### 1. INDICATIONS
- Respiratory and neurologic depression due to opiate intoxication unresponsive to O2 and support of ventilation.

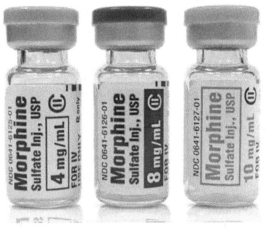

Fig. 3.5.6. Morphine Sulfate

### 2. PRECAUTIONS
- May cause opiate withdrawal.
- Half-life shorter than narcosis, repeat dosing may be needed.
- Monitor for recurrent respiratory depression.
- Rare anaphylactic reactions have been reported.
- Assist ventilation before naloxone administration, avoid sympathetic stimulation.
- Avoid in Meperidine-induced seizures.

### 3. DOSAGE
- Typical dose 0.4 to 2 mg, titrate until ventilation adequate.
- Use higher doses for complete narcotic reversal.
- Can administer up to 6 to 10mg over short period (<10minutes)
- IM/SQ 0.4 to 0.8 mg
- For chronic opioid-addicted patients, use smaller dose and titrate slowly.
- Can be given by endotracheal route if IV/IO access not available (other routes preferred)

## C. CODEINE PHOSPHATE
### 1. Mechanism of action
- Narcotic agonist analgesic with antitussive activity,
- MU receptor agonist.

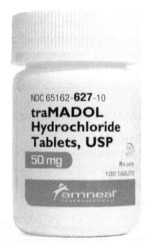

Fig. 3.5.7. Tramadol tablet

### 2. ADVERSE EFFECTS
- Constipation
- Drowsiness

### 3. CONTRAINDICATIONS & CAUTIONS
- Respiratory depression and death reported in children who received codeine following tonsillectomy and/or adenoidectomy that were also ultra-rapid metabolizers of codeine due to CYP2D6 polymorphism.

### 4. CONTRAINDICATIONS
- **Absolute**: Acute abdominal condition, diarrhea associated with toxins, pseudomembranous colitis, respiratory depression, postoperative use in children following tonsillectomy and/or adenoidectomy.
- **Relative:** Asthma (acute), inflammatory bowel disease, respiratory impairment.

### 5. CAUTIONS
- Cardiac arrhythmias, drug abuse/dependence, Emotional lability, gallbladder disease, head injury,
- Hepatic impairment, hypothyroidism, increased ICP, Prostatic hypertrophy, renal impairment, seizures with epilepsy, urethral stricture, urinary tract surgery. Do NOT give IV, because of severe adverse reactions
- Risk of life-threatening side effects in nursing infants, especially if mother is an ultra-rapid metabolizer of codeine

## POSTOPERATIVE PAIN IN CHILDREN
- *Deaths have occurred in children with obstructive sleep apnea who received codeine for postoperative pain following tonsillectomy and/or adenoidectomy.*
- *Codeine is converted to morphine by the liver; these children had evidence of being ultra-rapid metabolizers (via CYP2D6) of codeine, which is an inherited (genetic) ability that causes codeine to be converted rapidly into life-threatening or fatal amounts of morphine.*

## D. TRAMADOL

### 1. MECHANISM OF ACTION
* Non-opioid-derived synthetic opioid;
* centrally acting analgesic, but may act at least partially by binding to opioid Mu receptors, causing inhibition of ascending pain pathways.

### 2. ADVERSE EFFECTS
* Constipation (24-46%), Nausea (24-40%),
* Dizziness (10-33%), Vertigo (26-33%),
* Headache (18-32%), Somnolence (7-25%),
* Vomiting (9-17%), Agitation (7-14%),
* Anxiety (7-14%), Emotional lability (7-14%),
* Euphoria (7-14%), Hallucinations (7-14%),
* Nervousness (7-14%), Spasticity (7-14%),
* Dyspepsia (5-13%), Asthenia (6-12%),

### 3. CONTRAINDICATIONS
* Hypersensitivity to tramadol or opioids.

### 4. CAUTIONS
* Renal impairment (reduce dose).
* Anaphylactoid/fatal reactions including pruritus, hives, angioedema, epidermal necrolysis, and Stevens-Johnson syndrome reported with use; Use caution when administering with other respiratory depressants and monoamine oxidase inhibitors (MAOIs); risk of respiratory depression or increased ICP.
* Increased risk of respiratory depression in patients with respiratory disorders including COPD, hypercapnia, cor pulmonale, or hypoxia.
* Seizure risk even at recommended dosage, epilepsy patients, or recognized risks.
* Not recommended for obstetric preoperative medication or for postdelivery analgesia in nursing mothers.
* Increased risk of serotonin syndrome if coadministered with serotonergic drugs.
* Avoid use in patients who are suicidal; Use caution in patients taking tranquilizers and/or antidepressants.

## E. PARACETAMOL/ ACETAMINOPHEN

### 1. MECHANISM OF ACTION
* Acts on hypothalamus to produce antipyresis.
* May work peripherally to block pain impulse generation;
* May also inhibit prostaglandin synthesis in CNS.

### 2. PHARMACOKINETICS
* Peak Plasma Time: 6 hr (PO 500 mg, conventional tablet)
* Onset: 1 hr
* Metabolism: Liver (microsomal enzyme systems); conjugation (glucuronic/sulfuric acid).
* Metabolites: N-acetyl-p-benzoquinoneimine, N-acetylimidoquinone, NAPQI; further metabolized via conjugation with glutathione.
* Half-life elimination: 1.25-3 hr (adolescents); 2-5 hr (children); 4 hr (infants); 7 hr (neonates); 2-3 hr (adults).
* Excretion: urine (principally as acetaminophen glucuronide with acetaminophen sulfate/mercaptate).

### 3. CONTRAINDICATIONS
* Hypersensitivity
* Severe active liver disease

### 4. CAUTIONS
* Repeated administration in patients with anemia or cardiac, pulmonary, or renal disease.
* Risk of hepatotoxicity is higher in alcoholics, chronic high dose, or use of more than one acetaminophen-containing product.
* Use with caution in patients with G6PD deficiency.
* Risk for rare, but serious skin reactions that can be fatal; these reactions include Stevens - Johnson syndrome (SJS), toxic epidermal necrolysis (TEN), and acute generalized exanthematous pustulosis (AGEP); symptoms may include skin redness, blisters and rash.

| ANALGESICS | PHARMACOLOGY OF PAIN |
| --- | --- |
| Aspirin, NSAIDS | Reduce nociceptive stimulation by reducing inflammation |
| Local Anaesthetics | Block transmission nociceptive nerve fibres |
| Opiates | Stimulate antinociceptive pathways which modify pain transmission |
| Morphine, Antidepressants | Central action to reduce emotional component pain |

# F. ANTIEPILEPTICS

## I. CARBAMAZEPINE

### 1. MECHANISM OF ACTION
- Stabilizes inactivated state of sodium channels, thereby making neurons less excitable.
- May reduce activity of nucleus ventralis of the thalamus or decrease synaptic transmission or summation of temporal stimulation leading to neuronal discharge.

### 2. INDICATIONS
- Epilepsy
- Trigeminal Neuralgia
- Bipolar Mania
- Restless Legs Syndrome
- Postherpetic Neuralgia

### 3. ADVERSE EFFECTS
- Ataxia (15%), Dizziness (44%), Drowsiness (32%), Nausea (29%), Vomiting (18%),
- Dry mouth (8%).
- Rare: MI, Stevens-Johnson syndrome, Hepatic failure, punctate cortical lens opacities, Syndrome of inappropriate antidiuretic hormone secretion.

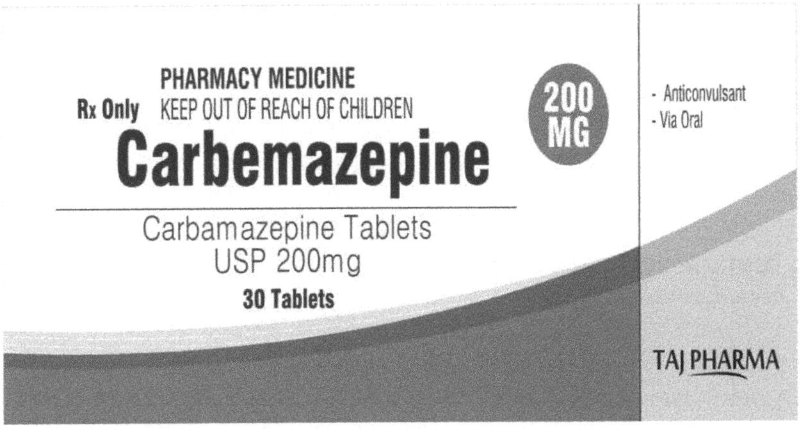

PHARMACY MEDICINE
Rx Only    KEEP OUT OF REACH OF CHILDREN
**Carbemazepine**
Carbamazepine Tablets
USP 200mg
**30 Tablets**
200 MG
- Anticonvulsant
- Via Oral
TAJ PHARMA

*Fig. 3.5.8. Carbamazepine tablets*

### 4. CONTRAINDICATIONS
Documented hypersensitivity.
- History of bone marrow suppression.
- Administration of MAO inhibitors within last 14 days
- Coadministration with:
  - *Nefazodone: Carbamazepine decreases plasma levels of nefazodone and its active metabolite.*
  - *NNRTIs (e.g., delavirdine, efavirenz, etravirine, nevirapine, rilpivirine): Carbamazepine induces CYP3A4 and may substantially reduce NNRTI serum concentration.*
- Jaundice, hepatitis.
- Pregnancy (especially first trimester: risk of fetal carbamazepine syndrome).

### 5. HEPATIC EFFECTS
- Slight elevations in liver enzymes.
- Rare cases of hepatic failure.
- Immunoallergenic syndromes.

## II. PHENYTOIN

### 1. MECHANISM OF ACTION
- Promotes Na+ efflux or decreases Na+ influx from membranes in motor cortex neurons.
- Stabilizes neuronal membrane.
- Slows conduction velocity.

### 2. CONTRAINDICATIONS & CAUTIONS
- Cardiovascular risk associated with rapid infusion rates
- Risk of hypotension and arrhythmias with infusion rates that exceed 50 mg/min in adults and 1-3 mg/kg/min (or 50 mg/min, whichever is slower) for pediatric patients.
- Careful cardiac monitoring is needed during and after IV administration.

### 3. CONTRAINDICATIONS
- Hypersensitivity, Sinus bradycardia, Heart block,
- Sinoatrial block, Second and third-degree A-V block,
- Adams-Stokes syndrome
- Pregnancy & Lactation
- Coadministration with Delavirdine; potential for loss of virologic response and possible resistance to delavirdine and to other nonnucleoside reverse transcriptase inhibitors (NNRTIs)

### 4. CAUTIONS
- Decreased bone mineral density reported with chronic use.

- Use caution in cardiovascular disease, hypoalbuminemia, hepatic impairment, hypothyroidism, porphyria, or seizures.
- Hematologic effects reported with use including agranulocytosis, leukopenia, pancytopenia, neutropenia, thrombocytopenia, and anaemias. Phenytoin is a potent inducer of hepatic drug-metabolizing enzymes.
- Increased risk of suicidal thoughts or behavior reported. May render OCPs ineffective because of induction of hepatic metabolism.
- Risk of gingival hyperplasia.

## III. VALPROIC ACID

### 1. MECHANISM OF ACTION
- May increase levels of the inhibitory neurotransmitter gamma-aminobutyric acid (GABA) in brain;
- May enhance or mimic action of GABA at postsynaptic receptor sites; May also inhibit sodium and calcium channels.

### 2. ADVERSE EFFECTS
- Nausea (31%), Headache (<31%), Increased bleeding time (26-30%), Thrombocytopenia (26-30%),
- Tremor (25%), Alopecia (<24%), Asthenia (16-20%), Infection (16-20%), Somnolence (16-20%), Amblyopia (11-15%), Diarrhea (11-15%)
- Diplopia (11-15%), Dizziness (11-15%), Dyspepsia (11-15%),
- Nystagmus (11-15%), Tinnitus (11-15%), Vomiting (11-15%)

### 3. CONTRAINDICATIONS & CAUTIONS
#### Hepatotoxicity
- Hepatic failure.
- Children younger than 2 years are at increased risk for fatal hepatotoxicity,
- Increased risk of valproate-induced acute liver failure and resultant deaths in patients with hereditary neurometabolic syndromes caused by DNA mutations of the mitochondrial DNA polymerase-gamma (POLG) gene (e.g., Alpers Huttenlocher Syndrome).
- If used in children with these conditions, it should be administered with extreme caution as a sole agent.
- Hepatotoxicity usually occurs during the first 6 months of treatment and may be preceded by malaise, weakness, lethargy, facial edema, anorexia, and vomiting.

#### Teratogenicity
- Do not use in women of childbearing age unless the drug is essential to the management of the medical condition;
- May cause neural tube defects.
- Children exposed in utero have increased risk for lower cognitive test scores compared with those exposed in utero to other antiseizure medications.

#### Pancreatitis
- Cases of life-threatening pancreatitis have been reported in children and adults.

### 4. CONTRAINDICATIONS
- Hypersensitivity
- Liver disease, significant hepatic impairment
- Urea cycle disorder
- Mitochondrial disorders
- Migraine
- Pregnancy

### 5. CAUTIONS
- Probability of thrombocytopenia increases significantly at total trough valproate plasma concentrations exceed 110 mcg/mL in females and 135 mcg/mL in males.
- Bleeding and other hematopoietic disorders may occur; monitor platelet counts and coagulation tests.
- Hepatotoxic (age <2 years, higher risk of fatal hepatotoxicity).
- Porphyria may occur.
- May produce false-positive urine ketone test and alter TFTs.
- May cause CNS depression, which may impair physical or mental to perform tasks requiring mental alertness.
- Drug reaction with eosinophilia and systemic symptoms (DRESS)/multiorgan hypersensitivity reaction reported; discontinue therapy; monitor for possible disparate manifestations associated with lymphatic, renal, hepatic, and/or hematologic organ systems.
- Not recommended for post-traumatic seizure prophylaxis in patients with acute head trauma (may increase mortality.
- Hypothermia reported during valproate therapy with or without associated hyperammonemia; this adverse reaction can also occur in patients using concomitant topiramate.
- Somnolence in the elderly can occur; valproic acid dosage should be increased slowly and with regular monitoring for fluid and nutritional intake.

# SECTION 6: INFECTIONS
## I. ANTIBACTERIAL DRUGS

### A. BASIC MECHANISMS OF ANTIBIOTIC ACTION AND RESISTANCE
- Five Basic Mechanisms of Antibiotic Action against Bacterial Cells:
  - Inhibition of Cell Wall Synthesis
  - Inhibition of Protein Synthesis (Translation)
  - Alteration of Cell Membranes
  - Inhibition of Nucleic Acid Synthesis
  - Antimetabolite Activity

### 1. INHIBITION OF CELL WALL SYNTHESIS          2BAV
- **Beta-Lactams:**
  - Inhibition of peptidoglycan synthesis (bactericidal)
- **Bacitracin**
  - Disrupts movement of peptidoglycan precursors (topical use).
- **Antimycobacterial agents**
  - Disrupt mycolic acid or arabinoglycan synthesis (bactericidal).
- **Vancomycin**
  - Disrupts peptidoglycan cross-linkage.

### 2. INHIBITION OF PROTEIN SYNTHESIS (Translation)
- ➤ **30S Ribosome site**          30 AM T
  - **Aminoglycosides**
    - Irreversibly bind 30S ribosomal proteins (bactericidal).
  - **Tetracyclines**
    - Block tRNA binding to 30S ribosome-mRNA complex (bacteriostatic).
- ➤ **50S Ribosome site**          50 CMC
  - **Chloramphenicol**
    - Binds peptidyl transferase component of 50S ribosome, blocking peptide elongation (bacteriostatic).
  - **Macrolides**
    - Reversibly bind 50S ribosome, block peptide elongation (bacteriostatic).
  - **Clindamycin**
    - Binds 50S ribosome, blocks peptide elongation; Inhibits peptidyl transferase by interfering with binding of amino acid-acyl-tRNA.

### 3. ALTERATION OF CELL MEMBRANES          POLYBAC
- **Polymyxins (topical)**
  - Cationic detergent-like activity (topical use).
- **Bacitracin (topical)**
  - Disrupt cytoplasmic membranes.

### 4. INHIBITION OF NUCLEIC ACID SYNTHESIS
- ➤ **DNA Effects**          QUIMET
  - **Quinolones**
    - Inhibit DNA gyrases or topoisomerases required for supercoiling of DNA; bind to alpha subunit.
  - **Metronidazole**
    - Metabolic cytotoxic by products disrupt DNA.
- ➤ **RNA Effects (Transcription)**          RIFBAC
  - **Rifampin**
    - Binds to DNA-dependent RNA polymerase inhibiting initiation & Rifabutin of RNA synthesis.
  - **Bacitracin (topical)**
    - Inhibits RNA transcription.

### 5. ANTIMETABOLITE ACTIVITY          SULTRIM
- **Sulfonamides & Dapsone**
  - Compete with p-aminobenzoic acid (PABA) preventing synthesis of folic acid.
- **Trimethoprim**
  - Inhibit dihydrofolate reductase preventing synthesis of folic acid.

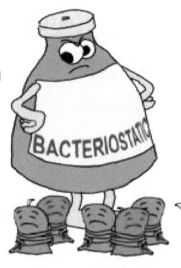
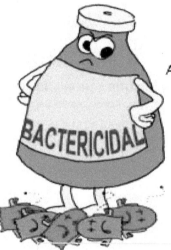

**EXAMPLES:**
Chloramphenicol
Erythromycin
Clindamycin
Sulfonamides
Trimethoprim
Tetracyclines

**EXAMPLES:**
Aminoglycosides
Beta-lactams
Vancomycin
Quinolones
Rifampin
Metronidazole

*Fig. 3.6.1. Bacteriostatic vs Bactericidal*

## B. ANTIMICROBIAL AGENTS COMMONLY USED

- **In the treatment of anaerobic infections are**:
  - ß-lactam antibiotics (carbapenems),
  - Metronidazole
  - ß-lactam compounds (ampicillin, amoxicillin, ticarcillin and piperacillin) in combination with a ß-lactamase inhibitor, such as clavulanic acid, sulbactam, or tazobactam.
- **Antibiotics that cover methicillin-resistant Staphylococcus aureus (MRSA):**
  - Ceftobiprole (> 5th generation)
  - Ceftaroline (5th generation)
  - Clindamycin
  - Daptomycin
  - Linezolid
  - Mupirocin (topical)
  - Tigecycline
  - Vancomycin

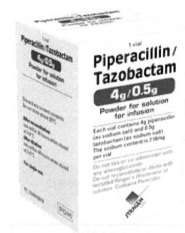

Piperacillin/ Tazobactam 4g/0.5g

*Fig. 3.6.2. Tazocin*

- **Antibiotics that cover Pseudomonas aeruginosa:**
  - Aminoglycosides
  - Carbapenems
  - Ceftazidime (3rd generation)
  - Cefepime (4th generation)
  - Ceftobiprole (5th generation)
  - Fluoroquinolones
  - Piperacillin/ Tazobactam (Tazocin)
  - Ticarcillin
- **Antibiotics that cover vancomycin- resistant Enterococcus (VRE):**
  - Linezolid
  - Streptogramins

## C. ANTIBACTERIAL DRUGS

## 1. PENICILLINS

- **Mechanism**
  - Interfere with bacterial cell wall synthesis
- **Subclassification**
  - Natural
    - Penicillin G
  - Penicillinase-resistant
    - Methicillin
    - Aminopenicillins
    - Ampicillin

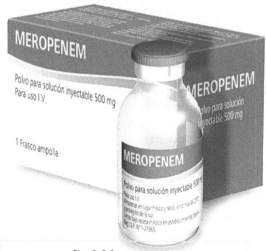

MEROPENEM

Polvo para solución inyectable 500 mg
Para uso I.V.

1 Frasco ampolla

*Fig. 3.6.3. meropenem*

## 2. CEPHALOSPORINS

- **Overview:** Bactericidal
- **Mechanism**
  - Disrupts the synthesis of the peptidoglycan layer of bacterial cell walls.
    - Does so through competitive inhibition on PCB (penicillin binding proteins).
    - Peptidoglycan layer is important for cell wall structural integrity.
  - Same mechanism of action as beta-lactam antibiotics (such as penicillins).

- **SUBCLASSIFICATION**
  - **First Generation**
    - Cefazolin (Ancef, Kefzol)
    - Cephalexin (Keflex, Keftabs)
  - **Second Generation**
    - Cefaclor (Ceclor)
    - Cefuroxime (Ceftin, Zinacef)
  - **Third Generation**
    - Ceftriaxone (Rocephin)
    - Cefixime (Suprax)
    - Cefotaxime (Claforan)
  - **Fourth Generation**
    - Cefepime (Maxipime)
    - Cefozopran (Firstein)
    - Cefpirome (Cefrom, Keiten, Broact, Cefir)
  - **Fifth-Generation**
    - Ceftaroline fosamil (Teflaro)
    - Ceftobiprole (Zeftera, Zevtera)

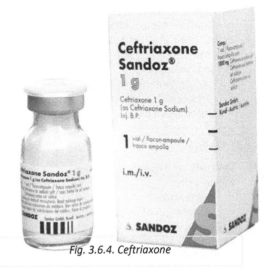

Fig. 3.6.4. Ceftriaxone

## 3. FLUOROQUINOLONES

- **Mechanism**
  - Blocks DNA replication via inhibition of DNA gyrase.
- **Side effects**
  - Inhibit early fracture healing through toxic effects on chondrocytes.
  - Increased rates of tendinitis, with special predilection for the Achilles tendon.
    - Tenocytes in the Achilles tendon have exhibited degenerative changes when viewed microscopically after fluoroquinolone administration.

- **Subclassification**
  - Ciprofloxacin (Cipro)
  - Levofloxacin (Levaquin)

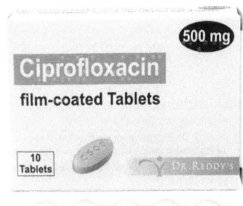

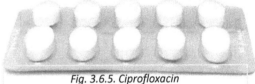

Fig. 3.6.5. Ciprofloxacin

## 4. AMINOGLYCOSIDES

- **Mechanism**
  - Bactericidal
  - Inhibition of bacterial protein synthesis:
    - Work by binding to the 30s-ribosome subunit, leading to the misreading of mRNA.
    - This misreading results in the synthesis of abnormal peptides that accumulate intracellularly and eventually lead to cell death.
- **Subclassification**
  - Gentamicin (Garamycin)
- **Contraindications**
  - Prior aminoglycoside toxicity or hypersensitivity

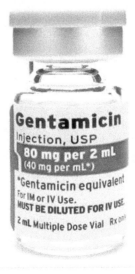

Fig. 3.6.6. Gentamycin

- **Cautions**
  - Risk of ototoxicity, neurotoxicity, nephrotoxicity
  - Narrow therapeutic index (not intended for long-term therapy).
  - Caution in renal failure (not on dialysis), myasthenia gravis, hypocalcemia, and conditions that depress neuromuscular transmission.
  - Adjust dose in renal impairment.
  - Endocarditis prophylaxis (GI, GU procedure): AHA Guidelines recommend only for high-risk patients.

## 5. VANCOMYCIN

- **Coverage:** Gram-positive bacteria.
- **Mechanism**
  - Bactericidal
  - An inhibitor of cell wall synthesis.
- **Resistance**
  - Increasing emergence of vancomycin-resistant enterococci has resulted in the development of guidelines for use by the CDC.
  - **Indications for vancomycin:**
    - Serious allergies to penicillins or beta-lactam antimicrobials.
    - Serious infections caused by susceptible organisms resistant to penicillins (MRSA, MRSE).
    - Surgical prophylaxis for major procedures involving implantation of prostheses in institutions with a high rate of MRSA or MRSE.

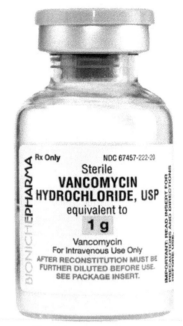

Fig. 3.6.7. Vancomycin

## 6. RIFAMPIN

- Pregnancy category: C
- Inhibits DNA-dependent RNA polymerase by binding to beta subunit, which in turn blocks RNA transcription; potent enzyme inducer.
- Most effective against intracellular phagocytized Staphylococcus aureus in macrophages:
  - Tuberculosis: May be given in conjunction with isoniazid or with isoniazid and pyrazinamide.
  - Neisseria Meningitidis Carrier.
  - Haemophilus Influenzae Type B Infection.
  - Prophylaxis.
- Absorption: PO well absorbed; food may delay or slightly reduce peak.
- Peak plasma time: PO, 2-4 hr
- Metabolized by liver; undergoes enterohepatic recirculation.
- Half-life: 3-4 hr (prolonged in hepatic impairment)
- Excretion: Feces (60-65%) and urine (~30%) as unchanged drug.
- **Side effects:**
  - Elevated LFT, Rash, Epigastric distress, Pseudomembranous colitis, Vomiting, Diarrhea, Anorexia, Nauseas, Pancreatitis

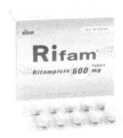

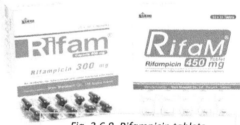

Fig. 3.6.8. Rifampicin tablets

## 7. LINEZOLID

- Linezolid binds to the 23S portion of the 50S subunit and acts by preventing the formation of the initiation complex between the 30S and 50S subunits of the ribosome.

## 8. TETRACYCLINE

- **Indication:** in chlamydia infections (urethritis), Rickettsia (Q fever), Brucella and the spirochaete Borrelia burgdorferi (Lyme disease).
- **Side effect:** they bind to Ca++ in growing bones and teeth, therefore not recommended in children under 12 years of age.
- **Route:** They are usually given orally and none of the commonly used tetracyclines is available in intravenous form.

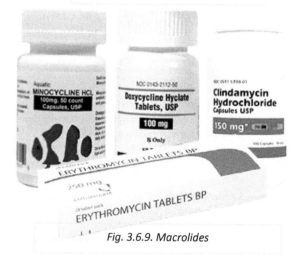

Fig. 3.6.9. Macrolides

# II. ANTIMALARIALS

- These agents inhibit growth by concentrating within acid vesicles of the parasite, increasing the internal pH of the organism.
- They also inhibit hemoglobin utilization and parasite metabolism.

## A. CHLOROQUINE PHOSPHATE

- Chloroquine phosphate is effective against P vivax, P ovale, P malariae, and drug-sensitive P falciparum. It can be used for prophylaxis or treatment.
- This is the prophylactic drug of choice for sensitive malaria.

## B. QUININE

- Quinine is used for malaria treatment only; it has no role in prophylaxis.
- It is used with a second agent in drug-resistant P falciparum.
- For drug-resistant parasites, the second agent is Doxycycline, Tetracycline, Pyrimethamine Sulfadoxine, or Clindamycin.

## C. QUINIDINE GLUCONATE

- Quinidine gluconate is indicated for severe or complicated malaria and is used in conjunction with Doxycycline, Tetracycline, or Clindamycin.
- Quinidine gluconate can be administered IV.

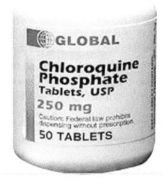

Fig. 3.6.10. Chloroquine phosphate

## D. DOXYCYCLINE

- Doxycycline is used for malaria prophylaxis or treatment.
- When it is administered for treatment of P falciparum malaria, this drug must be used as part of combination therapy (eg, typically with quinine).

## E. TETRACYCLINE

- Tetracycline may specifically impair the progeny of apicoplast genes, resulting in their abnormal cell division.
- Loss of apicoplast function in progeny of treated parasites leads to slow, but potent, antimalarial effect.

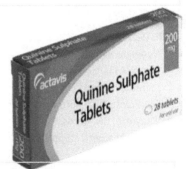

Fig. 3.6.11. Quinine Sulphate

## F. CLINDAMYCIN

- Clindamycin is part of combination therapy for drug-resistant malaria (eg, typically with quinine or quinidine).
- It is a good second agent in pregnant patients.

## G. MEFLOQUINE

- Mefloquine acts as a blood schizonticide. It may act by raising intravesicular pH within the parasite's acid vesicles. Mefloquine is structurally similar to quinine.
- It is used for the prophylaxis or treatment of drug-resistant malaria.
- It may cause adverse neuropsychiatric reactions and should not be prescribed for prophylaxis in patients with active or recent history of depression, generalized anxiety disorder, psychosis, or schizophrenia or other major psychiatric disorders.

## H. PRIMAQUINE

- Primaquine is not used to treat the erythrocytic stage of malaria.
- Administer the drug for the hypnozoite stage of P vivax and P ovale to prevent relapse.

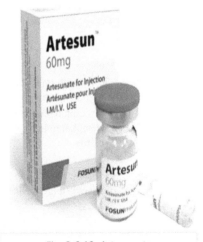

Fig. 3.6.12. Artesunate

## I. ARTEMETHER AND LUMEFANTRINE (Coartem)

- This drug combination is indicated for the treatment of acute, uncomplicated P falciparum malaria. It contains a fixed ratio of 20 mg artemether and 120 mg lumefantrine (1:6 parts). Both components inhibit nucleic acid and protein synthesis.
- Artemether is rapidly metabolized into the active metabolite dihydroartemisinin (DHA), producing an endoperoxide moiety.
- Lumefantrine may form a complex with hemin, which inhibits the formation of beta hematin.

## J. ARTESUNATE

- Artesunate, a form of artemisinin that can be used intravenously.

# SECTION 7: ENDOCRINE PHARMACOLOGY

## A. DIABETIS

## I. INSULIN

### 1. MECHANISM OF ACTION

- Glucose metabolism.
- Insulin and its analogs lower blood glucose by stimulating peripheral glucose uptake, especially by skeletal muscle and fat, and by inhibiting hepatic glucose production.
- Insulin inhibits lipolysis and proteolysis, and enhances protein synthesis.
- Insulin Neutral Protamine Hagedorn (NPH) and insulin regular is a combination insulin product with intermediate duration that has more rapid onset than that of insulin NPH alone.

| Glycogenesis | It is the formation of glycogen from glucose. |
|---|---|
| Glycolysis (aerobic) | It is the breaks down glucose and forms pyruvate with the production of two molecules of ATP. |
| Glycogenolysis | It is the biochemical breakdown of glycogen to glucose |
| Gluconeogenesis | It is the process of synthesizing glucose from non-carbohydrate sources. |

## FACTORS AFFECTING INSULIN SECRETION

| INCREASED INSULIN SECRETION | DECREASED INSULIN SECRETION |
|---|---|
| • Hyperglycaemia | • Hypoglycaemia |
| • Increase in blood free fatty acids | • Fasting |
| • Increase in blood amino acids | • Somatostatin |
| • Gastrointestinal hormones: Gastrin, CCK, Secretin and GIP | • Alpha-adrenergic activity |
| • Glucagon, GH, Cortisol | • Leptin |
| • Parasympathetic stimulation; | |
| • Acetyl choline | |
| • Beta-adrenergic stimulation | |
| • Insulin resistance | |
| • Obesity | |
| • Sulfonyl urea drugs (Glyburide, Tolbutamide) | |

### 2. DOSING FORMS

#### a. Type 1 Diabetes Mellitus

- Typically, 50-75% of total daily dose is given as intermediate- or long-acting insulin
- May use this combination product if the dosage ratio of NPH (isophane) to regular is 2:1

#### b. Type 2 Diabetes Mellitus

Morning

- Give 2/3rds of daily insulin SC
- Ratio of regular insulin to NPH (isophane) insulin 1:2

Evening

- Give 1/3 of daily insulin SC

### 2. ADVERSE EFFECTS

- Hypoglycemia, Insulin resistance, Lipodystrophy,
- Lipohypertrophy, Local allergic reaction
- Hypokalemia

### 3. CONTRAINDICATIONS

- Hypoglycemia
- Systemic allergic reactions

### 4. CAUTIONS

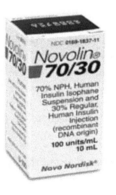
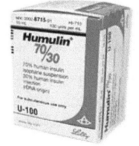
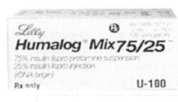
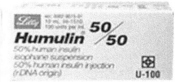

*Fig. 3.7.1. Insulin*

- Intermediate-acting insulin, do not use for circumstances that require rapid-acting insulin.
- Caution with decreased insulin requirements (eg, diarrhea, nausea/vomiting, malabsorption, hypothyroidism, renal impairment, hepatic impairment).
- Caution with increased insulin requirements (eg, fever, hyperthyroidism, trauma, infection, surgery).

## I. GLUCAGON

### 1. Mechanism of action

- Adjuvant treatment of toxic effects of calcium channel blocker or beta-blocker.
- Antagonist, stimulates cAMP synthesis to accelerate hepatic glycogenolysis and gluconeogenesis.
- Glucagon also relaxes smooth muscles of GI tract.

| FACTORS AFFECTING GLUCAGON SECRETION | |
|---|---|
| **INCREASED GLUCAGON SECRETION** | **DECREASED GLUCAGON SECRETION** |
| o  Amino acids | o  Hyperglycaemia |
| o  CCK, gastrin | o  Following meals |
| o  Cortisol | o  Insulin |
| o  Exercise | o  Somatostatin |
| o  Infection | o  Secretin |
| o  Beta adrenergic stimulants | o  Free fatty acids |
| o  Theophylline | o  Blood ketones |
| o  Acetylcholine | |
| o  Hypoglycaemia | |
| o  Fasting | |

### 2. DOSING FORMS

#### a. Hypoglycemia

- Indicated for severe hypoglycemic reactions in patients with diabetes treated with insulin: 1 mg (1 unit) IM/SC/IV if no IV for dextrose.
- Repeat q20min once or twice; give dextrose if no response.
- Administer supplemental carbohydrate to replete glycogen stores.

#### b. Radiography of GI

- Indicated as diagnostic aid for decreased GI motility.

#### c. Beta-Blocker & Calcium Channel Blocker Toxicity

- 3mg initially followed by infusion at 3mg/hour as necessary

### 3. ADVERSE EFFECTS

- Occasional nausea and vomiting, Rash, Hypotension, Tachycardia.

### 4. CONTRAINDICATIONS:

- Hypersensitivity & Pheochromocytoma.

### 5. CAUTIONS

- Do not administer to patients with history suggestive of insulinoma, pheochromocytoma, or both.
- Effective in treating hypoglycemia only if sufficient liver glycogen is present.
- Awaken patient following administration to provide oral glucose if possible, otherwise IV dextrose is required to replete glycogen stores.

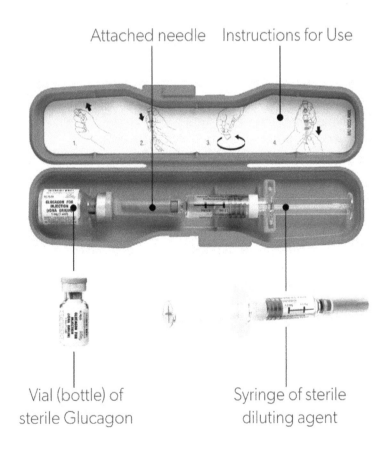

Attached needle    Instructions for Use

Vial (bottle) of sterile Glucagon

Syringe of sterile diluting agent

*Fig. 3.7.2. Glucagon kit*

# B. THYROID DISEASE

## I. LEVOTHYROXINE

### 1. MECHANISM OF ACTION

- Synthetic T4; thyroid hormone increases basal metabolic rate.
- Increases utilization and mobilization of glycogen stores.
- Promotes gluconeogenesis.
- Involved in growth development and stimulates protein synthesis.

### 2. PHARMACOLOGY
**Absorption:**

- 40-80% from GI tract (PO)
- Duration: Hypothyroidism, several weeks.

**Onset, hypothyroidism**

- Initial response: 3-5 days (PO); 6-8 hr (IV)
- Maximum effect: Several weeks
- Peak effect: 24 hr (IV)

**Onset, myxedema coma**

- Initial response: 6-12 hr (IV)
- Peak effect: 24 hr

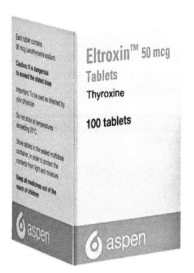
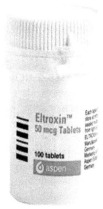

*Fig. 3.7.3. Eltroxin tablet*

**Metabolism**

- Deiodinated in blood and then 50% converted to active metabolite, triiodothyronine (T3), also by liver.
- Metabolites: T3 (active)

**Elimination**

- Half-life: 9-10 days (hypothyroid); 3-4 days (hyperthyroid); 6-7 days (euthyroid).
- Total body clearance: 0.8-1.4 L/day
- Excretion: Urine (major), feces (20%)

### 3. CONTRAINDICATIONS

- Hypersensitivity to thyroid hormone or other ingredients.
- Acute MI, thyrotoxicosis, untreated adrenal insufficiency.
- Treatment of obesity or infertility.

### 4. CAUTIONS

- Avoid undertreatment or overtreatment, which may result in adverse effects.
- Use caution in cardiovascular disease, HTN, endocrine disorders, osteoporosis, or myxedema.
- Initiate lower dose in elderly, those with angina pectoris, cardiovascular disease, or in those with severe hypothyroidism.
- Symptoms may be exacerbated or aggravated in patients with diabetes mellitus and insipidus
- Not recommended for TSH suppression in patients with thyroid nodules.
- Avoid use in patients with large thyroid nodules or long-standing goiters, or low-normal TSH levels.
- Long-term therapy decreases bone mineral density; use lowest dose in postmenopausal women and women using suppressive doses.

| In the treatment of thyrotoxic crisis | |
|---|---|
| Propranolol is the β-blocker of choice to use | T |
| Oral potassium iodide blocks release of thyroid hormones | T |
| Propythiouracil or carbimazole are given only once the patient is stable | F |
| Hydrocortisone is | F |
| **True or False:** | |
| • Hartmann's solution contains 2mmol/l of calcium | T |
| • Normal saline 0.9% contains 100mmol/l of Na | F |
| • 8.4% sodium Bicarbonate contains 500mmol/l of sodium | F |

# SECTION 8: VITAMIN B & IV FLUIDS

## I. THIAMINE

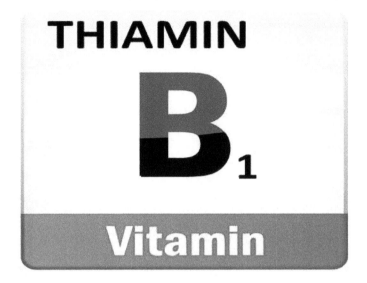

### 1. MECHANISM OF ACTION
- Forms thiamine pyrophosphate by combining with adenosine triphosphate; essential coenzyme in carbohydrate metabolism.

### 2. ADVERSE EFFECTS
- Warmth, Anaphylaxis, Cyanosis, Diaphoresis.
- Restlessness, Angioneurotic edema, Pruritus.
- Urticaria, Pulmonary edema, Weakness, Tightness of the throat, Nausea.

### 3. CONTRAINDICATIONS: Hypersensitivity

### 4. CAUTIONS
- In pregnancy
- Acute thiamine deficiency reported with dextrose administration; use caution when thiamine status uncertain.
- Hypersensitivity reactions reported following repeated parenteral doses.
- Parenteral products may contain aluminum; use caution in patients with impaired renal function.
- Evaluate for additional vitamin deficiencies if patient diagnosed with thiamine deficiency; single vitamin deficiencies are rare.

## II. COMPOSITION OF IV FLUIDS

| | TYPE | Na$^+$ | K$^+$ | Cl$^-$ | Ca$^{2+}$ | Glu | HCO3$^-$ | Osm |
|---|---|---|---|---|---|---|---|---|
| **0.9% NS** | Crystalloid | 154 | 0 | 154 | 0 | 0 | 0 | 308 |
| **5% Dextrose** | Crystalloid | 0 | 0 | 0 | 0 | 50 | 0 | 250 |
| **Hartmann's slt** | Crystalloid | 131 | 5 | 111 | 2 | 0 | 0 | 280 |
| **Gelofusine** | Colloid | 154 | <0.5 | 125 | <0.5 | 0 | 0 | 274 |
| **Extracellular fluid** | | 142 | 4 | 103 | 5 | 0.9-1.1 | 26 | 280-310 |
| **Intracellular fluid** | | 10 | 160 | 3 | 0.0001 | 0 | 10 | 280-310 |

# SECTION 9: MUSCULOSKELETAL SYSTEM

## I. NONSTEROIDAL ANTI-INFLAMMATORY DRUGS

- **Cyclooxygenase (COX) 1**: promotes synthesis of prostoglandins, keeps GI mucosa intact.
- **COX 2**: promotes synthesis of prostoglandins that are further involved in the inflammatory process.

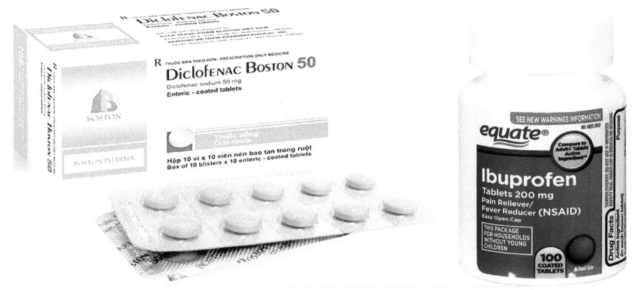

*Fig. 3.9.1. NSAIDs drugs*

### 1. MECHANISMS OF ACTION
- NSAIDs inhibit prostaglandin pathway, block COX.
- Most NSAIDs block COX 2 only, limiting GI ulcers.

### 2. MECHANISM OF COX INHIBITION BY NSAIDS
- All NSAIDs variably inhibit COX-1 and COX-2 and the mechanisms of inhibition fall into three broad categories, although there are exceptions. The three categories are:
  - **Category 1:** rapid competitive reversible binding of COX-1 and COX-2 (e.g., ibuprofen, piroxicam, mefenamic acid).
  - **Category 2:** rapid, lower-affinity reversible binding followed by time-dependent, higher-affinity, slowly reversible binding of COX-1 and COX-2 (e.g., diclofenac, flurbiprofen, indomethacin).
  - **Category 3:** rapid reversible binding followed by covalent modification of COX-1 and COX-2 (e.g., aspirin).
- The COX-2 inhibitors lack a carboxyl group and binding of these drugs within the COX active site does not require the charged interaction with Arg120.

### 3. SIDE EFFECTS
- Stomach problems like bleeding, ulcer and stomach upset
- High blood pressure
- Fluid retention
- Kidney problems
- Rashes

## ARACHIDONIC ACID (AA)
- It is a key intermediate in inflammatory pathways. It is produced from phospholipid by phospholipase in response to tissue damage and is converted to a number of potent inflammatory mediators by the action of cyclooxygenase enzyme (COX 1 and 2).
- These include:
  - **Prostaglandins** (increase vessel permeability as well as vasodilatation of renal arterioles).
  - **Prostacyclin** (vasodilatation and platelet inhibition)
  - **Thromboxane** (promotes platelet activation and aggregation)
- AA is also converted by 5-lipoxygenase enzyme to **Leukotrienes** (bronchoconstriction).
  - COX is inhibited by aspirin and NSAIDS, hence their role as anti-platelet and anti-inflammatory drugs.
  - *Serotonin is released from activated mast and other immune cells;*
  - *Bradykinin is synthesised from its circulating precursor Kallikrein.*

# Prostaglandins & Arachidonic Metabolism

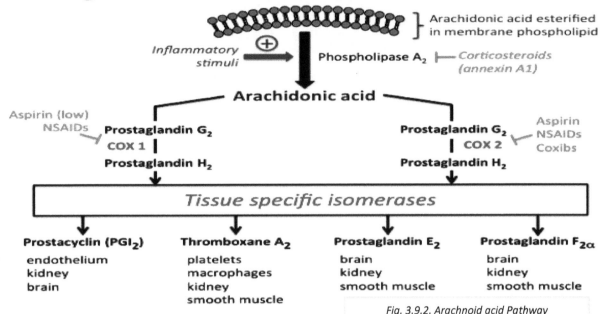

Fig. 3.9.2. Arachnoid acid Pathway

| Inflammatory mediators derived from arachidonic acid include | |
|---|---|
| Bradykinin | F |
| Prostaglandin E | T |
| Serotonin | F |
| Leukotrienes | T |

# II. DRUGS USED IN GOUT & HYPERURICAEMIA

## A. COLCHICINE

### 1. MECHANISMS OF ACTION

- Gout: Disruption of cytoskeletal functions through inhibition of β-tubulin polymerization into microtubules.
- This prevents activation, degranulation, and migration of neutrophils thought to mediate some gout symptoms.

### 2. ADVERSE EFFECTS

- Gastrointestinal (GI) effects (eg, diarrhea, nausea, cramping, abdominal pain, vomiting) (26-77%).

### 3. CONTRAINDICATIONS

- Coadministration with P-gp or strong CY3A4 inhibitors in patients with hepatic or renal impairment.
- Life-threatening and fatal colchicine toxicity has been reported with therapeutic dosages.
- Hypersensitivity

### 4. CAUTIONS

- Not to be used to treat pain from other causes; drug is not analgesic.
- Blood dyscrasias (eg, leukopenia, myelosuppression, thrombocytopenia, pancytopenia, granulocytopenia, aplastic anemia) have been reported at therapeutic dosages.
- Rhabdomyolysis and neuromuscular toxicity have been reported with long-term treatment.
- Acute gout: Dosages >1.8 mg/day provide no additional efficacy.

### 5. PREGNANCY & LACTATION

- Pregnancy category: C

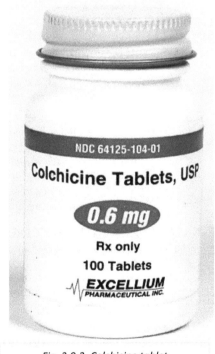

Fig. 3.9.3. Colchicine tablet

# SECTION 10: IMMUNOLOGICAL PRODUCTS & VACCINES

## I. ACTIVE IMMUNITY

- This is the stimulation of the immune mechanism to produce antibodies by giving an antigen as a vaccine.

## A. TYPES OF VACCINES

| LIVE ATTENUATED VACCINES | KILLED/INACTIVATED VACCINES | TOXOID VACCINES (INACTIVATED BACTERIAL TOXINS) | SUBUNIT VACCINES (GENETICALLY ENGINEERED) |
|---|---|---|---|
| o  Measles, Mumps, Rubella (MMR vaccine)<br>o  Varicella (chickenpox)<br>o  Influenza (nasal spray)<br>o  Rotavirus.<br>o  BCG<br>o  Polio (sabin)<br>o  Other:<br>  ▪  Zoster (shingles) and Yellow fever | o  Polio (IPV Salk)<br>o  Hepatitis A<br>o  Rabies | o  Diphtheria<br>o  Tetanus.<br>o  Botulism | o  Hepatitis B<br>o  Influenza (injection)<br>o  Haemophilus influenza type b (Hib)<br>o  Pertussis (part of DTaP)<br>o  Pneumococcal<br>o  Meningococcal<br>o  Human papillomavirus (HPV) |

**A**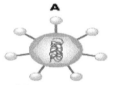

**B**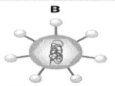

**C**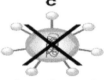

**D**

**E**

**Live attenuated vaccine**

**Chimeric live attenuated vaccine**

**Inactivated vaccine**

**Subunit vaccine**

**Nucleic acid-based vaccine**

*Fig. 3.10.1. Types of vaccine*

## B. ADVANTAGES AND DISADVANTAGES OF VACCINES

### 1. TOXOID VACCINES:

- o  *Advantages of toxoid vaccines*.
    - ▪  Safe because they cannot cause the disease they prevent and there is no possibility of reversion to virulence.
    - ▪  Because the vaccine antigens are not actively multiplying, they cannot spread to unimmunized individuals.
    - ▪  They are usually stable and long lasting as they are less susceptible to changes in temperature, humidity and light which can result when vaccines are used out in the community.

- o  *Disadvantages*
    - ▪  They usually need an adjuvant and require several doses.
    - ▪  Local reactions at the vaccine site are more common—this may be due to the adjuvant or a type III (Arthus) reaction—the latter generally start as redness and induration at the injection site several hours after the vaccination and resolve usually within 48–72 h.
    - ▪  The reaction results from excess antibody at the site complexing with toxoid molecules and activating complement by the classical pathway causing an acute local inflammatory reaction.

### 2. KILLED/INACTIVATED VACCINES

- ▪  The term killed generally refers to bacterial vaccines, whereas inactivated relates to viral vaccines.
    - o  *Advantages*
        - ▪  Killed/inactivated vaccines share the same advantages as toxoid vaccines with the additional one that all the antigens associated with infection are present and will result in antibodies being produced against each of them.

    - o  *Disadvantages*
        - ▪  They usually require several doses because the microbes are unable to multiply in the host and so one dose does not give a strong signal to the adaptive immune system; approaches to overcome this include the use of several doses and giving the vaccine with an adjuvant.
        - ▪  Local reactions at the vaccine site are more common—this is often due to the adjuvant.

- Using killed microbes for vaccines is inefficient because some of the antibodies will be produced against parts of the pathogen that play no role in causing disease.
- Some of the antigens contained within the vaccine, particularly proteins on the surface, may actually down-regulate the body's adaptive response—presumably, their presence is an evolutionary development that helps the pathogen overcome the body's defences.
- And finally, killed/inactivated vaccines do not give rise to cytotoxic T cells which can be important for stopping infections by intracellular pathogens, particularly viruses.

## 3. SUBUNIT VACCINES
- *Advantages*
  - Same as toxoid vaccines with the added benefit that one can distinguish vaccinated people from infected people.
  - For example, with hepatitis B vaccination, only an adaptive immune response to the surface antigen is possible whereas with infection core and e responses occur.
- *Disadvantages*
  - Subunit vaccines share the same disadvantages as toxoid vaccines, namely the need for an adjuvant, together with the frequent occurrence of local reactions at the injection site.

## 4. LIVE ATTENUATED
- *Advantages*
  - Activates all phases of the immune system.
  - Provides more durable immunity;
  - Boosters are required less frequently.
  - Low cost
  - Quick immunity
  - Easy to transport/administer: OPV (sabin) for Polio can be taken orally, rather than requiring a sterile injection by a trained healthworker, as the inactivated form IPV (Salk) does.
  - Vaccines have strong beneficial non-specific effects (go beyond the specific protective effects against the targeted diseases).
- *Disadvantages*
  - Secondary mutation can cause a reversion to virulence.
  - Can cause severe complications in immunocompromised patients.
  - Can be difficult to transport due to requirement to maintain conditions (e.g. temperature).

# II. IMMUNOGLOBULINS

## 1. INTRODUCTION
- The four most commonly used immunoglobulin preparations are as follows.
  - ✓ Human Hepatitis B Immunoglobulin
  - ✓ Human Rabies Immunoglobulin
  - ✓ Human Tetanus Immunoglobulin.
  - ✓ Human Varicella-Zoster Immunoglobulin
- There are 2 broad types of immunoglobulin preparations, "normal" and "specific".
- *Normal intravenous immunoglobulin (IVIG)* preparations are used in the treatment of patients who have no, or very low levels of, antibody production.
- This may be due to a genetic disorder, to disease, or to treatment such as chemotherapy.
- They are also used in the treatment of certain auto-immune conditions.
- *Specific immunoglobulins* are preparations that contain a high concentration of antibodies to particular viruses or bacteria.

## 2. SPECIFIC Ig

### A. HUMAN HEPATITIS B IMMUNOGLOBULIN
- Hepatitis B immunoglobulin (HBIG) is given as a prophylactic measure to people at increased risk of exposure to hepatitis B.
- People may have no symptoms at all but can still pass on the virus to others.
- It is possible to have contracted hepatitis B and not have symptoms for many years until it develops into long-term disease.
- Hepatitis B can be passed on in the following ways:
  - Sexually with an infected partner,
  - During delivery from an infected mother to her newborn baby,
  - Sharing needles: users of injected drugs who can infect others,
  - Blood transfusion: in a country where blood is not tested for the hepatitis B virus.

- People who have had hepatitis B but haven't recovered fully can remain infectious all their lives.
- Specific hepatitis B immunoglobulin (HBIG) is available for passive protection and is normally used in combination with hepatitis B vaccine to confer immediate cover (passive immunity) and long-lasting protection (active immunity) after exposure.
- Whenever immediate protection is required, immunization with the vaccine should be combined with the simultaneous administration of HBIG at a different injection site. It has been shown that passive immunization with HBIG does not suppress an active immune response. A single dose of HBIG is sufficient for healthy individuals.
- If infection has already occurred at the time of immunization, virus multiplication may not be inhibited completely, but severe illness and, most importantly, the development of the carrier state may be prevented.

**Groups requiring post-exposure prophylaxis:**
- Babies born to mothers, who are HBeAg positive carriers, who are HBsAg positive without e markers, or who have had acute hepatitis during pregnancy.
- Persons who are accidentally inoculated, or who contaminate the eye and mouth or fresh cuts or abrasions of the skin with blood from a known HBsAg positive person.
- Sexual partners of individuals suffering from acute hepatitis B, and who are seen within one week of onset of jaundice.

**HBeAg (hepatitis B "e" antigen):**
- This antigen is a protein from the hepatitis B virus that circulates in infected blood when the virus is actively replicating.

**HBsAg (hepatitis B surface antigen):**
- When blood is tested to determine if someone is infected with the hepatitis B virus, one thing looking for is HBsAg in the blood.
- If it is found, along with other specific antibodies, it means the person has a hepatitis B infection.

**Hep. B vaccine for neonates**

| Vaccination Program for Neonates | Baby should receive | |
|---|---|---|
| There is no contraindication to breast-feeding of a carrier mother when the baby begins immunization at birth. | Hepatitis B vaccine | HBIG single dose |
| Mother is HBsAg positive and HBeAg positive | Yes | Yes |
| Mother is HBsAg positive without e markers (or where they have not been determined) | Yes | Yes |
| Mother has acute hepatitis B during pregnancy | Yes | Yes |
| Mother is HBsAg positive and anti-HBe positive | Yes | No |

## B. HUMAN TETANUS IMMUNOGLOBULIN

- In the UK, vaccination against tetanus infection is part of the childhood immunization schedule.
- The first dose is given to babies at 2 months old followed by two additional doses at one-month intervals.
- Booster doses are also given at age 3-5 years (3 years after the primary course) and at age 13-18 years.
- Human tetanus immunoglobulin contains antibodies against tetanus.
- Booster doses in addition to 5 doses is not recommended except in the case of the treatment of a tetanus-prone wound.
  - *The following are considered tetanus-prone wounds:*
    - *Any wound or burn sustained more than 6 hours.*
    - *Any wound or burn at any interval after injury that shows one or more of the following: significant degree of dead tissue, puncture-type wound, contact with soil or manure (both likely to harbour tetanus organisms) and any clinical evidence of sepsis.*

## C. HUMAN VARICELLA ZOSTER IMMUNOGLOBULIN

- **Varicella:** the primary infection that causes chicken pox.
- **Herpes zoster:** the reactivation of the virus that causes shingles.
- Chicken pox is a common childhood disease with symptoms of slight fever, physical discomfort, uneasiness and skin rashes that blister into itching sores which eventually scab. In adults, a chicken pox infection is more severe than in children; many infected adults can develop pneumonia. Shingles is a recurring disease that appears in older adults who were previously infected with the virus.
- The virus lies dormant in the spinal cord for years.
- When reactivated it affects the nervous system and causes inflammation of the nerve fibres of the skin.
- The virus has properties that allow it to hide from the immune system for years, often for a lifetime. This inactivity is called latency.
- *Shingles is more common after the age of 50 and the risk increases with advancing age.*
- In many cases, the immune system has become impaired or suppressed from certain conditions such as AIDS or other immunodeficient diseases or from certain cancers or drugs that suppress the immune system.
- *Aging itself may increase the risk of shingles.*

# SECTION 11: ANAESTHESIA

## I. SEDATION AGENTS

### 1. MIDAZOLAM

- A short acting water-soluble benzodiazepine which at higher doses causes intense **sedation** (anaesthesia) and **retrograde amnesia.**
- The initial dose is **0.02-0.1mg/Kg** in adults older than 60 and the chronically ill or debilitated
- Onset of action: **30-60 seconds** with Peak action at **12min.**
- Half life: **2hrs;** Risk: May cause **hypotension.**
- Antidote: **Flumazenil** (caution!!! must be taken as it may have a shorter duration of action than the sedative agent, resulting in re-sedation.)

### 2. PROPOFOL

- Propofol is now used for procedural sedation in many EDs worldwide.
- **Has no analgesic property**
- Its mechanism of action is unclear but is thought to act by potentiating the inhibitory neurotransmitters GABA and glycine, which enhances spinal inhibition during anaesthesia.

### DOSAGE:

- For induction of anaesthesia **is 1 mg/kg initially then 0.5mg/kg every 1-2min.**
- For maintenance of anaesthesia is **4-12 mg/kg/hour.**
- Following intravenous injection propofol acts within **30 seconds** and its duration of action is **5-10 minutes.**

### SIDE EFFECTS OF PROPOFOL

- *Pain on injection (in up to 30%)*
- *Hypotension, Hyperventilation*
- *Transient apnoea*
- *Headache, Coughing and hiccup*
- *Thrombosis and phlebitis*

### CONTRAINDICATIONS

- **Absolute**
  - Known hypersensitivity to propofol or any of its components
  - Allergies to egg, egg products, soybeans or soy products (not Milk allergy)
  - Disorders of fat metabolism
- **Relative:**
  - Known case of epilepsy
  - Untreated HTN
  - Compromises left ventricular function
  - Hepatic or Renal impairment
  - Pregnant and lacting mother
  - Paediatric age <3 yrs

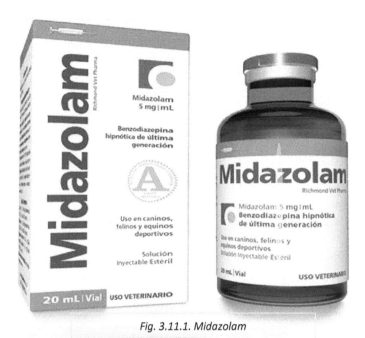

Fig. 3.11.1. Midazolam

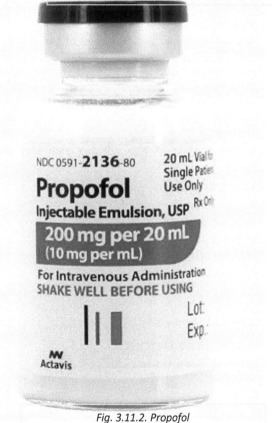

Fig. 3.11.2. Propofol

## 3. KETAMINE

- Ketamine is the only anaesthetic agent available that has **analgesic, hypnotic, and amnesic properties**. When used correctly it is a very useful and versatile drug. Ketamine acts by non-competitive antagonism of the NMDA receptor $Ca^{2+}$ channel pore and also inhibits NMDA receptor activity by interaction with the phenylcyclidine binding site.

- **DOSAGE AND ROUTES:**
  - Ketamine can be used intravenously and intramuscularly.
  - **10 mg/kg IM:** when used by this route it acts within **2-8 minutes** and has a duration of action of **10-20 minutes**.
- **1.5-2 mg/kg IVI:** administered over a period of 60 seconds. When used intravenously it acts within **30 seconds** and has a duration of action of **5-10 minutes** Ketamine is also effective when administered orally, rectally, and nasally.
- Baroreceptor function is well maintained and arrhythmias are uncommon.

## SIDE EFFECTS OF KETAMINE

- *Tachycardia*
- *Nausea and vomiting*
- *Increase BP, CVP, Cardiac Output*
- *Nystagmus*
- *Diplopia*
- *Rash*

- *Ketamine **1 – 2 mg/kg IV** is the ideal induction agent in asthmatic patients due to its **bronchodilatory effects**.*
- *Intravenous ketamine given in a dissociative dose may be an effective temporizing measure to avoid mechanical ventilation in adult patients with severe asthma exacerbations.*

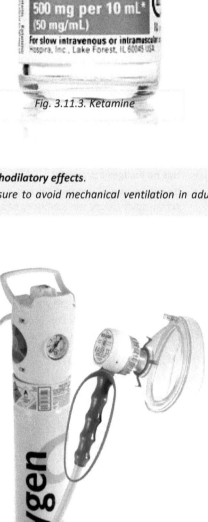

Fig. 3.11.3. Ketamine

## 4. ENTONOX

- Entonox is a **50/50 mix of oxygen and nitrous oxide**.
- Its main actions are **analgesia and depression of the central nervous system.**
- It is not known for certain how it works but it is postulated that it acts via the modulation of enkephalins and endorphins within the central nervous system.
- It takes approximately **30 seconds** to act and continues for approximately **60 seconds** after inhalation has ceased.
- Entonox is stored in **white or blue cylinders with blue and white shoulders.**

## INDICATIONS OF ENTONOX

- As an adjuvant to general anaesthesia
- As an analgesic during labour
- As an analgesic during painful procedures

## SIDE EFFECTS OF ENTONOX

- *Nausea and vomiting (15% of patients)*
- *Dizziness*
- *Euphoria*
- *Inhibition of vitamin B12 synthesis*

## CONTRAINDICATIONS OF ENTONOX

- **Entonox should be avoided in patients with:**
  - *Head injuries,*
  - *Chest injuries,*
  - *Suspected bowel obstruction,*
  - *Middle Ear disease,*
  - *Early pregnancy and*
  - *B12 or folate deficiency.*

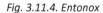

Fig. 3.11.4. Entonox

# II. INTRAVENOUS INDUCTION AGENTS

## 1. THIOPENTONE

- Thiopental sodium is a very short acting barbiturate that is primarily used for the induction of anaesthesia. Barbiturates are thought to act primarily at synapses by depressing post-synaptic sensitivity to neurotransmitters and by impairing pre-synaptic neurotransmitter release. The dose for **induction of anaesthesia** is **2-7 mg/kg.**
- Following intravenous injection thiopental sodium rapidly reaches the brain and causes unconsciousness within **30-45 seconds** and the effects last **5-15 minutes.**
- Its effects are cumulative with repeated administration.
- Thiopental sodium is negatively inotropic, **decreases cardiac output by approximately 20%.** It also **decreases systemic vascular resistance.**
- It is potent respiratory depressant and a period of apnoea may occur after administration. It also decreases renal blood flow and increases vasopressin secretion, resulting in a **fall in urine output.**
- **INDICATIONS**
  - o *Induction of anaesthesia*
  - o *Treatment of status epilepticus*
  - o *Brain protection*

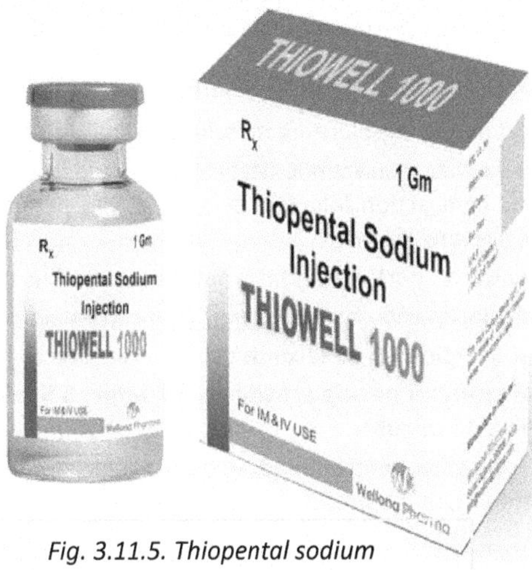

*Fig. 3.11.5. Thiopental sodium*

**SIDE EFFECTS OF THIOPENTAL SODIUM**

| | | |
|---|---|---|
| Hypersensitivity reactions | Negative inotrope | Accumulation -> inability to assess neurology in a timely manner |
| Laryngospasm | Arrhythmias | |
| Bronchospasm | Hypokalemia, Hyponatraemia | Extravasation -> necrosis |
| Increased infection risk | Myocardial depression | Porphyriogenic |
| | | Cough and Headache |

## 2. ETOMIDATE

- It is an intravenous induction agent associated with a **rapid recovery.** The dose for induction of anaesthesia is **0.3 mg/kg.**
- Following intravenous injection etomidate acts in **10-65 seconds** and its duration of action is **6-8 minutes.**
- Its effects are non-cumulative with repeated administration. Etomidate is notable for its relative **cardiovascular stability.** It causes less hypotension than thiopental sodium and propofol during induction. It is also associated with rapid recovery without a hangover effect.
- Etomidate is a potent inhibitor of steriodogenesis. Adrenal 11 beta-hydroxylase and cholesterol cleavage enzymes are inhibited by the drug, resulting in depression of cortisol and aldosterone synthesis for 24 hours after administration. *Because of this adrenocortical suppression it should not be used for maintenance of anaesthesia.*
- **SIDE EFFECTS:**
  - o *Adrenocortical suppression, Nausea and vomiting*
  - o *Pain on injection (in up to 50%)*
  - o *Phlebitis and venous thrombosis*
  - o *Arrhythmias and heart block, Hyperventilation*
  - o *Respiratory depression and apnoea*
  - o *Can cause both hypo- and hypertension*
  - o *Increased mortality in critically ill patients*

| Drug | Induction and recovery | Main unwanted effects | Notes |
|---|---|---|---|
| Thiopental | Fast onset (accumulation occurs, giving slow recovery), Hangover | CVS and Resp depression | Used as induction agent declining. ↓CBF and O2 consumption<br>Injection pain |
| Etomidate | Fast onset<br>Faily fast recovery | Excitatory effects during induction<br>Adrenocortical suppression | Less CVS and resp depression than Thiopenthal.<br>Injection pain |
| Propofol | Fast onset<br>Fast recovery | CVS and Resp depression<br>Pain at injection site | Most common induction agent<br>Rapidily metabolized<br>Possible to use as continuous infusion<br>Injection pain<br>Antiemetic |
| Ketamine | Slow onset<br>After effects common during recovery | Psychotomimetic effets following recovery<br>Postop Nausea-vomiting | Produces good analgesia and amnaesia<br>No injection site pain |
| Midazolam | Slower onset than other agents | Minimal CVS and resp depression | Little Resp and CVS depressions,<br>No pain, good amnaesia |

# III. MUSCLE RELAXATION

- If intubation is required, it may be necessary to paralyse the patient using:
  - ○ **Depolarizing muscle relaxants** (e.g. suxamethonium)
  - ○ **Non-depolarizing muscle relaxants** (Rocuronium, Cistracurium, Vecuronium or Atracurium).

## 1. SUXAMETHONIUM

- A short acting **depolarising muscle relaxant** with a rapid onset of action
- Binds to the postsynaptic acetylcholine receptors, resulting in transient receptor agonism and muscle contraction followed by a refractory period of muscle relaxation within **30–60 seconds** lasting several minutes.
- Its relatively short-lived effects are the result of its metabolism by **Plasma Cholinesterase.**
- Dosage intravenously is **0.5-2 mg/kg.** If second dose required – **consider atropine pre-treatment.**
- Onset of action **45-60 seconds** usually preceded by fasciculation within 15 seconds.
- Initial return of muscle activity occurs within **3-5 minutes** and adequate spontaneous ventilation within **8-10 minutes**.
- May cause hypotension and bradycardia (after second dose, in younger children (atropine pre-treatment), in the presence of hypoxia).

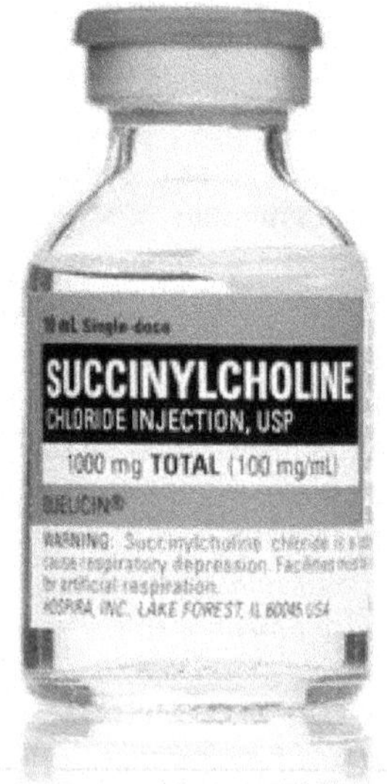

### SIDE EFFECTS OF SUXAMETHONIUM

- *Hyperkalemia*
- *Malignant hyperthermia*
- *Muscle pain*
- *Cardiac arrhythmias*
- Rapid increase in intraocular pressure

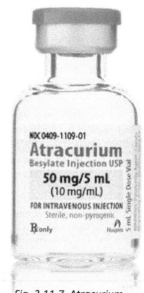

Fig. 3.11.6. Succinylcholine

### CONTRAINDICATIONS

- **Recent burns** but can be given in the first 24 hours following the burn.
- **Spinal cord trauma** causing paraplegia. It can be given immediately after the injury but should be avoided from approximately day-10 to day-100 after the injury.
- Other contraindications to the use of suxamethonium include:
  - ○ *Severe muscle trauma*
  - ○ *Hyperkalaemia*
  - ○ *History of malignant hyperthermia*

## 2. ATRACURIUM

- Atracurium is a **non-depolarising neuromuscular blocker** that is used to induce muscle relaxation and paralysis to facilitate intubation and controlled ventilation.
- Atracurium competes with acetylcholine for nicotinic (N2) receptor binding sites at the post-synaptic membrane of the neruomuscular junction. This prevents acetylcholine from stimulating the receptors. Because the blockade is competitive muscle paralysis occurs gradually.
- In order to enhance neuromuscular recovery post nondepolarizing relaxation at the end of surgery, the amount of acetylcholine in the synapse is increased by inhibiting the **acetylcholinesterase enzyme** using a reversal agent such as **Neostigmine.**
- The 'intubating' dose of atracurium is **0.3-0.6 mg/kg** and subsequent doses are one-third of this amount. Satisfactory intubating conditions are produced within **90 seconds** of administration.
- There is a linear relationship between the dose and the duration of action and atracurium is non-cumulative with repeated administration.
- **The duration of action of atracurium is prolonged by the following factors:**
  - ○ *Hypocalcaemia*
  - ○ *Hypokalaemia*
  - ○ *Hypoproteinaemia*
  - ○ *Hypercapnia*
  - ○ *Hypermagnesaemia*
  - ○ *Dehydration*
- *Acidosis* **Histamine release** may occur if doses > 600 µg/kg are used. This can result in cutaneous flushing, hypotension and bronchospasm.
- **Bradycardia** has also been reported.

Fig. 3.11.7. Atracurium

# IV. REVERSAL OF MUSCLE RELAXANTS

## 1. ANTICHOLINESTERASE AGENTS

- **Neostigmine, Edrophonium, and Pyridostigmine** are used to reverse neuromuscular blockade.
- **Edrophonium** has a rapid onset, but is not as effective as neostigmine for deep blocks.
- **Pyridostigmine** has a slow onset, which makes it ill-suited to the reversal of intermediate-acting neuromuscular agents.

### 1. NEOSTIGMINE

- Remains the most commonly used anticholinesterase agent, although many principles can also apply to edrophonium and pyridostigmine.
- Reduces the intensity of neuromuscular blockade in a dose-dependent manner up to **0.04-0.05 mg/kg**, but higher doses have little if any additional benefit. The agent must be injected only when sufficient spontaneous recovery is observed.
- It is recommended to wait until there are four visible twitches following TOF stimulation before administering neostigmine.
- If no fade is visible, significant residual blockade is possible, but adequate reversal requires only **0.02- 0.03 mg/kg of neostigmine**.
- If three or fewer twitches are visible, it is preferable to maintain anesthesia until there are four visible twitches and then give neostigmine at the usual **0.04-0.05 mg/kg doses.**
- *When the reversal agent is administered too early, **recovery might be incomplete**, and residual paralysis difficult to diagnose, as human senses cannot detect fade when the TOF ratio is 0.4 or greater.*

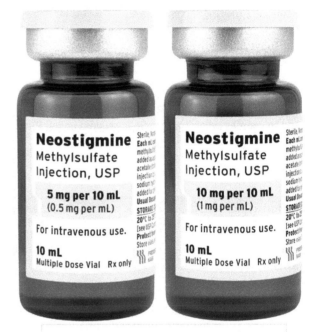

*Fig. 3.11.8. Neostigmine methylsulfate*

### 2. SUGAMMADEX

- Selective relaxant binding agent; forms a complex with the neuromuscular blocking agents **Rocuronium and Vecuronium**, and it reduces the amount of neuromuscular blocking agent available to bind to nicotinic cholinergic receptors in the neuromuscular junction.
- As a result, sugammadex inactivates rocuronium molecules and indirectly decreases the intensity of neuromuscular blockade.
- Once bound, the kidney excretes the sugammadex-rocuronium complex.
- To a lesser extent, sugammadex also shows an affinity for **Vecuronium an**
- **Pancuronium**; however, it has no affinity for other neuromuscular blockers such as Succinylcholine, Atracurium, Cistracurium, and Doxacurium.
- The recovery time following sugammadex administration is exceptionally fast, ie, approximately **2 minutes**.

### DOSAGE

- **For Rocuronium and Vecuronium**
  - A dose of **4 mg/kg** is recommended if spontaneous recovery of the twitch response has reached 1-2 post-tetanic counts (PTC) and there are no twitch responses to train-of-four (TOF) stimulation following rocuronium- or vecuronium-induced neuromuscular blockade

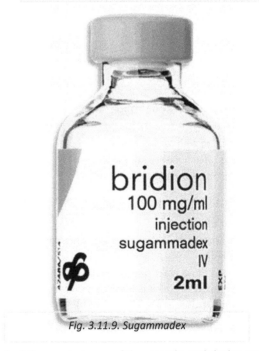

*Fig. 3.11.9. Sugammadex*

  - A dose of **2 mg/kg** is recommended if spontaneous recovery has reached the reappearance of the second twitch (T2) in response to TOF stimulation following rocuronium- or vecuronium-induced neuromuscular blockade
- **For Rocuronium only**
  - A dose of **16 mg/kg** is recommended if there is a clinical need to reverse neuromuscular blockade soon (~3 minutes) after administration of a single dose of **1.2 mg/kg** of rocuronium.
  - The efficacy of the **16 mg/kg** dose following administration of vecuronium has not been studied

# V. ADJUNCTS TO ANAESTHESIA

## 1. FENTANYL

- A potent synthetic opiate with a rapid onset of action and short half life.
- **Used to blunt sympathetic reflexes to laryngoscopy** and **the rise in ICP** associated with intubation.
- Dosage intravenously of **0.05-1mcg/kg**.
- May cause significant **respiratory depression, rigid chest syndrome** if given too rapidly and **hypotension.**

## 2. ATROPINE

- A competitive muscarinic antagonist, which causes vagal inhibition at the SA and AV nodes resulting in increased heart rate.
- Used **to counter reflex bradycardia** in children under 10 yrs or after repeat dose suxamethonium.
- Dosage intravenously of **0.02mg/kg** **3 minutes before** administration of Suxamethonium.

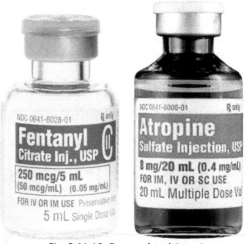

*Fig. 3.11.10. Fentanyl and Atropine*

| Drug | Dose | Precautions |
|------|------|-------------|
| Morphine | 0.05-0.20mg/Kg | Resp depression<br>Histamine release with hypotension, N&V, itching, bronchospasm, |
| Ketofol 10mg/ml sol | IV 1:1 ratio; 1-3ml every 2 min until desired effect achieved | |
| Naloxone | 1-2mg IV<br>Additional 2-3min to a total 10mg | Clinical duration shorter than longer acting opioids |
| Flumazenil | 0.02mg/kg -2mg over 15 sec<br>Additional 0.2mg doses at 1min interval until desired state of consciousness achieved | Contraindicated in patients taking benzodiazepines for an extended amount of time<br>Underlying seizure disorder<br>In Patients on TCA |

# E. LOCAL ANAESTHETICS

## 1. BUPIVICAINE
**0.25% (2.5mg/ml); 0.5% (5mg/ml)**

- Longer duration of action: **3-8 hrs**
- Most associated with cardiac toxicity
- Slower onset of action than adrenaline
- **Max. dose: 2mg/Kg (plain and adrenaline)**

## 2. PRILOCAINE  0.5%; 1%

- Used in **Bier's Blocks**
- **Max.dose: 6mg/kg plain (Not used with adrenaline)**
- Half-life: **1 hour**
- Prilocaine can cause **Methaemoglobinaemia** as one of its metabolites O-toluidine is a strong oxidizing agent which converts the $Fe^{2+}$ (ferrous iron) of normal haemoglobin to $Fe^{3+}$ (ferric iron) of methaemoglobin.
- Prilocaine is also used in topical anaesthetics such as EMLA (Eutectic Mixture of Local Anaesthetics - eutectic means that mixture has lower melting temperature than its individual constituents.)
- EMLA cream contains 2.5% prilocaine and 2.5% lidocaine.

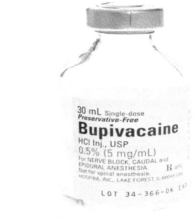

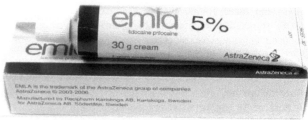

*Fig. 3.11.11. Bupivacaine and Prilocaine*

## 3. LIGNOCAINE   0.5%; 1%, 2%

- Plain or with adrenaline 1:200,000
- Duration of action:
  - **Plain: 30-60 minutes**
  - **Adrenaline: 90 minutes**
- Max. dose:
  - **Plain: 3mg/Kg**
  - **With Adrenaline: 7mg/Kg**
- IV infusion of a 20% Lipid Emulsion (eg, Intralipid 20%) has become an accepted part of treatment for systemic toxicity from local anesthetics
- *Lidocaine 0.5% (5mg/ml>>>mg= mls X 5)*
  - *Each 1 ml contains 5 mg of lidocaine hydrochloride*
- *Lidocaine 1% (10mg/ml>>>mg= mls X 10)*
  - *Each 1 ml contains 10.0 mg of lidocaine hydrochloride,*
  - *Each 20 ml solution contains 200 mg Lidocaine Hydrochloride*
- *Lidocaine 2% (20mg/ml>>>mg= mls X 20)*
  - *Each 1 ml contains 20.0 mg of lidocaine hydrochloride,*
  - *Each 2 ml solution contains 40 mg Lidocaine Hydrochloride E.P.*
  - *Each 5 ml solution contains 100 mg Lidocaine Hydrochloride E.P.*

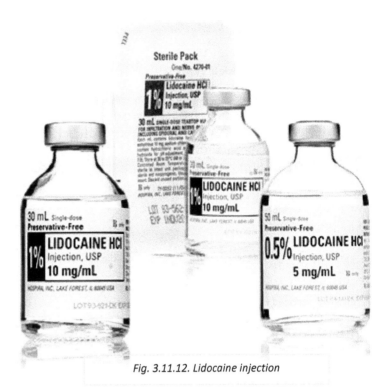

*Fig. 3.11.12. Lidocaine injection*

| True and False | |
| --- | --- |
| Propofol has strong analgesic property | F |
| Propofol is contraindicated with cow milk allergy? | F |
| Scoline is a non-depolarizing drug | F |
| Scoline needs reversal for prolonged action | F |
| Ipratropium is a muscuranic receptor antagonist | T |
| **True and False** | |
| The duration of action of propofol is appr. 20min | F |
| Anterograde amnaesia is usual feature of midazolam | T |
| 0.5% lignocaine has 50mg Lignocaine in 10mls | T |
| Bupivicaine is the agent of choice for regional anaesthesia | F |
| Ketamine is contraindicated in asthmatic | F |
| A child weighing 20kg can safely receive 6 mls of 1% plain lignocaine | T |
| Bupivicaine has at least twice the duration of action of lignocaine | T |
| Constricted pupils are associated with TCA overdose | F |
| Lignocaine Toxicity can be treated using IV lipid emulsion | T |
| Diltiazem overdose can be treated with glucagon | F |
| Oxidative phosphorylation is inhibited in salicylate poisoning | |
| TCA overdose causes urinary retention | T |
| Atropine is useful in organophosphate poisoning | T |
| 50g of activated charcoal should not be exceeded in salicylate poisoning | F |
| Methemoglobumaemia is associated with Local anaesthetic toxicity | T |
| **The following are true of the local anaesthetic prilocaine** | |
| It is amide group local anaesthetic | T |
| It has a half life of 4 hours | F |
| It's maximum safe dose is 5mg/kg | F |
| It can cause methaemoglobinaemia | T |

# SECTION 12: TOXICOLOGY

## I. DIGOXIN TOXICITY

**Digoxin (digitalis) is highly toxic in overdose.**

- Clinical features of acute toxicity include:
  - GI distress, nausea, vomiting and abdominal pain
  - Hyperkalaemia, Dysrhythmia (all kinds of tachycardia and bradycardias as well as ventricular fibrillation!)
  - Hypotension, Lethargy and confusion
  - (Visual disturbances, reduced visual acuity and yellow vision, are more a feature of chronic digitalis toxicity)

### ECG FEATURES OF DIGOXIN TOXICITY:
  - Prolonged PR interval
  - QT Shortened
  - T wave inversion
  - ST depression

- While peak serum levels of digoxin occur at 6hrs, the life threatening cardiovascular complications often occur later at 8-12 hours post-ingestion.
- **Digoxin cardiotoxicity** is resistant to normal supportive measures and is best treated with digoxin specific Fab fragments (Digibind).
- **Digoxin induced hyperkalaemia** is treated with insulin and glucose therapy.

## DIGOXIN IMMUNE FAB

- It is an antidote for overdose of digitalis: It is made from immunoglobulin fragments from sheep that have already been immunized with a digoxin derivative, digoxin dicarboxymethoxylamine.
- Its brand names include Digibind (GlaxoSmithKline) and DigiFab (BTG plc)

## II. LIDOCAINE TOXICITY

- There are several conditions that increase the potential for lidocaine toxicity:
  - *Liver dysfunction increases the risk of toxicity due to lidocaine being metabolized by the liver.*
  - *Low protein increases the risk of toxicity because lidocaine is protein bound.*
  - *Acidosis can also increase the risk of toxicity since acidosis increase the potential of lidocaine to dissociate from plasma proteins.*
- **Signs of severe toxicity:**
  - Sudden alteration in mental status, severe agitation or LOC +/- convulsions
  - Cardiovascular collapse: bradycardia, conduction blocks, asystole and VT may occur
  - Local anaesthetic (LA) toxicity may occur some time after an initial injection
- **IMMEDIATE MANAGEMENT**
  - Stop injecting the LA and Call for help
  - Maintain the airway and, if necessary, secure it with a tracheal tube
  - Give 100% oxygen and ensure adequate lung ventilation
  - Confirm or establish intravenous access
  - Control seizures: a benzodiazepine, thiopental or Propofol in small incremental doses
  - Assess cardiovascular status throughout
  - Consider drawing blood for analysis, but do not delay definitive treatment to do this

**TREATMENT:**

- **In circulatory arrest**
  - Start CPR using standard protocols
  - Manage arrhythmias using the same protocols
  - Give **intravenous Lipid Emulsion (Intralipid)**
  - Continue CPR throughout treatment with lipid emulsion
  - Recovery from LA-induced cardiac arrest may take >1 h
  - Propofol is not a suitable substitute for lipid emulsion
  - Lidocaine should not be used as an anti-arrhythmic therapy
- **Without circulatory arrest**
  - Use conventional therapies to treat hypotension, bradycardia, tachyarrhythmia
  - Consider intravenous lipid emulsion

## III. SALICYLATE TOXICITY

- Salicylate poisoning is a relatively common cause of poisoning and effective early treatment can prevent organ damage and death.
- Poisoning can be classified as mild, moderate or severe depending upon the plasma salicylate level:
  - *Mild poisoning = < 450 mg/L*
  - *Moderate poisoning = 450-700 mg/L*
  - *Severe poisoning = > 700 mg/L*

- **CLINICAL FEATURES INCLUDE:**
  - Nausea and Vomiting
  - Tinnitus and Deafness
  - Sweating and Dehydration
  - Hyperventilation
  - Cutaneous flushing
  - Hyperpyrexia (particularly children)
  - Hypoglycaemia (particularly children)
  - Severe poisoning can cause convulsions, cerebral oedema, coma, renal failure, non-cardiogenic pulmonary oedema and cardiovascular instability.

- **INVESTIGATIONS SHOULD INCLUDE:**
  - Plasma salicylate level
  - Arterial blood gas: **Primary respiratory alkalosis** may occur, followed by concomitant **primary metabolic acidosis (RALMAC)**
  - Blood glucose level
  - Urea and electrolytes
  - Clotting profile
  - ECG

## ECG ABNORMALITIES IN SALICYLATE OVERDOSE:

- *Widening of the QRS complex*
- *AV Block*
- *Ventricular Arrhythmias*

## TREATMENT

- Involves stabilization of the ABCs as necessary, limiting absorption, enhancing elimination, correcting metabolic abnormalities, and providing supportive care.
- No specific antidote is available for salicylates.
- **Gastric lavage** and **activated charcoal** (50 g) are indicated if greater than 4.5g has been ingested in the previous hour (or > 2 g in a child).
- Activated charcoal both reduces absorption and increases elimination of salicylate.
- Severe cases usually require **aggressive intravenous fluids** to correct dehydration and **1.26% sodium bicarbonate administration**, which increases elimination of the salicylate.
- **The urine pH** should be maintained at greater **than 7.5** and ideally should be between **8.0-8.5.**
- There is, however, no longer any role for **forced alkaline diuresis.**
- Life-threatening cases will require intensive care admission, intubation and ventilation and possibly **haemodialysis.**

## IV. PARACETAMOL/ACETAMINOPHEN TOXICITY

- Leads to Hepatic necrosis
- 90% is metabolised in the Liver to inactive metabolite
- Metabolism of the reminder is via CYP450:
  - NAPQI
  - NAPQI is bound by Glutathione and excreted
  - Glutathione stores are exhausted
  - Then NAPQI binds to other proteins in the Liver
- Paracetamol overdose is the most common overdose in the U.K. and is also the commonest cause of acute liver failure.
- The liver damage is caused by a metabolite of paracetamol, **N-acetyl-p-benzoquinoneimine (NAPQI),** which depletes the livers stores of **Glutathione** and directly damages liver cells.
- An overdose of greater than **12 g or > 150 mg/kg body weight** may cause severe liver damage and death. Acute renal tubular damage and necrosis may also occur.
- **Do NOT take plasma levels within 4 hours of ingestion as they are unreliable.**
- Patients may give inaccurate histories or if there is doubt about the timing or the need for treatment: **treat with NAC.**

- **Methionine** is ineffective in patients who have been given **oral activated charcoal.**
- **NAC** is the treatment of choice when patients are vomiting or present **more than 8 hours after ingestion.**

### SIGNS AND SYMPTOMS
- Initially asymptomatic
- End-organ toxicity often does not manifest until 24-48 hours after an acute ingestion.
- **Minimum toxic doses:**
  - Adults: 7.5-10 g
  - Children: 150 mg/kg; 200 mg/kg in healthy children aged 1-6 years

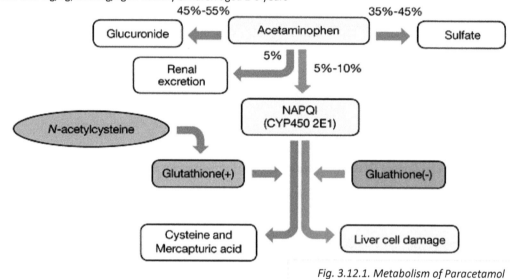

Fig. 3.12.1. Metabolism of Paracetamol

## HIGH RISK PATIENTS (RISK OF LIVER DAMAGE)
- *Regular alcohol ingestion*
- *Other enzyme (liver microsomal oxidases) inducers (e.g. carbamazepine, phenytoin, phenobarbitone, primidone and rifampicin)*
- *Glutathione depletion (e.g. malnutrition and HIV)*
- The earliest and most sensitive indicator of liver damage is a **prolonged INR**, which starts to rise at around **24 hours after overdose.**
- **LFTs** are usually normal **until around 16 hours after overdose.**
- **AST and ALT levels** then sharply rise and can reach > 10,000 units/L by **72-96 hours** after overdose.
- **Bilirubin** levels rise more slowly and reach their maximum at around **5 days**.

## MANAGEMENT OF PARACETAMOL OD IN THE ED
### 1. Management of Adult patients who present within 1-4 hour of ingestion
- Consider **charcoal** if more than 150 mg/kg body weight taken, presentation within 1 hour of ingestion and able to control the airway.
- **Take blood for plasma paracetamol concentration at 4 hours post ingestion.**
- Assess whether at high risk of severe liver damage (see above).
- Confirm timings of ingestion

### 2. Management of Adult patients who present within 4-8 hours of ingestion
- **Do not** start NAC immediately.
- Wait until 4 hours post ingestion and take Paracetamol/salicylates levels.
- Start NAC if level taken at 4 hours is in the appropriate treatment range.
- If the paracetamol concentration result is not available within 8 hours of ingestion (> 150 mg/kg or > 12 g in total) **start NAC immediately.**
- It can be stopped later if subsequent level well below treatment line.

### 3. Mx of all patients who present 8-15 hours after ingestion.
- Urgent action is required (antidote efficacy drops sharply).
- **Give NAC immediately** without waiting for the result of the plasma paracetamol concentration measurement if it is thought that more than 150 mg/kg body weight or a total of 12 g or more has been ingested.
- **Take Paracetamol/Salicylates levels, INR, Creatinine and ALT.**
- If the paracetamol concentration result is not available within 8 hours of ingestion (> 150 mg/kg or > 12 g in total) **start NAC immediately.**

- In patients already receiving NAC, only discontinue NAC if the plasma paracetamol concentration is below the treatment line on the graph and there is no abnormality of the INR, plasma creatinine or ALT and the patient is asymptomatic.
- Continue the infusion if there is any doubt as to the timing of the overdose.
- At the end of NAC infusion **check INR and plasma creatinine concentration**.
- Patients who are symptomatic or in whom the INR and/or plasma creatinine are abnormal require further monitoring. **Vitamin K** should be given if the INR is increased.
- **FFP / clotting factors** are only indicated **for active bleeding.**

### 4. Mx of patients who present 15-24 hours after ingestion:

- **Start NAC immediately.**
- Measure the plasma paracetamol concentration on admission.
- The infusion may be stopped and the patient discharged from medical care if each of the following criteria is met:
  - The patient is asymptomatic.
  - The INR and plasma creatinine are normal.
  - The plasma paracetamol concentration is **less than 10 mg/L** (0.07 mmol/L) 24 hours after ingestion.
- Patients in whom the INR and/or plasma creatinine are abnormal or whose plasma paracetamol concentrations exceed 10 mg/L at 24 hours after ingestion require further monitoring and contact with a hepatologist.

### 5. Mx of patients who present longer than 24 hours after ingestion:

- All should have their **INR, Plasma Creatinine concentration, ALT and Venous pH** (or hydrogen ion / bicarb concentration) determined.
- We recommend that they **all** be discussed with a poisons information centre or a specialist liver or poisons unit.

### 6. Specialist advice on those with liver disease.

- Liver transplantation is occasionally needed for liver failure secondary to paracetamol overdose for patients who presented or were treated late.

*WHEN TO TRANSFER PATIENTS TO A LIVER TRANSPLANT CENTRE*

- *High-risk features mandating admission to a liver transplant centre are:*
  - *INR >3.0 at 48 hours or >4.5 at any time*
  - *Oliguria or creatinine > 200 micromol/L*
  - *Acidosis with pH < 7.3 after resuscitation*
  - *Systolic hypotension with BP < 80mmHg*
  - *Hypoglycaemia*
  - *Severe thrombocytopenia*
  - *Encephalopathy of any degree*

## 1. N- ACETYLCYSTEINE (NAC)

- **NAC increases Gluthathione availability** leading to direct binding to NAPQI.
- NAC is nearly 100% hepatoprotective when it is **given within 8 hours** after acute acetaminophen ingestion, but can be beneficial in patients who present more than 24 hours after ingestion loading dose of 140 mg/kg.
- Acetylcysteine should be administered by intravenous infusion preferably using Glucose 5% as the infusion fluid. Sodium Chloride 0.9% solution may be used if Glucose 5% is not suitable.
- The full course of treatment with acetylcysteine comprises of 3 consecutive intravenous infusions.
- **Methionine P.O. 2.5 g 4 hourly to a total dose of 10 g.** is a useful alternative in patients who refuse treatment.
- Doses should be administered sequentially with no break between the infusions.
- The patient should receive a total dose of **300 mg/kg body weight over a 21-hour** period as follows (**Each ampoule = 200mg/mL acetylcysteine**):
  - **Adults:**
    - **Loading dose:** 150 mg/kg IV; mix in 200 mL of 5% dextrose in water (D5W) and infuse over 1 h.
    - **Dose 2:** 50 mg/kg IV in 500 mL D5W over 4 h.
    - **Dose 3:** 100 mg/kg IV in 1000 mL D5W over 16 h.
  - In patients who weigh more than 100 kg, limited data suggest a loading dose of 15,000 mg infused IV over 1 hours, then a first maintenance dose of 5,000 mg IV over 4 hours and a second maintenance dose of 10,000 mg over 16 hours.
  - **Children**

# V. $Ca^{2+}$ CHANNEL BLOCKER & β- BLOCKERS TOXICITY

- Both cause AV blockade
- Results in myocardial depression and bradycardia
- **TREATMENT:**
  - **CCB:** Atropine, Calcium, High-dose Insulin-dextrose
  - **Beta-Blockers:** Atropine, IV Glucagon, High-dose Insulin-dextrose

## VI. TCA TOXICITY

- Any overdose of amitriptyline **> 10 mg/kg** is potentially life-threatening.
- An overdose **> 30 mg/kg** will result in severe toxicity, cardiotoxicity and coma.
- The toxic effects of TCAs are mediated by several pharmacological effects:
    - *Anticholinergic effects*
    - *Direct alpha-adrenergic blockade*
    - *Blockade of noradrenaline reuptake at the preganglionic synapse*
    - *Blockade of sodium channels*
    - *Blockade of potassium channels*

### CLINICAL EFFECTS

| | |
|---|---|
| **Anticholinergic** | Dry mouth, Dry Skin<br>Constipation,<br>Urinary retention<br>Mydriasis/Blurred vision<br>Aggravation narrow angle glaucoma |
| **Anti-alpha adrenergic** | Orthostatic hypotension |
| **Antihistaminic** | Sedation |
| **Cardiac** | Tachycardia, Hypotension<br>Palpitation, Chest pain. |
| **CNS** | Decrease mental status, Respiratory depression,<br>Drowsiness' Confusion, Convulsion, Coma. |

- The cardiotoxic effects of TCAs are mediated by the blockade of **Na channels,** which causes QRS broadening, and blockade of **K channels**, which causes QT interval prolongation.
- **The degree of QRS broadening correlates with adverse events:**
    - *QRS > 100 ms is predictive of **seizures***
    - *QRS > 160 ms is predictive of **ventricular arrhythmias***
- **The ECG changes seen in TCA overdose include:**
    - *Sinus tachycardia (very common)*
    - *Prolongation of the PR interval & Broadening of QRS complex*
    - *Prolongation of the QT interval & Ventricular arrhythmias (severe toxicity)*

- **MANAGEMENT**
    - **Gastric lavage** may be helpful in recovering and identifying the TCA ingested.
    - **Activated charcoal** reduces the absorption of TCAs. It may also be beneficial in cases of multisubstance ingestion. It should be administered only in patients who are able to protect the airway.
    - **Endotracheal intubation** is indicated if the patient cannot adequately maintain a safe airway.
    - *Electrocardiography (ECG) is a highly sensitive tool, and a normal result can be used to rule out TCA toxicity. However, ECG is not specific enough to be used alone to diagnose TCA overdose.*

### ECG FEATURES OF TCA TOXICITY

- Sinus tachycardia
- Right-Axis Deviation
- Prolongation of the PR, QRS, and QTC intervals
- Nonspecific ST-segment and T-wave changes
- AV block
- Brugada pattern (downsloping ST-segment elevation in leads V1-V3 in association with right bundle branch block)
- Wide QRS (>100 milliseconds) is the basis for treatment with bicarbonate (alkalinization).
    - **QRS < 100 ms**: seizures and arrhythmias are unlikely
    - **QRS > 100 ms**: 34% chance of developing seizures and up to a 14% chance of developing a life-threatening cardiac arrhythmia.
    - **QRS complex > 160 ms**: 50% chance of ventricular arrhythmias.
- Early recognition of conduction disturbances is important in suspected TCA poisoning.

## VII. ACTIVATED CHARCOAL

- Effective within 1 hour
- **Not effective against:**
  - Iron
  - Lithium
  - Alcohols
  - Petroleum or Pesticides
  - Cyanide
- **Repeated doses can be useful in:**
  - Carbamazepine
  - Phenobarbitone (tal)
  - Quinine
  - Theophylline
  - Salicylate

## VIII. METHANOL AND ETHYLENE GLYCOL

- Metabolites cause toxic effects
- **Features:**
  - Similar to alcohol (without the smell)
  - **Methanol:** Blindness due to retinal injury, latent
  - **Ethylene Glycol:** renal failure with rapid progression
  - High Anion gap for both
- **Treatement:**
  - **Antidote:** Ethanol, Fomepizole
  - Dialysis

## IX. CHOLINERGIC SYNDROME

- **NMJ:** weakness, Flaccid paralysis
- **Parasympathetic:** miosis, increased secretions, Diarrhoea, increased urination, decreased HR
- **Sympathetic:** Mydriasis, sweating, increased HR and BP
- **CNS:** agitation, confusion, Fits
- **DUMBELS:** **D**iarrhoea, **U**rination, **M**iosis, **B**ronchospasm, **E**mesis, **L**acrimation, **S**alivation
- **Agents:**
  - Organophosphates
  - Nerve agents
  - Neostigmine and Physostigmine
  - Donepezil
- **Treatment:**
  - Personal Protective Equipment
  - Supportive: Secretion Management
  - **Antidote:** Atropine, Pralidoxime

## X. ANTICHOLINERGIC SYNDROME

Due to inhibition of ACh
- **Muscarinic Blockade:**
  - Dry mouth
  - Urinary retention
  - Constipation
  - Mydriasis
  - Tachycardia
  - Hyperthermia
- **Agitated Delirium**
  - Confusion
  - Fluctuating GCS
- **Agents**
  - Antipsychotics
  - TCA
  - Atropine
  - Antihistamines
  - Amphetamines
- **Treatment:**
  - Supportive
  - Benzodiazepines
  - Physostigmine

## XI. NEUROLEPTIC MALIGNANT SYNDROME

- **Characteristics:**
  - Neuromuscular rigidity
  - Autonomic disturbances
  - Altered mental status
- **Treatement:**
  - Cooling
  - GTN or Nitroprusside
  - **Antidotes:** Bromocryptine, Dantrolene

## XII. SYMPATHOMIMETIC SYNDROME

- Anxiety, delusions, paranoia
- Diaphoresis, Piloerection, Mydriasis
- Increased HR, BP, Arrhythmias
- Hyperreflexia, tremors, seizures
- **Agents:**
  - Amphetamines, Cocaine
  - MDMA
  - Ephedrine and Pseudoephedrine
  - MAOI and SSRI
- **Treatment:**
  - Supportive

## XIII. SEROTONIN SYNDROME

- **Characteristics:**
  - Neuromuscular rigidity
  - Autonomic disturbances
  - Altered mental status
- **Treatment:**
  - Supportive, may need cooling/ paralysis
  - **Antidote:** Cyproheptadine and Chlorpromazine

## XIV. ANTIPSYCHOTICS

- **Typical: Haloperidol, Chlorpromazine**
  - **Adverse reaction:**
    - Extrapyramidal
    - Anticholinergic
    - Histamine
    - NMS
- **Atypical: Clozapine, Quetiapine, Olanzapine**
  - **Adverse reaction:**
    - Same as above but less likely
    - Sexual dysfunction

## XVI. CYANIDE

- **Binding to Cytochrome Fe3+:**
  - Inhibits oxidative phosphorylation
  - Leads to acidosis
- **Features:**
  - N&V, headaches, seizures, coma
  - Can lead to hypotension and CV collapse
  - Profound acidosis
- **Treatement:**
  - **High flow O2**
  - **Antidotes:** Hydroxycobalamin, Na Thiosulphate, Dicobalt EDTA, Amyl/Na nitrite
  - **Supportive**

## VII. DRUGS AND THEIR ANTIDOTES

| 01 | Paracetamol | N-Acetylcysteine or Mucomyst/ Methionine |
|---|---|---|
| 02 | Warfarin | Prothrombin Complex Concentrate (PCC) or Vit K |
| 03 | Benzodiazepines | Flumazenil (Romazicon) |
| 04 | Beta-Blocking | Glucagon |
| 05 | Calcium Channel Blockers | Calcium; Anticholinergics |
| 06 | Dabigatran (Pradaxa) | Idarucizumab, Dialysis |
| 07 | Cyanide | Hydroxycobalamin, Na/Amyl Nitrite Dicobalt Edetate, Na Thiosulfate |
| 08 | Digoxin | Digoxin Immune Fab (Digibind) |
| 09 | Opioid (Heroin) | Naloxone (Narcan) |
| 10 | Iron | Deferoxamine |
| 11 | Heparin | Protamine Sulfate |
| 12 | Organophosphates | Atropine, Pralidoxime |
| 13 | Potassium | Insulin + Glucose, Kayexalate |
| 14 | Sodium channel blockers (TCAs), Salicylates | Sodium Bicarbonate |
| 15 | Ethylene glycol & Methanol | Ethanol / Fomepizole/ Dialysis / Thiamine |
| 16 | Local anesthetics | Intralipid/ Fat emulsion |
| 17 | Carbone Monoxide | Oxygen/Hyperbaric Oxygen |
| 18 | Heavy metals | Dimercaprol, Penicillamine, Na channel edetate |
| 19 | Paraquat | Charcoal, Fuller's earth |
| 20 | Antidepressants | Diazepam for convulsion, Bicarbonate for arrhythmia |
| 21 | Aspirin | Hemodialysis |
| 22 | Lithium | Gut decontamination, Hydration, Dialysis |
| 23 | Methaemoglobin | Methylene Blue |

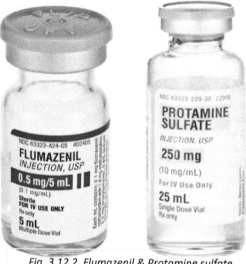

Fig. 3.12.2. Flumazenil & Protamine sulfate

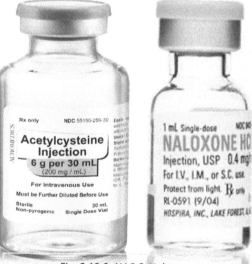

Fig. 3.12.3. NAC & Naloxone

# Part Four:
# Microbiology

Compiled and Edited by:
Dr Moussa Issa
MBChB MRCEM
Senior ED Registrar

# PART A: PRINCIPLES OF MICROBIOLOGY
# Section 1: Natural & Innate Immunity

## I. INTRODUCTION

- Innate (natural) immunity: Immunity present at birth and does not have to be learned through exposure to an invader. It thus provides an immediate response to foreign invaders. However, its components treat all foreign invaders in much the same way.
- They recognize only a limited number of identifying substances (antigens) on foreign invaders. However, these antigens are present on many different invaders.
- Innate immunity, unlike acquired immunity, has no memory of the encounters, does not remember specific foreign antigens, and does not provide any ongoing protection against future infection.
- The white blood cells involved in innate immunity are:
  - Monocytes (which develop into macrophages)
  - Neutrophils
  - Eosinophils
  - Basophils
  - Natural killer cells
- Other participants in innate immunity are
  - The complement system
  - Cytokines

## 1. MONOCYTES AND MACROPHAGES

- Macrophages develop from a type of white blood cell called monocytes.
- Monocytes become macrophages when they move from the bloodstream to the tissues. Monocytes move to the tissues when infection occurs.
- There, over a period of about 8 hours, monocytes enlarge greatly and produce granules within themselves, becoming macrophages.
- The granules are filled with enzymes and other substances that help kill and digest bacteria and other foreign cells.
- Macrophages stay in the tissues. They ingest bacteria, foreign cells, and damaged and dead cells.
- The process of a cell ingesting a microorganism, another cell, or cell fragments is called phagocytosis, and cells that ingest are called phagocytes.
- Macrophages secrete substances that attract other white blood cells to the site of the infection. They also help T cells recognize invaders neutrophils.

## 2. NEUTROPHILS

- The most common type of white blood cell in the bloodstream, are among the first immune cells to defend against infection. They ingest bacteria and other foreign cells.
- Neutrophils contain granules that release enzymes to help kill and digest these cells.
- Neutrophils circulate in the bloodstream and must be signalled to leave the bloodstream and enter tissues.
- The signal often comes from the bacteria themselves, from complement proteins, or from damaged tissue, all of which produce substances that attract neutrophils to a trouble spot. (The process of using substances to attract cells to a particular site is called chemotaxis.)
- Neutrophils also release substances that produce fibers in the surrounding tissue. These fibers may trap bacteria, thus keeping them from spreading and making them easier to destroy.

## 3. EOSINOPHILS

- Eosinophils can ingest bacteria but also target foreign cells that are too large to ingest.
- Eosinophils contain granules that release enzymes and other toxic substances when foreign cells are encountered.
- These substances make holes in the target cell's membranes.
- Eosinophils circulate in the bloodstream. However, they are less active against bacteria than are neutrophils and macrophages.
- One of their main functions is to attach to and thus help immobilize and kill parasites.
- Eosinophils may help destroy cancer cells. They also produce substances involved in inflammation and allergic reactions.

## 4. BASOPHILS

- Basophils do not ingest foreign cells.

- They contain granules filled with histamine, a substance involved in   important in the initial defense against viral infections.
- Also, natural killer cells produce cytokines that regulate some of the functions of T cells, B cells, and macrophages.

## 5. COMPLEMENT SYSTEM

- The complement system consists of more than 30 proteins that act in a sequence: One protein activates another and so on.
- This sequence is called the complement cascade.
- Complement proteins have many functions in acquired immunity as well as innate:
  - Killing bacteria directly and Helping destroy bacteria by attaching to them and thus making the bacteria easier for neutrophils and macrophages to identify and ingest.
  - Attracting macrophages and neutrophils to a trouble spot.
  - Neutralizing viruses and Helping immune cells remember specific invaders.
  - Promoting antibody formation and enhancing the effectiveness of antibodies.
  - Helping the body eliminate dead cells and immune complexes (which consist of an antibody attached to an antigen).

## 6. CYTOKINES

- Cytokines are the messengers of the immune system.
- White blood cells and certain other cells of the immune system produce cytokines when an antigen is detected.
- There are many different cytokines, which affect different parts of the immune system:
  - Some cytokines stimulate activity. They stimulate certain white blood cells to become more effective killers and to attract other white blood cells to a trouble spot.
  - Other cytokines inhibit activity, helping end an immune response.
  - Some cytokines, called interferons, interfere with the reproduction (replication) of viruses.
- Cytokines also participate in acquired immunity.

# II. BARRIERS TO INFECTION

## 1. PHYSICAL BARRIERS

- The first line of defence (or outside defence system) includes physical and chemical barriers that are always ready and prepared to defend the body from infection.
- These include the skin, tears, mucus, cilia, stomach acid, urine flow, 'friendly' bacteria and neutrophils.
- Pathogenic microorganisms must make it past this first line of defence.
- If this defence is broken, the second line of defence within the body is activated.

**THE SKIN:**
- Prevents invasion by microorganisms unless it is damaged—for example, by an injury, insect bite, or burn.
- Other effective physical barriers are mucous membranes, such as the lining of the mouth, nose, and eyelids.

**THE AIRWAYS:**
- Filter out particles that are present in the air that is inhaled.
- The walls of the passages in the nose and airways are coated with mucus.

**THE DIGESTIVE TRACT:**
- Has a series of effective barriers, including stomach acid, pancreatic enzymes, bile, and intestinal secretions.
- The contractions of the intestine (peristalsis) and the normal shedding of cells lining the intestine help remove harmful microorganisms.

**THE BLADDER:**
- It is protected by the urethra that drains urine from the body.
- In males older than 6 months, the urethra is long enough that bacteria are seldom able to pass through it to reach the bladder, unless the bacteria are unintentionally placed there by catheters or surgical instruments.
- In females, the urethra is shorter, occasionally allowing external bacteria to pass into the bladder.
- In both sexes, when the bladder empties, it flushes out any bacteria that reach it.

**THE BLOOD:**
- The body also defends against infection by increasing the number of certain types of white blood cells (neutrophils and monocytes), which engulf and destroy invading microorganisms.

## 2. INFLAMMATION

- A response triggered by damage to living tissues.

- The inflammatory response is a defense mechanism that evolved in higher organisms to protect them from infection and injury.
- Its purpose is to localize and eliminate the injurious agent and to remove damaged tissue components so that the body can begin to heal. The response consists of changes in blood flow, an increase in permeability of blood vessels, and the migration of fluid, proteins, and white blood cells (leukocytes) from the circulation to the site of tissue damage.
- An inflammatory response that lasts only a few days is called **acute inflammation**, while a response of longer duration is referred to as **chronic inflammation**.
- Although acute inflammation is usually beneficial, it often causes unpleasant sensations, such as the pain of a sore throat or the itching of an insect bite.
- In some instances, inflammation can cause harm. Tissue destruction can occur when the regulatory mechanisms of the inflammatory response are defective or the ability to clear damaged tissue and foreign substances is impaired.
- In other cases, an inappropriate immune response may give rise to a prolonged and damaging inflammatory response.
- The 4 cardinal signs of inflammation are: redness (rubor), heat (*calor*), swelling (*tumor*), and pain (*dolor*).
  - **Redness** is caused by the dilation of small blood vessels in the area of injury.
  - **Heat** results from increased blood flow through the area and is experienced only in peripheral parts of the body such as the skin.
  - Fever is brought about by chemical mediators of inflammation and contributes to the rise in temperature at the injury.
  - **Swelling** (edema) is caused primarily by the accumulation of fluid outside the blood vessels.
  - **The pain** associated with inflammation results in part from the distortion of tissues caused by edema, and it also is induced by certain chemical mediators of inflammation, such as bradykinin, serotonin, and the prostaglandins.
  - A fifth consequence of inflammation is the **loss of function** of the inflamed area which may result from pain that inhibits mobility or from severe swelling that prevents movement in the area.

# III. NORMAL BACTERIAL FLORA

## 1. SIGNIFICANCE OF THE NORMAL FLORA

### A. SKIN FLORA:
- The varied environment of the skin results in locally dense or sparse populations, with Gram-positive organisms (e.g., staphylococci, micrococci, diphtheroids) usually predominating.

### B. ORAL AND UPPER RESPIRATORY TRACT FLORA:
- A varied microbial flora is found in the oral cavity, and streptococcal anaerobes inhabit the gingival crevice.
- The pharynx can be a point of entry and initial colonization for Neisseria, Bordetella, Corynebacterium, and Streptococcus spp.

### C. GASTROINTESTINAL TRACT FLORA:
- Organisms in the stomach are usually transient, and their populations are kept low by acidity (H. pylori).
- In normal hosts the duodenal flora is sparse.
- The ileum contains a moderately mixed flora ($10^6$ to $10^8$/g of contents).
- The flora of the large bowel is dense ($10^9$ to $10^{11}$/g of contents) and is composed predominantly of anaerobes.
- These organisms participate in bile acid conversion and in vitamin K and ammonia production in the large bowel.
- They can also cause intestinal abscesses and peritonitis.

### D. UROGENITAL FLORA:
- The vaginal flora changes with the age of the individual, the vaginal pH, and hormone levels.
- Transient organisms (e.g., Candida spp.) frequently cause vaginitis.

### E. CONJUNCTIVAL FLORA:
- The conjunctiva harbors few or no organisms.
- Haemophilus and Staphylococcus are among the genera most often detected.

### F. HOST INFECTION:
- Many elements of the normal flora may act as opportunistic pathogens, especially in hosts rendered susceptible by rheumatic heart disease, immunosuppression, radiation therapy, chemotherapy, perforated mucous membranes, etc.
- The flora of the gingival crevice causes dental caries in about 80 percent of the population.

# SECTION 2: MECHANISMS OF DISEASE

## I. BASIC TERMINOLOGY:

- **Colonisation** is a normal state and is not pathological
- **Pathogen** is an organism capable of causing an infection
- **Infection** describes a microbe-induced state of disease

## II. TYPES OF BACTERIAL PATHOGENS

o   There are three categories of bacterial pathogens: obligate, opportunistic and accidental pathogens.

### 1. OBLIGATE PATHOGENS

- Must cause disease in order to be transmitted from one host to another.
- These bacteria must also infect a host in order to survive, in contrast to other bacteria that are capable of survival outside of a host.

| OBLIGATE ANAEROBES | OBLIGATE AEROBES | FACULTATIVE ANAEROBIC BACTERIA |
|---|---|---|
| • live and grow in the absence of oxygen: BC TAP | • that require oxygen to grow: BMNP | • make ATP via aerobic respiration and are also capable of switching to fermentation: LESS |
| o Bacteroides spp<br>o Clostridium spp<br>o Treponema spp<br>o Actinomyces spp<br>o Peptostreptococcus spp | o Bacillus spp<br>o Mycobacterium tuberculosis<br>o Nocardia spp<br>o Pseudomonas aeruginosa | o Listeria spp<br>o Escherichia coli<br>o Staphylococcus spp and Streptococcus spp<br>o Shewanella oneidensis |

### 2. OPPORTUNISTIC PATHOGENS

- Can be transmitted from one host to another without having to cause disease. However, in a host whose immune system is not functioning properly, the bacteria can cause an infection that leads to a disease. In those cases, the disease can help the bacteria spread to another host.
- **Examples of opportunistic pathogens** include Vibrio cholera, Pneumocystitis sp, Pseudomonas aeruginosa, CMV, M. tuberculosis, C. albicans, Isospora belli, Kaposi sarcoma, Clostridium difficile...

### 3. ACCIDENTAL PATHOGENS

- Some bacterial pathogens cause disease only accidentally. Indeed, the disease actually limits the spread of the bacteria to another host.
- Examples of these "accidental' pathogens include Neisseria meningitides and Bacteroides fragilis...

# III. MECHANISMS OF BACTERIAL PATHOGENICITY

## A. COLONIZATION

- The first stage of microbial infection is colonization: the establishment of the pathogen at the appropriate portal of entry.
- Pathogens usually colonize host tissues that are in contact with the external environment.
- Sites of entry in human hosts include the urogenital tract, the digestive tract, the respiratory tract and the conjunctiva.
- Organisms that infect these regions have usually developed tissue adherence mechanisms and some ability to overcome or withstand the constant pressure of the host defenses at the surface.

## B. BACTERIAL ADHERENCE TO MUCOSAL SURFACES

- In its simplest form, bacterial adherence or attachment to a eucaryotic cell or tissue surface requires the participation of two factors: a receptor and a ligand.
- The receptors so far defined are usually specific carbohydrate or peptide residues on the eucaryotic cell surface.
- The bacterial ligand, called an adhesin, is typically a macromolecular component of the bacterial cell surface which interacts with the host cell receptor.
- Adhesins and receptors usually interact in a complementary and specific fashion.

## SPECIFIC ADHERENCE OF BACTERIA TO CELL AND TISSUE SURFACES:

- **Tissue tropism:**
  - o particular bacteria are known to have an apparent preference for certain tissues over others,
  - o e.g. S. mutans is abundant in dental plaque but does not occur on epithelial surfaces of the tongue; the reverse is true for S. salivarius which is attached in high numbers to epithelial cells of the tongue but is absent in dental plaque.

- **Species specificity:**
  - o certain pathogenic bacteria infect only certain species of animals,
    e.g. N. gonorrhoeae infections are limited to humans;
  - o Enteropathogenic E. coli K-88 infections are limited to pigs; E. coli CFA I and CFA II infect humans; E. coli K-99 strain infects calves.
  - o Group A streptococcal infections occur only in humans.

- **Genetic specificity within a species:**
  - o Certain strains or races within a species are genetically immune to a pathogen,
  - o e.g. Certain pigs are not susceptible to E. Coli K-88 infections;
  - o Susceptibility to Plasmodium vivax infection (malaria) is dependent on the presence of the Duffy antigens on the host's red blood cells.

## MECHANISMS OF ADHERENCE TO CELL OR TISSUE SURFACES:

- o **Nonspecific adherence**: reversible attachment of the bacterium to the eucaryotic surface (sometimes called "docking")
- o **Specific adherence**: irreversible permanent attachment of the microorganism to the surface (sometimes called "anchoring").
- Nonspecific adherence involves nonspecific attractive forces which allow approach of the bacterium to the eucaryotic cell surface.
- Specific adherence involves permanent formation of many specific lock-and-key bonds between complementary molecules on each cell surface.
- Complementary receptor and adhesin molecules must be accessible and arranged in such a way that many bonds form over the area of contact between the two cells.
- Once the bonds are formed, attachment under physiological conditions becomes virtually irreversible.
- Specific adherence involves complementary chemical interactions between the host cell or tissue surface and the bacterial surface.
- In the language of medical microbiologist, a bacterial "adhesin" attaches covalently to a host "receptor" so that the bacterium "docks" itself on the host surface. The adhesins of bacterial cells are chemical components of capsules, cell walls, pili or fimbriae. The host receptors are usually glycoproteins located on the cell membrane or tissue surface.
- Adhesion (of the bacterium to the eucaryotic cell surface) is inhibited by:
  - o Isolated adhesin or receptor molecules
  - o Adhesin or receptor analogs
  - o Enzymes and chemicals that specifically destroy adhesins or receptors
  - o Antibodies specific to surface components (i.e., adhesins or receptors)

### Examples of Attachments:

- Influenza virus: Attaching via a haemagglutinin antigen
- Giardia lamblia: Attaching to gut mucosa via a specialised sucking disc
- P. falciparum: Causing red cell protein expression facilitating cerebral malaria
- HIV: Binding strongly to CD4 antigen

# IV. FACTORS FACILITATING MICROBIAL INVASION

- Microbial invasion can be facilitated by:
  - o Virulence factors
  - o Microbial adherence
  - o Resistance to antimicrobials
  - o Defects in host defense mechanisms.

## A. VIRULENCE FACTORS

- Virulence factors assist pathogens in invasion and resistance of host defenses; these factors include:
  - o Capsule
  - o Enzymes
  - o Toxins

## CAPSULE

- Some organisms (eg, certain strains of pneumococci, meningococci, type B Haemophilus influenzae) have a capsule that prevents opsonic antibodies from binding and thus are more virulent than nonencapsulated strains.

## ENZYMES

- Bacterial proteins with enzymatic activity (eg, protease, hyaluronidase, neuraminidase, elastase, and collagenase) facilitate local tissue spread.
- Invasive organisms (eg, Shigella flexneri, Yersinia enterocolitica) can penetrate and traverse intact eukaryotic cells, facilitating entry from mucosal surfaces.
- Some bacteria (eg, Neisseria gonorrhoeae, H. influenzae, Proteus mirabilis, clostridial species, Streptococcus pneumonia...) produce IgA-specific proteases that cleave and inactivate secretory IgA on mucosal surfaces.

## TOXINS

- Organisms may release toxins (called exotoxins), which are protein molecules that may cause the disease (eg, diphtheria, cholera, tetanus, botulism) or increase the severity of the disease.
- Endotoxin triggers humoral enzymatic mechanisms involving the complement, clotting, fibrinolytic, and kinin pathways and causes much of the morbidity in gram-negative sepsis.

## OTHER FACTORS

- Many microorganisms have mechanisms that impair antibody production by inducing suppressor cells, blocking antigen processing, and inhibiting lymphocyte mitogenesis.
- Resistance to the lytic effects of serum complement confers virulence.
- Among species of N. gonorrhoeae, resistance predisposes to disseminated rather than localized infection.
- Some organisms resist the oxidative steps in phagocytosis.
- For example, Legionella and Listeria either do not elicit or actively suppress the oxidative step.
- Whereas other organisms produce enzymes (eg, catalase, glutathione reductase, superoxide dismutase) that mitigate the oxidative products.

## DIFFERENCE BETWEEN EXOTOXINS AND ENDOTOXINS

| CHARACTERISTICS | EXOTOXINS | ENDOTOXINS |
|---|---|---|
| Source | Living gram positive and gram-negative bacteria | Lysed gram-negative bacteria |
| Location | Released from the cell | Part of cell |
| Chemical Composition | Protein | Lipopolysaccharide |
| Heat Sensitivity | Labile (60-80°C) | Stable |
| Immune Reactions | Strong | Weak |
| Conversion to Toxoids | Possible | Not possible |
| Fever | No | Yes |
| Enzyme Activity | None | Yes |
| Molecular Weight | 10KDa. | 50-1000KDa. |
| Denaturing on Boiling | Yes | No |
| Specificity | Specific to particular bacterial strain | Non-specific |
| Antigenicity | High | Poor |
| Examples | Staphylococcus aureus, Streptococcus pyogenes Bacillus cereus, Bacillus anthracis Diphtheria, Tetanus, Botulism. | E. coli, Salmonella typhi, Shigella, Vibrio cholera. |

## B. MICROBIAL ADHERENCE

- Adherence to surfaces helps microorganisms establish a base from which to penetrate tissues.
- Among the factors that determine adherence are **adhesins** (microbial molecules that mediate attachment to a cell) and host receptors to which the adhesins bind.
- Host receptors include cell surface sugar residues and cell surface proteins (eg, fibronectin) that enhance binding of certain gram-positive organisms (eg, staphylococci).
- Other determinants of adherence include fine structures on certain bacterial cells (eg, streptococci) called **fibrillae**, by which some bacteria bind to human epithelial cells.
- Other bacteria, such as Enterobacteriaceae (eg, Escherichia coli), have specific adhesive organelles called **fimbriae or pili**.
- Fimbriae enable the organism to attach to almost all human cells, including neutrophils and epithelial cells in the genitourinary tract, mouth, and intestine.

### Biofilm

- *Biofilm is a slime layer that can form around certain bacteria and confer resistance to phagocytosis and antibiotics.*
- *It develops around Pseudomonas aeruginosa in the lungs of patients with cystic fibrosis and around coagulase-negative staphylococci on synthetic medical devices, such as IV catheters, prosthetic vascular grafts, and suture material.*
- *Factors that affect the likelihood of biofilm developing on such medical devices include the material's roughness, chemical composition, and hydrophobicity.*

## C. ANTIMICROBIAL RESISTANCE

- Resistant bacterial strains have acquired genes that are encoded on plasmids or transposons and that enable the microorganisms to synthesize enzymes that:
  - o Modify or inactivate the antimicrobial agent
  - o Change the bacterial cell's ability to accumulate the antimicrobial agent
  - o Resist inhibition by the antimicrobial agent

## D. DEFECTS IN HOST DEFENSE MECHANISMS

### 1. PRIMARY IMMUNE DEFICIENCIES

- Are genetic in origin;
- Most primary immune deficiencies are recognized during infancy; however, up to 40% are recognized during adolescence or adulthood.

### 2. ACQUIRED IMMUNE DEFICIENCIES:

- Are caused by another disease (eg, cancer, HIV infection, chronic disease) or by exposure to a chemical or drug that is toxic to the immune system.
- Mechanisms: Defects in immune responses may involve Cellular immunity, Humoral immunity, Phagocytic system and Complement system.

### a. CELLULAR DEFICIENCIES

- Are typically T-cell or combined immune defects.
- T cells contribute to the killing of intracellular organisms.
- Patients with T-cell defects can present with opportunistic infections such as Pneumocystis jirovecii or cryptococcal infections.
- Chronicity of these infections can lead to failure to thrive, chronic diarrhoea, and persistent oral candidiasis.

### b. HUMORAL DEFICIENCIES

- Are typically caused by the failure of B cells to make functioning immunoglobulins.
- Patients with this type of defect usually have infections involving encapsulated organisms (eg, H. influenzae, streptococci).
- Patients can present with poor growth, diarrhoea, and recurrent sinopulmonary infections.

### c. A DEFECT IN THE PHAGOCYTIC SYSTEM

- Affects the immediate immune response to bacterial infection and can result in development of recurrent abscesses, severe pneumonias, or delayed umbilical cord separation.

### d. PRIMARY COMPLEMENT SYSTEM

- Defects are particularly rare. Patients with this type of defect may present with recurrent infections with pyogenic bacteria (eg, encapsulated bacteria, Neisseria sp) and have an increased risk of autoimmune disorders (eg, SLE).

# SECTION 3: CONTROLLING INFECTION

- Any molecule or substance that reacts to a product of a specific immune response and stimulates antibody generation is considered as an **antigen**.
- The antibody generation by an antigen is called antigenicity of that particular molecule. Antigens can be either a protein or a polysaccharide.
- The antigen uptake, antigen processing, and antigen presentation are mediated by antigen presenting cells (APCs), such as dendritic cells.
- Depending on the immune activity, antigens can be classified as immunogens, tolerogens, or allergens.
- Antigens may also be classified according to their origin as exogenous or endogenous.

| EXOGENOUS ANTIGENS | ENDOGENOUS ANTIGENS |
|---|---|
| Foreign compounds entered the body from outside | Compounds have been generated within the body. |
| Actively taken up into antigen presenting cells | Are already present within the cytoplasm of antigen presenting cells. |
| Active phagocytosis required | Active phagocytosis is not requiered |
| Can be a product of viruses or bacterial cells that are processed by antigen presenting cells. | Can be a tumor- or virus-derived product |
| Are recognized in association of MHC class II. | Are recognized in association of MHC class I |
| Recognized by Helper T cells (TH cells). | Recognized by cytotoxic T cells (Tcyt cells) |

**MHC= Major Histocompatibility Complex or Human Leukocyte Antigen (HLA)**

## Antigens generated by endogenous and exogenous antigen processing activate different effector functions

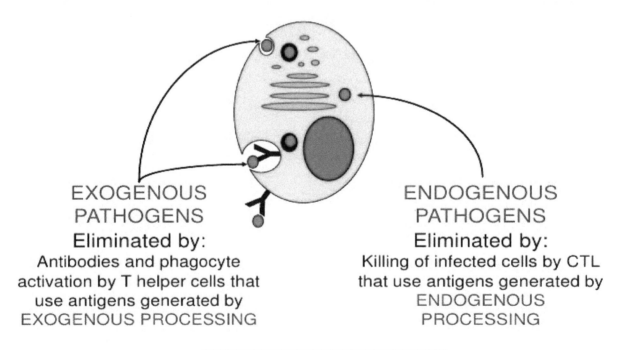

EXOGENOUS PATHOGENS
Eliminated by:
Antibodies and phagocyte activation by T helper cells that use antigens generated by EXOGENOUS PROCESSING

ENDOGENOUS PATHOGENS
Eliminated by:
Killing of infected cells by CTL that use antigens generated by ENDOGENOUS PROCESSING

*Fig. 4.1.3.1. Exogenous vs Endogenous antigens*

# HOSPITAL-ACQUIRED INFECTION

- **Nosocomial infections** are infections acquired in hospitals and other healthcare facilities.
- To be classified as a nosocomial infection, the patient must have been admitted for reasons other than the infection and must also have shown no signs of active or incubating infection.
- These infections occur:
  - up to 48 hours after hospital admission
  - up to 3 days after discharge
  - up to 30 days after an operation
  - In a healthcare facility when a patient was admitted for reasons other than the infection.
- Hospital-acquired infections are caused by viral, bacterial, and fungal pathogens; The most common types are:
  - **BSI**       : Bloodstream infection
  - **VAP**      : Pneumonia (e.g., ventilator-associated pneumonia)
  - **UTI**       : Urinary tract infection
  - **SSI**       : Surgical site infection
- *Gram-positive bacteria are the commonest cause of nosocomial infections with Staphylococcus aureus being the predominant pathogen.*
- Gram-positive bacteria have overtaken Gram-negative organisms as the predominant cause of nocosomial infections.
- Inadequate antibiotic therapy is associated with poor outcome and particularly with bacterial resistance.
- There has been an increase in the rate of antibiotic resistant bacteria associated with nosocomial infections in ICU.
- **Methicillin-resistant *S. aureus* (MRSA)** causes up to 60% of nocosomial infection in ICU. A broad-spectrum antibiotic such as **vancomycin** is usually prescribed for treatment.
- However, **vancomycin-resistant enterococci** and isolated cases of vancomycin-resistant *S. aureus* have been reported.
- This highlights the need for the use of appropriate antibiotics and some centres now discourage the use of vancomycin as first line treatment for *Clostridium difficile* diarrhoea.
- **Ventilator-associated pneumonia (VAP)** affects up to 20% of patients admitted to intensive care units (ICU). VAP is the most common and fatal infection of ICU. The presence of invasive medical devices is an important contributor to the pathogenesis and development of VAP.

## CONTROL OF HOSPITAL-ACQUIRED INFECTION

- Infection control measures are important for the effective control, prevention and treatment of infection.
- Knowledge of emerging pathogens and resistance profile is essential for treatment against nocosomial infections.
- Shorter duration of treatment and correct dosage of antibiotic therapy is recommended to reduce the selection pressure for resistant isolates.
- *Hand washing is the single most important measure to prevent nocosomial infections.*
- *Poor hand hygiene is responsible for 40% of infections transmitted in hospitals.*
- Accessibility of the hand washing stations and the use of alcohol gels improve compliance with hand washing.
- Gloves must not be used as a substitute for hand washing; they must be washed on glove removal.

- **Other measures:**
  - Isolation of patients: Importance of aprons, gloves, sink &alcohol gel.
  - Disinfection: As a reduction in the number of infectious particles.
  - Disinfectants: As substances, which kill or inhibit microbes.
  - Iodine: As a slow-acting skin anti-bacterial disinfectant.
  - Chlorhexidine: As an anti-staphylococcal agent.
  - Sterilisation: As the inactivation of all infectious agents.
  - Autoclaving and irradiation: As the main methods used.

## HEALTHCARE ASSOCIATED INFECTIONS (HCAI)

- Healthcare-associated infections (HCAIs) can develop either as a direct result of healthcare interventions such as medical or surgical treatment, or from being in contact with a healthcare setting.
- Alcohol gel dries quickly, and is bactericidal, fungicidal and virucidal.
- The term HCAI covers a wide range of infections.
- The most well-known include those caused by methicillin-resistant Staphylococcus aureus (MRSA) and Clostridium difficile (C. difficile).

# Section 4: Principles of Investigation

## 1. MICROBIOLOGIC EXAMINATION

- *Direct Examination and Techniques*
  - o   Microscopy
  - o   Immunofluorescence,
  - o   immuno-peroxidase staining, and other immunoassays
  - o   Genetic probes identify genus- or species-specific DNA or RNA sequences.
- *Culture*
  - o   Isolation of infectious agents frequently requires specialized media. (see below)
  - o   Nonselective (noninhibitory) media permit the growth of many microorganisms.
  - o   Selective media contain inhibitory substances that permit the isolation of specific types of microorganisms.
- *Microbial Identification*
  - o   Colony and cellular morphology may permit preliminary identification.
  - o   Growth characteristics under various conditions, utilization of carbohydrates and other substrates, enzymatic activity, immunoassays, and genetic probes are also used.
- *Serodiagnosis*
  - o   A high or rising titer of specific IgG antibodies or the presence of specific IgM antibodies may suggest or confirm a diagnosis.
- *Antimicrobial Susceptibility*
  - o   Microorganisms, particularly bacteria, are tested in vitro to determine whether they are susceptible to antimicrobial agents.
- *Molecular techniques*
  - o   Nucleic acid amplification as a technique used for diagnosis where the microbe is slow growing (eg M. tuberculosis, C trachomatis).

## 2. COMMON MEDIA IN ROUTINE USE

- **Nutrient Broth**
  - o   Used as a basal media for the preparation of other media and to study soluble products of bacteria.

- **Peptone Water**
  - o   It is used as base for sugar media and to test indole formation.

- **Blood Agar:**
  - o   Most commonly used medium.
  - o   5-10% defibrinated sheep or horse blood is added to melted agar at 45-50°C.
  - o   Certain bacteria when grown in blood agar produce hemolysis around their colonies.
  - o   Certain bacteria produce no hemolysis.
  - o   Types of changes:
    - ▪ **Beta hemolysis**:
      - o   The colony is surrounded by a clear zone of complete hemolysis.
      - o   E.g. Streptococcus pyogenes is a beta haemolytic streptococci, S agalactiae
    - ▪ **Alpha hemolysis**:
      - o   The colony is surrounded by a zone of greenish discoloration due to formation of biliverdin
      - o   e.g. Viridans streptococci, S pneumoniae
    - ▪ **Gamma hemolysis** or **No hemolysis**:
      - o   There is no change in the medium surrounding the colony.

- **Chocolate Agar or Heated Blood agar**
  - o   Prepared by heating blood agar.
  - o   It is used for culture of pneumococcus, gonococcus, meningococcus and Haemophilus.
  - o   Heating the blood inactivates inhibitor of growths.

- **MacConkey Agar**
  - o   Most commonly used for Enterobacteriaceae.
  - o   It contains agar, peptone, sodium chloride, bile salt, lactose and neutral red.
  - o   It is a selective and indicator medium:
    - ▪ **Selective medium:** As bile salt does not inhibit the growth of Enterobacteriaceae but inhibits growth of many other bacteria.
    - ▪ **Indicator medium**
      - o   As the colonies of bacteria that ferment lactose take a pink colour due to production of acid.
      - o   Acid turns the indicator neutral red to pink.

- These bacteria are called *'lactose fermenter'*, e.g. Escherichia coli.
- Colorless colony indicates that lactose is not fermented, i.e. the bacterium is non-lactose fermenter, e.g. Salmonella, Shigella, and Vibrio.

- **Lowenstein-Jensen Medium**
  - It is used to culture tubercle bacilli.
  - It contains egg, malachite green and glycerol.
    - Egg is an enrichment material which stimulates the growth of tubercle bacilli,
    - Malachite green inhibits growth of organisms other than mycobacteria,
    - Glycerol promotes the growth of Mycobacterium tuberculosis but not Mycobacterium bovis.

- **Other tests**
- **Heterophil Antibody Tests**
  - Heterophil antibody tests such as the **Paul Bunnell or Monospot tests** may be used in the diagnosis of infectious mononucleosis due to Epstein–Barr virus (EBV) or glandular fever.
  - Heterophil antibodies have the ability to agglutinate red blood cells of different animal species.
  - The Paul-Bunnell test uses sheep erythrocytes; the Monospot test, horse red cells.
  - In infectious mononucleosis, IgM heterophil antibodies are usually detectable for the ***first 3 months of infection.***
  - Generally, it will not be positive during *the 4-6-week incubation period before the onset of symptoms*.
  - It will also not be positive *after active infection has subsided*, even though the virus persists in the same cells in the body for the rest of the carrier's life.
  - Characteristically, they are able to agglutinate sheep erythrocytes; *it is absorbed by ox red blood cell but not guinea-pig kidney cells.*

# SECTION 5: IMMUNISATION

**Normal childhood immunization schedule (UK immunization schedules)**

| 2 months | 3 months | 4 months | 12-13 months |
|---|---|---|---|
| • 5-in-1 (DTaP/IPV/Hib) vaccine<br>• Pneumococcal (PCV) vaccine<br>• Rotavirus vaccine<br>• Men B vaccine<br><br>**DTaP: Diphtheria-Tetanus-Pertussis**<br>**IPV : Inactivated Poliovaccine**<br>**Hib : H. influenza vaccine**<br>**Men B: Meningococcal group B vaccine** | • 5-in-1 (DTaP/IPV/Hib) vaccine, second dose<br>• Men C vaccine<br>• Rotavirus vaccine, second dose | • 5-in-1 (DTaP/IPV/Hib) vaccine, third dose<br>• Pneumococcal (PCV) vaccine, second dose<br>• Men B vaccine second dose | • Hib/Men C booster, given as a single jab containing meningitis C (second dose) and Hib (fourth dose)<br>• Measles, mumps and rubella (MMR) vaccine, given as a single jab<br>• Pneumococcal (PCV) vaccine, third dose<br>• Men B vaccine third dose |

| 2, 3 and 4 years plus school years one and two | From 3 years and 4 months (up to starting school) | 12-13 years (girls only) | 13-18 years |
|---|---|---|---|
| • Children's flu vaccine (annual) | • Measles, mumps and rubella (MMR) vaccine, second dose<br>• 4-in-1 (DTaP/IPV) pre-school booster, given as a single jab containing vaccines against diphtheria, tetanus, whooping cough (pertussis) and polio | • HPV (Human papilloma virus) vaccine, which protects against cervical cancer – two injections given between six months and two years apart. | • 3-in-1 (Td/IPV) teenage booster, given as a single jab and contains vaccines against diphtheria, tetanus and polio<br>• Men ACWY vaccine (Meningococcal A, C, W and Y diseases).<br>• There are two Men ACWY vaccines called Nimenrix and Menveo. They are very similar and both work equally well. |

| 19-25 years (first-time students only) | 65 and over | 70 years (and 78 and 79-year-olds as a catch-up) |
|---|---|---|
| • Men ACWY vaccine. | • Flu (every year)<br>• Pneumococcal (PCV) vaccine | • Shingles vaccine |

## VACCINES FOR SPECIAL GROUPS

- There are some vaccines that aren't routinely available to everyone on the NHS, but that are available for people who fall into certain risk groups, such as pregnant women, people with long-term health conditions and healthcare workers.
- Additional ones include hepatitis B vaccination, TB vaccination and chickenpox vaccination.

## TRAVEL VACCINES

- There are some free travel vaccines on the NHS from any local surgery.
- These include the hepatitis A vaccine, the typhoid vaccine and the cholera vaccine.
- Other travel vaccines, such as yellow fever vaccination, are only available privately.

| VACCINES | N° DOSES | EXPECTED AGE |
|---|---|---|
| Diphtheria | 5 | Months 2,3,4 & Age 3,13 |
| Tetanus | 5 | Months 2,3,4 & Age 3,13 |
| IPV | 5 | Months 2,3,4 & Age 3,13 |
| Pertussis | 4 | Months 2,3,4 & Age 3 |
| Hib | 4 | Months 2,3,4 & Age 1 (Age1= Months 12) |
| PCV | 4 | Months 2,4 & Age 1,65 |
| Shingles | 3 | Age 70, 78, 79 |
| Men B | 3 | Months 2,4 & Age 1 |
| Men C | 2 | Month 3 & Age 1 |
| Men ACWY | 2 | Age 13,19 |
| MMR | 2 | Age 1,3 |
| Rotavirus | 2 | Months 2,3 |

Source: http://www.nhs.uk/conditions/vaccinations/pages/childhood-vaccination-schedule.aspx

# PART B: SPECIFIC PATHOGENS

## I. GRAM POSITIVE vs GRAM NEGATIVE

### DIFFERENCE BETWEEN GRAM POSITIVE AND GRAM NEGATIVE

| CHARACTERISTICS | GRAM POSITIVE | GRAM NEGATIVE |
|---|---|---|
| Gram Reaction | Retain crystal violet dye and stain blue or purple | Can be decolorized to accept counterstain and stain pink or red |
| Cell Wall | 20-30 nm thick. The wall is Smooth. | 8-12 nm thick. The wall is wavy. |
| Peptidoglycan Layer | Thick (multilayered) | Thin (single-layered) |
| Teichoic Acids | Present in many | Absent |
| Periplasmic Space | Absent | Present |
| Outer Membrane | Absent | Present |
| Porins | Absent | Occurs in Outer Membrane |
| Lipopolysaccharide (LPS) Content | Virtually None | High |
| Lipid and Lipoprotein Content | Low (acid-fast bacteria have lipids linked to peptidoglycan) | High (because of presence of outer membrane) |
| Mesosomes | Quite Prominent | Less Prominent |
| Flagellar Structure | 2 rings in basal body | 4 rings in basal body |
| Toxin Produced | Exotoxins | Endotoxins or Exotoxins |
| Resistance to Physical Disruption | High | Low |
| Cell Wall Disruption by Lysozyme | High | Low |
| Susceptibility to Penicillin and Sulfonamide | High | Low |
| Susceptibility to Streptomycin, Chloramphenicol and Tetracycline | Low | High |
| **Pathogens** | Staphylococcus, corynebacterium diphtheriae, streptococcus, enterococcus, bacillus, clostridium, chlamydia, mycobacterium, listeria, nocardia asteroids, rickettsia, actinomyces, | Bacteroides, coxiella, legionella, francisella, proteus Klebsiella, shigella, salmonella, yersinia, moraxella, Neisseria acinetobacter, pseudomonas, bordetella, brucella, haemophilus, pasteurella, serratia |

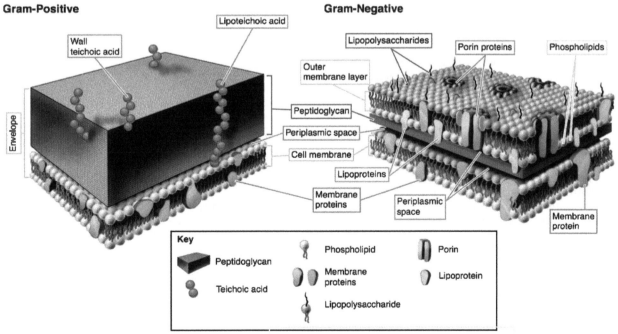

Fig. 4.2.1.1. Gram positive vs Gram negative

# Section 1: Streptococci & Staphylococci

# A. Streptococci

## I. α-HEMOLYTIC: STREPTOCOCCUS PNEUMONIAE

**INFECTIOUS AGENT**
- The gram-positive coccus streptococcus pneumoniae (Pneumococcus).

**TRANSMISSION**
- Person to person through close contact via respiratory droplets.
- It can infect the upper respiratory tracts of adults and children and can spread to the blood, lungs, middle ear, or nervous system.

**EPIDEMIOLOGY**
- Streptococcus pneumoniae is the most common cause of community-acquired pneumonia worldwide.
- The prevalence is higher in developing than in industrialized countries.
- It is commonly a disease of healthy young to middle-aged adults, is rare in infants, and the elderly, and is considerably more common in men than in women. Alcoholics appear to be particularly vulnerable.

**TYPES OF PNEUMONIA**
- **Aspiration Pneumonia**
  - Aspiration Pneumonia results when food, drink, vomit, secretions or other foreign material is inhaled and causes an inflammatory response in the lungs and bronchial tubes.
  - Aspiration Pneumonia occurs predominantly in the right lung because its total capacity is greater than that of the left lung.
- **Atypical Pneumonia**
  - This term refers of Pneumonia caused by the following bacteria: Legionella pneumophila, Mycoplasma pneumoniae, and Chlamydophila pneumoniae.
  - Atypical pneumonia is caused by bacteria and does not respond to the normal antibiotics used for treatment.

- **Bacterial Pneumonia**
  - Bacterial Pneumonia occurs when pneumonia-causing bacteria masses and multiplies in the lungs.
  - The alveoli become inflamed and pus is produced, which spreads around the lungs. The bacteria that caused Bacterial Pneumonia are: streptococcus pneumonia, staphylococcus aureus, hemophilus influenza, and legionella pneumophilia.

- **Bronchial Pneumonia**
  - Bronchopneumonia is a descending infection starting around the bronchi and bronchioles.
  - The terminal bronchioles become blocked with exudates and form consolidated patches. This results in atelectasis.

- **Community-acquired Pneumonia**
  - This means the infection was acquired at home.
  - With this type of pneumonia, the most common cause is 'Streptococcus Pneumonia'.

- **Hospital-acquired Pneumonia**
  - Patients develop features after being in hospital for 24 hours or longer.
  - Infectious agent is often Gram-negative bacteria such as 'Escherichia coli or Klebsiella'.

- **Mycoplasmal Pneumonia (walking pneumonia)**
  - It is similar to bacterial pneumonia, whereby the mycoplasmas proliferate and spread - causing infection.

- **Pneumocystis carinii Pneumonia**
  - Pneumocystis carinii pneumonia is the result of a fungal infection in the lungs caused by the Pneumocystis carinii fungus.
  - This fungus does not cause illness in healthy individuals, but rather in those with a weakened immune system.

- **Ventilator Associated Pneumonia (VAP)**
  - This type of pneumonia usually occurs two days after a hospitalised patient has been intubated and been receiving mechanical ventilation. This is especially a life-threatening infection as patients who require mechanical support are already critically ill.

- **Viral Pneumonia**
  - Viral Pneumonia is believed to be the cause of half of all pneumonias.
  - The viruses invade the lungs and then multiply- causing inflammation.

**CLINICAL PRESENTATION**
- Pneumococcal pneumonia is commonly seen in young adults after exposure to cold or after previous respiratory infection.

- It typically follows a viral infection, often influenza.
- The onset of the disease is sudden with fever and chills and ends in crisis after 9-10 days.
- Sudden onset of fever and malaise, cough, pleuritic chest pain, or purulent or blood-tinged sputum.
- In the elderly, fever, shortness of breath, or altered mental status may be initial symptoms.
- Pneumococcal meningitis may present as a stiff neck, headache, lethargy, or seizures.

## DIAGNOSIS
- Isolation from blood or cerebrospinal fluid, but most patients do not have detectable bacteremia.
- Pneumococcal urine antigen test may be useful.
- Radiologic examination shows alveolar filling in large areas of lung, producing a solid appearance that extend to entire lobes or segments.
- High white blood cell counts should raise suspicion for bacterial infection.

## SEQUENCE OF STAGES
- It is described in 4 phases:
  - **Congestion (Day 1):**
    - Occurs in the first 24 hours
    - Cellular exudates containing neutrophils, lymphocytes and fibrin replaces the alveolar air.
    - Capillaries in the surrounding alveolar walls become congested.
    - The infections spread to the hilum and pleura fairly rapidly
    - Pleurisy occurs, marked by coughing and deep breathing
  - **Red hepatization (Day 2-3)**
    - Occurs in the 2-3 days after consolidation
    - The consistency of the lungs resembles that of the liver
    - The lungs become hypeaemic
    - Alveolar capillaries are engorged with blood
    - Fibrinous exudates fill the alveoli
    - This stage is characterized by the presence of many **erythrocytes**, **neutrophils**, **desquamated epithelial cells**, and **fibrin** within the alveoli.
  - **Gray hepatization (Day 4-8):**
    - Occurs in the 2-3 days after Red Hepatization
    - This is an avascular stage
    - The lung appears gray-brown to yellow because of fibrinopurulent exudates, disintegration of red cells, and hemosiderin.
    - The pressure of the exudates in the alveoli causes compression of the capillaries.
    - **Leukocytes** migrate into the congested alveoli.
  - **Resolution (after Day 8):**
    - This stage is characterized by the resorption and restoration of the pulmonary architecture.
    - A large number of **macrophages** enter the alveolar spaces.
    - Phagocytosis of the bacteria-laden leucocytes occurs.
    - Consolidation tissue re-aerates and the fluid infiltrate causes sputum.
    - Fibrinous inflammation may extend to and across the pleural space, causing a rub heard by auscultation, and it may lead to resolution or to organization and pleural adhesions

## COMPLICATIONS OF PNEUMONIA:
- Delayed resolution.
- Pleural effusion
- Empyema
- Lung abscess
- Bacteremia
- Septicemia
- Meningitis
- Septic arthritis
- Endocarditis or pericarditis

## TREATMENT
- Many strains are resistant to penicillin, Cephalosporins, and macrolides.
- In countries where β-lactam resistance is common, the initial regimen for pneumococcal meningitis might include vancomycin or a fluoroquinolone, plus a third-generation cephalosporin.

## PREVENTION
- Pneumococcal Vaccine (PCV) available in UK at months 2, 4 and 12-13 and age 65+.

# II. β-HEMOLYTIC: STREPTOCOCCUS PYOGENES

## CLINICAL MANIFESTATIONS

- **Acute Streptococcus pyogenes infections**:
    o Pharyngitis, scarlet fever (rash), impetigo, cellulitis, or erysipelas.
    o Necrotizing fasciitis, Myositis
    o Streptococcal toxic shock syndrome.
    o Acute Rheumatic Fever
    o Acute Glomerulonephritis.
- **S agalactiae**:
    o **In neonates**: Meningitis, Neonatal Sepsis and Pneumonia.
    o **In adults**: Vaginitis, Puerperal Fever, Urinary Tract Infection, Skin Infection, and Endocarditis.

## ANOTHER STREPTOCOCCUS CAUSE:

- **Viridans streptococci**: Endocarditis
- **Enterococcus**: Urinary tract and Biliary tract infections.
- **Anaerobic streptococci** participate in mixed infections of the abdomen, pelvis, brain, and lungs.

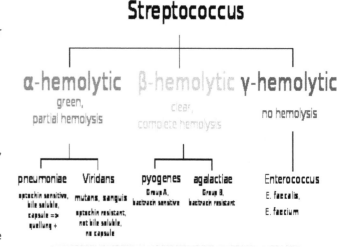

Fig. 4.2.1.2. Classes of streptococcus

## STRUCTURE

- Streptococci are Gram-positive, nonmotile, nonsporeforming, catalase-negative cocci that occur in pairs or chains.
- Older cultures may lose their Gram-positive character.
- Most streptococci are facultative anaerobes, and some are obligate (strict) anaerobes.
- Most require enriched media (blood agar).
- Group A streptococci have a hyaluronic acid capsule

## CLASSIFICATION AND ANTIGENIC TYPES

- Streptococci are classified on the basis of colony morphology, hemolysis, biochemical reactions, and (most definitively) serologic specificity.
- They are divided into three groups by the type of hemolysis on blood agar:
    o β-hemolytic: clear, complete lysis of red cells.
    o α hemolytic: incomplete, green hemolysis.
    o γ hemolytic: no hemolysis.
- Serologic grouping is based on antigenic differences in cell wall carbohydrates (groups A to V), in cell wall pili-associated protein, and in the polysaccharide capsule in group B streptococci.

## PATHOGENESIS

- Streptococci are members of the normal flora.
- Virulence factors of group A streptococci include:
    o M protein and lipoteichoic acid for attachment;
    o A hyaluronic acid capsule that inhibits phagocytosis.
    o Other extracellular products, such as pyrogenic (erythrogenic) toxin, which causes the rash of scarlet fever; and Streptokinase, streptodornase (DNase B), and streptolysins.
- Some strains are nephritogenic.
- Immune-mediated sequelae do not reflect dissemination of bacteria.
- Non-group A strains have no defined virulence factors.

## HOST DEFENSES

- Antibody to M protein gives type-specific immunity to group A streptococci.
- Antibody to erythrogenic toxin prevents the rash of scarlet fever.
- Immune mechanisms are important in the pathogenesis of acute rheumatic fever.
- Maternal IgG protects the neonate against group B streptococci.

## EPIDEMIOLOGY

- Group A β-hemolytic streptococci (S pyogenes) are spread by respiratory secretions and fomites.
- The incidence of both respiratory and skin infections peaks in childhood.
- Infection can be transmitted by asymptomatic carriers.
- Acute rheumatic fever was previously common among the poor; susceptibility may be partly genetic.
- Group B streptococci (S agalactiae) are common in the normal vaginal flora and occasionally cause invasive neonatal infection.

**DIAGNOSIS**

- Diagnosis is based on cultures from clinical specimens.
- Serologic methods can detect group A or B antigen; definitive antigen identification is by the precipitin test.
- Bacitracin sensitivity presumptively differentiates group A from other β-haemolytic streptococci (B, C, G); group B streptococci typically show hippurate hydrolysis; group D is differentiated from other viridans streptococci by bile solubility and optochin sensitivity.
- Acute glomerulonephritis and acute rheumatic fever are identified by anti-streptococcal antibody titers.
- In addition, acute rheumatic fever is diagnosed by clinical criteria.

**CONTROL**

- Prompt penicillin treatment of streptococcal pharyngitis reduces the antigenic stimulus and therefore prevents glomerulonephritis and acute rheumatic fever.
- Vancomycin resistance among the enterococci is an emerging microbial threat.

# CLINICAL RELEVANCE:
# INFECTIVE ENDOCARDITIS

- **Infective endocarditis (IE)** is infection of the endocardium (inner lining of the heart) almost always affecting the heart valves.
- It is notoriously difficult to diagnose.

## DUKE CRITERIA FOR INFECTIVE ENDOCARDITIS

- For diagnosis the requirement is:
  - 2 major and 1 minor criteria or
  - 1 major and 3 minor criteria or
  - 5 minor criteria

## MAJOR CRITERIA

- Positive blood cultures for infective endocarditis
- typical microorganism for infective endocarditis from 2 separate blood cultures
  - **Viridans streptococci, Streptococcus bovis**, and HACEK group or
  - Community-acquired **Staphylococcus aureus** or **enterococci** in the absence of a primary focus or
  - Persistently positive blood cultures, defined as recovery of a microorganism consistent with infective endocarditis from:
    - 2 blood cultures drawn 12 hours apart or all of 3 or most of 4 or more separate blood cultures, with first and last drawn at least 1 hour apart
- Evidence of endocardial involvement
  - Positive echocardiogram for infective endocarditis
    - Oscillating intracardiac mass on valve or supporting structures or in the path of regurgitant jets or on implanted material in the absence of an alternative anatomical explanation or
    - Abscess or
    - New partial dehiscence of prosthetic valve or
  - New valvular regurgitation

## MINOR CRITERIA

- Predisposing heart condition or intravenous drug use
- Fever: 38°c
- Vascular phenomena: major arterial emboli, septic pulmonary infarcts, mycotic aneurysm, intracranial hemorrhage, conjunctival hemorrhages, and janeway lesions
- Immunologic phenomena:
  - Glomerulonephritis
  - Osler nodes
  - Roth spots
  - Rheumatoid factor
- Microbiologic evidence: positive blood culture but not meeting major criterion as noted previously or serologic evidence of active infection with organism consistent with infective endocarditis
- Echocardiography findings consistent with infective endocarditis but not meeting major criterion as noted previously

- There are two recognised forms if IE:
  - **Sub-acute IE** usually affects structurally abnormal heart valves and runs an indolent course over weeks to months due to the less virulent nature of the common pathogens – **Strep. viridans (60% or cases) and enterococci**
  - **Acute IE** affects structurally normal heart valves by particularly virulent or invasive organisms, e.g. **S aureus and group B Streptococcus.**

- o Acute IE causes more valve damage and carries a higher mortality (10-30%) then sub-acute IE.
- o In order from most commonly affected to least: Mitral valve, Aortic valve, Tricuspid valve and rarely the pulmonary valve.
- *In stable patients with suspected chronic or subacute IE, three sets of blood cultures should be taken 6 hours apart before starting antibiotics.*
- *In septic and/or unwell patients this should all be done within the first hour.*
  - o In either case, the bacteraemia of IE is continuous so that timing of blood cultures is unrelated to any clinical features including fever.

### 1. ETIOLOGY
- People with the following cardiac conditions are at increased risk:
  - o Acquired valvular heart disease with stenosis or regurgitation.
  - o Valve replacement.
  - o Structural congenital disease (excluding ASD or fully repaired VSD or PDA).
  - o Previous infective endocarditis.
  - o Hypertrophic cardiomyopathy.

## A. NATIVE VALVE ENDOCARDITIS
- The following are the main underlying causes of NVE:
  - o **Rheumatic valvular disease (30% of NVE)** - Primarily involves the mitral valve followed by the aortic valve
  - o **Congenital heart disease (15% of NVE)** - Underlying etiologies include a patent ductus arteriosus, ventricular septal defect, tetralogy of Fallot, or any native or surgical high-flow lesion.
  - o **Mitral valve prolapse** with an associated murmur (20% of NVE)
  - o **Degenerative heart disease** - Including calcific aortic stenosis due to a bicuspid valve, Marfan syndrome, or syphilitic disease
- Approximately 70% of infections in NVE are caused by Streptococcus species, including **S viridans, Streptococcus bovis, and enterococci.**
- Staphylococcus species cause 25% of cases and generally demonstrate a more aggressive acute course.
- Treatment: **Penicillin G and Gentamicin.**

## B. PROSTHETIC VALVE ENDOCARDITIS
- **Early PVE** may be caused by a variety of pathogens, including S aureus and S epidermidis. These nosocomially acquired organisms are often methicillin-resistant (eg, MRSA).
- **Late disease** is most commonly caused by streptococci.
- Overall, CoNS (Coagulase Negative Staphylococcus) are the most frequent cause of PVE (30%).
- S aureus causes 17% of early PVE and 12% of late PVE.
- Corynebacterium, nonenterococcal streptococci, fungi (eg, C albicans, Candida stellatoidea, and Aspergillus species), Legionella, and the **HACEK** (ie, Haemophilus aphrophilus, Actinobacillus actinomycetemcomitans, Cardiobacterium hominis, Eikenella corrodens, Kingella kingae) organisms cause the remaining cases.
- Treatment: **Vancomycin and Gentamicin** may be used for treatment, despite the risk of renal insufficiency.
- **Rifampin** is necessary in treating individuals with infection of prosthetic valves or other foreign bodies because it can penetrate the biofilm of most of the pathogens that infect these devices. However, it should be administered with vancomycin or gentamicin. Substitution of **Linezolid for Vancomycin** should be considered in patients with unstable renal function.

## C. I.V.D.A. INFECTIVE ENDOCARDITIS
- Infective Endocarditis in IntraVenous Drug Abusers can be difficult and requires a high index of suspicion.
- Two thirds of patients have no previous history of heart disease or murmur on admission.
- A murmur may be absent in those with tricuspid disease, owing to the relatively small pressure gradient across this valve.
- Pulmonary manifestations may be prominent in patients with tricuspid infection: ⅓ has pleuritic chest pain, and ¾ demonstrate chest radiographic abnormalities.
- **S aureus** is the most common (< 50% of cases) etiologic organism in patients with IVDA IE.
- MRSA accounts for an increasing portion of S aureus infections and has been associated with previous hospitalizations, long-term addiction, and nonprescribed antibiotic use.
- Groups A, C, and G streptococci and enterococci are also recovered from patients with IVDA IE.
- Currently, gram-negative organisms are involved infrequently.
- P aeruginosa and the HACEK family are the most common examples.
- Treatment: **Nafcillin and Gentamicin.**The emergence of methicillin-resistant S aureus (MRSA) and penicillin-resistant streptococci has led to a change in empiric treatment with liberal substitution of **Vancomycin** in lieu of a penicillin antibiotic.

## D. NOSOCOMIAL / HOSPITAL ASSOCIATED I.E.

- Endocarditis may be associated with central or peripheral intravenous catheters, rhythm control devices such as pacemakers and defibrillators, hemodialysis shunts and catheters, and chemotherapeutic and hyperalimentation lines.
- These patients tend to have significant comorbidities, more advanced age, and predominant infection with S aureus.
- The mortality rate is high in this group.
- The organisms that cause NIE/HCIE obviously are related to the type of underlying bacteremia.
- The gram-positive cocci (ie, S aureus, CoNS, enterococci, nonenterococcal streptococci) are the most common pathogens.

## E. FUNGAL ENDOCARDITIS

- Fungal endocarditis is found in intravenous drug users and intensive care unit patients who receive broad-spectrum antibiotics.
- Blood cultures are often negative, and diagnosis frequently is made after microscopic examination of large emboli.

### 2. APPROACH CONSIDERATIONS

- The criterion standard test for diagnosing infective endocarditis (IE) is the documentation of a continuous bacteremia (>30 min in duration) based on blood culture results. Because of the ability of S aureus to produce an endotheliosis, the presence of a continuous bacteremia does not necessarily imply an infected valvular vegetation.
- The major goals of therapy for infective endocarditis (IE) are to eradicate the infectious agent from the thrombus and to address the complications of valvular infection. The latter includes both the intracardiac and extracardiac consequences of IE.
- Some of the effects of IE require surgical intervention.
- General measures include the following:
  - Treatment of congestive heart failure
  - Oxygen
  - Hemodialysis (may be required in patients with renal failure)
- In most cases, the etiologic microbial agent is not known while the patient is in the ED.
- Antibiotics remain the mainstay of treatment for IE.
- In the setting of acute IE, institute antibiotic therapy as soon as possible to minimize valvular damage.
- Three to 5 sets of blood cultures are obtained within 60-90 minutes, followed by the infusion of the appropriate antibiotic regimen.
- Empiric antibiotic therapy is chosen based on the most likely infecting organisms. In the case of subacute IE, treatment may be safely delayed until culture and sensitivity results are available.
- Waiting does not increase the risk of complications in this form of the disease.

# B. Staphylococci

## I. STAPHYLOCOCCUS AUREUS AND EPIDERMIDIS

### CLINICAL MANIFESTATIONS

- **S aureus causes:**
  - ○ Superficial skin lesions: boils, styes
  - ○ Localized abscesses
  - ○ Deep-seated infections: osteomyelitis, endocarditis and furunculosis.
  - ○ Hospital acquired (nosocomial) infection of surgical wounds and, with S epidermidis, causes infections associated with indwelling medical devices.
  - ○ Food poisoning by releasing **enterotoxins into food.**
  - ○ Toxic shock syndrome
- ***Staphylococcus saprophiticus***
  - ○ It is implicated in 5-15% of UTIs.
  - ○ It is the second commonest cause of UTI in young sexually active women and is often referred to as **'honeymooner's' cystitis**.
- Other species of staphylococci (S lugdunensis, S haemolyticus, S warneri, S schleiferi, and S intermedius) are infrequent pathogens.

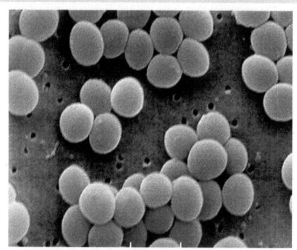

### STRUCTURE

- Staphylococci are Gram-positive cocci 1μm in diameter.
- ***They form clumps.***

### CLASSIFICATION

- S aureus and S intermedius are coagulase positive.
- All other staphylococci are coagulase negative.
- They are salt tolerant and often hemolytic.
- Identification requires biotype analysis.

### NATURAL HABITAT

- *S aureus* colonizes the nasal passage and axillae.
- *S epidermidis* is a common human skin commensal.
- Other species of staphylococci are infrequent human commensals.
- Some are commensals of other animals.

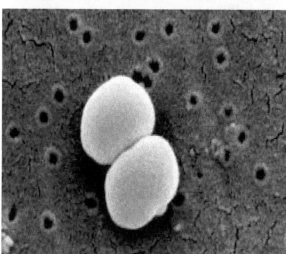

*Fig. 4.2.1.3. Staphylococcus aureus and epidermidis*

### PATHOGENESIS

- S aureus expresses many potential virulence factors. Surface proteins that promote colonization of host tissues.
- Factors that probably inhibit phagocytosis (capsule, immunoglobulin binding protein A).
- Toxins that damage host tissues and cause disease symptoms.
- Coagulase-negative staphylococci are normally less virulent and express fewer virulence factors.
- S epidermidis readily colonizes implanted devices.

### HOST DEFENSES

- Phagocytosis is the major mechanism for combatting staphylococcal infection.
- Antibodies are produced which neutralize toxins and promote opsonization.
- The capsule and protein A may interfere with phagocytosis. Biofilm growth on implants is impervious to phagocytosis.

### TREATMENT

- Infections acquired outside hospitals can usually be treated with penicillinase-resistant β-lactam: Methicillin, Flucloxacillin, Cloxacillin, Oxacillin, Nafcillin, Dicloxacillin
- Hospital acquired infection is often caused by antibiotic resistant strains and can only be treated with **Vancomycin.**
- Infection control programs are used in most hospitals.

# CLINICAL RELEVANCE:

## 1. MRSA

### CAUSAL AGENT

* Methicillin Resistant Staphylococcus Aureus, a bacterium commonly found on human skin and mucosa, which are resistant to methicillin and other commonly used antibiotics including oxacillin, penicillin and amoxicillin.

### COMMON CLINICAL FEATURES

* Ranging from minor skin sepsis to more life-threatening infections.
* Refer to clinical manifestations of S aureus above.

### EPIDEMIOLOGY

* Worldwide: A major cause of nosocomial infection.
* Community acquired infection may occur when hospital patients are discharged.
* In England and Wales MRSA as a proportion of total *S. aureus* increased from 2% in 1990 to 42% in 2000 and is attributed to the emergence of new strains, failure to maintain good hospital hygiene including hand washing, heavier usage of hospitals, and reductions in hospital staffing.

### RESERVOIR

* Colonized or infected humans. Rarely animals. The bacterium lives harmlessly on the skin and in the nose of up to 30% of the general population.

### MODE OF TRANSMISSION

* Person to person, through contact with secretions from infected skin lesions, nasal
* Directly on the hands
* Indirectly on equipment and the environment.

### INCUBATION PERIOD

* Variable: **4-10 days.**

### PERIOD OF COMMUNICABILITY

* While the infection or the carrier state persists.

### PREVENTION AND CONTROL

* Thorough **hand washing** and drying between caring for people, and whenever necessary, has been shown to be the single most important measure in reducing cross-infection. Basic infection control practices are key to the prevention and control of MRSA in health care settings.

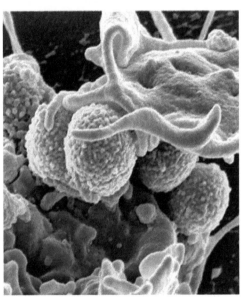

*Fig. 4.2.1.4. MRSA*

## 2. OSTEOMYELITIS

* Acute osteomyelitis is pyogenic infection of the bone and bone marrow.
* It may be acute or chronic (occurring over months to years).
* It may be caused by haematogenous spread of organisms (e.g. seeding from remote infections) or from direct contact with an adjacent infected tissue (e.g. the diabetic foot) an exogenous source of infection (e.g. open fracture).
* **Common organisms:**
  o Staphylococcus aureus accounts for 80-90% of cases
  o E coli, Pseudomonas, Klebsiella: Osteomyelitis arise from haematological spread in patients with chronic UTI or who use intravenous drugs.
  o Salmonella causes 50% of osteomyelitis in Sickle cell patients (but is very rare outside this group)
  o H influenzae and Group B streptococcus are less common.

### SITE OF OSTEOMYELITIS

  o **Neonates:** Metaphysis, epiphysis or both
  o **Children:** Metaphysis of long bones (particularly the distal femur and proximal tibia)
  o **Adults:** Epiphysis and sub-chondral region

* **PATHOGENESIS OF ACUTE OSTEOMYELITIS:**
  o Organism penetration of the bone marrow -> acute inflammation -> necrosis of bones within 48 hours -> infection spreads along Haversian canals towards the cortex and periosteum -> abscess formation -> dead piece of bone (sequestrum) formation -> rupture of periosteum -> draining sinus.
  o After weeks to months, chronic osteomyelitis may develop
  o Characterised by infiltration of chronic inflammatory cells and deposition of a layer of new bone outside the periosteum called an **involucrum.**

# SECTION 2: TUBERCULOSIS

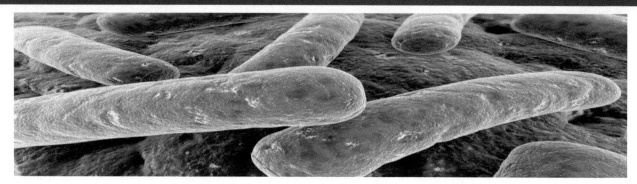

## STRUCTURE

- *Mycobacterium tuberculosis* is an obligate pathogenic bacterial species in the family **Mycobacteriaceae** and the causative agent of tuberculosis. First discovered in **1882 by Robert Koch**, *M. tuberculosis* has an unusual, waxy coating on its cell surface primarily due to the presence of mycolic acid. This coating makes the cells impervious to Gram staining, and as a result, *M. tuberculosis* can appear either Gram-negative or Gram-positive. Acid-fast stains such as **Ziehl-Neelsen, or fluorescent stains** such as auramine are used instead to identify *M. tuberculosis* with a microscope. The physiology of *M. tuberculosis* is highly aerobic and requires high levels of oxygen.
- Primarily a pathogen of the mammalian respiratory system, it infects the lungs. The most frequently used diagnostic methods for tuberculosis are the tuberculin skin test, acid-fast stain, culture, and polymerase chain reaction. Mycobacteria are **slender, curved rods that are acid fast and resistant to acids, alkalis, and dehydration.** The cell wall contains complex waxes and glycolipids.

## CLINICAL MANIFESTATIONS

- Tuberculosis primarily affects the lower respiratory system and is characterized by a chronic productive cough, fever, night sweats, and weight loss. Multiplication on enriched media is very slow, with doubling times of 18 to 24 hours; clinical isolates may require 4 to 6 weeks to grow.

## CLASSIFICATION AND ANTIGENIC TYPES

- On the basis of growth rate, catalase and niacin production, and pigmentation in light or dark, mycobacteria are classified into members of the Mycobacterium tuberculosis complex (M tuberculosis, M bovis, M africanum, M microtii) and nontuberculous species.
- Gene probe technology now facilitates this distinction.

## PATHOGENESIS

- Tuberculous mycobacteria enter the alveoli by airborne transmission.
- They resist destruction by alveolar macrophages and multiply, forming the primary lesion or tubercle; they then spread to regional lymph nodes, enter the circulation, and reseed the lungs. Tissue destruction results from cell-mediated hypersensitivity.

## HOST DEFENSES

- Susceptibility is influenced by genetic and ethnic factors.
- Acquired resistance is mediated by T lymphocytes, which lyse infected macrophages directly or activate them via soluble mediators (e.g., gamma interferon) to destroy intracellular bacilli; antibodies play no protective role.

## EPIDEMIOLOGY

- M tuberculosis is contagious, but only 5–10 percent of infected normal individuals develop active disease.
- Tuberculosis is most common among the elderly, poor, malnourished, or immunocompromised, especially persons infected with human immunodeficiency virus (HIV).
- Persistent infection may reactivate after decades owing to deterioration of immune status; exogenous reinfection also occurs.

## DIAGNOSIS

- Recent infection with M tuberculosis results in conversion to a positive Mantoux skin test with purified protein derivative (PPD).
- A diagnosis of active disease is based on clinical manifestations, an abnormal chest radiograph, acid-fast bacilli in sputum or bronchoscopic specimens and recovery of the organism. Assays based upon amplification of mycobacterial genes.

## TREATMENT AND CONTROL

- Therapy consists of a 6 to 9-month course of isoniazid, rifampin, pyrazinamide and ethambutol.
- Additional drugs may be used if drug resistance is suspected.
- If the patient is HIV-positive, treatment for longer periods (9–12 months) is recommended.
- PPD conversion without other signs or symptoms may warrant prophylactic isoniazid therapy for 6 months.
- M bovis BCG vaccine is used in more than 120 countries, but its efficacy is controversial.

# SECTION 3: CLOSTRIDIAL INFECTION

## I. TETANUS AND CLOSTRIDIUM TETANI

- Clostridium tetani, a spore-forming, anaerobic, gram-positive bacterium.
- Tetanus is different from other vaccine-preventable diseases because it does not spread from person to person.
- The bacteria are usually found in soil, dust, and manure and enter the body through breaks in the skin — usually cuts or puncture wounds caused by contaminated objects. Bacteria are ubiquitous in the environment.

### TRANSMISSION
- Contact with nonintact skin, usually via injuries from contaminated objects. **"Tetanus-prone" wounds** include those contaminated with dirt, human or animal excreta, or saliva; punctures; burns; crush injuries; or injuries with necrotic tissue.

### EPIDEMIOLOGY
- Distributed worldwide; more common in rural and agricultural regions, areas where contact with soil or animal excreta is likely, and areas where immunization is inadequate. Tetanus can affect any age group.

### CLINICAL PRESENTATION
- Incubation period is **3-21 days, range 1 day to several months.**
- **Most cases occur within 14 days.**
- Acute symptoms typically include muscle rigidity and spasms, often in the jaw and neck.
- Symptoms of less common forms of tetanus (localized or cephalic) can include muscle spasms confined to the injury site, head or face lesions, and flaccid cranial nerve palsies. Progression from these forms to generalized tetanus may occur.
- Severe tetanus can lead to respiratory failure and death.
- Case-fatality ratios are high even where modern intensive care is available.

### DIAGNOSIS
- Diagnosis is made clinically; no confirmatory laboratory tests are available.

### TREATMENT
- Tetanus requires hospitalization, treatment with human tetanus immune globulin (TIG), a tetanus toxoid booster, and agents to control muscle spasm, aggressive wound care, and antibiotics.
- **Metronidazole** is the most appropriate antibiotic.
- The wound should be **debrided widely** and excised if possible.

### PREVENTION
- Ensure adequate immunity to tetanus by completing the childhood primary vaccine series with tetanus toxoid, a booster dose during adolescence, and at 10-year intervals thereafter during adulthood.
- For heavily contaminated wounds, a booster dose may be given if more than 5 years have elapsed since the last dose.

> - In general, Human Anti-Tetanus Immunoglobulin **"HATI"** is only given for untreated infected or tetanus prone wounds such as:
>    - Heavily soiled wounds
>    - Punctured wounds and animal bites
>    - Wounds with devitalized tissue
> - **UK schedule of tetanus immunization is:**
>    - Course of 3 IM injections of inactivated Tetanus toxoid given with diphteria, pertussis, Polio and Hib at ages TWO, THREE and FOUR MONTHS.
>    - Tetanus Booster at 3.5-5YEARS
>    - Last Booster at 14-5YEARS (before leaving school)
>    - Full 5 doses course give lifelong immunity

## OPISTHOTONUS
- It is a state of severe hyperextension and spasticity in which an individual's head, neck and spinal column enter into a complete "bridging" or "arching" position. This abnormal posturing is an extrapyramidal effect and is caused by spasm of the axial muscles along the spinal column.
- It is seen in some cases of severe cerebral palsy and traumatic brain injury or as a result of the severe muscular spasms associated with tetanus. It can be a feature of severe acute hydrocephalus. Opisthotonus in the neonate may be a symptom of meningitis, tetanus, severe kernicterus, or the rare Maple syrup urine disease. Opisthotonos can sometimes be seen in lithium intoxication.
- It is a rare extrapyramidal side effect of phenothiazines, haloperidol, and metoclopramide. Opisthotonus with the presence of the risus sardonicus is also a symptom of strychnine poisoning.

# II. CLOSTRIDIUM DIFFICILE

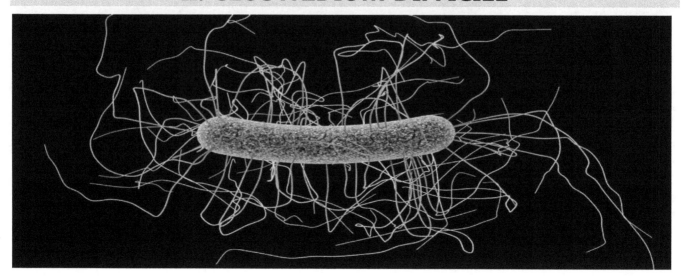

## EPIDEMIOLOGY

- **Clostridium difficile**, a spore-forming bacterium, is a component of the normal intestinal flora of a small percentage of healthy adults (3%) and of a relatively large percentage (2/3) of healthy neonates.
- It also may be found in the environment, especially in hospitals.
- Antibiotic therapy is the key factor that alters the colonic flora.
- C difficile infection (CDI) occurs primarily in hospitalized patients.

## SIGNS AND SYMPTOMS

- Mild to moderate watery diarrhea that is rarely bloody
- Cramping abdominal pain, Anorexia, Malaise...
- Physical examination may reveal the following in patients with the disorder:
  - Fever: Especially in more severe cases
  - Dehydration
  - Lower abdominal tenderness
  - Rebound tenderness: Raises the possibility of colonic perforation and peritonitis

## DIAGNOSIS

- The presence of antibiotic therapy, diarrhea, and pseudomembranes by colonoscopy help establish the severity of disease, coupled with the demonstration of organisms and/or toxin in feces.

## CONTROL

- **Metronidazole** and **Vancomycin** should be used therapeutically.
- However, relapses can occur.
- Supportive therapy may be needed.

# III. OTHER PATHOGENIC CLOSTRIDIA

- **CLOSTRIDIUM PERFRINGENS**
  - Food poisoning, Necrotizing enteritis, Gas Gangrene

- **C SORDELLII**
  - Causes bacteremia, Endometritis
  - Nonbacteremic infections.

- **C SEPTICUM**
  - Correlated with the presence of cancer.

- **C TERTIUM**
  - Associated with bacteremia.

# SECTION 4: NEISSERIA

# I. MENINGOCOCCAL DISEASE

## CAUSAL AGENT
- Meningococcal meningitis and meningococcal septicaemia are systemic infections caused by the bacteria *Neisseria meningitidis* (a gram-negative diplococcus bacterium).
- The infection may present as meningitis, septicaemia or a combination of both.
- Meningococci are divided into at least 13 distinct serogroups. The most common are serogroups A, B, C, Y and W135.
- Most disease in the UK is caused by group B.

## COMMON CLINICAL FEATURES
- The early symptoms are non-specific and are often mistaken for a viral infection.
- Meningococcal infection progresses rapidly, with the clinical picture changing hourly.
- In infant's symptoms, can include the sudden onset of fever, floppiness, high-pitched crying, neck retraction with arching of the back and sometimes vomiting.
- In infants, there is progressive irritability, altered consciousness and sometimes convulsions.
- Common symptoms in children and adults can include the sudden onset of fever, malaise, increasing headache, nausea, photophobia, neck stiffness and often vomiting.
- In meningococcal septicaemia, a rash may develop along with signs of advancing shock and isolated limb and/or joint pain.
- The rash may be non-specific early on but as the disease progresses the rash may become petechial or purpuric and may not blanch.
- Meningococcal sepsis occurs without meningitis in 5-10% of invasive meningococcal infections.
- In the UK, Meningococcal disease has a case fatality rate of approximately **10%**.
- Case fatality ratios increase with age and is higher in those with septicaemia than in those with meningitis alone.
- Of patients who recover **11-19%** develop permanent sequelae, including hearing loss, brain damage, seizures and loss of limb.

## EPIDEMIOLOGY
- Endemic worldwide.
- The highest burden of meningococcal disease occurs in sub-Saharan Africa (**the Meningitis Belt**).
- *N. meningitides* A, C and W135 are the main serogroups involved in the meningococcal activity in Africa.
- In 2005 1,462 laboratories confirmed cases of *N. meningitidis* were reported in England and Wales.
- The majority of meningococcal infections occur in children under 5 years, with a peak incidence at 6 months of age.
- There is a smaller, secondary peak in incidence among young adults aged between 15-19 years of age.
- Meningococcal disease shows a marked seasonal variation with the highest incidence occurring during the **winter**.
- Most cases of meningococcal disease occur sporadically, with <5% of cases occurring in clusters.
- Outbreaks are more common among teenagers and young adults and outbreaks have been reported in schools and universities.
- Since the introduction of Men C vaccine into the UK routine immunisation programme the number of laboratory confirmed group C cases have fallen by over 90% among all age groups immunised.
- Cases among other age groups have fallen by two-thirds as a result of reduced carriage rates.
- In the UK serogroup B is now responsible for >85% of laboratory confirmed cases.

## MODE OF TRANSMISSION
- Person to person, transmitted by droplet aerosol or secretions from the nasopharynx of colonized persons.
- Transmission usually requires either frequent or prolonged close contract.
- Risk factors for the development of disease is not fully understood but may include age, season, smoking, preceding influenza A infection and living in closed or semi-closed communities such as military barracks.

## INCUBATION PERIOD
- **2-10 days**, commonly 3-4 days.

## PERIOD OF COMMUNICABILITY
- While live meningococci are present in discharges from nose and mouth.
- Meningococci usually disappears from the nasopharynx within 24 hours of appropriate antimicrobial treatment.
- **Up to 10%** of people may be asymptomatic carriers with nasopharyngeal colonization by *N. meningitidis*. However, **less than 1%** of those colonized will progress to invasive disease.
- High carriage rates of **up to 25%** have been observed in 15-19-year olds.
- Carriage confers natural immunity.

**TREATMENT**
- An immediate dose of **Benzyl Penicillin** for suspected meningococcal infection should be given.
  - *Children aged < 1 year - 300mg*
  - *Children aged 1-9 years - 600mg*
  - *Adults and children aged >10 years - 1200mg*

**PREVENTION AND CONTROL**
- In the UK immunisation against meningococcal group C is recommended for persons under the age of 25 years and for all first-year university students.
- Public health action is indicated for confirmed or suspected cases.
- There are 4 key actions in response to a suspected case as outlined by Hawker et al:
  - Ensure rapid admission to hospital and pre-admission benzyl penicillin.
  - Ensure appropriate laboratory investigations are undertaken.
  - Arrange for chemoprophylaxis for close contact and immunisation if infection is due to a vaccine preventable strain.
  - Provide information about meningococcal disease to parents, GPs and educational establishments.

**CHEMOPROPHYLAXIS**
- Chemoprophylaxis should be offered to close contacts of cases, irrespective of vaccination status.
- **Close Contacts:**
  - Close contact are those who have had prolonged close contact with the case in a household type setting during the seven days before the onset of illness.
  - These include; those living and/or sleeping in the same household (including extended household), pupils in the same dormitory, boy/girlfriends, or university students sharing a kitchen in a hall of residence.
  - Those who have had transient close contact with a case only if they have been directly exposed to large particle droplets/secretions from the respiratory tract of a case around the time of admission to hospital.
- *Chemoprophylaxis is recommended for health care workers whose mouth or nose has been directly exposed to droplets or secretions within a distance of 3 feet from a probable or confirmed case.*
- *In the case of a pregnant patient, ceftriaxone or a similar cephalosporin should be used.*

| RECOMMENDED CHEMOPROPHYLAXIS | |
|---|---|
| Adults and children aged > 12 years | Rifampicin: 600mg twice daily for 2 days |
| Children aged 1-12 years | Rifampicin: 10mg/kg twice daily for 2 days |
| Infants aged < 12 months | Rifampicin: 5mg/kg twice daily for 2 days |
| OR | |
| Adults | Ciprofloxacin: 500mg single dose (unlicensed for this use) |
| Children aged 5 - 12 years | Ciprofloxacin: 250mg single dose (unlicensed for this use) |

# II. GONORRHOEAE

**CAUSAL AGENT**
- Gonorrhea is a purulent infection of the mucous membrane surfaces caused by **Neisseria gonorrhoeae**.
- N gonorrhoeae is a gram-negative, intracellular, aerobic diplococcus; more specifically, it is a form of diplococcus known as the **gonococcus**.
- Cells are Gram-negative cocci, usually seen in pairs with the adjacent sides flattened.

**CLINICAL MANIFESTATIONS**
- N gonorrhoeae is spread by sexual contact or through vertical transmission from the mother's genital tract to the newborn during birth, causing **ophthalmia neonatorum** and **systemic neonatal infection.**
- In women, the cervix is the most common site of gonorrhoea, resulting in **endocervicitis** and **urethritis**, which can be complicated by pelvic inflammatory disease (**PID**). In men, gonorrhea causes **anterior urethritis**.
- Disseminated infections occur either by extension to adjacent organs (pelvic inflammatory disease, epididymitis) or by bacteremic spread (skin lesions, tenosynovitis, septic arthritis, endocarditis, and meningitis).

**PATHOGENESIS**
- Gonorrhea is usually acquired by sexual contact.
- Gonococci adhere to columnar epithelial cells, penetrate them, and multiply on the basement membrane.
- Adherence is facilitated through pili and opa proteins.
- Gonococcal lipopolysaccharide stimulates the production of tumor necrosis factor, which causes cell damage.
- Gonococci may disseminate via the bloodstream.
- Strains that cause disseminated infections are usually resistant to serum and complement.

## HOST DEFENSES

- Infection stimulates inflammation and local immunity; however, it is not known whether the secretory immune response is protective.
- Serum antibodies also appear.
- Individuals with genetic defects in late-acting complement components are at increased risk for disseminated infections.
- Protection, if it exists, may be strain specific.

## EPIDEMIOLOGY

- Gonorrhoea is a sexually transmitted disease of worldwide importance.
- The highest attack rate in both men and women occurs between 15 and 29 years of age.
- Host-related factors such as the number of sexual partners, contraceptive practices, sexual preference, and population mobility contribute to the incidence of gonorrhoea.

## DIAGNOSIS

- Gonorrhoea cannot be diagnosed solely on clinical grounds.
- For men, a Gram-stained smear of urethral exudate showing intracellular Gram-negative diplococci is diagnostic.
- For women, and for men when a direct smear is not definitive, culturing on selective medium is often required.
- N gonorrhoeae must be differentiated from other Neisseria species.
- Where appropriate, isolates should be examined for antibiotic resistance.
- A non-amplified DNA probe test is commercially available. This test does not require viable organisms and is useful where maintenance of viability during specimen transport is a problem; however, it is not as sensitive as culture.
- Serologic tests are not recommended for uncomplicated infections.

## CONTROL

- Although penicillin is no longer the first-line antibiotic used in the treatment of Neisseria gonorrhoeae, approximately 85% of cases are still sensitive to penicillin.
- The current first-line treatment for Neisseria gonorrhoeae is a **third-generation cephalosporin** with **azithromycin** (possible coinfection with Chlamydia trachomatis), which is effective in over 99% of cases.
- Sex partner(s) should be referred and treated.
- No effective vaccine yet exists.
- Condoms are effective in preventing gonorrhea.
- The Centers for Disease Control (CDC) recommends that all patients with gonorrheal infection also be treated for presumed co-infection with Chlamydia trachomatis.

# SECTION 5: PSEUDOMONAS

## CLINICAL MANIFESTATIONS

- Pseudomonas species are Gram-negative, aerobic bacilli measuring 0.5 to 0.8 μm by 1.5 to 3.0 μm. Motility is by a single polar flagellum.
- Pseudomonas aeruginosa and P maltophilia account for 80 percent of opportunistic infections by pseudomonas.
- Other infections caused by Pseudomonas species include endocarditis, pneumonia, and infections of the urinary tract, central nervous system, wounds, eyes, ears, skin, and musculoskeletal system.

  *Pseudomonas aeruginosa infection is a serious problem in patients hospitalized with cancer, cystic fibrosis, and burns; the case fatality is 50 %.*

## EPIDEMIOLOGY

- Pseudomonas species normally inhabit soil, water, and vegetation and can be isolated from the skin, throat, and stool of healthy persons. They often colonize hospital food, sinks, taps, mops, and respiratory equipment.
- Spread is from patient to patient via contact with fomites or by ingestion of contaminated food and water.

## DIAGNOSIS

- Pseudomonas can be cultured on most general-purpose media and identified with biochemical media.

## CONTROL

- The spread of Pseudomonas is best controlled by cleaning and disinfecting medical equipment.
- In burn patients, topical therapy of the burn with antimicrobial agents such as silver sulfadiazine, coupled with surgical debridement, has markedly reduced sepsis.
- Antibiotic susceptibility testing of clinical isolates is mandatory because of multiple antibiotic resistance; however, the combination of **Gentamicin** and **Carbenicillin** can be very effective in patients with acute P aeruginosa infections.

# Section 6: Pertussis (Whooping Cough)

**CAUSAL AGENT**
- An acute bacterial respiratory infection caused by *Bordetella pertussis*.

**COMMON CLINICAL FEATURES**
- Characterized by 3 stages:
  - **The catarrhal stage**: onset of coryza, sneezing, low-grade fever, and a mild cough (1-2 weeks).
  - **Paroxysmal stage**: bouts of coughing ending with a high-pitched inspiratory whoop or vomiting (lasting 1-6 weeks but may persist for up to 10 weeks).
  - **Convalescence stage**: recovery is gradual and the cough becomes less paroxysmal and disappears in 2-3 weeks (recovery may take weeks to months).
- The most severe infections are in infants of which over 50% are hospitalized
- In adult's symptoms range from mild respiratory infection to paroxysmal cough episodes.

**COMPLICATIONS**
- Pneumonia, seizure, encephalopathy, weight loss and death.
- Complications are most likely to occur in young infants among who the most common cause of pertussis related deaths is secondary bacterial pneumonia.
- Pertussis can occur in previously immunized and infected individuals, but immunization and prior infection attenuate the clinical picture.

**EPIDEMIOLOGY**
- Endemic worldwide.
- Pertussis is a major cause of childhood morbidity and mortality in developing countries, where an estimated 50 million cases and 300,000 deaths occur each year.
- In the UK notifications, have declined significantly since the introduction of pertussis immunization.

**RESERVOIR**
- Humans

**MODE OF TRANSMISSION**
- Droplets spread from an infectious case.

**INCUBATION PERIOD**
- Average **9-10 days** with a range of 6-20 days.

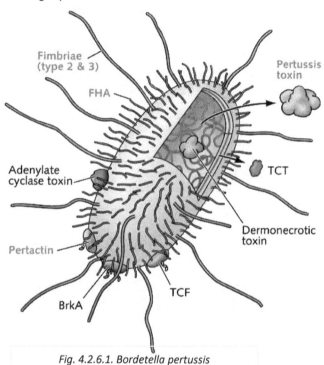

Fig. 4.2.6.1. *Bordetella pertussis*

**PERIOD OF COMMUNICABILITY**
- *Persons with pertussis are highly infectious during the catarrhal stage and during the first 2 weeks of the paroxysmal stage.*
- *A case is normally not infectious 3 weeks after the onset of the paroxysmal stage, though in up to 20% of cases infectivity may persist for up to 6 weeks.*
- *When treated with erythromycin patients are no longer contagious after 5 days of treatment.*

**PREVENTION AND CONTROL**
- Maintain high immunization coverage
- In the UK accellular pertussis vaccine is given in the primary course with diphtheria, tetanus, polio and Hib (as DtaP/IPV/Hib), given at aged 2, 3, & 4 months of age.
- A further booster dose is given with the preschool boosters between the ages of 3 and 5.
- Respiratory isolation for cases until at least 5 days (or until 14-day course of erythromycin completed).
- Arrange for laboratory confirmation.
- Vaccination of unvaccinated household contacts and exclusion from school.
- Antibiotic prophylaxis may be of value for unvaccinated household contacts of cases, particularly in infants <6 months of age, **if given within 21 days of onset of the first case.**

**TREATMENT**
- **Macrolide antibiotics** (azithromycin, clarithromycin, and erythromycin) are recommended for the treatment of pertussis in people aged ≥1 month.
- For infants aged <1-month, **Azithromycin** is the preferred antibiotic.
- Antimicrobial therapy with a macrolide antibiotic administered <3 weeks after cough onset can limit transmission to others.

# SECTION 7: ENTEROBACTERIACEAE

- **Common characteristics of Enterobacteriaceae family:**
  - Large family of Gram-negative bacteria that includes: Salmonella, Escherichia coli, Yersinia pestis, Klebsiella and Shigella, Proteus, Enterobacter, Serratia, and Citrobacter.
  - Several are present in the human intestinal tract (normal part of the gut flora).
  - They are gram negative, short rods.
  - They are non-spore forming.
  - They are facultative anaerobes.
  - They are catalase positive.
  - Some strains produce highly toxic endotoxins.
  - These organisms have simple nutritional requirements and MacConkey agar is used to isolate and differentiate them.
  - Motile by peritrichous flagella, except Shigella and Klebsiella which are non-motile.
  - Cytochrome C oxidase negative.

# I. KLEBSIELLA

## CLINICAL MANIFESTATIONS

- Common klebsiellae infections in humans include:
  - **Community-acquired pneumonia**: Pulmonary diseases caused by *K pneumoniae* are in the form of bronchopneumonia or bronchitis.
  - **Nosocomial infection:** Important manifestations of klebsiellae infection in the hospital setting include UTI, pneumonia, bacteremia, wound infection, cholecystitis, and catheter-associated bacteriuria.
  - **Rhinoscleroma and ozena:** caused by *K rhinoscleromatis* and *K ozaenae* respectively.
  - **Chronic genital ulcerative disease:** *K granulomatis* infection can result in granuloma inguinale or donovanosis.
  - **Colonization:** It is a common problem in patients with indwelling catheters.

## STRUCTURE

- The genus *Klebsiella* belongs to the tribe Klebsiellae, facultative anaerobic, rod shaped bacteria **with a prominent polysaccharide capsule**, a member of the family Enterobacteriaceae.
- Three species in the genus *Klebsiella* are associated with illness in humans: *Klebsiella pneumoniae, Klebsiella oxytoca and Klebsiella granulomatis*.
- Organisms known as *Klebsiella ozaenae* and *Klebsiella rhinoscleromatis* are considered nonfermenting subspecies of *K pneumoniae* that have characteristic clinical manifestations.

## PATHOGENICITY

- Klebsiella is found in the normal flora of the mouth, skin and intestines.
- The bacteria overcome innate host immunity through a polysaccharide capsule, which is the main determinant of their pathogenicity.
- The capsule is composed of complex acidic polysaccharides.

## EPIDEMIOLOGY

- *K pneumoniae* is an important cause of **community-acquired pneumonia:**
  - Community-acquired *Klebsiella* (Friedländer) pneumonia is a disease of debilitated middle-aged and older men with alcoholism.
  - *The mortality rate may be 50%, regardless of treatment.*
- Klebsiellae are also important in **nosocomial infections:**
  - Nosocomial infections may affect adults or children, and they occur more frequently in premature infants, patients in neonatal intensive care units, and hospitalized individuals who are immunocompromised
- Klebsiellae account for approximately 8% of all hospital-acquired infections.
- Klebsiellae cause as many as 14% of cases of primary bacteremia, second only to *Escherichia coli* as a cause of gram-negative sepsis.
- The mortality rate approaches 100% for persons with alcoholism and bacteremia.

## CONTROL

- *Klebsiella* organisms are resistant to multiple antibiotics. In general, initial therapy of patients with possible bacteremia is empirical.
- Agents with high intrinsic activity against *K pneumoniae* should be selected for severely ill patients.
- Examples of such agents include:
  - **Third-generation Cephalosporins:** Cefotaxime,
  - **Carbapenems:** Imipenem/Cilastatin.
  - **Aminoglycosides:** Gentamicin, Amikacin
  - **Quinolones.**
- These agents may be used as monotherapy or combination therapy.

# II. ESCHERICHIA

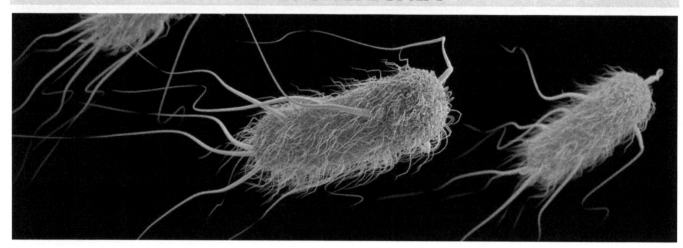

## CLINICAL MANIFESTATIONS

- **Neonatal meningitis**
  - ○ **Group B streptococci (GBS)** are the most commonly identified causes of bacterial meningitis, implicated in roughly 50% of all cases.
  - ○ **Escherichia coli** accounts for another 20%. Thus, identification and treatment of maternal genitourinary infections is an important prevention strategy.
  - ○ **Listeria monocytogenes** is the third most common pathogen, accounting for 5-10% of cases; it is unique in that it exhibits transplacental transmission.
  - ○ Pregnant women are at a higher risk of colonization with the **K1 capsular antigen strain of** *E coli*.
  - ○ This strain is also commonly observed in neonatal sepsis, which carries a mortality rate of 8%; most survivors have subsequent neurologic or developmental abnormalities.
  - ○ In adults, *E coli* meningitis is rare but may occur following neurosurgical trauma or procedures or complicating *Strongyloides stercoralis* hyperinfection involving the CNS.

- **Pneumonia**
  - ○ *E coli* respiratory tract infections are uncommon and are almost always associated with *E coli* UTI.

- **Intra-abdominal infections**
  - ○ *E coli* intra-abdominal infections often result from a perforated viscus (eg, appendix, diverticulum) or may be associated with intra-abdominal abscess, cholecystitis, and ascending cholangitis.
  - ○ Patients with diabetes mellitus are also at high risk of developing pylephlebitis of the portal vein and liver abscesses.

- **Enteric infections:**
  - ○ 6 different varieties of *E coli* have been reported:
  - ○ **Enterotoxigenic *E coli* (ETEC):** causes traveler's diarrhea.
    - ▪ ETEC produces LT toxin and ST toxin. These toxins act on the enterocyte to stimulate fluid secretion, resulting in diarrhoea.
    - ▪ LT toxin is heat **L**abile and increases local cAMP in the enteric cell.
    - ▪ ST toxin is heat **S**table toxin and increases cGMP.
  - ○ **Enteropathogenic *E coli* (EPEC):** causes of childhood diarrhea.
  - ○ **Enteroinvasive *E coli* (EIEC):** causes a *Shigella* -like dysentery.
  - ○ **Enterohemorrhagic *E coli* (EHEC):** causes hemorrhagic colitis or hemolytic-uremic syndrome (HUS, 6% of patients).
  - ○ **Enteroaggregative *E coli* (EAggEC):** associated with persistent diarrhea in children in developing countries.
  - ○ **Enteroadherent *E coli* (EAEC):** childhood diarrhea and traveler's diarrhea in Mexico & North Africa.
  - ○ **ETEC, EPEC, EAggEC, and EAEC** colonize the small bowel.
  - ○ **EIEC and EHEC** preferentially colonize the large bowel prior to causing diarrhea.
  - ○ **Shiga toxin–producing *E coli* (STEC)** is among the most common causes of foodborne diseases.
  - ○ This organism is responsible for several GI illnesses, including nonbloody and bloody diarrhea.
  - ○ Patients with these diseases, especially children, may be affected by neurologic and renal complications, including HUS.
  - ○ **Strains of STEC serotype O157-H7** have caused numerous outbreaks and sporadic cases of bloody diarrhea and HUS (also Thrombotic thrombocytopaenic purpura)
  - ○ In enteric infections, the causative organism is suggested based on the clinical presentation and the characteristic of the patient's stool:
    - ▪ **ETEC, EPEC, EAggEC and EAEC** infections produce watery stools without inflammatory cells.
    - ▪ **EIEC** infection produces dysentery-type stools,
    - ▪ **EHEC** infection produces hemorrhagic-type stools.

- **Urinary tract infections**
  - The urinary tract is the most common site of *E coli* infection, and more than 90% of all uncomplicated UTIs are caused by *E coli* infection.
  - *E coli* causes a wide range of UTIs:
    - Uncomplicated urethritis/cystitis,
    - symptomatic cystitis, pyelonephritis,
    - Acute prostatitis, prostatic abscess, Urosepsis.
- Uncomplicated cystitis occurs primarily in females who are sexually active and are colonized by an uropathogenic strain of *E coli*.
- **Uropathogenic strains** of *E coli* have an adherence factor called **P fimbriae, or pili**, which binds to the P blood group antigen.
- **Complicated** UTI and pyelonephritis are observed in elderly patients with structural abnormalities or obstruction such as prostatic hypertrophy or neurogenic bladders or in patients with urinary catheters.

## STRUCTURE

- *Escherichia* organisms are gram-negative bacilli that exist singly or in pairs. ***E coli* is facultatively anaerobic** with a type of metabolism that is both fermentative and respiratory. They are either nonmotile or motile by peritrichous flagella.
- *E coli* is a major facultative inhabitant of the large intestine.

## EPIDEMIOLOGY

- *The incubation period is **3-4 days**.*
- *90% of both community-acquired and nosocomial UTI (leading cause).*
- *20% of Neonatal meningitis (second to GBS). E coli neonatal meningitis carries a mortality rate of 8%, and most survivors have neurological or developmental abnormalities. E coli causes 12-50% of nosocomial infections and 4% of cases of diarrheal disease (Leading cause of diarrhoea is Nontyphoidal salmonella).*
- Up to 50% of females eventually experience at least one episode of UTI.
- Men older than 45 years with prostatic hypertrophy are at an increased risk of UTI due to related bladder stasis.
- Among neonates, *E coli* UTI is more common in boys than in girls, but circumcision reduces the risk.

## CONTROL

- **E coli meningitis:** Third-Generation Cephalosporins
- **E coli pneumonia**
  - Respiratory support and adequate oxygenation
  - Third-Generation Cephalosporins or Fluoroquinolones.
- **E coli cholecystitis/cholangitis**
  - Third-Generation Cephalosporins that cover E coli and Klebsiella organisms.
  - Empiric coverage should also include anti– E faecalis coverage.
- **E coli intra-abdominal abscess**
  - Anaerobic coverage: ampicillin and sulbactam or cefoxitin.
  - In severe infection: piperacillin and tazobactam, imipenem and cilastatin, or meropenem may be used.
- **E coli enteric infections**
  - Fluid replacement with solutions containing appropriate electrolytes.
- **Traveler's diarrhea:**
  - Doxycycline, trimethoprim/sulfamethoxazole (TMP/SMZ)
  - Fluoroquinolones, rifaximin.
  - They shorten the duration of diarrhea by 24-36 h.
- **Uncomplicated E coli cystitis**
  - Single dose of antibiotic or 3-day course of a fluoroquinolone, TMP/SMZ, or nitrofurantoin.
- **Recurrent E coli cystitis** (ie, >2 episodes/yr.)
  - Continuous or postcoital prophylaxis with a fluoroquinolone, TMP/SMZ, or nitrofurantoin.
- **Patients with complex cases** (diabetes, >65yr, or recent history of UTI):
  - 7- to 14-days course of levofloxacin,
  - Third-generation Cephalosporins, or aztreonam.
- **Acute uncomplicated E coli pyelonephritis**
  - In young women: fluoroquinolone or TMP/SMZ x 14/7
  - Patients with vomiting, nausea, or underlying illness (eg, diabetes) should be admitted to the hospital.
  - If fever and flank pain persist for more than 72 hrs, ultrasonography or CT scanning may be performed.
- **E coli perinephric abscess or prostatitis**
  - At least 6 wk of antibiotics.
- **E coli sepsis**
  - At least 2 wk of antibiotics and identification of the source of bacteremia based on imaging study results.
- Azithromycin significantly reduced Shiga toxin levels even when O157:H7 viability remained high.

*Antibiotics are not useful in EHEC infection and may predispose to development of HUS. Antimotility agents are contraindicated in children and in persons with enteroinvasive E coli (EIEC) infection.*

# III. SHIGELLOSIS

**CAUSAL AGENT**
- Acute bacterial illness caused by four species of Shigella: dysenteriae, flexneri, boydii and sonnei.
- Shigella sonnei is the most common species in Western Europe and causes a relatively mild illness.

**COMMON CLINICAL FEATURES**
- Watery or bloody diarrhoea, abdominal pain, fever and malaise.
- S. boydii and S. dysenteriae, and most S. flexneri infections, originate outside the UK and present clinically as dysentery (diarrhoea with blood, mucus, and pus).
- S. dysenteriae may be associated with serious disease, including **toxic megacolon and the haemolytic uraemic syndrome.**

**EPIDEMIOLOGY**
- Worldwide shigellosis causes an estimated 600,000 deaths per year, the majority in young children.
- In the UK Shigella infection has decreased dramatically since the peak incidence period of 1950-1969 when 20,000 - 40,000 cases were reported each year.

**RESERVOIR**
- Humans

**MODE OF TRANSMISSION**
- Person to person via the faecal-oral route.
- From contaminated food or water.

**INCUBATION PERIOD**
- **1-3 days** with a range of 12-96 hours
- Up to 1 week for S. dysenteriae type 1.

**PERIOD OF COMMUNICABILITY**
- As long as organism is excreted in the stool, usually within 4 weeks after illness.

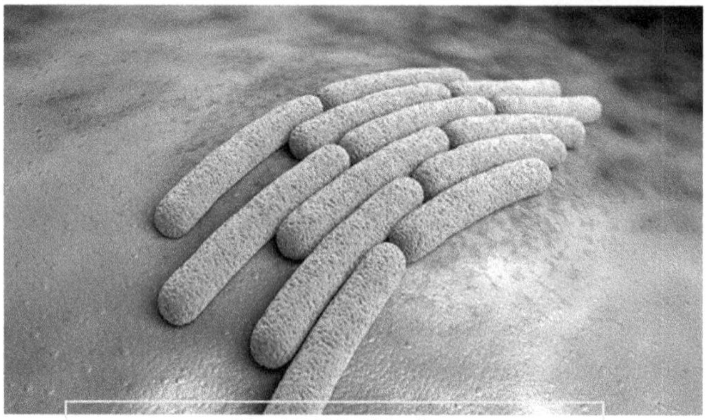

*Fig. 4.2.7.1. Shigella*

**PREVENTION AND CONTROL**
- Follow correct food hygiene practices for food preparation and cooking in domestic and commercial kitchens as described by the WHO Five keys to safer food.

# IV. SALMONELLA (NONTYPHOIDAL)

**INFECTIOUS AGENT**
- *SALMONELLA ENTERICA* subspecies *ENTERICA* is a gram-negative, rod-shaped bacillus.
- Nontyphoidal salmonellosis refers to illnesses caused by all serotypes of *SALMONELLA* except for Typhi, Paratyphi A, Paratyphi B (tartrate negative), and Paratyphi C.

**TRANSMISSION**
- Usually through fecal-oral route.
- Transmission can also occur through direct contact with infected animals or their environment and directly between humans.

**EPIDEMIOLOGY**
- Nontyphoidal salmonellae are a leading cause of bacterial diarrhea worldwide; they are estimated to cause 94 million cases of gastroenteritis and 115,000 deaths globally each year.

**CLINICAL PRESENTATION**
- Gastroenteritis is the most common clinical presentation of nontyphoidal *SALMONELLA* infection.
- The incubation period **is 6–72 hours**, but illness usually occurs within **12–36 hours** after exposure.
- Illness is commonly manifested by acute diarrhoea, abdominal pain, fever, and sometimes vomiting.
- The illness usually **lasts 4–7 days**, and most people recover without treatment.
- Approximately 5% of people develop bacteremia or focal infection (such as meningitis or osteomyelitis).
- Salmonellosis outcomes differ by serotype.
- Infections with some serotypes, including Dublin and Choleraesuis, are more likely to result in invasive infections.
- Rates of invasive infections and death are generally higher among infants, older adults, and people with immunosuppressive conditions (including HIV), hemoglobinopathies, and malignant neoplasms.

## DIAGNOSIS
- Diagnosis is based on isolation of **SALMONELLA** organisms.
- About 90% of isolates are obtained from routine stool culture, but isolates are also obtained from blood, urine, and material from sites of infection. Isolates of salmonellae are needed for serotyping and antimicrobial susceptibility testing.

## TREATMENT
- Supportive therapy and no antimicrobial agents: recommended for most patients with uncomplicated **SALMONELLA** infection.
- Antimicrobial therapy: indicated for complicated cases
    - Fluoroquinolones are often employed for empiric treatment of patients with moderate to severe travelers' diarrhoea;
    - Azithromycin and Rifaximin are also commonly used.

## PREVENTION
- No vaccine is available against nontyphoidal **SALMONELLA** infection.
- Preventive measures are aimed at:
    - Avoiding foods and drinks at high risk for contamination;
    - Frequent handwashing, especially after contacting animals or their environment.

# V. TYPHOID & PARATYPHOID FEVER

## INFECTIOUS AGENT
- Typhoid fever is a potentially severe and occasionally life-threatening febrile illness caused by the bacterium *Salmonella enterica* serotype Typhi.
- Paratyphoid fever is a similar illness caused by *S. enterica* serotype Paratyphi A, B (tartrate negative), or C.

## TRANSMISSION
- Humans are the only source of these bacteria; no animal or environmental reservoirs have been identified.
- Transmission: Fecal-oral route. Transmission through sexual contact, especially among men who have sex with men, has been documented rarely.

## EPIDEMIOLOGY
- Areas of risk include East and Southeast Asia, Africa, the Caribbean, and Central and South America.

## CLINICAL PRESENTATION
- The incubation period of typhoid infections is Range **1-3 weeks, commonly 8-14 days**, depending on infective dose.
- For paratyphoid, the range is **1-10 days.**
- The onset of illness is insidious, with gradually increasing fatigue and a fever that increases daily from low-grade to as high as 38°C–40°C by the third to fourth day of illness.
- Headache, malaise, and anorexia are nearly universal and abdominal pain, diarrhea, or constipation are common.
- Hepatosplenomegaly can often be detected. A transient, macular rash of rose-colored spots can occasionally be seen on the trunk.
- *Fever is commonly lowest in the morning, reaching a peak in late afternoon or evening.* The serious complications of typhoid fever generally occur after 2–3 weeks of illness and may include intestinal hemorrhage or perforation, which can be life threatening.

## DIAGNOSIS
- Infection with typhoid or paratyphoid fever results in a low-grade septicemia. Although blood culture is the mainstay of diagnosis in typhoid fever, a single culture is positive in only approximately 50% of cases.
- Multiple cultures increase the sensitivity and may be required to make the diagnosis.
- Bone marrow culture increases the diagnostic yield to approximately 80% of cases.
- Stool culture is not usually positive during the earliest phase of the disease.
- **The Widal test** is unreliable but is widely used in developing countries because of its low cost.
- Because there is no definitive serologic test for typhoid or paratyphoid fever, the initial diagnosis often has to be made clinically.
- The combination of a history of risk for infection and a gradual onset of fever that increases in severity over several days should raise suspicion of typhoid or paratyphoid fever.

## TREATMENT
- A fluoroquinolone, most often **ciprofloxacin**, is used for empiric treatment in most parts of the world.
- **Injectable third-generation Cephalosporins** are often the empiric drug of choice when the possibility of fluoroquinolone resistance is high.
- **Azithromycin** is increasingly used to treat typhoid fever or paratyphoid fever because of the emergence of multidrug-resistant strains, although increasing resistance to azithromycin in *Salmonella* Typhi strains has already been documented.
- Patients treated with an antibiotic may remain febrile for 3–5 days, although the height of the fever generally decreases each day.

## PREVENTION
- Safe food and water precautions and frequent handwashing are important in preventing typhoid and paratyphoid fever.
- Vaccines: recommended to prevent typhoid fever (not 100% effective).

# Section 8: Gram-Negative Gastrointestinal Disease

## I. CAMPYLOBACTER SPECIES

**CLINICAL MANIFESTATIONS**

- Mild to severe diarrhoea (frequently with bloody stools).
- Abdominal pain, cramping, fever, headache, nausea and/or vomiting.
- Infection with campylobacter can cause serious illness among the immuno-compromised.
- Illness typically lasts about **1 week** in healthy persons.
- Most infections are self-limiting and are not treated with antibiotics.
- However, treatment with erythromycin reduces the length of time that infected individuals shed the bacteria in their faeces.
- *Recently, Campylobacter infections have been identified as the most common antecedent to an acute neurological disease, the Guillain-Barré syndrome.*
- *C jejuni antigens that cross-react with one or more neural structures may be responsible for triggering the Guillian-Barre syndrome.*
- *Campylobacter infection can rarely cause a reactive Arthritis, Pancreatitis and Endocarditis*

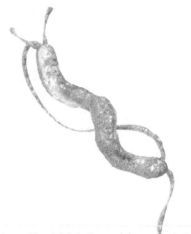

*Fig. 4.2.8.1. Campylobacter pylori*

**STRUCTURE**

- Campylobacter are Gram-negative, microaerophilic, non-fermenting, motile rods with a **single polar flagellum**.
- They are oxidase-positive and grow optimally at 37° or 42°C.

**RESERVOIR**

- Animals: Poultry, cattle, pigs, sheep and shellfish.
- Most raw poultry meat is contaminated with C. jejuni.

**MODE OF TRANSMISSION:**

- Ingestion of infected undercooked meats and meat products, especially poultry.
- Ingestion of unpasteurized or contaminated milk, contaminated ice and water.
- While person to person spread occurs, most cases are thought to be single, sporadic cases.
- In the UK, approximately 5% of cases are thought to occur through contact with infected pets.

**EPIDEMIOLOGY**

- *The incubation period is 2-5 days with a range of 1-10 days.*
- *Campylobacter is a major cause of diarrhoeal disease in humans.*
- *Infection with campylobacter is the most common cause of bacterial infectious intestinal disease in England and Wales, with approximately 50,000 cases reported each year.*
- *In temperate zones, including England and Wales infection with Campylobacter occurs more frequently during the early spring and summer.*
- Laboratory confirmed cases in England and Wales have been shown to be high among children.

**CONTROL**

- Campylobacter is generally sensitive to macrolide antibiotics such as **Erythromycin** and **Azithromycin**.
- **Notify**: In the UK Campylobacter infection is notifiable as 'suspected food poisoning', of which it is the most commonly reported cause.
- Follow correct food hygiene practices for food preparation and cooking in domestic and commercial kitchens.
- Prevent cross contamination of raw and cooked food by washing hands before, during and after food preparation.
- Wash and sanitize all equipment, surfaces and utensils used for food preparation.
- Separate raw and cooked food, and use separate equipment and utensils for handling raw food.
- Cook food thoroughly (until centre of food reaches at least 70°C), especially poultry, meat, eggs and seafood.
- Reheat cooked food thoroughly, and store cooked and raw food at a safe temperature.
- Use safe water and raw materials, e.g. pasteurized milk and water.
- Wash fruit and vegetables.

# II. HELICOBACTER PYLORI

**CLINICAL MANIFESTATIONS**

- Helicobacter pylori is associated with chronic superficial gastritis and plays a role in the pathogenesis of peptic ulcer disease.
- Increasing evidence indicates that H pylori infection is important in causing gastric carcinoma and lymphoma.
- Acute infection may cause vomiting and upper gastrointestinal pain; hypochlorhydria and intense gastritis develop.
- Chronic infection usually is asymptomatic.

**STRUCTURE**

- This Gram-negative curved or spiral rod is distinguished by **multiple, sheathed flagellae** (highly motile) and abundant urease.

**CLASSIFICATION AND ANTIGENIC TYPES**

- The antigenic structures are not completely defined and no universal typing scheme has been developed; strains may be differentiated by genotypic methods including restriction endonuclease analysis, and polymerase chain reaction (PCR).

**PATHOGENESIS**

- Helicobacter pylori is sheltered from gastric acidity in the mucus layer and a small proportion of cells adheres to the gastric epithelium.
- The microorganism does not appear to invade tissue.
- Production of urease, a vacuolating cytotoxin, and the cagA-encoded protein is associated with injury to the gastric epithelium
- *Colonization with Helicobacter pylori confers a 10-20% lifetime risk of developing peptic ulcers and a 1-2% lifetime risk of developing gastric cancer.*

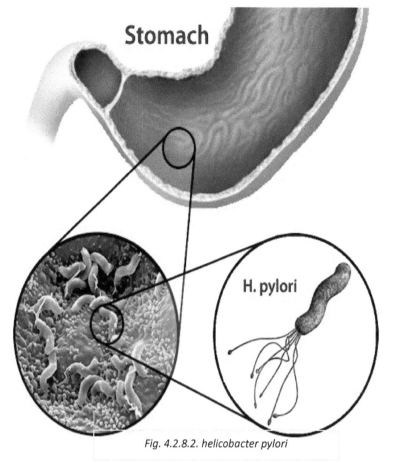

Fig. 4.2.8.2. helicobacter pylori

**HOST DEFENSES**

- Local and systemic humoral immune responses are essentially universal, but are not able to clear infection.

**EPIDEMIOLOGY**

- H pylori infection has a worldwide distribution; about 1/3 of the world's population is infected.
- The prevalence of infection increases with age.
- The major, if not exclusive, reservoir is humans but the exact modes of transmission are not known.
- H pylori has now been isolated from feces and dental plaque.

**DIAGNOSIS**

- Examination of gastric biopsy or stained smears allows presumptive diagnosis; definitive diagnosis is made by culture.
- Recently, non-invasive techniques such as the **Urea Breath Test** and serologic tests have been developed to diagnose H pylori infection, with accuracy exceeding 95 %.
- Serum antibody levels fall slowly and therefore cannot be used to accurately assess eradication.
- Either of the 13C-urea breath test or the stool antigen test are viable options for assessing successful eradication.

**CONTROL**

- Several indications have emerged for the use of antimicrobial therapies that eradicate H pylori infection.
- No vaccine is yet available.

# SECTION 9: LEGIONELLA

**INFECTIOUS AGENT**
- Gram-negative bacteria of the genus *legionella*.
- Most cases of legionellosis are caused by *legionella pneumophila*, but all species of *legionella* can cause disease.

**TRANSMISSION**
- Inhalation of a water aerosol containing the bacteria.
- The bacterium grows in *warm freshwater* environments.
- *Person-to-person transmission does not occur with either Legionnaires' disease or Pontiac fever.*

**EPIDEMIOLOGY**
- Legionellae are ubiquitous worldwide.
- Disease occurs after exposure to aquatic settings that promote bacterial growth:
  - The aquatic environment is somewhat stagnant,
  - The water is warm (**25°c–42°c**).
  - The water must be aerosolized so that the bacteria can be inhaled into the lungs.
- These 3 conditions are met almost exclusively in developed or industrialized settings.
- Disease does not occur in association with natural freshwater settings such as waterfalls, lakes, or streams.
- Legionellosis has been reported worldwide.
- **Risk factors:**
  - Aged >50 years,
  - Current or former smokers,
  - Chronic lung conditions.
  - Immunocompromised.

**CLINICAL PRESENTATION**
- **Legionnaires' disease**
  - Typically presents **with pneumonia**, which usually requires hospitalization and can be fatal in 10%–15% of cases.
  - Symptom onset occurs **2–14 days** after exposure.
  - In outbreak settings, <5% of people exposed to the source of the outbreak develop Legionnaires' disease.
- **Pontiac fever**
  - Is milder than Legionnaires' disease and presents as an influenzalike illness, with fever, headache, and muscle aches, **but no signs of pneumonia.**
  - Pontiac fever can affect healthy people, as well as those with underlying illnesses, and symptoms occur within **72 hours of exposure.**
  - Up to 95% of people exposed in outbreak settings can develop symptoms of Pontiac fever.

**DIAGNOSIS**
- Isolation of *legionella* from respiratory secretions, lung tissue, pleural fluid, or a normally sterile site is an important method for diagnosis of Legionnaires' disease.
- Clinical isolates are often necessary to interpret the findings of an investigation through comparison with isolates obtained from environmental sources.
- The most used diagnostic method is the *legionella* **urinary antigen assay.**
- Other diagnostic tests include direct fluorescent antibody and PCR.

**TREATMENT**
- Appropriate antibiotics include **Fluoroquinolones** and **Macrolides**.
- Treatment may be necessary for up to 3 weeks.
- In severe cases, patients may have prolonged stays in intensive care units.
- *Pontiac fever is a self-limited illness that requires supportive care only; antibiotics have no benefit.*

**PREVENTION**
- There is no vaccine for legionellosis, and antibiotic prophylaxis is not effective.

- *Because of differences in mechanism of disease, Legionella cannot be isolated in people who have Pontiac fever.*
- *The most used diagnostic method is the legionella Urinary Antigen Assay.*
- *There is no vaccine for Legionellosis, and antibiotic prophylaxis is not effective.*

# SECTION 10: CHLAMYDIA

**CAUSAL AGENT**
- Chlamydia trachomatis
- Chlamydiae are obligate intracellular bacteria.

**COMMON CLINICAL FEATURES**
- In women symptoms, may present as cervicitis and urethritis, which may be complicated by pelvic inflammatory disease, tubal damage, infertility and ectopic pregnancy. Up to 70% of infections in women are asymptomatic.
- Endocervical chlamydial infection has been associated with increased risk of acquiring HIV infection.
- In men symptoms, may present as urethritis, which may be complicated by epididymitis.
- Asymptomatic infection may be found in up to 50% of sexually active men.
- Can also infect the eye and cause trachoma: a common cause of blindness in the developing world.

**EPIDEMIOLOGY**
- Occurs worldwide.
- Genital Chlamydia infection is the most commonly sexually transmitted infection (STI) diagnosed in genitourinary medicine (GUM) clinics in the UK (Health Protection Agency). The number of uncomplicated Chlamydia diagnoses in GUM clinics has risen steadily since the mid 1990s. In 2005 there were 109,832 newly diagnosed cases of uncomplicated genital Chlamydia infections reported in the UK.
- In the UK the highest rates of Chlamydia are seen among females aged 16-19 years and among males aged 20-24 years (HPA).
- Genital chlamydial infection is an important reproductive health problem. An estimated 10-30% of infected women develop pelvic inflammatory disease (PID).

**MODE OF TRANSMISSION**
- Direct sexual contact.

**INCUBATION PERIOD**
- Probably **7-14 days.**

**PERIOD OF COMMUNICABILITY**
- Until treated. Limited short-term immunity occurs.

**TREATMENT**
- Treatment is with 7 days of doxycycline or erythromycin or a single dose of azithromycin. Infected individuals should abstain from sexual intercourse until they and their sexual partners have completed treatment to avoid re-infection.

**PREVENTION AND CONTROL**
- The use of condoms reduces the risk of infection. In the UK screening for genital Chlamydia is offered to all sexually active women

## PELVIC INFLAMMATORY DISEASE (PID)
- PID is initiated by infection that ascends from the vagina and cervix into the upper genital tract. ***Chlamydia trachomatis is the predominant sexually transmitted organism associated with PID.***
- Other organisms implicated in the pathogenesis of PID include Neisseria gonorrhoeae, Gardnerella vaginalis, Haemophilus influenzae, and anaerobes such as Peptococcus and Bacteroides species.
- In 30-40% of cases, PID is polymicrobial. The diagnosis of acute PID is primarily based on historical and clinical findings.

**CLINICAL MANIFESTATIONS**
- Vary widely, however; many patients exhibit few or no symptoms, whereas others have acute, serious illness.
- The most common presenting complaint is lower abdominal pain. Many women report an abnormal vaginal discharge.
- The differential diagnosis includes appendicitis, cervicitis, urinary tract infection, endometriosis, and adnexal tumors.

**RISK FACTORS**
- Multiple sexual partners, a history of prior STIs, and a history of sexual abuse. Frequent vaginal douching has been considered a risk factor for PID, but studies reveal no clear association.
- Gynecologic surgical procedures such as endometrial biopsy, curettage, and hysteroscopy break the cervical barrier, predisposing women to ascending infections. Younger age has been found to be associated with an increased risk of PID.
- Likely reasons include increased cervical mucosal permeability, a larger zone of cervical ectopy, a lower prevalence of protective antichlamydial antibodies, and increased risk-taking behaviors.

# SECTION 11: HERPES & VARICELLA

## I. HERPES SIMPLEX VIRUSES

**CAUSAL AGENT**
- Two serotypes of herpes simplex virus have been identified: Herpes simplex virus type 1 (HSV-1) and Herpes simplex virus type 2 (HSV-2).

**COMMON CLINICAL FEATURES**
- Infection with HSV is characterized by a localised primary infection, latency and recurrence.
    o Herpes simplex virus type 1 (HSV-1) is typically associated with gingivostomatitis (**orally transmitted**).
    o Herpes simplex virus type 2 (HSV-2) is **sexually transmitted**. Symptoms include genital ulcers or sores.
- The virus may also lead to meningoencephalitis or cause infection of the eye.
- Both HSV-1 and HSV-2 can affect the genital tract and HSV-2 can cause primary infection of the mouth.
- Complications include eczema herpeticum, Bell's palsy, encephalitis, meningitis, ocular herpes and erythema multiforme.

**EPIDEMIOLOGY**
- Worldwide 50-90% of adults possess circulating antibodies against HSV-1 and initial infection usually occurs before age 5.
- There is also a secondary peak among young adults.
- HSV-2 infection usually begins with sexual activity and is rare before adolescence.
- Genital herpes simplex virus infection is the most common ulcerative sexually transmitted disease in the UK.

**RESERVOIR**
- Humans.

**MODE OF TRANSMISSION**
- Direct contact with oral secretions.
- Unprotected vaginal or anal sex, genital contact or through oral sex.

**INCUBATION PERIOD**
- **1-6 days**. The virus may be shed in the saliva for 1-8 weeks after primary infection and for about 3 days in recurrent infections.

**PERIOD OF COMMUNICABILITY**
- HSV can be isolated for 2 weeks and up to 7 weeks after primary infection.
- HSV may be shed intermittently for years and possible lifelong in the presence or absence of clinical manifestations.

**TREATMENT**
- Oral antivirals for primary infection and reactivation.
- Topical antivirals may be used for reactivation.

**PREVENTION AND CONTROL**
- Sunscreen and oral antiviral may be considered to prevent reactivation.
- Personal hygiene to limit spread.

## II. CHICKENPOX AND SHINGLES

**CAUSAL AGENT**
- **Chickenpox:** a systemic viral infection caused by infection with human varicella-zoster virus (VZV), a member of the herpesvirus family.
- VZV is a double-stranded DNA virus.
- Herpes Zoster (**shingles**) is caused by reactivation of latent varicella infection whose genomes persist in sensory root ganglia of the brain stem and spinal cord.

**COMMON CLINICAL FEATURES**
- Generally, a mild disease in children lasting 4-7 days, sometimes characterized by a short prodromal period (low-grade fever, malaise)
- Followed by a vesicular rash (usually on the trunk) lasting 3-4 days which become granular scabs.
- There are successive crops of vesicles over several days.
- The most common complications from varicella infection are bacterial infections of the skin and soft tissues in children and pneumonia in adults.
- Severe complications include, septicaemia, toxic shock syndrome, necrotizing fiscilitis, osteomyelitis, bacterial pneumonia and septic arthritis.
- **Congenital varicella syndrome** occurs following infection during pregnancy (first 5 months), although most risk appears to be in weeks 13-20.
- Herpes zoster (shingles) is more prevalent among older age groups.

## EPIDEMIOLOGY

- Endemic worldwide, occurring mainly in children.
- The incidence in older children and adults is rising in the UK and other Western countries.
- In temperate climates, 90% of individuals have been infected by age 15 and 95% by young adulthood.
- In tropical climates a higher proportion of cases occur in adults.

## RESERVOIR

- Humans.

## MODE OF TRANSMISSION

- Direct person to person contact, by droplet or airborne spread of vesicular fluid or respiratory secretions.
- Also by contact with articles recently contaminated by discharges from vesicles and mucous membranes from an infected person.
- Highly contagious infecting up to 90% of those exposed.

## INCUBATION PERIOD

- **2-3 weeks,** commonly **14-16 days**.
- Longer following passive immunization or in the immunodeficient.

## PERIOD OF COMMUNICABILITY

- Commonly 1-2 days following onset of rash and until all lesions are crusted (usually 5 days).

## PREVENTION AND CONTROL

- Exclude children with chickenpox from school until 5 days from the onset of rash. Infected healthcare workers should be excluded from work for the same period.
- *Primary varicella-zoster virus infection causes chickenpox.*
- *Reactivation of latent Herpes-zoster virus causes shingles.*

## MANAGEMENT OF SHINGLES

- Conservative therapy includes the following:
  - Nonsteroidal anti-inflammatory drugs (NSAIDs)
  - Wet dressings with 5% aluminum acetate (Burrow solution)
  - Lotions (e.g., calamine)
- Primary medications for acute zoster–associated pain include the following:
  - Narcotic and nonnarcotic analgesics (both systemic and topical)
  - Neuroactive agents (e.g., tricyclic antidepressants [TCAs])
  - Anticonvulsant agents
  - Steroid treatment for herpes zoster is traditional but controversial. A substantial dose (e.g., 40-60 mg of oral prednisone every morning) is typically administered as early as possible in the course of the disease and is continued for 1 week, followed by a rapid taper over 1-2 weeks.
  - Antiviral therapy
  - Vaccine at **70 years (and 78 and 79-year-olds as a catch-up)**

# III. CYTOMEGALOVIRUS

## CLINICAL MANIFESTATIONS

- Cytomegalovirus causes three clinical syndromes:
  - **Congenital cytomegalovirus infection** causes hepatosplenomegaly, retinitis, rash and central nervous system involvement.
  - In about 10% of older children and adults, **primary cytomegalovirus** infection causes a mononucleosis syndrome with fever, malaise, atypical lymphocytosis and pharyngitis.
  - **Immunocompromised hosts** (transplant recipients and human immunodeficiency virus [HIV]-infected individuals) may develop life-threatening disseminated disease involving the lungs, gastrointestinal tract, liver, retina and central nervous system.

## PATHOGENESIS

- Cytomegalovirus replicates mainly in the salivary glands and kidneys and is shed in saliva and urine. Replication is slow, and the virus induces characteristic giant cells with intranuclear inclusions.

## EPIDEMIOLOGY

- Transmission is via intimate contact with infected secretions.
- Cytomegalovirus infections are among the most prevalent viral infections worldwide.

# IV. EPSTEIN-BARR VIRUS

**CLINICAL MANIFESTATIONS**
* Epstein-Barr virus causes classic **Mononucleosis.** In immunocompromised hosts, the virus causes a **Lymphoproliferative Syndrome.**
* In some families, Epstein Barr virus causes **Duncan's Syndrome.**

**PATHOGENESIS**
* Epstein Barr virus replicates the epithelial cells of the oropharynx and in β lymphocytes.

**EPIDEMIOLOGY**
* Epstein Barr virus is transmitted by intimate contact, particularly via the exchange of saliva.

# V. HUMAN HERPESVIRUS 6 AND 7

**CLINICAL MANIFESTATIONS**
* Human herpes viruses 6 and 7 are associated with **exanthem subitem (roseola)** and with **rejection of transplanted kidneys.**

**PATHOGENESIS**
* The pathogenesis is poorly understood.

**EPIDEMIOLOGY**
* Antibodies to this virus are present in almost everyone by age 5.

# VI. HUMAN HERPESVIRUS 8 (KAPOSI SARCOMA)

**CLINICAL MANIFESTATIONS**
* Human herpesvirus 8 has been found associated with **Kaposi's sarcoma** in AIDS patients as well as intra-abdominal solid tumors.

**PATHOGENESIS AND EPIDEMIOLOGY**
* Virtually nothing is known about the pathogenesis and epidemiology of this newly described herpesvirus.

# VII. B VIRUS

**CLINICAL MANIFESTATIONS**
* In humans, B virus causes **encephalitis** that is usually fatal; survivors have brain damage.

**PATHOGENESIS**
* B virus is transmitted to humans by the bite of infected **rhesus monkeys** and is transported up neurons to the brain.

**EPIDEMIOLOGY**
* The reservoir for the disease is latent infection in rhesus monkeys, particularly those from Southeast Asia and India.
* In stressed or unhealthy animals, the virus may reactivate and appear in saliva.

# VIII. FIFTH DISEASE

* Fifth disease is a mild rash illness caused by **parvovirus B19.**
* This disease, also called **erythema infectiosum**, got its name because it was fifth in a list of historical classifications of common skin rash illnesses in children.
* It is more common in children than adults.
* A person usually gets sick with fifth disease within 4 to 14 days after getting infected with **parvovirus B19.**

**SIGNS & SYMPTOMS**
* The first symptoms of fifth disease are usually mild and may include fever, runny nose, and Headache.
* After several days, there is a red rash on the face called **"slapped cheek" rash.** (MRCEM 09 DEC 2015)
* This rash is the most recognized feature of fifth disease.
* It is more common in children than adults.
* Some people may get a second rash a few days later on their chest, back, buttocks, or arms and legs.
* The rash may be itchy, especially on the soles of the feet.

- It can vary in intensity and usually goes away in 7 to 10 days, but it can come and go for several weeks. As it starts to go away, it may look lacy.
- People with fifth disease can also develop pain and swelling in their joints (polyarthropathy syndrome). This is more common in adults, especially women.
- Some adults with fifth disease may only have painful joints, usually in the hands, feet, or knees, and no other symptoms.
- The joint pain usually lasts 1 to 3 weeks, but it can last for months or longer.
- It usually goes away without any long-term problems.

## COMPLICATIONS
- Fifth disease is usually mild for children and adults who are otherwise healthy.
- But for some people fifth disease cause serious health complications.
- People with weakened immune systems caused by leukemia, cancer, organ transplants, or HIV infection are at risk for serious complications from fifth disease.
- It can cause chronic anemia that requires medical treatment.

## TRANSMISSION
- Parvovirus B19, which causes fifth disease, spreads through respiratory secretions (such as saliva, sputum, or nasal mucus) when an infected person coughs or sneezes.
- The patient is most contagious when it seems like "just a cold" and before the start of the rash or joint pain and swelling.
- After the rash the patient is not likely to be contagious.
- People with fifth disease who have weakened immune systems may be contagious for a longer amount of time.

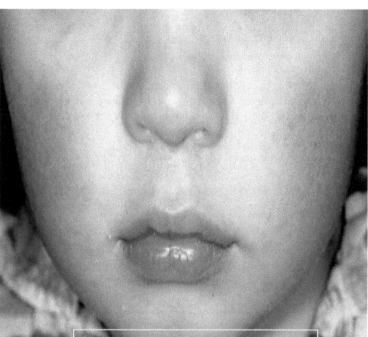

*Fig. 4.2.11.1. Slapped cheek syndrome*

- Parvovirus B19 can also spread through blood or blood products.
- A pregnant woman who is infected with parvovirus B19 can pass the virus to her baby.
- Once the patient recovers from fifth disease, he develops immunity that generally protects from parvovirus B19 infection in the future.

## DIAGNOSIS
- Healthcare providers can often diagnose fifth disease just by seeing "slapped cheek" rash on a patient's face.
- A blood test can also be done to determine the susceptibility or immunity to parvovirus B19 infection or recently infected.
- The blood test may be particularly helpful for pregnant women who may have been exposed to parvovirus B19 and are suspected to have fifth disease.

## PREVENTION
- There is no vaccine or medicine that can prevent parvovirus B19 infection.
- washing hands often with soap and water
- covering mouth and nose when cough or sneeze
- not touching eyes, nose, or mouth
- avoiding close contact with people who are sick
- staying home when sick
- *After you get the rash, you are probably not contagious.*

## TREATMENT
- Fifth disease is usually mild and will go away on its own.
- Children and adults who are otherwise healthy usually recover completely.
  Treatment usually involves relieving symptoms, such as fever, itching, and joint pain and swelling.

# SECTION 12: HIV

**INFECTIOUS AGENT**
- HIV, **a single-stranded,** positive-sense, enveloped **RNA** virus in the genus *lentivirus.*

**TRANSMISSION**
- HIV can be transmitted through:
  - Sexual contact, needle- or syringe-sharing,
  - Medical use of blood or blood components,
  - Organ or tissue transplantation
  - Artificial insemination.
  - From mother to child during pregnancy, at birth, and postpartum through breastfeeding.
- HIV may be transmitted occupationally to health care workers who are exposed to blood and other potentially infectious bodily fluids via percutaneous injury or splash exposures to mucous membranes or non-intact skin.

**EPIDEMIOLOGY**
- HIV infection occurs worldwide.
- Sub-saharan Africa remains the most affected part of the world (25 million cases or 71% of all people living with HIV infection).
- Notable increases in HIV infection have occurred in Eastern Europe and central Asia.
- Most new infections come from low- and middle-income countries.

**DIAGNOSIS**
- Most people develop detectable antibodies within **2–8 weeks (mean, 25 days)**.
- 97% of people develop antibodies in the **first 3 months after infection**.
- In rare cases, it can take up to 6 months to develop antibodies to HIV.
- After being infected, a person remains antibody positive for life, except when people lose the capacity to mount detectable antibodies in the latest stages of the disease.
- The earliest time after exposure that HIV infection can be diagnosed is approximately 9 days, when HIV RNA becomes detectable in blood; however, tests needed to measure HIV RNA are costly and may not be available.
- Any person not known to be HIV-infected who is diagnosed with an aids-compatible illness, such as pneumocystis pneumonia, should be tested for HIV.

**TREATMENT**
- Prompt medical care and effective treatment with antiretrovirals can inhibit HIV from damaging the immune system and delay progression of disease.
- Effective treatment also substantially reduces the risk of HIV transmission to others.

**PREVENTION**
- No vaccine is available to prevent infection with HIV.
- Use condoms consistently and correctly, especially if engaging in vaginal, anal, or oral sex with a person who is HIV infected or whose HIV status is unknown
- Avoid injecting drugs
- Avoid sharing needles or other devices that can puncture skin.
- Avoid, if at all possible, blood transfusions or use of clotting factor concentrates from untested source.

## Risk of transmission of blood-borne viruses from patient to healthcare worker

| INFECTION | PATIENT TO HEALTHCARE WORKER |
|---|---|
| **Hepatitis B (HBV)** | Up to 30% |
| **Hepatitis C (HCV)** | 1-3% |
| **HIV** | 0.3% |

**Source:** http://www.hse.gov.uk/biosafety/blood-borne-viruses/risk-healthcare-workers.htm

# SECTION 13: HEPATITIS

## I. HEPATITIS A

**INFECTIOUS AGENT**
- Hepatitis A virus (HAV) is a **nonenveloped RNA virus** classified as a **picornavirus**.

**TRANSMISSION**
- Person to person, primarily through the **faecal-oral route:**
  - Contaminated food and water.
  - Contaminated raw shellfish harvested from sewage contaminated water.
- Blood exposure (rare).

**INCUBATION PERIOD**
- **15-50 days**, average 28-30 days.

**PERIOD OF COMMUNICABILITY**
- From 2 weeks before the onset of symptoms until 1 week after.
- Maximum infectivity occurs during latter half of the incubation period and for a few days after onset of jaundice.
- Infants and children can shed virus for up to 6 months after infection.

**EPIDEMIOLOGY**
- Endemic worldwide, prevalence is higher in countries with poor sanitation and hygiene.
- In developing countries with high endemicity the peak age of infection occurs largely in early childhood, among whom HAV infection is mostly asymptomatic.
- In countries where Hepatitis A is highly endemic, exposure to HAV is almost universal before the age of 10 years.
- In countries with low endemicity the peak age of infection occurs mainly among adults.
- The incidence of HAV has been decreasing in developed countries over the last 50 years.

**CLINICAL PRESENTATION**
- Infection with HAV may range from asymptomatic to symptoms of fever, malaise, abdominal pain, loss of appetite, nausea, vomiting and diarrhoea followed by dark urine and jaundice.
- In young children infection with HAV is usually asymptomatic whereas symptomatic disease occurs more commonly among adults.
  - **In children aged <6 years:**
    - 70% infections are asymptomatic;
    - If symptomatic, Jaundice is uncommon.
  - **Among older children and adults:**
    - The illness usually lasts <2 months,
    - Approximately **10%–15%** of infected people have prolonged or relapsing symptoms over a 6- to 9-month period.
- Case fatality is low, around **0.6%** increasing with age to **1.8%** in adults over 50 and **10%** in adults aged over 70.
- Protective antibodies develop in response to infection and confer lifelong immunity. Chronic infection does not occur.

**DIAGNOSIS**
- Demonstration of IgM antibodies to HAV (IgM anti HAV) in serum.
- *Diagnosis requires a positive test for **antibody to HAV (anti-HAV) IgM** in serum, detectable from 2 weeks before the onset of symptoms to approximately 6 months afterward.*

**TREATMENT**
- Supportive care.

**PREVENTION**
- Vaccination or immune globulin (IG)
- Food and water precautions,
- Maintaining standards of hygiene and sanitation (especially among children in child day care and in schools).
- Vaccination advised for travellers (aged 5 and above) to countries outside Western Europe, North America and Australasia.

---

- *People are most infectious 1–2 weeks before the onset of clinical signs and symptoms.*
- *A positive total anti-HAV result and a negative IgM anti-HAV result indicate past infection or vaccination and immunity.*
- *The presence of serum IgM anti-HAV usually indicates current or recent infection and does not distinguish between immunity from infection and vaccination.*

# II. HEPATITIS B

### HBV STRUCTURE
- Hepatitis B virus (HBV), a member of the **hepadnavirus** group, **double-stranded DNA viruses** which replicate, unusually, by reverse transcription.

### RESERVOIR
- Humans

### MODE OF TRANSMISSION
- Through direct contact with the bodily fluids of an infected person: blood, saliva, semen, vaginal secretions and to a lesser extent in breast milk, tears and urine.
- **The concentration of HBV is highest in blood.**
- In areas of high endemicity, the most common route of transmission is perinatal or is acquired in early childhood.
- Common modes of transmission:
  - *Perinatal transmission*
  - *Sexual transmission*
  - *Close household contact*
  - *Intravenous drug use*
  - *Child to child transmission*
  - *Contaminated needles or syringes*
  - *Skin penetrating procedures including acupuncture, body piercing and tattooing.*
  - *Needle stick injuries.*
- *The HBV virus is 50-100 times more infectious than HIV.*

### INCUBATION PERIOD
- **45-180 days**, average 60-90 days

### PERIOD OF COMMUNICABILITY
- All persons who are **HBsAg-positive** are potentially infectious.
- The infectivity of chronically infected individuals ranges from high to modest.

### COMMON CLINICAL FEATURES
- Many infections with HBV are asymptomatic or range from mild symptoms to fulminant hepatitis with fatigue, abdominal pain, loss of appetite, intermittent nausea, vomiting and jaundice.
- The development of chronic HBV infection is age dependant, with young children more likely to develop chronic infection.

## DISTINCTIVE PROPERTIES
- **Develop chronic hepatitis:**
  - 90% of infants infected perinatally
  - 30-50% among children between ages 1 and 5 years.
  - 5 to 10% of immunocompetent adults
- 60-65% show subclinical disease and recover fully.
- 20-25% that contract HBV develop acute hepatitis.
- The risk of death from HBV related liver cancer or cirrhosis is approximately 25% for persons who become chronically infected during childhood.
- The risk of acquiring Hep B in a needlestick from a Hep B positive donor is 30%.

### HOST DEFENSES
- **Hepatitis B surface antigen (HBsAg):**
  - The presence of HBsAg indicates that the person is infectious.
  - HBsAg is the antigen used to make Hepatitis B vaccine.
  - This is the first detectable marker of infection and is present as early as the incubation period.
  - **Persistent carriage** of hepatitis B is defined by the presence of hepatitis B surface antigen (HBsAg) in the serum for more than six months.

- **Hepatitis B surface antibody (anti-HBs):**
  - The presence indicates the person has recovered from and has immunity to Hepatitis B.
  - Anti-HBs also develops in a person who has been successfully vaccinated against Hepatitis B.

- **Hepatitis B core antibody (anti-HBc):**
  - This serological marker appears at the onset of symptoms in acute Hepatitis B and persists for life.
  - The presence indicates previous or ongoing infection with Hepatitis B in an undefined timeframe.

- **IgM antibody to Hepatitis B core antigen (IgM anti-HBc)**:
  - Indicates a recent, acute infection with the virus.

- **IgG antibody to Hepatitis B core antigen (IgG Anti-HBc)**:
  - Is indicative of chronic infection.

- **Hepatitis B envelope antigen (HBeAg)**:
  - Hepatitis B envelope antigen is found in the blood during acute and chronic Hepatitis B infection.
  - A positive HBeAg test indicates that the virus is replicating and the infected person has high levels of the Hepatitis B virus.

- **Hepatitis B envelope antibody (HBeAb or anti-HBe)**:
  - This substance is produced by the immune system temporarily during acute HBV infection or consistently during or after a burst in viral replication.
  - A person who converts from positive HBeAg to HBeAB is more likely to achieve long-term clearance of the virus.

## DIAGNOSIS
- Laboratory evaluation for HBV disease consists of:
  - Liver enzyme tests, Hematologic and coagulation studies
  - Platelet count and a complete blood count (CBC).
  - *Serologic tests for HBsAg and anti-HBc IgM are required for the diagnosis of acute HBV.*
- To evaluate the patient's level of infectivity, quantification of HBV DNA is essential, and the presence of hepatitis B e antigen (HBeAg) should be determined. *Indeed, the best indication of active viral replication is the presence of HBV DNA in the serum.*

## PROTECTION OF HEPATITIS B
- Hepatitis B **vaccine**
- Antiviral treatment may be effective in approximately 95% of the patients who are treated with first-line oral therapy, as defined by undetectable HBV DNA.
- For those who are treated with **interferon**, about 17% have persistent HBV DNA suppression.
- For selected candidates, **liver transplantation** currently seems to be the only viable treatment for the later stages of hepatitis B infection, with a posttransplantation viral control of greater than 90-95%.

## HBV AND HEPATOCELLULAR CARCINOMA
- Chronic hepatitis B infection is the major contributor to the development of approximately 50% of cases of hepatocellular carcinoma (HCC) worldwide.
- Studies indicate that the level of hepatitis B virus (HBV) DNA, which indicates viral replication, is a strong predictor for cirrhosis and HCC regardless of other viral factors.
- Approximately 9% of patients in Western Europe who have cirrhosis develop HCC due to hepatitis B infection at a mean follow-up of 73 months.
- The probability of HCC developing 5 years after the diagnosis of cirrhosis has been established is 6%, and the probability of decompensation is 23%.

# III. HEPATITIS C

### INFECTIOUS AGENT
- Hepatitis C virus (HCV), a spherical, **enveloped, positive-strand RNA virus.**

### RESERVOIR
- Humans

### MODE OF TRANSMISSION
- Contact with infected blood or bodily fluids. ***The primary mode of transmission is through contaminated blood.***
- Other less efficient modes of transmission include; mother to child transmission (vertical transmission), sexual transmission, exposure to contaminated medical and dental procedures abroad, tattooing or skin piercing with blood contaminated equipment and patient to health care worker and vice versa. The highest risk groups are current and past injecting drug users, those who received blood products before 1986 and recipients of blood transfusions before 1991.

### INCUBATION PERIOD
- Range **2-6 weeks**, commonly 6-9 weeks.

### PERIOD OF COMMUNICABILITY
- From 1 week or more before onset of first symptoms.
- May persist indefinitely

**EPIDEMIOLOGY**

- Endemic worldwide.
- *HCV is a major cause of liver disease worldwide.*
- The World Health Organisation estimate that 180 million people are infected with HCV worldwide, 130 million of whom are chronic HCV carriers at risk of developing liver cirrhosis and/or cancer.
- In England the prevalence of HCV is estimated to be **0.5%.**
- Amongst diagnosed infections, injecting drug use is the single biggest risk factor, accounting for more than 90% of infections.
- Most people diagnosed with hepatitis C infection are men aged between 25 and 45 years, reflecting the fact that men are more likely to be injecting drug users.

- **The prevalence of hepatitis C in injecting drug users in contact with health services is estimated at 38%.**
- The risk of acquiring Hep C in a needlestick from a Hep C positive patient is 3%.

**CLINICAL PRESENTATION**

- **80%** with acute HCV infection have no symptoms.
- If symptoms occur, they may include loss of appetite, abdominal pain, fatigue, nausea, dark urine, and **jaundice.**
- **10%–20%** develop severe liver disease, but progression to end-stage liver disease is slow and typically does not occur until ≥20 years after infection.
- Nonetheless, *HCV is a major cause of cirrhosis and hepatocellular cancer and is the leading reason for liver transplantation.*

**DIAGNOSIS**

- Two major types of tests are available:
  - IgG assays for HCV antibodies
  - Nucleic acid amplification testing to detect HCV RNA in blood (viremia).
- 75%–85% of people who seroconvert to anti-HCV, indicative of acute infection, will progress to chronic infection and persistently detectable viremia.
- False-negative antibody test results, while rare, may occur early in acute infection, usually in the first 15 weeks after exposure and infection.

**TREATMENT**

- Interferon
- The new treatments offer all-oral regimens, short duration of therapy (from 6–12 weeks to 24–48 weeks), few side effects, and high cure rates (>90%).
- *No therapies for HCV postexposure prophylaxis are available.*

**PREVENTION**

- No vaccine is available to prevent HCV infection, nor does immune globulin provide protection.

| Name of virus | Hepatitis A virus | Hepatitis B virus | Hepatitis C virus | Hepatitis D virus | Hepatitis E virus |
|---|---|---|---|---|---|
| **Classification** | Picornavirus | Hepadnavirus | Flavivirus | Deltavirus | Hepevirus |
| **Viral genome** | ssRNA | dsDNA | ssRNA | -ssRNA (-ve) | ssRNA |
| **Transmission** | Enteric | Parenteral | Parenteral | Parenteral | Enteric |
| **Incubation period** | 15-45 days | 45-160 days | 15-150 days | 30-60 days | 15-60 days |
| **Chronic Hepatitis** | No | Yes<br><br>10% chance | Yes<br><br>> 50% chance | Yes<br><br>< 5% of infectious<br><br>> 80% of superinfection | No |
| **Cure?** | No cure.<br><br>Treatments usually tackle the symptoms | No cure.<br><br>Treatments usually tackle the symptoms | No cure.<br><br>Treatments usually tackle the symptoms | No cure.<br><br>Treatment: Alpha interferon for 12 months | No cure.<br><br>Treatments usually tackle the symptoms |

# IV. HEPATITIS E

## INFECTIOUS AGENT
- Infection is caused by hepatitis E virus (HEV), a **single-stranded, RNA virus** belonging to the Hepeviridae family.

## TRANSMISSION
- HEV is transmitted primarily by the **fecal-oral route.**
- In regions with poor sanitation and limited access to safe drinking water, epidemics and interepidemic occurrences of hepatitis E are largely waterborne.
- Transmission to fetuses and neonates by women infected during pregnancy is common.

## EPIDEMIOLOGY
- Clinical attack rates are highest in young adults aged 15–49 years.
- In outbreak-prone areas, interepidemic disease is sporadically encountered.
- In these areas, pregnant women (whether infected sporadically or during an epidemic) are at risk of their HEV disease progressing to liver failure and death.
- *Miscarriages and neonatal deaths are common complications of HEV infection*.
- Symptomatic disease is observed most frequently in adults aged >50 years.
- Primary infection acquired by people who are immunosuppressed, particularly recipients of solid-organ allografts, may progress to chronic infection.

## CLINICAL PRESENTATION
- The incubation period of acute HEV is **2–9 weeks** (mean 6 weeks).
- Signs and symptoms of disease during acute infection include **jaundice**, fever, loss of appetite, abdominal pain, and lethargy.
- A wide range of neurologic manifestations have been associated with HEV.
- For most people, HEV infection and disease is self-limited.
- Pregnant women (especially those infected during the second or third trimester) may present with or progress to liver failure, and their fetuses are at risk of spontaneous abortion and premature delivery.
- People with preexisting liver disease may undergo further hepatic decompensation with HEV infection.
- Recipients of organ transplants tend to have no symptoms associated with acute and chronic HEV infection.

## DIAGNOSIS
- The diagnosis of acute hepatitis E is established by detecting **anti-HEV IgM and IgG in serum.**
- Detecting **HEV RNA** in serum or stools further confirms the serologic diagnosis but is seldom required.
- Longer-term, serial detection of HEV RNA in serum or stools, regardless of the HEV antibody serostatus, suggests chronic HEV infection.

## TREATMENT
- Treatment is supportive.
- Oral **ribavirin** has been used to treat chronic hepatitis E in solid-organ transplant recipients.

## PREVENTION
- No vaccine is available, nor are drugs for preventing infection.

| VIRUSES | |
|---|---|
| **DNA VIRUSES (CH³AKS)** | **RNA VIRUSES** |
| • CMV | • Hepatitis A, C, E |
| • **H**epatitis B virus | • Influenza virus |
| • **H**erpes viruses | • Measles, Mumps, Rubella |
| • **H**PV | • Picornaviruses |
| • **A**denovirus | • Rabies virus |
| • **K**aposi sarcoma | • Retroviruses: HIV, T-cell leukaemia |
| • **S**mall Pox virus | |

# Section 14: Mumps, Measles & Rubella

## I. MUMPS

**CAUSAL AGENT**

- An enveloped, **negative-strand RNA** virus (a paramyxovirus) of the genus Rubulavirus.

**COMMON CLINICAL FEATURES**

- Acute viral illness characterized by fever, headache, tenderness and swelling in one or both parotid salivary glands.
- Swelling commonly peaks between **1-3 days** following infection.
- **In 25%** of cases swelling occurs only on one side.
- Up to **75%** cases, mumps parotitis is bilateral.
- **30%** of cases in children are asymptomatic.

**COMPLICATIONS:** rare but can include:

- Aseptic meningitis,
- Orchitis (occurs in about **25%** of adolescent and adult males and is rare in prepubescent males),
- Oophoritis (occurs in **5%** of post pubertal females, mastitis may also occur.
- Less common complications include pancreatitis, myocarditis, arthritis, thyroiditis, deafness and spontaneous abortion.

**EPIDEMIOLOGY**

- In the UK infections with mumps peaks during the **winter and spring**.
- Prior to the introduction of vaccination in 1988 mumps caused epidemics every 3 years with the highest attack rates occurring among children aged 5-9 years.
- In 2004 90% of confirmed cases of mumps occurred among children and young adults over 15 years (an age-group who did not receive the MMR).

**RESERVOIR**

- Humans

**MODE OF TRANSMISSION**

- Person to person via airborne transmission or droplet spread.
- Also, direct contact with the saliva of an infected person.

**INCUBATION PERIOD**

- **16-18 days** - range 14-25 days.

**PERIOD OF COMMUNICABILITY**

- Identified in saliva - 7 days before to 9 days after the onset of parotid swelling.
- Maximum infectiousness occurs 2 days before to 4 days after the onset of illness.
- Subclinical infections can be communicable.

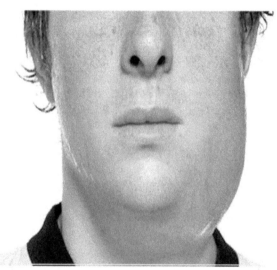

Fig. 4.2.14.1. Mumps

**IDENTIFICATION**

- Serology.
- The mumps virus can be isolated from saliva, blood, urine and CSF in acute phase.

**PREVENTION AND CONTROL**

- Routine MMR vaccination, 2 doses at 12-15 months and at 4 years of age.
- There is no upper age limit and where required, two doses can be given separated by at least a one month interval (HPA).
- Exclusion from school for 5 days from onset of parotid swelling and arrange for laboratory confirmation.
- There is no single antigen mumps vaccine licensed in the UK.
- Laboratory diagnosis by oral fluid testing is offered by the Health Protection Agency.

## II. MEASLES

## INFECTIOUS AGENT

- Measles virus is a member of the genus Morbillivirus of the family Paramyxoviridae (**RNA paramyxovirus**).

## COMMON CLINICAL FEATURES

- Prodromal illness with high fever, coryza, respiratory infection, conjunctivitis and **Koplik's spots** in the mouth.
- Characteristic rash (raised red blotches) appears on the 3-7th day, initially on the face and then becoming generalized lasting 4-7 days.

## COMPLICATIONS

- An estimated **20%** of measles cases experience one or more complications including:
  - o Otitis media,
  - o Pneumonia,
  - o Corneal scarring,
  - o Croup,
  - o Diarrhoea
  - o Encephalitis.
- Complications are more common in children under 5 years and in adults over 20 years.
- Case fatality rates range from **3-5%** increasing to **10-30%** among the immunocompromised, malnourished and children suffering from clinical or subclinical vitamin A deficiency.

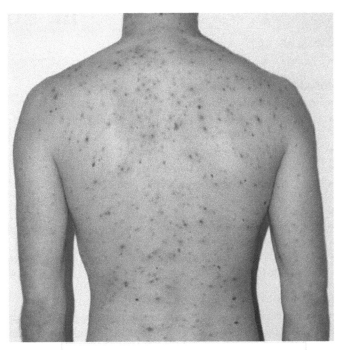

*Fig. 4.2.14.2. Measles*

- Measles infection among pregnant women can lead to a higher risk of spontaneous abortion, premature labour and low birth weight.

## EPIDEMIOLOGY

- Endemic worldwide;
- Measles is the leading cause of death among young children.
- Measles is the leading cause of blindness among children in Africa.
- Since the introduction of the MMR vaccine in 1998 and increases in coverage rates were achieved (over 90%) measles transmission has been significantly reduced.

## RESERVOIR

- Humans; no known animal reservoir.

## MODE OF TRANSMISSION

- Person to person via droplet infection or direct contact with nose and throat secretions of infected persons.
- Almost all non-immune children exposed to the measles virus will become infected.

## INCUBATION PERIOD

- From exposure to prodrome average **10-12 days**.
- From exposure to rash onset average **14 days** (range of 7-18 days).

## PERIOD OF COMMUNICABILITY

- From 1 day before the beginning of the prodromal period until 4 days after the appearance of rash.

## TREATMENT

- Treatment is supportive.
- Vitamin A for all children: Vitamin A is administered once a day for 2 days at the following doses:
  - o 50,000 IU for infants aged <6 months
  - o 100,000 IU for infants aged 6–11 months
  - o 200,000 IU for children aged ≥12 months

## PREVENTION AND CONTROL

- Routine MMR vaccination, 2 doses at 12-15 months and at 4 years of age.
- There is no upper age limit and where required, two doses can be given separated by at least a one month interval.

# III. RUBELLA

**CAUSAL AGENT**

- Rubella virus, a member of the togaviridae.

**COMMON CLINICAL FEATURES**

- A mild viral illness. Children may develop few or no symptoms.
- Infection with rubella among adults is characterized by mild fever, sore throat, conjunctivitis, headache, joint aches for 2-3 days followed by a maculopapular rash, which lasts about 3 days.
- Swollen lymph glands around the ears and back of head.
- **Up to 50%** of rubella infections are subclinical.
- The main differential diagnosis is parvovirus or measles.

**COMPLICATIONS**

- Risk of intrauterine transmission among susceptible pregnant women infected in the **first trimester is >90%,** declining to **50% in the second trimester** to no increased risk >20 weeks.
- Congenital rubella infection may lead to miscarriage, stillbirth and a range of severe birth defects known as **congenital rubella syndrome (CRS)**: low birth weight, cataracts, heart defects, hearing impairment, small head size and developmental delay.

**EPIDEMIOLOGY**

- In the UK infections with mumps peaks during the **winter and spring**.
- Prior to the introduction of immunization against rubella, epidemics occurred in 6-year cycles.

**MODE OF TRANSMISSION**

- Person to person via airborne transmission or droplet spread.
- Direct contact with nasopharyngeal secretions of an infected person.

**INCUBATION PERIOD**

- **14-17 days**, with a range of 14-21 days.

**PERIOD OF COMMUNICABILITY**

- From 1 week before the onset of rash to 1 week after the onset of rash.

**PREVENTION AND CONTROL**

- Routine MMR vaccination, 2 doses at 12-15 months & at 4 years of age.
- There is no upper age limit and where required, two doses can be given separated by at least a one-month interval.
- Rubella vaccine is also available as a single antigen vaccine. It is offered to previously unimmunised and seronegative post-partum women. Unless MMR is contraindicated, this may be used in place of rubella vaccine (HPA).
- Screen all women in early pregnancy and immunize post-partum if found to be susceptible.

# IV. PARAINFLUENZA VIRUSES

**CLINICAL MANIFESTATIONS**

- Parainfluenza viruses cause mild or severe upper and lower respiratory tract infections, particularly in children.

**CLASSIFICATION AND ANTIGENIC TYPES**

- Human parainfluenza viruses are divided into types 1, 2, 3, and 4.
- Type 4 consists of A and B subtypes.

**PATHOGENESIS**

- Transmission is by droplets or direct contact.
- The virus disseminates locally in the ciliated epithelial cells of the respiratory mucosa.

**HOST DEFENSES**

- Nonspecific defences, including interferon, are followed by the appearance of secretory and humoral antibodies and cell-mediated immune responses.

### EPIDEMIOLOGY

- Parainfluenza virus diseases occur worldwide; they are usually endemic but sometimes epidemic.
- Primary infections occur in young children; reinfection is common but results in milder disease.

### DIAGNOSIS

- Clinical symptoms are nonspecific.
- Laboratory diagnosis is made by detecting viral antigen, by isolating the virus, or by detecting a rise in antibody titer or elevated IgG- and IgA- (IgM-) antibodies in a single serum.

### CONTROL

- No vaccine is available.

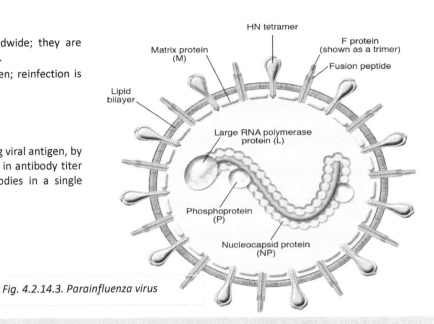

*Fig. 4.2.14.3. Parainfluenza virus*

# V. RESPIRATORY SYNCYTIAL VIRUS

### CLINICAL MANIFESTATIONS

- This virus causes upper and lower respiratory tract disease; the latter is most frequent in young children and is also significant in the elderly.

### CLASSIFICATION AND ANTIGENIC TYPES

- Respiratory syncytial viruses are divided into types A and B.

### PATHOGENESIS

- Transmission is by droplets or direct contact.
- The virus infects the ciliated epithelial cells of the respiratory mucosa and disseminates locally.
- Disease is caused partly by immunopathologic antibody-dependent cellular cytotoxicity.

### HOST DEFENSES

- Nonspecific immune defences, including interferon, are followed by the appearance of secretory and serum antibody and cell-mediated responses.
- Reinfection occurs, but the frequency and severity of disease decrease with age.

### EPIDEMIOLOGY

- This disease is found worldwide; in temperate climates, epidemics occur in **winter and early spring** and affect mainly infants and young children.

### DIAGNOSIS

- Clinical symptoms are nonspecific;
- Laboratory diagnosis is made by detecting viral antigen, by isolating the virus or by detecting RNA with polymerase chain reaction (PCR), or by detecting a rise in antibody titer or elevated IgM antibodies in a single serum.

### CONTROL

- There is no vaccine.
- Aerosolized ribavirin can be used for treatment if necessary.
- In hospital wards, infected patients may be isolated

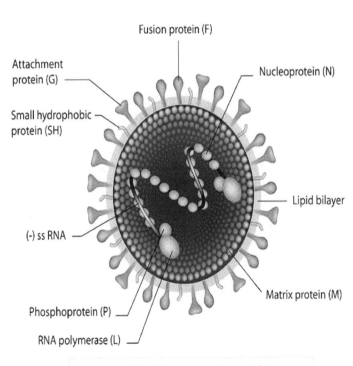

Respiratory Syncytial Virus

*Fig. 4.2.14.4. Respiratory Syncytial virus*

# SECTION 15: RESPIRATORY VIRUSES

## I. UPPER RESPIRATORY INFECTIONS

### COMMON COLD, SINUSITIS, PHARYNGITIS, EPIGLOTTITIS AND LARYNGOTRACHEITIS

**ETIOLOGY**
- Most URIs are viral in origin.
- Typical viral agents that cause URIs include the following: **CRAC**
  - Rhinoviruses: 50-75% of cases
  - Coronaviruses: 15% of cases
  - Adenoviruses: 5% of cases
  - Coxsackieviruses
- For the most part, similar agents cause URI in adults and children; however, Moraxella catarrhalis and bocavirus cause URIs more commonly in children than in adults.

**PATHOGENESIS**
- Organisms gain entry to the respiratory tract by inhalation of droplets and invade the mucosa.
- Epithelial destruction may ensue, along with redness, edema, hemorrhage and sometimes an exudate.

**CLINICAL MANIFESTATIONS**
- Initial symptoms of a cold are runny, stuffy nose and sneezing, usually without fever.
- Other upper respiratory infections may have fever.
- Children with epiglottitis may have difficulty in breathing, muffled speech, drooling and stridor.
- Children with serious laryngotracheitis (croup) may also have tachypnoea, stridor and cyanosis.

**MICROBIOLOGIC DIAGNOSIS**
- Common colds can usually be recognized clinically.
- Bacterial and viral cultures of throat swab specimens are used for pharyngitis, epiglottitis and laryngotracheitis.
- Blood cultures are also obtained in cases of epiglottitis.

**PREVENTION AND TREATMENT**
- Viral infections are treated symptomatically.
- Streptococcal pharyngitis and epiglottitis caused by H influenzae are treated with antibacterials.
- Haemophilus influenzae type b vaccine is commercially available and is now a basic component of childhood immunization program.

## 1. NASOPHARYNGITIS
- Of the more than 200 viruses known to cause the symptoms of the common cold, the principal ones are as follows:
  - **Rhinoviruses**: These cause approximately 30-50% of colds in adults; they grow optimally at temperatures near 32.8°C (91°F), which is the temperature inside the human nares.
  - **Coronaviruses**: While they are a significant cause of colds, exact case numbers are difficult to determine because, unlike rhinoviruses, coronaviruses are difficult to culture in the laboratory.
  - **Enteroviruses**, including coxsackieviruses, echoviruses, and others
- Other viruses that account for many URIs include the following:
  - Adenoviruses
  - Orthomyxoviruses (including influenza A and B viruses)
  - Paramyxoviruses (e.g., parainfluenza virus [PIV])
  - Respiratory Syncytial Virus (RSV)
  - Epstein-Barr Virus (EBV)
  - Human metapneumovirus (hMPV)
- Bocavirus: Commonly associated with nasopharyngeal symptoms in children·

## 2. PHARYNGITIS
- This is most often viral in origin.
- Recognition of group A streptococcal pharyngitis (Streptococcus pyogenes, the sole species) is vital because serious complications may follow untreated disease.
- Viral causes of pharyngitis include the following:
  - Adenovirus: May also cause laryngitis and conjunctivitis
  - Influenza viruses

- o   Coxsackievirus
- o   Herpes simplex virus (HSV)
- o   EBV (infectious mononucleosis)
- o   Cytomegalovirus (CMV)
- Bacterial causes of pharyngitis include the following:
  - o   Group A streptococci (approximately 5-15% of all cases of pharyngitis in adults; 20-30% in children)
  - o   Group C and G streptococci
  - o   Neisseria gonorrhoeae
  - o   Arcanobacterium (Corynebacterium) hemolyticum
  - o   Corynebacterium diphtheriae
  - o   Atypical bacteria (e.g., Mycoplasma pneumoniae and Chlamydia pneumoniae; absent lower respiratory tract disease, the clinical significance of these pathogens is uncertain)
  - o   Anaerobic bacteria

## 3. RHINOSINUSITIS

- Viral causes are similar to those of viral nasopharyngitis and include the following: Rhinovirus, Enterovirus, Coronavirus, Influenza A and B virus, PIV, RSV, and Adenovirus.
- Bacterial causes are similar to those seen in otitis media.
- Bacterial pathogens isolated from maxillary sinus aspirates of patients with acute bacterial rhinosinusitis include the following:
  - o   *Streptococcus pneumoniae*: 38% in adults, 21-33% in children
  - o   *Haemophilus influenzae*: 36% in adults, 31-32% in children
  - o   *Moraxella catarrhalis*: 16% in adults; 8-11% in children
  - o   *Staphylococcus aureus*: 13% in adults, 1% in children
- Other pathogens include group A streptococci and other streptococcal species.
- Uncommon causes include C pneumoniae, Neisseria species, anaerobes, and gram-negative rods.
- Nosocomial sinusitis often involves pathogens that colonize the upper respiratory tract and migrate into the sinuses. Prolonged endotracheal intubation places patients at increased risk for nosocomial sinusitis.
- *Methicillin-resistant* S aureus *(MRSA)* is less common than sensitive staphylococci.
- Gram-negative bacilli (e.g., Escherichia coli, Pseudomonas aeruginosa) are other causes.
- Aspergillus species are the leading causes of noninvasive fungal sinusitis. Although fungi are part of the normal flora of the upper airways, they may cause acute sinusitis in patients with immunocompromise or diabetes mellitus.

## 4. EPIGLOTTITIS

- This is a bacterial infection.
- In the vast majority of children, H influenzae type b (Hib) is isolated from blood or epiglottal cultures.
- Since the routine use of the Hib conjugate vaccine began, case rates in children younger than 5 years have declined by more than 95%.
- The prevalence of invasive Hib disease is approximately 1.3 cases per 100,000 children.
- Rates in adults have remained low and stable.
- Other bacteria, found more commonly in adults than in children, include group A streptococci (GAS), S pneumoniae, and M catarrhalis.
- In adults, cultures are most likely to be negative.

## 5. CROUP OR LARYNGOTRACHEOBRONCHITIS

- o   **Viral causes:**
  - It is typically caused by parainfluenza virus (PIV) type 1, 2, or 3.
    - o   PIVs account for up to 80% of croup cases.
    - o   PIV type 1 is the leading cause of croup in children.
  - Other viruses include influenza viruses and RSV.
  - Uncommon causes include hMPV (human metapneumovirus), adenovirus, rhinovirus, enterovirus (including coxsackievirus and enteric cytopathic human orphan [ECHO] viruses), and measles virus.
- o   **Bacterial causes:**
  - Approximately 95% of all cases of whooping cough are caused by the *gram-negative Bordetella pertussis*.
  - The remaining cases result from B parapertussis.
  - Other forms of laryngitis and laryngotracheitis are typically caused by viruses similar to those that cause nasopharyngitis, including rhinovirus, coronavirus, adenovirus, influenza virus, parainfluenza virus, and RSV.
  - Candida species may cause laryngitis in immunocompromised hosts.

- Bacterial laryngitis is far less common than viral laryngitis.
- Other Bacterial causes include the following:
  - Group A streptococci
  - Corynebacterium diphtheriae, an aerobic gram-positive rod that may infect only the larynx or may represent an extension of nasopharyngeal infection
  - Chlamydia pneumoniae, Mycoplasma pneumoniae
  - Moraxella catarrhalis, H influenzae, S aureus, M tuberculosis

| INCUBATION PERIODS | |
|---|---|
| Rhinoviruses and group A streptococci | **1-5 days** |
| Influenza and parainfluenza | **1-4 days** |
| Respiratory syncytial virus | **1 week** |
| Pertussis | **7-10 days** |
| Diphtheria | **1-10 days.** |
| Epstein-Barr virus (EBV) | **4-6 weeks.** |

# II. LOWER RESPIRATORY INFECTIONS

## BRONCHITIS, BRONCHIOLITIS AND PNEUMONIA

### ETIOLOGY

- Causative agents of lower respiratory infections are viral or bacterial.
- Viruses cause most cases of bronchitis and bronchiolitis.
- *In community-acquired pneumonias, the most common bacterial agent is Streptococcus pneumoniae.*
- Atypical pneumonias are cause by such agents as *Mycoplasma pneumoniae, Chlamydia spp, Legionella, Coxiella burnetti and viruses.*
- Nosocomial pneumonias and pneumonias in immunosuppressed patients have protean aetiology with *gram-negative organisms and staphylococci* as predominant organisms.

### PATHOGENESIS

- Organisms enter the distal airway by inhalation, aspiration or by hematogenous seeding.
- The pathogen multiplies in or on the epithelium, causing inflammation, increased mucus secretion, and impaired mucociliary function; other lung functions may also be affected.
- In severe bronchiolitis, inflammation and necrosis of the epithelium may block small airways leading to airway obstruction.

### CLINICAL MANIFESTATIONS

- Symptoms include cough, fever, chest pain, tachypnoea and sputum production. Patients with pneumonia may also exhibit non-respiratory symptoms such as confusion, headache, myalgia, abdominal pain, nausea, vomiting and diarrhoea.

### MICROBIOLOGIC DIAGNOSIS

- Sputum specimens are cultured for bacteria, fungi and viruses.
- Culture of nasal washings is usually sufficient in infants with bronchiolitis.
- Fluorescent staining technic can be used for legionellosis.
- Blood cultures and/or serologic methods are used for viruses, rickettsiae, fungi and many bacteria.
- Enzyme-linked immunoassay methods can be used for detections of microbial antigens as well as antibodies.
- Detection of nucleotide fragments specific for the microbial antigen in question by DNA probe or polymerase chain reaction.

### PREVENTION AND TREATMENT

- Symptomatic treatment is used for most viral infections.
- Bacterial pneumonias are treated with antibacterials.
- Vaccine

# Section 16: Gastrointestinal Viruses

## I. ROTAVIRUSES

**CAUSAL AGENT**
- Rotaviruses belong to the reoviridae family.
- There are 3 serogroups of which group A is the most common.

**COMMON CLINICAL FEATURES**
- Characterized by sudden onset of watery diarrhoea (occasionally with blood in the stool), vomiting, abdominal pain and mild fever.
- Occasionally associated with severe dehydration and death in young children.

**EPIDEMIOLOGY**
- Endemic Worldwide
- The most common cause of gastroenteritis in infants and young children in developed and developing countries.
- Most children are infected by rotavirus by age 3, with peak incidence of clinical disease in the 6-24-month age group.
- The WHO estimate that rotavirus accounts for almost **40% of all cases of severe diarrhoea worldwide** and approximately 600,000 deaths each year (mostly in developing countries among children <2 years).
- **Rotavirus is a major cause of nosocomial diarrhoea in newborns and infants.**
- In the UK it is estimated that approximately 18,000 children are hospitalised in England and Wales due to rotavirus-related illness.
- Outbreaks are common, especially in child day care setting such as nurseries and in hospitals.
- In temperate climates such as the UK, the incidence is higher during the **winter** months.

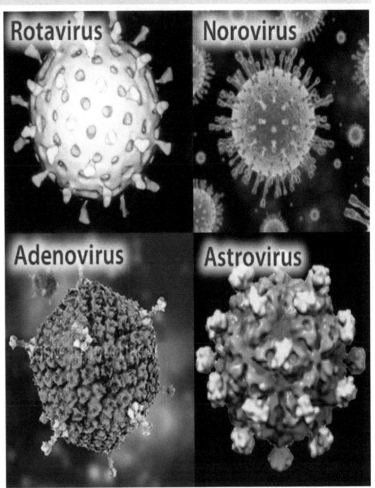

*Fig. 4.2.16.1. Gastrointestinal viruses*

**RESERVOIR**
- Gastrointestinal tract of humans.

**MODE OF TRANSMISSION**
- Person to person via the faecal-oral route.
- Ingestion of contaminated food or water.
- Although rotaviruses do not effectively multiply in the respiratory tract, they may be spread from respiratory secretions. (MRCEM Part A)
- Environmental contamination (contaminated surfaces).

**INCUBATION PERIOD**
- **1-3 days.**

**PERIOD OF COMMUNICABILITY**
- During acute stage and for a short period after afterwards (usually < 1 week in healthy children).

**PREVENTION AND CONTROL**
- Vaccine: 2 doses at 2 and 3 months old
- Exclude from nursery or school (or risk occupations) until 48 hours after the resolution of diarrhoea and vomiting.
- Follow correct food hygiene practices for food preparation and cooking in domestic and commercial kitchens.
- Good standard of infection control in hospitals and nursing homes.

# II. NOROVIRUSES

## INFECTIOUS AGENT
- Norovirus infection is caused by nonenveloped, **single-stranded RNA viruses** of the genus *norovirus*, which have also been referred to as "**Norwalk-like viruses**," **Norwalk viruses**, and small round-structured viruses.
- Norovirus gastroenteritis is sometimes incorrectly referred to as "stomach flu"; however, there is no biologic association with influenza or influenza viruses.

## TRANSMISSION
- Transmission occurs primarily through the **fecal-oral route**, either through direct person-to-person contact or indirectly via contaminated food or water.
- Norovirus is also spread through **aerosols** of vomitus and contaminated environmental surfaces and objects.

## EPIDEMIOLOGY
- Norovirus infections are common throughout the world, and globally most children will have experienced ≥1 infection by the age of 5 years.
- Norovirus infections can occur year-round, but in temperate climates, norovirus activity peaks during the **winter**.
- Norovirus is a cause of travelers' diarrhea; prevalence ranges from 3% to 17% of travelers returning with diarrhea.
- Risk for infection is present anywhere food is prepared in an unsanitary manner and may become contaminated, or where drinking water is inadequately treated.
- Of particular risk are "ready-to-eat" cold foods, such as sandwiches and salads. Raw shellfish, especially oysters, are also a frequent source of infection, because virus from contaminated water concentrates in the gut of these filter feeders. Contaminated ice has also been implicated in outbreaks.
- Large norovirus outbreaks are associated with settings where people live in close quarters and can easily infect each other, such as hotels, cruise ships, camps, dormitories, and hospitals.
- Viral contamination of inanimate objects or environmental surfaces (fomites) may persist during and after outbreaks and be a source of infection.

## CLINICAL PRESENTATION
- Acute onset of vomiting with **nonbloody** diarrhea.
- The incubation period is **12–48 hours**.
- Other symptoms include abdominal cramps, nausea, and sometimes a low-grade fever.
- Illness is generally self-limited, and full recovery can be expected in 1–3 days.
- In some cases, dehydration, especially in patients who are very young or elderly, may require medical attention.

## DIAGNOSIS
- Norovirus infection is generally diagnosed based on symptoms.
- The most common diagnostic test used RT-PCR, which rapidly and reliably detects the virus in stool specimens.

## TREATMENT
- Supportive care:
  - Oral or intravenous rehydration.
  - Antimotility agents should be avoided in children aged <3 years, but may be a useful adjunct to rehydration in older children and adults.
  - Antiemetic agents should generally be reserved for adults.
  - Antibiotics are not useful in treating patients with norovirus disease.

## PREVENTION
- No vaccine is currently available.
- Frequent and proper handwashing.
- Avoiding possibly contaminated food and water.
- In addition to handwashing, measures to prevent transmission of noroviruses between people traveling together include carefully cleaning up fecal material or vomit and disinfecting contaminated surfaces and toilet areas.
- Soiled articles of clothing should be washed at the maximum available cycle length and machine-dried at high heat.
- To help prevent the spread of noroviruses, ill people have been isolated on cruise ships and in institutional settings.

# SECTION 17: YEASTS AND FUNGI

# I. CANDIDA

- Candida is a genus of yeasts and is the most common cause of fungal infections worldwide.
- Many species are harmless commensals or endosymbionts of hosts including humans; however, when mucosal barriers are disrupted or the immune system is compromised they can invade and cause disease.
- Candida albicans is the most commonly isolated species, and can cause infections (candidiasis or thrush) in humans and other animals.
- In winemaking, some species of Candida can potentially spoil wines.
- Many species are found in gut flora, including C. albicans in mammalian hosts, whereas others live as endosymbionts in insect hosts.
- Antibiotics promote yeast infections, including gastrointestinal Candida overgrowth, and penetration of the GI mucosa.
- While women are more susceptible to genital yeast infections, men can also be infected.
- Certain factors, such as prolonged antibiotic use, increase the risk for both men and women.
- People with diabetes or impaired immune systems, such as those with HIV, are more susceptible to yeast infections.
- Candida antarctica is a source of industrially important lipases.

## STRUCTURE
- Grown in the laboratory, Candida appears as large, round, white or cream colonies with a yeasty odor on agar plates at room temperature.
- C albicans ferments glucose and maltose to acid and gas, sucrose to acid, and does not ferment lactose, which help to distinguish it from other Candida species.
- Many species of Candida use a non-standard genetic code in the translation of their nuclear genes into the aminoacid sequences of polypeptides.

## PATHOGENESIS
- Candidas are almost universal in low numbers on healthy adult skin and albicans is part of the normal flora of the mucous membranes of the respiratory, gastrointestinal, and female genital tracts.
- In the case of skin, the dryness of skin compared to other tissues prevents the growth of the fungus, but damaged skin or skin in intertriginous regions is more amenable to rapid growth of fungi.
- Overgrowth of several species including albicans can cause superficial infections such as oropharyngeal candidiasis (thrush) and vulvovaginal candidiasis (vaginal candidiasis). Oral candidiasis is common in elderly denture wearers.
- In otherwise healthy individuals, these infections can be cured with topical or systemic antifungal medications (commonly over-the-counter antifungal treatments like miconazole or clotrimazole).
- In debilitated or immunocompromised patients, or if introduced intravenously, candidiasis may become a systemic disease producing abscess, thrombophlebitis, endocarditis, or infections of the eyes or other organs.
- Typically, relatively severe neutropenia is a prerequisite for the Candida to pass through the defenses of the skin and cause disease in deeper tissues; in such cases, mechanical disruption of the infected skin sites is typically a factor in the fungal invasion of the deeper tissues.
- Colonization of the gastrointestinal tract by C. albicans after antibiotic therapy may not cause symptoms and may also result from taking antacids or antihyperacidity drugs.

## CLINICAL FEATURES OF NAPKIN DERMATITIS
- **Irritant napkin dermatitis**: well-demarcated variable erythema, oedema, dryness and scaling. Affected skin is in contact with the wet napkin and tends to spare the skin folds
- **Chafing:** erythema and erosions where the napkin rubs, usually on waistband or thighs
- *Candida albicans*: erythematous papules and plaques with small satellite spots or superficial pustules
- **Impetigo** (*Staphylococcus aureus* and/or *Streptococcus pyogenes*): irregular blisters and pustules
- **Infantile seborrhoeic dermatitis**: cradle cap and bilateral salmon pink patches, often desquamating, in skin folds
- **Atopic dermatitis**: bilateral scratched, dry plaques anywhere, but uncommon in nappy area; family history common.
- **Psoriasis:** persistent, well-circumscribed, symmetrical, shiny, red, scaly or macerated plaques; other sites may be involved; family history common.
- **Disseminated secondary eczema or autoeczematisation:** rash in distal sites associated with severe napkin rash.

# II. CRYPTOCOCCUS

## CRYPTOCOCCUS MENINGITIS

- Infection with the encapsulated yeast Cryptococcus neoformans can result in harmless colonization of the airways, but it can also lead to meningitis or disseminated disease, especially in persons with defective cell-mediated immunity.
- Cryptococcosis represents a major life-threatening fungal infection in patients with severe HIV infection and may also complicate organ transplantation, reticuloendothelial malignancy, corticosteroid treatment, or sarcoidosis.

### DIAGNOSIS

- The workup in patients with suspected cryptococcosis includes the following:
  - Cutaneous lesions: Biopsy with fungal stains and cultures
  - Blood: Fungal culture, cryptococcal serology, and cryptococcal antigen testing
  - Cerebrospinal fluid: India ink smear, fungal culture, and cryptococcal antigen testing
  - Urine and sputum cultures, even if renal or pulmonary disease is not clinically evident
  - In AIDS patients with cryptococcal pneumonia, culture of bronchoalveolar lavage washings
  - With possible CNS cryptococcosis, especially in patients who present with focal neurologic deficits or a history compatible with slowly progressive meningitis, consider obtaining a computed tomography or magnetic resonance imaging scan of the brain prior to performing a lumbar puncture. With pulmonary cryptococcosis, radiographic findings in patients who are asymptomatic and immunocompetent may include the following:
    - Patchy pneumonitis
    - Granulomas ranging from 2-7 cm
    - Miliary disease similar to that in tuberculosis

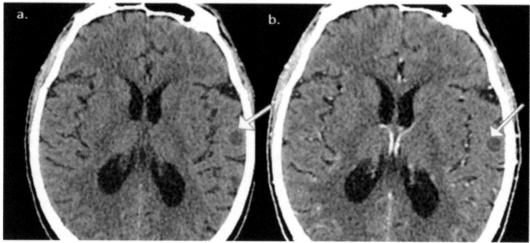

Fig. 4.2. 17.1.
A-66-year-old male patient diagnosed with cryptococcal meningitis and cryptococcoma in the left fronto-parietal region (arrow). A. CT axial cut without contrast shows hypodense lesion. B- In contrast-enhanced axial CT scans, the image does not exhibit contrast enhancement(arrow).

### MANAGEMENT

- Pulmonary cryptococcosis resolves without specific therapy in most immunocompetent patients.
- Antifungal therapy is necessary for the following:
  - Pulmonary cryptococcosis in immunosuppressed hosts.
  - CNS cryptococcosis
  - Disseminated nonpulmonary non-CNS cryptococcosis
- *Antifungal therapy requires the following:*
  - Amphotericin B with or without Flucytosine.
  - Flucytosine speeds clearance of viable yeast from CSF but is potentially toxic, especially in patients with renal dysfunction
  - After 2 weeks, fluconazole (400 mg/day) for a minimum of 8-10 weeks
- Monitor CSF pressure during the initial phase of therapy. If the opening pressure exceeds 250 mm $H_2O$, remove CSF to reduce the closing pressure to below 200 mm $H_2O$ or at least 50% of the elevated opening pressure.
- Consider weekly CSF examination until culture conversion is documented and cultures remain negative for 4 weeks.
- CSF protein abnormalities may persist for years despite successful therapy; thus, an elevated CSF protein as the only residual abnormality should not dictate prolonging therapy
- *Pulmonary cryptococcosis can be treated with observation only, if the following criteria are met:*
  - CSF chemistry parameters are normal
  - CSF culture, India ink preparation, and serology results are negative.
  - Urine culture results are negative.
  - The pulmonary lesion is small and stable or shrinking.
  - The patient has no predisposing conditions for disseminated disease.

# Section 18: Worms

## I. ASCARIS LUMBRICOIDES

**CLINICAL MANIFESTATIONS**
- Symptoms correlate with worm load: light loads are asymptomatic; heavier loads cause abdominal symptoms, diarrhea, and sometimes malnutrition.
- A bolus of worms may obstruct the intestine.
- Migrating larvae can cause pneumonitis and eosinophilia.

**STRUCTURE**
- Ascaris lumbricoides is the largest intestinal nematode of humans.
- Females are up to 30 cm long; males are smaller.
- Three types of eggs may appear in feces: fertilized, unfertilized, and decorticated.

**MULTIPLICATION AND LIFE CYCLE**
- Adults in the small intestine produce eggs that pass in feces, embryonate in soil, are ingested, and hatch.
- The larvae migrate from the intestine to the lung and back to the intestine, where they mature.

**PATHOGENESIS**
- Migrating larvae cause eosinophilia and sometimes allergic reactions.
- Erratic adult worms may invade other organs.
- Heavy infections can impair nutrition.

**HOST DEFENSES**
- Resistance increases with age; the mechanism is not clear.

**EPIDEMIOLOGY**
- Egg viability is supported by warm, moist soil.
- Transmission is favored by unsanitary disposal of feces. Prevalence is highest in children.

**DIAGNOSIS**
- Diagnosis is made most often by identifying eggs in stool; occasionally, erratic adults emerge from body orifices.

**CONTROL**
- **Anthelminthic** medications, such as **Albendazole** and **Mebendazole**, are the drugs of choice for treatment of Ascaris infections.
- Infections are generally treated for 1-3 days.

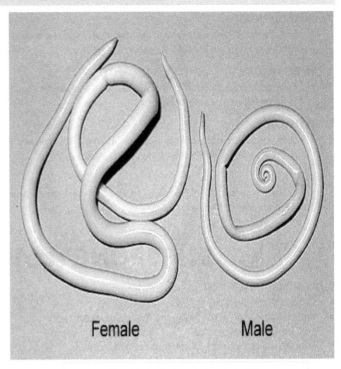

Female          Male

*Fig. 4.2.18.1. Ascaris lumbricoides*

## II. HOOKWORMS

**CLINICAL MANIFESTATIONS**
- Pneumonitis, cough, dyspnea and hemoptysis may mark the migration of larvae through the lungs.

**STRUCTURE**
- Two species of hookworms infect humans: Ancylostoma duodenale and Necator americanus.
- They are distinguished by the morphology of the mouth parts and male bursa.
- Females are larger. Eggs are oval, thin-shelled, and transparent. Eggs hatch to release rhabditiform larvae, which mature into filariform (infective stage) larvae.

**MULTIPLICATION AND LIFE CYCLE**
- Adults attach to the mucosa of the small intestine.
- Eggs passed in feces embryonate and hatch in soil; mature larvae penetrate the skin and migrate first to the lungs, and then to the intestine, where they mature into the adult stage.

### PATHOGENESIS

- Larvae entering skin often cause an erythematous reaction. Larvae in the lung may cause small haemorrhages, eosinophilic infiltration, and pneumonitis.
- Blood loss from sites of intestinal attachment may cause iron-deficiency anaemia.

### HOST DEFENSES

- Spontaneous self-cure may represent a hypersensitivity reaction. Infection induces high levels of IgE.

### EPIDEMIOLOGY

- Transmission is favored by poor sanitation and warm moist soil. Prevalence rises with age.

### DIAGNOSIS

- Diagnosis is by detection of eggs and (sometimes) larvae in stool. Low levels of hemoglobin are suggestive.

### CONTROL

- Control is by sanitary disposal of feces and by education and **Albendazole** or **Mebendazole.**

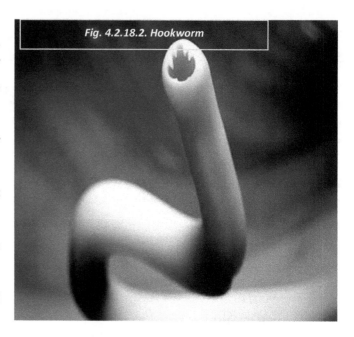

*Fig. 4.2.18.2. Hookworm*

# III. STRONGYLOIDES STERCORALIS

### CLINICAL MANIFESTATIONS

- Ground itch may occur where larvae penetrate the skin.
- Pneumonitis, epigastric pain, mucous diarrhoea, and eosinophilia may occur. In immunocompromised individuals, worms may disseminate to other organs.

### STRUCTURE

- Males are free-living; females may be free-living or parasitic.
- Eggs develop into rhabditiform and then filariform (infectious) larvae.

### MULTIPLICATION AND LIFE CYCLE

- Parasitic females parthenogenetically produce embryonated eggs, which hatch in the intestine.
- Rhabitiform larvae pass in the feces, mature to the infective filariform stage in soil, penetrate the skin, and migrate to the lungs and other organs, then the intestine.
- Autoinfection also occurs.
- Free-living worms reproduce sexually in soil.

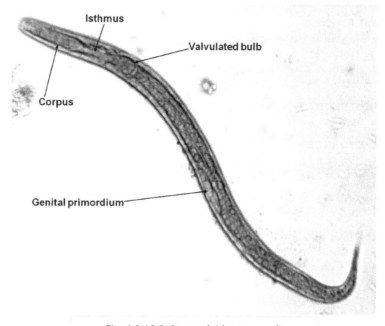

*Fig. 4.2.18.3. Strongyloides stercoralis*

### PATHOGENESIS

- Worms cause inflammation and ulceration of the intestines.
- Migrating larvae cause cutaneous pruritus and pneumonitis.
- Hyperinfection causes sloughing of mucosa, and disseminated infection occasionally leads to pulmonary hemorrhage, pneumonia, or meningitis and death.

### HOST DEFENSES

- Immunity is not well understood. Infection induces elevated IgE and eosinophilia.
- Impairment of cell-mediated immunity favours disseminated disease and autoinfection.

### EPIDEMIOLOGY

- Prevalence is usually low; the infection is more common in tropical countries with poor sanitation, especially Southeast Asia and parts of Africa.
- Dogs occasionally serve as a reservoir.

## DIAGNOSIS

- Epigastric pain, eosinophilia, and mucous diarrhea are suggestive; diagnosis is confirmed by detecting rhabditiform larvae in feces, duodenal aspirates, or sputum.
- Fecal cultures and serology may be helpful.

## CONTROL

- First line therapy: **Ivermectin**, in a single dose, 200 µg/kg orally for 1-2 days.
- **Albendazole** 400 mg orally two times a day for 7 days.
- **Ivermectin** 200 µg/kg per day orally until stool and/or sputum exams are negative for 2 weeks.
- More on: Handwashing.

# IV. TRICHURIS TRICHIURA

## CLINICAL MANIFESTATIONS

- Diarrhoea, anemia, weight loss, abdominal pain, nausea, vomiting, eosinophilia, tenesmus, rectal prolapse, stunted growth and finger clubbing may occur.

## STRUCTURE

- Adults are whip-shaped, slender anteriorly and broader posteriorly.
- Males are shorter than females and have a coiled posterior. The unembryonated eggs are barrel-shaped with bipolar plugs.

## MULTIPLICATION AND LIFE CYCLE

- Adults in the large intestine lay eggs which pass in feces and embryonate in soil. Eggs that are ingested hatch and larvae mature to adults in the gut.

## PATHOGENESIS

- Adults prefer the cecum but will also colonize the large intestine.
- Worms cause mucosal inflammation, eosinophilic infiltration, and minor blood loss; heavy infections may lead to anemia and nutrititional deficiency.

## HOST DEFENSES

- Defenses are little understood; resistance does not increase with age.

## EPIDEMIOLOGY

- Transmission is favored by poor sanitation and warm soil.

## DIAGNOSIS

- Diagnosis is by detection of eggs in feces.

## CONTROL

- Single doses of **Mebendazole** in the treatment of very light to heavy Trichuris infections all reduced egg output by over 80%.

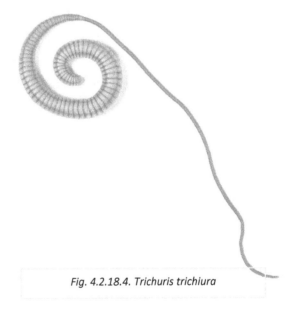

Fig. 4.2.18.4. Trichuris trichiura

# V. ENTEROBIUS VERMICULARIS

## CLINICAL MANIFESTATIONS

- Enterobiasis is most common in children, who usually manifest pruritus ani and sometimes insomnia, abdominal pain, anorexia, and pallor. Genitourinary infection may occur in females.

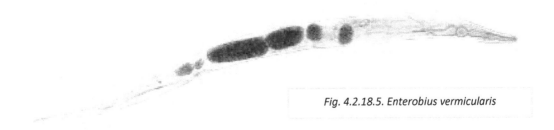

Fig. 4.2.18.5. Enterobius vermicularis

## STRUCTURE
- Worms are white and spindle-shaped with a large, bulbar esophagus.
- Males are smaller and have a curved posterior.
- Eggs are ovoid, thin-shelled, and flat on one side.

## MULTIPLICATION AND LIFE CYCLE
- Females usually migrate out the anus at night and deposit eggs on the perianal skin.
- The eggs embryonate quickly and, if ingested, hatch and mature in the intestines.

## PATHOGENESIS
- Intestinal lesions are rare; extraintestinal infection may lead to complications.

## HOST DEFENSES
- The defenses are little known. Most infections occur in children.

## EPIDEMIOLOGY
- Enterobius vermicularis is the most common helminth in the United States. Household and institutional epidemics occur, usually in children.
- Transmission is usually by hand to mouth transfer of infective eggs.

## DIAGNOSIS
- Eggs are rare in feces but are readily collected by Scotch-tape perianal swabs.

## CONTROL
- Control is by anthelmintic treatment and by improved personal hygiene, including washing the perianal region and changing night clothes.
- The medications used for the **treatment** of pinworm are either **Mebendazole, Pyrantel Pamoate**, or **Albendazole**

# VI. THE HELMINTHS

- The helminths are worm-like parasites.
- The clinically relevant groups are separated according to their general external shape and the host organ they inhabit.
- There are both hermaphroditic and bisexual species.
- The definitive classification is based on the external and internal morphology of egg, larval, and adult stages.

## 1.  FLUKES (TREMATODES)
- Adult flukes are leaf-shaped flatworms.
- Prominent oral and ventral suckers help maintain position in situ.
- Flukes are hermaphroditic except for blood flukes, which are bisexual.
- The life-cycle includes a snail intermediate host.

## 2. TAPEWORMS (CESTODES)
- Adult tapeworms are elongated, segmented, hermaphroditic flatworms that inhabit the intestinal lumen.
- Larval forms, which are cystic or solid, inhabit extraintestinal tissues.

## 3. ROUNDWORMS (NEMATODES)
- Adult and larval roundworms are bisexual, cylindrical worms.
- They inhabit intestinal and extraintestinal sites.

### Platyhelminthes (flatworms)

**Turbellaria (free-living)**

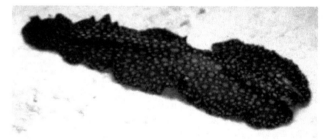

**Cestoda (tapeworms, parasites)**

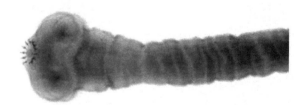

**Trematoda (flukes, parasites)**

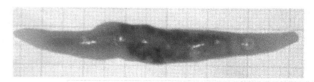

*Fig. 4.2.18.6. The Helminths*

# VII. ONCHOCERCIASIS (RIVER BLINDNESS)

### INFECTIOUS AGENT
- **Onchocerca volvulus**, *a filarial nematode.*

### TRANSMISSION
- Through **female blackflies** (genus *Simulium*), which typically bite during the day and breed near rapidly flowing rivers and streams.

### EPIDEMIOLOGY
- Endemic in much of sub-Saharan Africa.
- Small endemic foci are also present in the Arabian Peninsula (Yemen) and in the Americas (Brazil and Venezuela).

### CLINICAL PRESENTATION
- Highly pruritic, papular dermatitis; subcutaneous nodules; lymphadenitis; and ocular lesions, which can progress to visual loss and blindness.
- Symptoms begin after patent infections are established, which may take **18 months.**
- Nodules are more common in endemic populations.

### DIAGNOSIS
- Presence of microfilariae in superficial skin shavings or punch biopsy, adult worms in histologic sections of excised nodules, or characteristic eye lesions.
- Serologic testing is most useful for detecting infection when microfilariae are not identifiable.

### TREATMENT
- **Ivermectin** is the drug of choice.
- Repeated annual or semiannual doses may be required, as the drug kills the microfilariae but not the adult worms.
- Some experts recommend treating patients with 1 dose of ivermectin followed by 6 weeks of doxycycline to kill **WOLBACHIA**, an endosymbiotic rickettsialike bacterium that appears to be required for the survival of the **O. VOLVULUS** macrofilariae and for embryogenesis.
- **Diethylcarbamazine** is contraindicated in onchocerciasis, because it has been associated with severe and fatal posttreatment reactions.

### PREVENTION
- Avoid blackfly habitats (free-flowing rivers and streams) and use protection measures against biting insects.

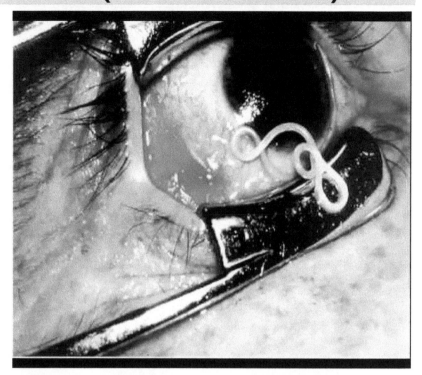

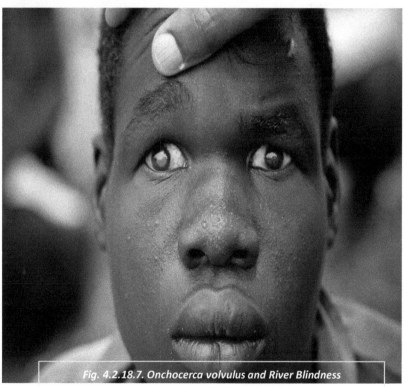

*Fig. 4.2.18.7. Onchocerca volvulus and River Blindness*

# SECTION 19: MALARIA

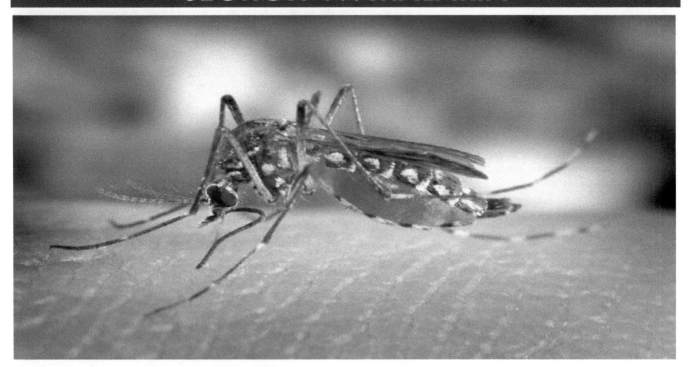

## INFECTIOUS AGENT

- Malaria is caused by protozoan parasites of the genus *plasmodium*: *p. falciparum, p. Vivax, p. Ovale & p. Malariae.*
- In addition, **p. Knowlesi**, a parasite of old world (eastern hemisphere) monkeys, has been documented as a cause of human infections and some deaths in Southeast Asia.

## THE LIFE CYCLE OF PLASMODIUM

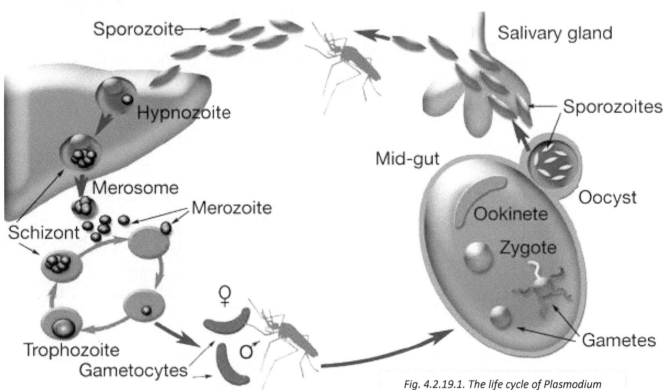

*Fig. 4.2.19.1. The life cycle of Plasmodium*

- Malaria is transmitted by the bite of a mosquito in which hundreds of **sporozoites** are released into the vertebrate host's bloodstream.

- The parasites eventually migrate to the liver, passing through some cell types such as Kupfer cells, and form parasitophorous vacuoles in hepatocytes.
- At this stage they can either remain dormant as a **hypnozoite form** (*P. vivax* or *P. ovale*), or initiate development that results in the production of thousands of **merozoites.**
- The parasites then induce detachment of the infected hepatocyte, allowing it to migrate to the liver sinusoid where budding of parasite-filled vesicles called **merosomes** occurs.
- The new merozoites quickly invade erythrocytes where they replicate, sometimes synchronously, in a cycle that may correspond to the cycle of fever and chills in malaria.
- In response to a cue that is not well understood, some parasites differentiate into **male and female gametocytes**, which are the forms taken up by the mosquito and which can live quiescently in the bloodstream for weeks.
- Once they enter the mosquito via a blood meal they rapidly undergo transition into activated **male and female gametes**.
- The motile and short-lived diploid parasite form, **the ookinete**, migrates out of the blood meal, across the peritrophic matrix to the mid-gut wall where an **oocyst** is formed.
- After a meiotic reduction in chromosome number **sporozoites** are formed within the oocyst.
- Eventually the oocyst ruptures and the sporozoites migrate to the salivary gland where they await transfer to the vertebrate host.

## TRANSMISSION
- All species are transmitted by the bite of an infective **female *anopheles* mosquito**.
- Injection or transfusion of contaminated blood may also transmit malaria. Congenital transmission is rare.
- The mosquitoes that can transmit malaria are found not only in malaria endemic areas, but are also found in areas where malaria has been eliminated.
- The latter areas are thus constantly at risk of re-introduction of the disease.

## EPIDEMIOLOGY
- Despite the apparent progress in reducing the global prevalence of malaria, many areas remain malaria endemic.
- Malaria transmission occurs in large areas of Africa, Latin America, parts of the Caribbean, Asia (including south Asia, Southeast Asia, and the Middle East), Eastern Europe, and the south pacific.

| INCUBATION PERIOD | | |
| --- | --- | --- |
| | **Prepatent period** (Time between infective bite and detection of the parasites in a blood smear) | **Incubation period** (Time between infective bite and the onset of clinical symptoms) |
| *P. falciparum* | 6-12 days | 9-14 days |
| *P. vivax* | 8-12 days | 12-18 days |
| *P. ovale* | 8-12 days | 12-18 days |
| *P. malariae* | 12-16 days | 18-40 days |

- *Some strains of P. vivax, may have an incubation period of 8-10 months or longer.*
- *Transfusion associated malaria (rare) has a shorter incubation period.*
- *G6PD deficiency confers partial protection against malaria*

## PERIOD OF COMMUNICABILITY
- Humans may infect mosquitoes as long as infective gametocytes are present in the blood.
- Anopheles mosquitoes remain infective for life.

## CLINICAL PRESENTATION
- Malaria typically produces a string of recurrent attacks, each of which has 3 stages - chills, followed by fever and then sweating.
- ***Plasmodium Falciparum*** is responsible for most malaria deaths worldwide. It is most prevalent in sub-Saharan Africa and in certain areas of South East Asia and the Western Pacific.
- *P. falciparum* may present with a varied clinical picture, including one or more of the following, fever, chills, sweats, anorexia, nausea, lassitude, headache, muscle and joint pain, cough and diarrhoea. If treated inadequately the disease may progress to severe malaria, of which the most important manifestations are; acute encephalopathy (cerebral malaria), severe anemia, icterus, renal failure, hypoglycaemia and respiratory distress.
- ***Plasmodium vivax,*** is the most geographically widespread of the species. Once found in temperate climates, *P. vivax* is now found mostly in the tropics, especially throughout Asia.
- *P. vivax* produces less severe symptoms including, a slowly rising fever of several days duration followed by a shaking chill and rapidly rising temperature, commonly accompanied by headache, nausea and profuse sweating.
- Following a fever free period this cycle of symptoms may recur daily, every other day or every third day. An untreated primary attack may last from a week to a month. Relapses can occur at irregular intervals for up to 5 years.

- *Plasmodium malariae,* infections produce typical malaria symptoms and can persist in the blood for very long periods (possibly for life) without producing symptoms.
- **Plasmodium ovale**, is less common and generally occurs in West Africa. It can cause relapses.
- **Pregnant women** are particularly vulnerable to malaria as pregnancy reduces a woman's immunity to malaria, making her more susceptible to malaria infection and increasing the risk of illness, severe anaemia and death.
- For the unborn child, maternal malaria increases the risk of spontaneous abortion, stillbirth, premature delivery and low birth weight; a leading cause of child mortality.
- Persons who are partially immune or who have been taking prophylactic drugs may show an atypical clinical picture and a prolonged incubation period.

### DIAGNOSIS

- *Smear microscopy* remains the gold standard for malaria diagnosis.
- Malaria parasites can be identified by examining under the microscope a drop of the patient's blood, spread out as a "blood smear" on a microscope slide.
- Prior to examination, the specimen is stained (most often with the **Giemsa stain**) to give the parasites a distinctive appearance.
- This technique remains the gold standard for laboratory confirmation of malaria.
- However, it depends on the quality of the reagents, of the microscope, and on the experience of the laboratorian.
- PCR tests are also available for detecting malaria parasites.

### TREATMENT

- Malaria can be treated effectively early in the course of the disease, but delay of therapy can have serious or even fatal consequences.
- Travelers who have symptoms of malaria should be advised to seek medical evaluation **as soon as possible**.

### PREVENTION

- Malaria prevention consists of a combination of mosquito avoidance measures and chemoprophylaxis.
- As outlined by Bradley et al. the A, B, C, D of malaria prevention, is essential to prevent the risk of malaria infection among UK travellers.

| Awareness | Know about the risk of malaria infection |
|---|---|
| Bites | Prevent or avoid |
| Compliance | With appropriate malaria chemoprophylaxis |
| Diagnose | Breakthrough malaria swiftly and obtain treatment promptly |

- Although efficacious, the recommended interventions are not 100% effective.
- **Mosquito avoidance measures:**
  - Using mosquito bed nets (preferably insecticide-treated nets).
  - Using an effective insecticide spray in living and sleeping areas during evening and nighttime hours.
  - Wearing clothes that cover most of the body.
- **Chemoprophylaxis:**
  - All recommended primary chemoprophylaxis regimens involve taking a medicine before, during, and after travel to an area with malaria.
  - Beginning the drug before travel allows the antimalarial agent to be in the blood before the traveler is exposed to malaria parasites.
  - In addition to primary prophylaxis, presumptive antirelapse therapy (also known as terminal prophylaxis) uses a medication toward the end of the exposure period (or immediately thereafter) to prevent relapses or delayed-onset clinical presentations of malaria caused by **hypnozoites** (dormant liver stages) of *p. Vivax or p. Ovale.*

## COMPLICATIONS OF FALCIPARUM

- Metabolic acidosis
- Hypoglycaemia
- Peripheral circulatory failure
- Cerebral malaria
- Respiratory failure/ ARDS
- Hepatitis
- DIC
- **Blackwater Fever**: acute intravascular hemolysis (G6PD, Quinine, High parasitemia, immune hemolysis)
- **Renal failure**: results from deposition of haemoglobin in renal tubules >>> decreased renal blood flow >>>acute tubular necrosis >>>ARF
  - Renal failure requires either peritoneal dialysis or hemodialysis

# INCUBATION PERIOD &
# LIST OF NOTIFIABLE DISEASES IN THE UK

| GRAM POSITIVE BACTERIA | |
|---|---|
| MRSA | 4-10d |
| Tetanus | 3-21d |
| Diphtheria | 2-5d |

| GRAM NEGATIVE BACTERIA | |
|---|---|
| N meningitidis | 2-10d |
| Bordetella | 9-10d |
| E coli | 3-4d |
| Shigella | 1-3d |
| Salmonella non-typhi | 6-72hrs |
| Salmonella typhi | 6-30d |
| Salmonella Paratyphi | 1-10d |
| Campylobacter | 2-5d |
| Legionella | 2-14d |
| Pontiac fever | 72hrs |
| Chlamydia | 7-14d |

| VIRUS | |
|---|---|
| Herpes simplex | 1-6d |
| Varicella zoster (chickenpox) | 13-17d |
| Smallpox | 12-14d |
| Measles | 9-12d |
| Mumps | 16-20d |
| Rubella | 14-17d |
| Enterovirus disease | 6-12d |
| Brucellosis | 2–4 weeks |
| Hep. A | 15-50d |
| Hep. E | 14-60d |
| Mononucleosis | 30-50d |
| Hep. B & C | 50-150d |
| Rabies | 30-100d |
| Papilloma (warts) | 50-150d |
| Aids | 1-10 years |

| PROTOZOA | |
|---|---|
| Plasmodium falciparum | 7-14d |
| Plasmodium ovale & vivax | 12-18d |
| Plasmodium malariae | 18-40d |

Diseases notifiable to local authority proper officers under the Health Protection (Notification) Regulations 2010:

- Acute encephalitis
- Acute infectious hepatitis
- Acute meningitis
- Acute poliomyelitis
- Anthrax
- Botulism
- Brucellosis
- Cholera
- Diphtheria
- Enteric fever (typhoid or paratyphoid fever)
- Food poisoning
- Haemolytic uraemic syndrome (HUS)
- Infectious bloody diarrhoea
- Invasive group A streptococcal disease
- Legionnaires' disease
- Leprosy
- Malaria
- Measles
- Meningococcal septicaemia
- Mumps
- Plague
- Rabies
- Rubella
- Severe Acute Respiratory Syndrome (SARS)
- Scarlet fever
- Smallpox
- Tetanus
- Tuberculosis
- Typhus
- Viral haemorrhagic fever (VHF)
- Whooping cough
- Yellow fever

Source: https://www.gov.uk/guidance/notifiable-diseases-and-causative-organisms-how-to-report

# Past Asked Questions

**The following are true regarding hospital acquired infections**

| | |
|---|---|
| Pseudomonas persists on hospital surfaces due to its ability to produce resistant spores    (they form Biofilm) | F |
| Urinary catheters are the most common cause of hospital bacteraemia | F |
| Alcohol gels are more effective than hand washing in preventing norovirus transmission | F |
| C. difficile is an opportunistic pathogen | T |

**In patients with a diagnosis of falciparum malaria**

| | |
|---|---|
| Schizogeny describes the dormant phase of the Tparasite life cycle | F |
| High parasitaemias (>2%) are only seen with falciparum malaria | T |
| Life threatening complications arise from plasmodium toxin release | F |
| Children below the age of 5yrs are at high risk or cerebral oedema and severe anaemia | T |

**Regarding mumps:**

| | |
|---|---|
| It is transmitted by respiratory droplets | T |
| Mumps parotitis is usually unilateral (75% bilateral) | F |
| Aseptic meningitis is the commonest extra salivary gland complication | T |
| Infertility is a common sequelae of mumps orchitis | F |

**Which statement regarding Infective endocarditis (IE) are true?**

| | |
|---|---|
| Fever is a major diagnostic criterion | F |
| The mitral valve is the most commonly affected valve | T |
| Strep. viridans is the most common cause of endocarditis affecting damaged heart valves | T |
| The bacteraemia of IE is intermittent and blood cultures have a higher yield when taken while the patent is febrile | F |

**Regarding osteomyelitis:**

| | |
|---|---|
| In otherwise healthy patients the most common causative organism is Staphylococcus epidermidis | F |
| Sickle cell disease predisposes to Salmonella osteomyelitis | T |
| In children the metaphysis of the distal femur and proximal tibia are the most common sites affected | T |
| An involucrum is a feature of chronic osteomyelitis | T |

**Regarding Tetanus**

| | |
|---|---|
| A complete course of tetanus vaccination consists of five doses | T |
| The second booster dose should be given before the age of 16 | T |
| The tetanus vaccine consists of live attenuated tetanus bacteria | F |
| Persons who have not completed a course of tetanus vaccination should be offered human anti-tetanus immunoglobulin if they suffered any kind of wound | F |

**Regarding Neisseria meningitides**

| | |
|---|---|
| It is a gram negative diplococcus bacterium | T |
| It is carried in the axilla and groin of asymptomatic individuals | F |
| It causes disease through release of a potent exotoxin | F |
| It may be seen on gram stain of petechial biopsies | T |

**Regarding meningococcal meningitis:**

| | |
|---|---|
| Neisseria meningitidis is a gram positive organism | F |
| Meningococcus is the most common organism causing bacterial meningitis in neonates | F |
| Meningococcal meningitis is rarely accompanied by systemic meningococcal sepsis | F |
| Vaccination against meningitis strains A, B, C, W and Y are now in clinical use in the UK. | T |

**Regarding Campylobacter jejuni**

| | |
|---|---|
| Campylobacter jejuni is a flagellated gram-positive bacterium | F |
| It is the most common reported bacterial cause of infectious gastroenteritis in the UK | T |
| Campylobacter enteritis is short lived, almost always lasting less than 48hrs | F |
| It can be transmitted via unpasteurised milk | T |

**Which statements regarding Chlamydia are true?**

| | |
|---|---|
| It is an obligate intracellular organism | T |
| Chlamydia induced genital infection is the most common STD throughout the world | T |
| Co-infection with Chlamydia trachomatis and Neisseria gonorrhoeae is common | T |
| Infection is frequently asymptomatic | T |

**Regarding hepatitis C virus which infects around 0.5% of the UK population:**

| | |
|---|---|
| Over 80% of cases of Hepatitis C infection result in chronic liver disease | F |
| Incubation period is typically 2-3 weeks | F |
| Most cases in the UK are acquired through intravenous drug use | T |
| The risk of acquiring Hep C in a needlestick from a Hep C positive donor is 0.3% | F |

# Part Five:
# Pathology
# &
# Haematology

Compiled and Edited by:
**Dr Moussa Issa**
MBChB MRCEM
Senior ED Registrar

# SECTION 1: INFLAMMATORY RESPONSE

## 1. THE COMPLEMENT SYSTEM

- The complement system is a set of over 20 different protein molecules always found in the blood.
- There are no cells in the system.
- With an infection, this system of molecules is activated, leading to a sequence of events on the surface of the pathogen that helps destroy the pathogen and eliminate the infection.

## A. ACTIVATION CASCADE

- The complement system can be activated in two main ways:
  - **Alternative pathway**: *First, the activation is part of the innate (natural) immune response.*
  - *It does not rely on pathogen-binding antibodies:*
    - Neither antibodies nor T cell receptors are involved.
    - For example, certain polysaccharides found on the surface of bacteria can activate the system.
    - This can occur immediately and does not require prior exposure to the molecules.
  - **Classic pathway**: *the second and most potent means occurs in an adaptive immune response:*
    - When antibodies (IgG or IgM) binds to antigen at the surface of a cell. It is triggered by activation of the C1-complex.
    - This exposes the Fc region of the antibody in a way that allows the first complement protein (C1) to bind.

## B. CASCADE PATHWAY

- In either case, a cascade of events follows, in which each step leads to the next.
- At the center of the cascade are steps in which the proteolysis of a complement protein leads to a smaller protein and a peptide.
- The smaller protein remains bound to the complex at the surface of the microorganism, while the peptide diffuses away.
- Complement C3 is cleaved into C3b andC3a.
- C3b remains bound to the complex at the surface of the microorganism.
- This not only activates the next step, but also C3b is a good opsonin.
- The small peptide, C3a diffuses away and acts as a chemotactic factor and an inflammatory paracrine.
- Next, complement protein C5 is cleaved into C5b and C5a. The C5b remains bound to complex on the surface of the cell while the C5a diffuses away and acts much like C3a.
- Then the complement proteins C6, C7, and C8 bind successively to the growing complex.
- Finally, a number of C9 complement proteins bind to the complex.
- These C9 proteins are elongated molecules that form a circle with a large hole in the middle.
- This structure, which is called a **Membrane Attack Complex** (MAC), pierces the membrane of the cell.
- This initiates a sequence of event leading to lysis (of a microbe) or apoptosis (of a cell of the body in pathologies and tissue transplants).
- Thus, the complement system triggers a constellation of effects that helps deal with an infection:
  - *Opsonization: pathogen is marked for ingestion and eliminated by a phagocyte*
  - *Chemotaxis*
  - *Inflammation*
  - *lysis, apoptosis*

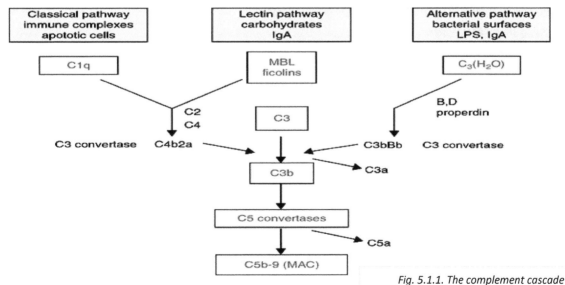

*Fig. 5.1.1. The complement cascade*

## 2. EFFECTS OF THE INFLAMMATORY RESPONSE

- The main symptoms of the inflammatory response are as follows.
  - The tissues in the area are red and warm, as a result of the large amount of blood reaching the site.
  - The tissues in the area are swollen, due to the increased amount of blood and proteins that are present.
  - The area is painful, due the expansion of tissues, causing mechanical pressure on nerve cells, and also due to the presence of pain mediators.
- Once the inflammatory process has begun, it continues until the infection that caused it has been eradicated.
- Phagocytes continue to consume and destroy bacteria, the acquired immune system binds and disposes of harmful toxins.
- Pus is produced, pus being the debris that is left over from the battle between the invader and the immune system.
- There are two main ways in which cells can commit Apoptosis.
  - *By receiving an Apoptosis signal*: When a chemical signal is received that indicates that the cell should kill itself, it does so.
  - *By not receiving a "stay-alive" signal*: Certain cells, once they reach an activated state, are primed to kill themselves automatically within a certain period of time, i.e. to commit Apoptosis, unless instructed otherwise. However, there may be other cells that supply them with a "stay-alive" signal, which delays the Apoptosis of the cell.
  - It is only when the primed cell stops receiving this "stay-alive" signal that it kills itself.
- The immune system employs method two above. The immune cells involved in the inflammatory response, once they become activated, are primed to commit Apoptosis. Helper T cells emit a stay-alive signal, and keep emitting that signal for as long as they recognise foreign antigens in the body, prolonging the inflammatory response.
- If foreign antigen is not eradicated from the body or the helper T cells do not recognise that fact, or if the immune cells receive the stay-alive signal from another source, then chronic inflammation may develop.

## 3. INFLAMMATORY MARKERS

### A. ACUTE-PHASE REACTANTS

- Acute-phase reactants are proteins whose plasma concentration increases (positive acute-phase proteins) or decreases (negative acute-phase proteins) by at least 25% during inflammatory states.
- The effect of inflammatory molecules such as interleukin (IL)-6, IL-1, tumor necrosis factor α (TNF-α), interferon gamma (IFN-γ), and transforming growth factor β (TGF-β) causes a change in hepatic protein synthesis collectively known as acute-phase response.
- ESR and CRP are the most widely measured acute-phase reactants in clinical practice.

### B. ERYTHROCYTE SEDIMENTATION RATE (ESR)

- ESR is a measure of the height of erythrocytes that fall through plasma in a Westergen or a Wintrobe tube **over a period of 1 hour.**
- ESR can be greatly influenced by the shape and number of red blood cells as well as other plasma constituents like fibrinogen, globulins, and albumins.
- In the presence of the certain diseases like inflammatory, malignancy, connective tissue and infection... the red cells become coated with surface proteins, causing them to stick together and sediment faster.
- In the absence of inflammation; ESR increases with Age, anemia, nephritic syndrome, hypergammaglobulinemia and the upper limit varies with sex:

$$ESR = Age/2 \text{ (men) or } (Age+10)/2 \text{ (women)}$$

- ESR can be spuriously normal in cryoglobulinemia and hemoglobinopathy.

### C. C- REACTIVE PROTEIN (CRP)

- Annular (ring-shaped), pentameric protein found in blood plasma, whose levels rise in response to inflammation.
- The concentration of CRP in serum is more sensitive than ESR to evaluate and monitor inflammation, and it is independent of factors that affect ESR.
- *CRP is synthesized by the liver in response to factors released by macrophages and fat cells (adipocytes).*
- *It is a member of the pentraxin family of proteins.*
- *It is not related to C-peptide (insulin) or protein C (blood coagulation).*
- *It is an acute-phase protein of hepatic origin that increases following interleukin-6 secretion   by   macrophages and T cells.*
- Its physiological role is to bind to **lysophosphatidylcholine** (from phosphocholine) expressed on the surface of dead or dying cells (and some types of bacteria) in order to activate the complement system via the C1Q complex.
- This activates the complement system, promoting phagocytosis by macrophages, which clears necrotic, apoptotic cells and bacteria.
- It plays a role in innate immunity as an early defense system against infections.
- *CRP rises within two hours of the onset of inflammation, up to a 50,000-fold, and peaks at 48 hours.*
- *Its half-life of 18 hours is constant, and therefore its level is determined by the rate of production and hence the severity of the precipitating cause.*
- *CRP is thus a screen for inflammation.*

# 4. ANTINUCLEAR FACTOR / ANTIBODIES

- Autoantibodies that bind to contents of the cell nucleus.
- In normal individuals, the immune system produces antibodies to foreign proteins (antigens) but not to human proteins (autoantigens). In some individuals, antibodies to human antigens are produced.
- They are found in many disorders including autoimmunity, cancer and infection, with different prevalences of antibodies depending on the condition.
- ANAs is used in the diagnosis of some autoimmune disorders:
  - SLE, Sjögren's Syndrome, Scleroderma,
  - Polymyositis, Dermatomyositis,
  - Autoimmune Hepatitis  and Drug Induced Lupus.
- The ANA test detects the autoantibodies present in an individual's blood serum.
- The common tests used for detecting and quantifying ANAs are *indirect immunofluorescence and enzyme-linked immunosorbent assay* (ELISA).
- Positive autoantibody titres at a dilution equal to or greater than 1:160 are usually considered as clinically significant.
- Positive titres of less than 1:160 are present in up to 20% of the healthy population, especially the elderly.
- Although positive titres of 1:160 or higher are strongly associated with autoimmune disorders, they are also found in 5% of healthy individuals.
- A positive ANA test is seldom useful if other clinical or laboratory data supporting a diagnosis are not present.
- The presence of ANAs in rheumatoid arthritis is suggestive of **Felty's syndrome**.
- A variety of different staining patterns are seen and each is suggestive of different disorders:
  - **Homogenous staining** is suggestive of lupus
  - **Speckled staining**: mixed connective tissue disease.
  - **Nucleolar staining** is suggestive of scleroderma.
  - **Centromere staining** is suggestive of CREST syndrome.
  - **Anti-double stranded DNA** is suggestive of SLE.
  - **Anti-histone antibodies** are highly suggestive of drug-induced lupus.

- **Antibodies associated with Autoimmunes diseases**:
  - **Anti-Ro**: Sjogren's syndrome, congenital heart block
  - **Anti-La:** Sjogren's syndrome
  - **Anti-Scl70**: progressive systemic sclerosis
  - **Anti-centromere**: CREST syndrome
  - **Anti-Sm**: SLE (with a high risk of renal lupus)
  - **Anti-RNP:** mixed connective disease, SLE
  - **Anti-Jo1**: polymyositis

- **Antibodies associated with gastrointestinal/ liver diseases**:
  - **Anti-mitochondrial antibodies:** primary biliary cirrhosis
  - **Anti-smooth muscle antibodies:** auto-immune hepatitis, cryptogenic cirrhosis
  - **Anti-gliadin antibodies**: coeliac disease
  - **Anti-endomysial antibodies**: coeliac disease
  - **Intrinsic factor antibodies:** pernicious anaemia
  - **Gastric parietal cell antibodies:** pernicious anaemia, gastric atrophy.

# SECTION 2:  IMMUNE RESPONSE

## 1. ANTIGEN

- Substance that stimulates an immune response, especially the production of antibodies.
- Antigens are usually proteins or polysaccharides but can be any type of molecule, including small molecules (haptens) coupled to a protein (carrier).
- Antigens induce immunity and usually involves the production of antibodies and of specific cells (cell-mediated immunity) whose purpose is to facilitate the elimination of foreign substances.
- The part of the antigen that antibody binds to is called the antigenic determinant, antigenic site or epitope.

## 2. NON SPECIFIC DEFENCES

- Innate, or non-specific, immunity is the immune system we are born with.
- There are three aspects of innate immunity:

| Anatomical barriers such as: | Humoral barriers such as: | Cellular barriers such as: |
|---|---|---|
| ✓ Cough reflex<br>✓ Enzymes in tears and skin oils<br>✓ Mucus<br>✓ Skin<br>✓ Stomach acid | ✓ The complement system<br>✓ Interleukin-1 | ✓ Neutrophils<br>✓ Eosinophils<br>✓ Basophils<br>✓ Monocytes and Macrophages<br>✓ Dendritic cells<br>✓ Natural killer cells |

## 3. SPECIFIC IMMUNITY

- **Passive immunity** is protection by products produced by an animal or human, and transferred to another human, usually by injection.
- Passive immunity often provides effective protection, but this protection is temporary.
- The most common form of passive immunity is that which an infant receives from its mother.
- **Active immunity** is protection that is produced by the person's own immune system. This type of immunity is usually permanent.
- Active immunity is stimulation of the immune system to produce antigen-specific humoral (antibody) and cellular immunity.
- One way to acquire active immunity is to have the natural disease. In general, once persons recover from an infectious disease, they will be immune to those diseases for the rest of their lives. **Pertussis is an exception.**
- The persistence of protection for many years after the infection is known as immunologic memory.
- Upon re-exposure to the antigen, these memory cells begin to replicate and produce antibody very rapidly to re-establish protection.
- Another way to produce active immunity is by **vaccination.**

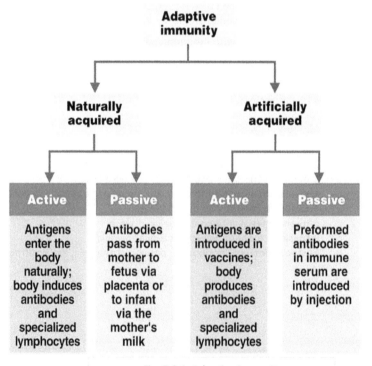

*Fig. 5.2.1. Adaptive immunity*

## 4. CELLS & MOLECULES OF THE IMMUNE SYSTEM

### A. GRANULOCYTES

### 1. NEUTROPHILS

- The most abundant, they defend against bacterial or fungal infection and other very small inflammatory processes.
- They are usually the first responders to microbial infection; their activity and death in large numbers forms pus.

### 2. EOSINOPHILS

- Primarily deal with parasitic infections.
- They are also the predominant inflammatory cells in allergic reactions.

### 3. BASOPHILS
- o Chiefly responsible for allergic and antigen response by releasing the chemical histamine, which causes dilation of the blood vessels.

## B. AGRANULOCYTES
### 1. MONOCYTES
- o Produced by the bone marrow from precursors called monoblasts.
- o Monocytes circulate in the bloodstream for about one to three days and then typically move into tissues throughout the body.
- o In the tissues, monocytes mature into different types of macrophages at different anatomical locations.
- o Monocytes are the largest corpuscles in the blood.

### 2. LYMPHOCYTES
### a. B-cells:
- Lymphocytes normally involved in the production of antibodies to combat infection.
- They are precursors to plasma cells.
- During infections, individual B-cell clones multiply and are transformed into plasma cells, which produce large amounts of antibodies against a particular antigen on a foreign microbe.
- This transformation occurs through interaction with the appropriate **CD4 T-helper cells**.

### b. T-cells:
- A class of lymphocytes, so called because they are derived from the thymus and have been through thymic processing.
- Involved primarily in controlling cell-mediated immune reactions and in the control of B-cell development.
- *The T-cells coordinate the immune system by secreting lymphokine hormones which is part of specific, or inducible immunity. There are 3 different types of T-cells:* **Helper, Killer,** and **Suppressor.**

## C. PHAGOCYTES
- o Neutrophils, Monocytes, Macrophages, Mast Cells, and Dendritic Cells.
- o These cells engulf foreign organisms or particles.
- **Dendritic cells** (DC) in the skin are called **Langerhans cells.**
- **Cells are seen in chronic infection:**
  - o Macrophages, Giant cells, Lymphocytes, Plasma cells, Mast cells and Basophils.

## 5. ANTIBODY (Ig GAMED)
- There are five classes of antibody: IgG, IgA, IgM, IgD and IgE.
- These are all structurally slightly different have a range of functions.
- Each B-cell can produce only one specific antibody to an antigen, each antibody is highly specific and will bind to only one antigen.
- **IgG:** This class of antibody is the most important class of immunoglobulin in secondary immune responses. IgG crosses the placenta, conferring protection to the new born and is able to activate the complement system through the classical pathway.
- **IgM:** is by far the largest antibody in the human circulatory system. **It is the first antibody to appear in response to initial exposure to an antigen**. It can also activate the classical pathway complement.
- **IgA:** is found primarily in secretions such as breast milk, tears, saliva and mucosal membranes.

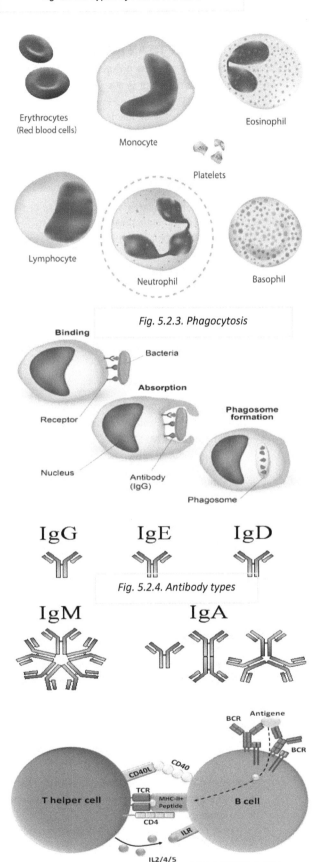

Fig. 5.2.2. Types of Red blood cells

Fig. 5.2.3. Phagocytosis

Fig. 5.2.4. Antibody types

Fig. 5.2.5. T helper and B cells

- **IgE:** evolved to provide protection against certain parasitic infections however in developed countries it is more commonly associated with allergic diseases such as asthma and hayfever.
- **IgD:** this is an antigen receptor on B cells that have not been exposed to antigens.

## 6. COMPLICATIONS DUE TO AN ALTERED IMMUNE RESPONSE

- An efficient immune response protects against many diseases and disorders.
- An inefficient immune response allows diseases to develop.
- Too much, too little, or the wrong immune response causes immune system disorders. An overactive immune response can lead to the development of autoimmune diseases, in which antibodies form against the body's own tissues.
- Complications from altered immune responses include:
  - Allergy or hypersensitivity, Anaphylaxis, Autoimmune disorders, Transplant rejection, Serum sickness, Graft versus host disease, Immunodeficiency disorders, etc.

## 7. HYPERSENSITIVITY TYPES

- The immune system is an integral part of human protection against disease, but the normally protective immune mechanisms can sometimes cause detrimental reactions in the host.
- The traditional classification for hypersensitivity reactions is that of **Gell and Coombs** and is currently the most commonly known classification system.
- It divides the hypersensitivity reactions into the following 4 types:
  - **Type I reactions or immediate hypersensitivity reactions (allergy):**
    - Involve immunoglobulin E (IgE) mediated release of histamine and other mediators from mast cells and basophils.
    - Examples: **4A**
      - Anaphylaxis
      - Allergic Rhinoconjunctivitis
      - Atopy
      - Asthma.

  - **Type II reactions or cytotoxic hypersensitivity reactions:**
    - Involve IgG or IgM antibodies bound to cell surface antigens, with subsequent complement fixation.
    - Examples: **DART MEGG**
      - Drug-induced hemolytic anemia.
      - Autoimmune hemolytic anemia (e.g. Rhesus)
      - Rheumatic Heart Disease
      - Thrombocytopenia
      - Myasthenia gravis
      - Erythroblastosis fetalis
      - Goodpasture's syndrome
      - Graves' disease

  - **Type III reactions or immune-complex reactions:**
    - Involve circulating antigen-antibody immune complexes that deposit in postcapillary venules, with subsequent complement fixation.
    - Examples: **SPERMALS**
      - Serum sickness
      - Post streptococcal glomerulonephritis
      - Extrinsic allergic alveolitis (hypersensitivity pneumonitis)
      - Rheumatoid arthritis
      - Membranous nephropathy
      - Arthus reaction
      - Lupus nephritis
      - Systemic lupus erythematosus

  - **Type IV reactions or delayed hypersensitivity reactions, cell-mediated immunity:**
    - Are mediated by T cells rather than by antibodies.
    - Examples: **2C 2M**
      - Contact dermatitis from poison ivy or nickel allergy.
      - Chronic transplant rejection
      - Mantoux test and Multiple sclerosis

# SECTION 3:  BASIC HUMAN PATHOLOGY

## I. NECROSIS TYPES
### 1. COAGULATIVE NECROSIS
- Seen in infarcts or ischemia in any tissue (except brain).
- Due to loss of blood
- **Gross:** tissue is firm
- **Micro:** Cell outlines are preserved (cells look ghostly), and everything looks red.

### 2. LIQUEFACTIVE OR COLLIQUATIVE NECROSIS
- Seen in infections and, for some unknown reason, in brain infarcts.
- Due to lots of neutrophils around releasing their toxic contents, "liquefying" the tissue.
- **White infarction** (anaemic infarction) occurs if there is occlusion in an end-arterial vessel system. It tends to affect solid organs such as the spleen and kidneys.
- **Red infarction** (haemorrhagic infarction) occurs in situations where there is a dual circulatory system, in veins and in reperfusion injury. It tends to affect organs such as the lungs and small intestine.
- **Venous infarcts** are rare since most veins have a good collateral supply. They can, however, occur in the kidney after renal vein thrombosis as the renal vein has no collateral.
- **Gross:** tissue is liquefied and creamy yellow (pus)
- **Micro:** lots of neutrophils and cell debris

### 3. CASEOUS NECROSIS
- Seen in tuberculosis
- Due to the body trying to wall off and kill the bug with macrophages.
- **Gross:** White, soft, cheesy-looking ("caseous") material.
- **Micro:** fragmented cells and debris surrounded by a collar of lymphocytes and macrophages (granuloma).

### 4. FAT NECROSIS
- Seen in acute pancreatitis (also salivary glands and Breast).
- Damaged cells release lipases, which split the triglyceride esters within fat cells.
- **Gross:** chalky, white areas from the combination of the newly-formed free fatty acids with calcium (**saponification**)
- **Micro:** shadowy outlines of dead fat cells; sometimes there is a bluish cast from the calcium deposits, which are basophilic.

### 5. FIBRINOID NECROSIS
- Seen in immune reactions in vessels.
- Complexes of antigens and antibodies (immune complexes) combine with fibrin.
- **Gross:** changes too small to see grossly.
- **Micro:** vessel walls are thickened and pinkish-red (called "fibrinoid" because it looks like fibrin but has other stuff in there too).
- Fibrinoid necrosis is characterised by the presence of an amorphous eosinophilic material that is reminiscent of fibrin, within the area of cell death.

### 6. GANGRENOUS NECROSIS
- Seen when an entire limb loses blood supply and dies (usually the lower leg)
- **Gross:** skin looks black and dead; underlying tissue is in varying stages of decomposition
- **Micro:** initially there is coagulative necrosis from the loss of blood supply (**dry gangrene**); if bacterial infection is superimposed, there is liquefactive necrosis (**wet gangrene**).

## 2. MYOCARDIAL INFARCTION
- Acute MI indicates irreversible myocardial injury resulting in necrosis of a significant portion of the myocardium (> 1 cm).
- Acute MI is usually initiated by the fissuring of an atheromatous plaque.
- This is followed by haemorrhage into the plaque and contraction of the smooth muscle within the artery wall.
- Thrombus then forms on the surface of the plaque causing further obstruction of the lumen of the artery.
- If such an occlusion persists for more than 20 minutes, irreversible myocardial cell damage and cell death will occur.
- The inflammatory infiltrate is primarily neutrophilic.
- A positive troponin test indicates myocyte necrosis.
- The sequence of events after a myocardial infarction is as follows:
  - **1-4 hours:** Myoglobin starts to rise and peaks at 6-7 hours.

- ○ **1.5 hrs:** Heart-type fatty acid binding protein (HFABP) starts to rise at and peaks at 5-10 hrs.
- ○ **4-8 hours:** Creatine kinase starts to rise at and peaks at 18 hours.
- ○ **12-24 hours:** Classic coagulative necrosis occurs.
- ○ **24-48 hours:** Invasion of neutrophils occurs (Liquefactive necrosis).
- ○ **3days - 1week:** Macrophages reabsorb dead cell debris. There is maximum wall weakness during this time.
- ○ **1-6 weeks:** Ingrowth of capillaries occurs. Granulation tissue forms which later matures in a dense non-contractile fibrous scar.

## 3. TRANSIENT ISCHEMIC ATTACKS (TIA)

- Transient ischaemic attacks (TIA) were traditionally defined as a sudden, focal neurological deficit of presumed vascular origin lasting less than 24hours.
- However, the 24hr time limit was quite arbitrary and with improved imaging, it became clear that many TIAs, particularly those that lasted longer than an hour, although appearing to clinically resolve would cause radiologically evident infarction of cerebral tissue.
- Thus, a better definition of TIA might be: brief episode of neurologic dysfunction resulting from focal temporary cerebral ischemia not associated with cerebral infarction.
- In reality, most true TIAs last less than 15 minutes.
- Much longer and brain tissue dies.
- **Amourosis fugax** (temporary monocular blindness) results from temporary occlusion of the central retinal artery which supplies the inner layers of the retina.
- The retinal artery is a branch of the ophthalmic artery, which in turn is the first branch of the internal carotid artery inside the skull.
- The anterior cerebral artery branches from the internal carotid more distally and supplies the frontal lobe.
- Hypertension is a significant risk factor for stroke and TIA, as are diabetes, smoking, alcohol abuse and atrial fibrillation.
- NICE guidance advises starting antiplatelet therapy (aspirin 300mg daily) after TIA has been clinically diagnosed.
- In the UK, patients are risk stratified using the ABCD2 score and most discharged on aspirin and with early clinic follow up where brain imaging is performed as well as further investigation for treatable causes of stroke

## 4. COLLAGEN TYPES

- **Type I collagen**
  - ○ Found throughout the body *except in cartilaginous tissues.*
  - ○ It is found in skin, tendon, vascular, ligature, organs and is the main component of bone.
  - ○ It is also synthesized in response to injury and in the fibrous nodules in fibrous diseases.
  - ○ Over 90% of the collagen in the body is type I.

- **Type II collagen**
  - ○ It is the main component of cartilage.
  - ○ It is also found in developing cornea and vitreous humour.
  - ○ These are formed from two or more collagens or co-polymers rather than a single type of collagen.

- **Type III collagen**
  - ○ It is found in the walls of arteries and other hollow organs and usually occurs in the same fibril with type I collagen.
  - ○ Mutations in genes associated with type III and type IV collagen are associated with connective tissue disorders such as **Ehlers-Danlos syndrome** and also with **aneurysm formation**.

- **Type IV** forms the bases of cell basement membrane.

- **Type V collagen** and **type XI collagen** are minor components of tissue and occur as fibrils with type I and type II collagen respectively. Type V forms cell surfaces, hair and placenta.

## 5. MULTINUCLEATE GIANT CELLS (MGC'S)

- **A typical granuloma** contains giant multinucleated cells (Langhan's cells) surrounded by epithelioid cell aggregates (activated macrophages), T lymphocytes and fibroblasts.
- MGCs are frequently present in granulomas and invariably present in bone (osteoclasts).
- They are polykaryons resulting from the fusion of mononuclear phagocytes under the influence of cytokines.
- Granulomas may or may not contain MGC's.
- Some granulomas consist entirely of MGC's whereas others may be completely devoid of giant cells.
- MGC's may be the only significant abnormal finding in bronchial and transbronchial biopsies from patients with sarcoidosis.
- The MGC's which are present in granulomas are classified as being either of Langhans or foreign body types.
- **The Langhans cell** (*Not Langerhan's Cells*) is characterized by location of the nuclei at the periphery of the cell in an arcuate configuration.
- **In the foreign body type** the nuclei are randomly distributed, often aggregating towards the center of the cell.
- Some giant cells exhibit features of both Langhans and foreign body types.

- **Touton giant cells** are seen in lesions with high lipid content such as xanthoma, xanthogranuloma, and fat necrosis. They are characterized by a ring of nuclei surrounding a central eosinophilic zone and surrounded by a zone of pallor extending to the periphery of the cell.
- **Epithelium-derived MGC's** may be prominent in certain viral infections such as measles (**Warthin-Finkeldey cells**), respiratory syncytial virus, herpes simplex-varicella-zoster, and parainfluenza.
- **Aschoff cells** are associated with rheumatic heart disease. They are found in Aschoff bodies surrounding centres of fibrinoid necrosis.
- Multinucleate giant cells derived from neoplastic cells may be formed in a variety of neoplasms.
- *MGC's retain phagocytic capability which is considered to be less than that of monocytes/macrophages*

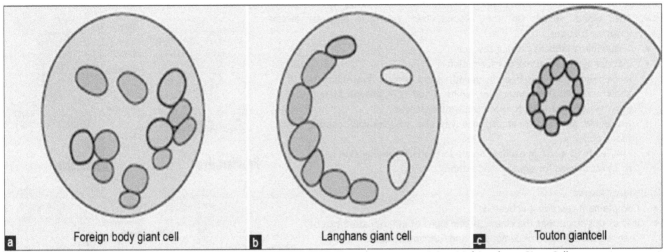

| a Foreign body giant cell | b Langhans giant cell | c Touton giantcell |

*Fig. 5.3.1. Multinucleate Giant Cells*

## 6. ANAPHYLAXIS

- A severe, life-threatening, generalised or systemic hypersensitivity reaction.
- It is characterised by rapidly developing, life-threatening problems involving the airway (pharyngeal or laryngeal oedema) and/or breathing (bronchospasm with tachypnoea) and/or circulation (hypotension and/or tachycardia). In most cases, there are associated skin and mucosal changes.
- It is a type I hypersensitivity reaction. Anaphylaxis requires pre-sensitisation.
- During the initial exposure to an antigen, antigen specific IgE is produced and attached to the surface of mast cells.
- During subsequent exposure(s), the antigen binds and crosslinks surface IgE triggering mast cell degranulation and release of inflammatory mediators most notably histamine but also serotonin, bradykinin and others.
- This may occur locally and cause a local inflammatory condition (allergic rhinitis for example) or systemically where the inflammatory response causes the life-threatening features of anaphylaxis.
- Mast cells are produced by the bone marrow from where they migrate to many different body tissues.
- They are found in high number in sub-epithelial (sub-cutaneous and sub-mucosal) tissues and around blood vessels and nerves.
- Hence, skin rashes (hives), swelling (angioedema), bronchospasm and vascular changes are prominent.
- In many cases of anaphylaxis, an initial immediate reaction is followed by a late phase reaction, usually 2-8 hours after the initial exposure (rarely up to 24 hours).
- This late phase reaction happens due to the infiltration of tissues with eosinophils, basophils, neutrophils, monocytes and CD4+ T cells.

## 7. CONTROL OF BODY TEMPERATURE

- **The hypothalamus** is the body's thermostat. It works with other higher brain centres and the autonomic nervous system to maintain core body temperature at around 37°C.
- **Interleukin 1** (IL-1) is an endogenous pyrogen, released as part of the acute phase response to inflammation and/or infection. It resets the thermoregulatory set point of the hypothalamus to a higher level.
- Core temperature can then rise to the new set point generating fever. This effect of IL-1 is probably mediated by **prostaglandins.**
- **Catecholamines** and sympathetic stimulation decrease heat loss and increase core temperature by:
  o vasoconstriction of cutaneous vessels;
  o increased metabolism of thermogenic brown fat; and
  o Piloerection which traps a layer of insulating warm air next to the skin.
- Rectal temperature tends to be around 0.5 – 1.0°C higher than oral temperature.
- For completeness, temperature measured in the axilla will be around 0.5 – 1.0°C lower than the corresponding oral temperature.

# SECTION 4:  WOUND & BONE HEALING

## I. HEALING PHASES

### PHASES & ACTIVITIES IN THE WOUND

**1. Haemostasis**

- The blood vessels in the wound bed contract (vascular vasoconstriction).
- Tissue injury induces clotting cascade
- Platelet aggregation >>> clot formation
- Once haemostasis has been achieved, blood vessels then dilate to allow essential cells; antibodies, white blood cells, growth factors, enzymes and nutrients to reach the wounded area.
- Histamine and serotonin increase vascular permeability causing tissue oedema.
- This leads to a rise in exudate levels so the surrounding skin needs to be monitored for signs of maceration.

**2. Inflammatory**

- Complement cascade is activated.
- It is at this stage that the characteristic signs of inflammation can be seen: erythema, heat, oedema, pain and functional disturbance.
- The predominant cells are: **'neutrophils and macrophages'**; autolysing any devitalized 'necrotic or sloughy' tissue.
- **Polymorphs** (PMBLs) migrate to the wound after a few hours and act for up to 4 days. PMNLs cleanse the wound environment
- Rectal temperature tends to be around 0.5 – 1.0°C higher than oral temperature.
- **Monocytes** migrate to the wound site and transform into **Macrophages** (48-72hrs) to promote and co-ordinate the later stages of repair through release of cytokines and growth factors.
- **Lymphocytes** infiltrate
- Febrile and Acute phase response

**3. Proliferative**

- **36hrs-2 weeks** after wounding.
- The wound is 'rebuilt' with new **granulation tissue** which is comprised of **collagen** and **extracellular matrix** and into which a new network of blood vessels develops, a process known as **'Angiogenesis'**.
- Healthy granulation tissue is dependent upon the fibroblast receiving sufficient levels of oxygen and nutrients supplied by the blood vessels.
- **Fibroblasts** appear between **2-4days** and lay down the new ECM (Collagen II & III, Fibronectin, Hyaluronan, GAGs).
- Epithelial cells finally resurface the wound, a process known as **'Epithelialisation'**

**4. Remodelling/ Maturation**

- This phase involves remodelling of **collagen from type III to type I**
- Cellular activity reduces and the number of blood vessels in the wounded area regress and decrease.
- Myofibroblasts promote wound contraction
- May last up to 300 days.
- Final product is **Avascular, Acellular scar.**

---

- *First 24hrs: wound fills with clots and exudates and neutrophils and monocytes as a result of inflammatory changes. Epithelial cells migrate to and proliferate in the wound. By the end of the first day: mitoses in the connective tissue are seen*
- *Day 3: capillary sprout is seen.*
- *Day 4-5: Reticulin fibres are present*
- *Day 8-10: fibres are strong enough to take any strain (most sutures are removed)*
- *A wound has less than 10% of its final healed strength at 2 weeks.*
- *Wound strength increases to 20% at 3 weeks and 50% by 4 weeks.*
- *A healed wound only reaches approximately 80% of the tensile strength of unwounded skin.*

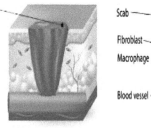

**Hemostasis**

Blood clot

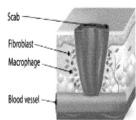

**Inflammatory**

Scab

Fibroblast

Macrophage

Blood vessel

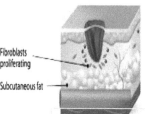

**Proliferative**

Fibroblasts proliferating

Subcutaneous fat

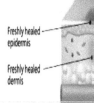

**Remodeling**

Freshly healed epidermis

Freshly healed dermis

*Fig. 5.4.1. Wound healing phases*

# II. CATEGORIES OF WOUND HEALING

## CATEGORY 1: PRIMARY WOUND HEALING

- Primary wound healing or healing by first intention occurs within hours of repairing a full-thickness surgical incision.
- This surgical insult results in the mortality of a minimal number of cellular constituents.

## CATEGORY 2: DELAYED PRIMARY HEALING

- If the wound edges are not reapproximated immediately, delayed primary wound healing transpires.
- This type of healing may be desired in the case of contaminated wounds.
- By the 4th day, phagocytosis of contaminated tissues is well underway, and the processes of epithelization, collagen deposition, and maturation are occurring. Usually the wound is closed surgically at this juncture, and if the "cleansing" of the wound is incomplete, chronic inflammation can ensue, resulting in prominent scarring.

## CATEGORY 3: SECONDARY HEALING

- Secondary healing or healing by secondary intention. In this type of healing, a full-thickness wound is allowed to close and heal.
- Secondary healing results in an inflammatory response that is more intense than with primary wound healing.
- In addition, a larger quantity of granulomatous tissue is fabricated because of the need for wound closure.
- Secondary healing results in pronounced contraction of wounds. Fibroblastic differentiation into myofibroblasts, which resemble contractile smooth muscle, is believed to contribute to wound contraction.
- These myofibroblasts are maximally present in the wound from the 10th-21st days.

**WOUND HEALING IS IMPAIRED BY THE FOLLOWING:**

- Poor blood supply
- Superimposed wound infection
- Foreign material in the wound
- Nutrient deficiency e.g. vitamin C deficiency
- Drugs e.g. corticosteroids

# III. FRACTURE HEALING

- **Within 48 hours**, chemotaxic signaling mechanisms attract the inflammation cells necessary to promote the healing process.
- **Within 7-14 days,** granulation tissue is formed between the fragments, leading to vascularisation of the haematoma.
- On radiographs, there may be increased translucency of the fracture during this stage, due to bone resorption.
- Cells within the granulation tissue proliferate and begin to differentiate into **fibroblasts** and **chondroblasts.**
- They produce an extracellular organic matrix of fibrous tissue and cartilage; wherein woven bone is deposited by osteoblasts.
- This stage usually **lasts 4-16 weeks.**
- The newly formed callus is still damageable by shear forces, whereas axial traction and pressure promote the matrix formation.
- The mesh of woven bone is then replaced by lamellar bone, which is organized parallel to the axis of the bone.
- Eventually, remodelling of the bone takes place, restoring its normal cortical structure depending on load distribution.
- This is an ongoing process that may last for several years.
- In children, remodelling occurs faster than in older people and may compensate malunion to some degree.

- **AVERAGE HEALING TIMES OF COMMON FRACTURES:**
  - Phalanges: 3 weeks
  - Metacarpals: 4-6 weeks
  - Distal radius: 4-6 weeks
  - Lower arm: 8-10 weeks
  - Humerus: 6-8 weeks
  - Femoral neck: 12 weeks
  - Femoral shaft: 12 weeks
  - Tibia: 10 weeks

| In a patient diagnosed with transient ischaemic attack (TIA) | |
|---|---|
| Most true TIA last less than 15 minutes | T |
| Amaurosis fugax results from transient occlusion of the anterior cerebral artery | F |
| Hypertension is a risk factor | T |
| A CT scan of the brain is necessary before antiplatelet therapy can | F |

# SECTION 5: HAEMATOLOGY

## I. ANAEMIA

| MACROCYTOSIS WITH MEGALOBLASTIC BONE MARROW: | MACROCYTOSIS WITH NORMOBLASTIC BONE MARROW: "PRALM" | CAUSES OF LYMPHOCYTOSIS: |
|---|---|---|
| o Folate deficiency<br>o Vitamin B12 deficiency<br>o Drugs: Methotrexate, azathioprine and hydroxyurea. | o **P**regnancy<br>o **R**eticulocytosis<br>o **A**lcohol<br>o **L**iver disease<br>o **M**yxoedema | o Acute viral infections<br>o Chronic infections e.g. TB, brucella, hepatitis, syphilis<br>o Thyrotoxicosis<br>o Chronic leukemias and lymphomas |
| **CAUSES OF LEUCOERYTHROBLASTIC BLOOD PICTURE** | **CAUSES OF NEUTROPHILIA:** | **CAUSES OF EOSINOPHILIA:** |
| o Bone marrow infiltration:<br>　• Gaucher's disease, Osteopetrosis<br>　• Metastatic cancer, Myelofibroma<br>　• Leukaemia, Myeloma, Lymphoma<br>o Acute severe illness:<br>　• Severe Haemolysis, Massive Trauma and Sepsis. | o Localised or generalized bacterial infections<br>o Inflammation e.g. MI, trauma, vasculitis<br>o Myeloproliferative disorders.<br>o Malignancy<br>o Metabolic disorders e.g. uraemia, gout, eclampsia, acidosis<br>o Drugs e.g. corticosteroids | o Allergy e.g. asthma and hayfever<br>o Skin disease e.g. eczema and psoriasis<br>o Parasitic infections e.g. filariasis, ascariasis and toxocariasis<br>o Hodgkins disease<br>o Tropical eosinophilia<br>o Sarcoidosis<br>o Polyarteritis nodosa |

## 1. IRON DEFICIENCY ANAEMIA

- Iron is a constituent of haemoglobin and is essential for erythropoiesis.
- Iron deficiency is often caused by long-term blood loss.
- Peripheral smear results in iron deficiency anaemia are as follows:
  - o RBCs are microcytic & hypochromic in chronic cases.
  - o Platelets usually are increased.
  - o In contrast to thalassemia, target cells are usually not present, and anisocytosis and poikilocytosis are not marked.
  - o In contrast to hemoglobin C disorders, intraerythrocytic crystals are not seen.
- **Results of iron studies are as follows:**
  - o Low serum iron, MCV, MCHC and ferritin levels
  - o Elevated TIBC (Total Iron Binding Capacity) are diagnostic of iron deficiency.
  - o A normal serum ferritin can be seen in patients who are deficient in iron and have coexistent diseases (e.g., hepatitis or anaemia of chronic disorders).

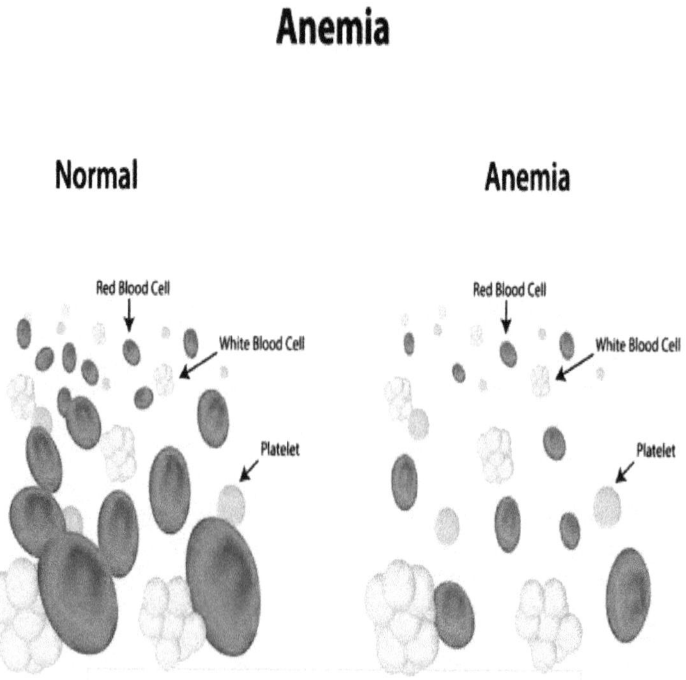

Fig. 5.5.1. Anaemia

## 2. MEGALOBLASTIC ANAEMIA

- The aetiology of vitamin B12 deficiency is: lack of intrinsic factor (IF), altered pH in the small intestine, and lack of absorption of B12 complexes in **the terminal ileum.**
- Vitamin B12 deficiency from any cause, as well as folic acid deficiency, can result in megaloblastic anaemia.
- Megaloblastic anaemia is a common cause of a macrocytic anaemia. In clinical practice it is almost always caused by deficiency of vitamin B12 or folate. Vitamin B12 deficiency normally arises from malabsorption, the classic clinical syndrome is the autoimmune disorder **pernicious anaemia.** Folate deficiency is more often due to frank dietary deficiency or increased dietary requirements as in pregnancy. *Vitamin B12 deficiency should be excluded or corrected before Folate is administered as subacute combined degeneration of the cord can be precipitated.*
- Vitamin B12 is available for therapeutic use parenterally (IV) as either cyanocobalamin or hydroxocobalamin.

# 3. HAEMOLYTIC ANAEMIA

- 'Haemolytic anaemias' are caused by abnormal destruction of red cells. Most inherited haemolytic disorders have a defect within the red cell whilst most acquired disorders have the defect outside the cell.
- Haemolysis causes characteristic clinical features and laboratory abnormalities. It may be intra- or extravascular.
- **Hereditary spherocytosis and hereditary elliptocytosis** are haemolytic disorders caused by a deficiency in the red cell membrane.
- **G6PD and Pyruvate Kinase** are key enzymes in red cell metabolism; inherited deficiency leads to haemolysis.
- **Autoimmune Haemolytic Anaemia (AIHA)** can be divided into 'warm' and 'cold' types dependent on the temperature at which the antibody reacts optimally with red cells.
- For each type of AIHA there are possible underlying causes which must be identified and treated.
- The term **'Microangiopathic Haemolytic Anaemia' (MAHA)** describes the intravascular destruction of red cells in the presence of an abnormal microenvironment.
- **Thrombotic Thrombocytopenic Purpura** (TTP)
  - It is a microangiopathic haemolytic anaemia (MAHA) that is predominantly seen in adults.
  - In TTP there is an excess of von Willebrand factor in the plasma causing platelets to adhere to the vascular endothelium.
  - This results in thrombocytopenia and the blockage of small capillaries in the brain and kidney by platelet thrombi.
  - Activation of the coagulation cascade causes fibrin strand deposition and destruction of passing red blood cells.
  - TTP is characterized by five features:
    - ✓ Fever
    - ✓ Thrombocytopenia
    - ✓ Microangiopathic haemolytic anaemia
    - ✓ Neurologic features including hallucinations, headaches, stroke and altered mental status.
    - ✓ Renal failure.
- **Haemolytic uraemic syndrome** (HUS), another example of MAHA, is predominantly seen in children.
- **Paroxysmal nocturnal haemoglobinuria (PNH)** is a rare example of acquired haemolysis caused by an intrinsic red cell defect.

# 4. G6PD DEFICIENCY

- Glucose-6-phosphate dehydrogenase (G6PD) deficiency is the most common enzyme deficiency in humans.
- It has a high prevalence in persons of African, Asian, and Mediterranean descent.
- It is inherited as an *X-linked recessive disorder*, with an inheritance pattern similar to that of hemophilia and color blindness: *males usually manifest the abnormality and females are carriers.*
- G6PD deficiency can present as **neonatal hyperbilirubinemia.** Jaundice usually appears within 24 hours after birth, at the same time as or slightly earlier than physiologic jaundice but later than in blood group alloimmunization.
- In addition, persons with this disorder can experience episodes of brisk **hemolysis** after ingesting fava beans or being exposed to certain infections or drugs. Hemolysis begins **24 to 72 hours** after exposure to oxidant stress. Many individuals with G6PD deficiency are asymptomatic.  When hemolysis is severe, patients present with weakness, tachycardia, jaundice & hematuria. Some patients have a history of chronic haemolytic anaemia. Acute hemolysis is self-limiting, resolving after **8 - 14 days**.
- Hemolytic episodes destroy aging red blood cells (RBCs) that have the lowest levels of G6PD, New RBCs produced to compensate for anaemia contain high levels of G6PD. Young RBCs are not vulnerable to oxidative damage and hence limit the duration of hemolysis.
- G6PD deficiency **confers partial protection against malaria**.
- Physical examination findings may be normal in patients with G6PD deficiency. Jaundice and splenomegaly may be present in patients with severe hemolysis. Patients may have right upper quadrant tenderness due to hyperbilirubinemia and cholelithiasis.
- Most individuals with G6PD deficiency do not need treatment. However, they should be taught to avoid drugs and chemicals that can cause oxidant stress. Transfusions are rarely indicated. Splenectomy is usually ineffective.
- Infants with prolonged neonatal jaundice as a result of G6PD deficiency should receive **phototherapy with a bili light.**
- **Exchange transfusion** may be necessary in cases of severe neonatal jaundice or hemolytic anemia caused by favism.
- Patients with chronic hemolysis or non-spherocytic anemia should be placed on **daily folic acid** supplements.

# 5. THE THALASSAEMIAS

➢ **Definition**
- Thalassemia also called **Mediterranean anemia**.
- A form of **inherited autosomal recessive** blood disorder characterized by abnormal formation of Hb resulting in improper oxygen transport and destruction of red blood cells.

➢ **Pathophysiology**
- Hemoglobin (Hb) consists of an iron-containing heme ring and four globin chains: **two α and two non-α.**
- The composition of the four globin chains determines the Hb type.
  - **Fetal Hb** (HbF) has two α and two γ chains ($\alpha 2\gamma 2$).
  - **Adult Hb** (HbA) has 2 α and 2 β chains ($\alpha 2\beta 2$),
  - **HbA2** has two α and two δ chains ($\alpha 2\delta 2$).

- At birth, HbF accounts for approximately 80% of Hb and HbA accounts for 20%.
- The transition from γ-globin synthesis (HbF) to β-globin synthesis (HbA) begins before birth.
- By approximately 6 months of age, healthy infants mainly have HbA, a small amount of HbA2, and negligible amounts of HbF.
- In thalassemia, patients have defects in either α or β globin chain, causing production of abnormal red blood cells.
- The thalassemias are classified according to which chain of the hemoglobin molecule is affected:
- **α-Thalassemia**
  - α globin chains are encoded by two closely linked genes on chromosome 16.
  - Deficient synthesis is usually due to a deletion of one or more of these genes:
    - A single gene deletion results in **α-thalassemia silent carrier status.**
    - A 2-gene deletion causes **α-thalassemia trait.**
    - A three-gene deletion leading to significant production of HbH, which has four β chains ($\beta_4$), results in **α-Thalassemia intermedia** or **HbH disease**.
    - A four-gene deletion results in significant production of **Hb Bart's**, which has four γ chains ($\gamma_4$).
  - α-Thalassemia is most common in individuals of African and Southeast Asian descent.
- **β-Thalassemia**
  - β-Thalassemia results from deficient or no synthesis of β-globin chains, leading to excess α chains.
  - β-thalassemia is most common in individuals of Mediterranean (Southern Europe), African, Middle East, and India descent.
  - β-Globin synthesis is controlled by one gene on each chromosome 11.
    - A single gene defect results in **β-thalassemia trait.**
    - Severely reduced or no synthesis from both genes results in **β-thalassemia major.**
    - Less severely reduced synthesis of β chains results in **β-thalassemia intermedia.**

> **Epidemiology**
  - Thalassemia affects men and women equally.
  - About 5% of the world's population has a globin variant, but only 1.7% has α- or β-thalassemia trait.
  - Thalassemia trait affects 5-30% of people in these ethnic groups.
  - The prevalence of β-thalassemia is highest in areas where malaria is (or was) endemic.
  - In Europe, the highest concentrations of the disease are found in Greece, coastal regions in Turkey, in parts of Italy.

> **CLINICAL MANIFESTATIONS AND COMPLICATIONS**
  - Mild or severe Microcytic Anaemia.
  - Megaloblastic Anaemia (Folate deficiency)
  - Iron overload.
  - Bone deformities.
  - Cardiovascular illness.
  - May confer a degree of protection against malaria (Plasmodium *falciparum*), which is or was prevalent in the regions where the trait is common.

# 6. SICKLE CELL SYNDROMES

- Sickle cell anaemia is an autosomal recessive genetic disorder that results from the substitution of valine for glutamic acid at position 6 of the b-globin gene, leading to production of a defective form of haemoglobin, haemoglobin S (HbS).
- Under physiological stress, deoxygenated HbS polymerizes, deforming the red blood cell (RBC) into the classic sickle shape. The sickled RBCs obstruct the microcirculation, causing tissue hypoxia, which in turn promotes further sickling.
- Patients who are homozygous for the HbS gene (HbSS) have full-blown sickle cell anaemia. Milder forms of disease are seen in patients with one HbS allele and a second allele that is also abnormal, for example with haemoglobin C (HbSC) or b-thalassaemia (HbSb+).
- Heterozygote carriers of the disease are mostly asymptomatic.
- The clinical manifestations of sickle cell anaemia are diverse, since any organ system can be affected. They are commonly divided into vaso-occlusive, haematological and infectious crises.

## A. VASO-OCCLUSIVE CRISIS

- Vaso-occlusive crisis occurs when sickled RBCs obstruct the microcirculation, causing ischaemic injury to tissues.
- Pain is the most frequent complaint during these episodes, and it is ischaemic in origin. Most crises of this type last between 3 days and a week.
- Bones (e.g. the femur, tibia, humerus and lower vertebrae) are frequently involved, giving rise to the painful 'bone crisis', while involvement of the femoral head may cause avascular necrosis.
- Vaso-occlusive crisis can involve the joints and soft tissue, and it may present as dactylitis or as hand-and-foot syndrome (painful and swollen hands and/or feet in children).
- **Acute chest syndrome** is a life-threatening complication of vaso-occlusion, with chest pain, fever, hypoxia and pulmonary infiltrates on the chest X-ray.
- The acute chest syndrome is difficult to diagnose in the emergency department setting, since radiological abnormalities lag symptoms.
- Pneumonia may coexist with acute chest syndrome, each condition exacerbating the other.
- Vaso-occlusion involving the abdominal organs can mimic **an acute abdomen**.

- With repeated episodes, the spleen autoinfarcts, rendering it fibrotic and functionless in most adults with sickle cell anaemia.
- Central nervous system (CNS) manifestations of vaso-occlusive crisis are myriad, including cerebral infarction (children), haemorrhage (adults), seizures, transient ischaemic attacks, cranial nerve palsies, meningitis, sensory deficits and acute coma. Cerebrovascular accidents are not uncommon in children, and they tend to be recurrent.
- These patients are often maintained on hypertransfusion programmes to suppress HbS.
- Skin ulceration, especially over bony prominences (malleoli), and retinal haemorrhages frequently complicate sickle cell disease.
- Finally, vaso-occlusion may involve the corpus cavernosum, preventing blood return from the penis and leading to **priapism**
- Vaso-occlusive crisis is often precipitated by the following:
  - *Dehydration (especially from exertion or during warm weather)*
  - *Cold weather (owing to vasospasm)*
  - *Hypoxia (flying in unpressurized aircraft)*
  - *Infection*
  - *Alcohol*
  - *Emotional stress*
  - *Pregnancy*

## B. HAEMATOLOGICAL CRISIS

- Haematological crisis is manifested by a sudden exacerbation of anaemia, with a corresponding drop in the haemoglobin level.
- This can be due to acute splenic sequestration, in which sickled cells block splenic outflow, leading to the pooling of peripheral blood in the engorged spleen (seen in young patients with functioning spleens).
- Less commonly, it is due to hepatic sequestration.
- Haematological crisis can also be caused by aplasia, in which the bone marrow stops producing new RBCs (*aplastic crisis*). This is most commonly seen in patients with parvovirus B19 infection or folic acid deficiency.

## C. INFECTIOUS CRISIS

- In most adults with sickle cell anaemia, infectious crisis is due to underlying functional asplenia leading to defective immunity against encapsulated organisms (e.g. *Haemophilus influenzae* and *Streptococcus pneumoniae*).
- Individuals with infectious crisis also have lower serum immunoglobulin M (IgM) levels, impaired opsonisation and sluggish alternative complement pathway activation.
- Accordingly, persons with sickle cell anaemia also exhibit increased susceptibility to other common infectious agents, including *Mycoplasma pneumoniae, Salmonella typhimurium, Staphylococcus aureus* and *Escherichia coli*.

# 7. DISSEMINATED INTRAVASCULAR COAGULATION

- The clinical scenario and blood tests indicate that the patient is suffering from disseminated intravascular coagulation (DIC) as a complication of meningococcal septicaemia. DIC results from pathological overactivation of the coagulation cascade, leading to the consumption of clotting factors as well as of fibrinogen and platelets.
- It is seen in association with a number of well-defined clinical situations, including sepsis, major trauma, malignancy and obstetric emergencies.
- The resultant widespread intravascular clotting causes:
  - Blood vessel occlusion, leading to tissue ischaemia and end-organ damage
  - Depletion of clotting factors, fibrinogen and platelets, leading to profuse and uncontrollable bleeding
  - Haemolysis of passing red cells by fibrin strands in the small vessels, leading to a microangiopathic haemolytic anaemia
- Clinically, DIC is characterized by bleeding from any site. Bleeding into the skin gives petechiae and/or widespread ecchymoses.
- Intracranial, pulmonary and gastrointestinal bleeding may be life-threatening. Early evidence of DIC is often seen at sites of iatrogenic trauma: as excessive bleeding from venepuncture sites or from the oropharynx after intubation or as haematuria following catheterization.
- Despite greater understanding and more aggressive therapy, the mortality from severe DIC remains high and early recognition and treatment is vital for any chance of survival.
- Diagnosis of DIC requires the presence of clinical manifestations of DIC – either haemorrhagic or thrombotic – and the following laboratory investigations:
  - Thrombocytopenia on the FBC
  - Raised International Normalized Ratio (INR), prothrombin time (PT) and activated partial thromboplastin time (APTT)
  - Elevated D-dimer
  - Reduced fibrinogen
  - Raised fibrinogen degradation products (FDPs)

# 8. ANAEMIA OF CHRONIC DISEASE (ACD)

- ACD is seen in a wide range of chronic, malignant, inflammatory and infective disorders.
- The pathogenesis of ACD is complex.
- There is a reduction in both red cell production and survival.
- Hepcidin is likely to be a key mediator.
- *The anaemia is usually of normochromic, normocytic type, non-progressive and is rarely severe.*
- Treatment is that of the underlying disorder.
- Blood transfusion and erythropoietin may help in selected cases.
- Iron supplementation has a limited role.

# 9. COMPLICATIONS OF BLOOD TRANSFUSION

- **Early:**
  - **Acute transfusion reactions:**
    - **Major life-threatening:**
      - Haemolysis (ABO incompatibility)
      - Gram-negative Bacteraemia
      - Anaphylaxis/Acute hypotension
      - Air embolism
      - Thrombophlebitis
      - Metabolic: *Metabolic alkalosis, Hyperkalaemia, Citrate toxicity, hypocalcaemia, Hypothermia*
    - **Minor:**
      - Urticaria
      - Febrile non-haemolytic transfusion reaction
  - **Transfusion related acute lung injury (TRALI)**

- **Delayed/Late:**
  - Delayed haemolytic transfusion reaction (Rhesus antigen)
  - Transfusion-associated graft vs host disease (TA-CVHD)
  - Transfusion-transmitted infections (TTI): Viral (*Hepatitis A, B, C, HIV, CMV*); Bacterial (*Treponema pallidum, Salmonella*); Parasites (*Malaria, Toxoplasma*)
  - Iron overload

## COMPLICATIONS OF  MASSIVE BLOOD TRANSFUSION

- Fluid overload
- Clotting abnormalities: Thrombocytopaenia
- Hypocalcaemia
- Hypothermia
- Decreased oxygen release by transfused red cells due to 2,3-Diphosphoglycerate (2,3-DPG) levels (Left shift in Hb-O2 curve).

| Which statements regarding anaphylaxis are true? | |
|---|---|
| It requires mast cell degranulation | T |
| It is mediated by IgM crosslinking | F |
| A late phase reaction may occur up to eight hours after the initial reaction | T |
| Mast cells are found only in the skin | F |
| **The following are true when considering the control of body temperature** | |
| Interleukin-1 mediates the febrile response | T |
| The pituitary is the main site for thermoregulatory control | F |
| Catecholamines increase heat loss | F |
| The rectal temperature is around 0.5 degrees below the oral T° | F |

# II. LEUKAEMIA

### 1. CLASSIFICATION
- Leukemias are a group of heterogeneous neoplastic disorders of white blood cells.
- Based on their origin, myeloid or lymphoid, they can be divided into two types.
- Acute leukemias usually present as hemorrhage, anaemia, infection, or infiltration of organs.
- Many patients with chronic leukemias are asymptomatic.
- Other patients present with splenomegaly, fever, weight loss, malaise, frequent infections, bleeding, thrombosis, or lymphadenopathy.

## 1. CHRONIC MYELOGENOUS LEUKEMIA (CML)
- It is characterized by an uncontrolled proliferation of granulocytes.
- An accompanying proliferation of erythroid cells and megakaryocytes is usually present.
- Many patients are asymptomatic but may present with splenomegaly, weight loss, malaise, bleeding or thrombosis.
- A blast crisis is diagnosed if any of the following features are present in a patient with CML:
  - > 20% myeloblasts or lymphoblasts in the blood or bone marrow.
  - Large clusters of blasts found on bone marrow biopsy.
  - The presence of a **chloroma** (a solid tumour comprised of myeloblasts that occurs outside of the bone marrow).
- CML can be treated with **tyrosine kinase inhibitors** such as **Imatinib** and **Dasatinib.**

## 2. CHRONIC LYMPHOCYTIC LEUKEMIA (CLL)
- Represents a monoclonal expansion of lymphocytes.
- In 95% of cases, CLL is a predominantly malignant clonal disorder of B lymphocytes.
- The remainder is secondary to a T-cell clone.
- There is primary involvement of the bone marrow and secondary release into the peripheral blood.
- The recirculating lymphocytes selectively infiltrate the lymph nodes, the spleen, and the liver.
- Most patients are asymptomatic at diagnosis.
- As the disease progresses, lymphadenopathy, splenomegaly, and hepatomegaly develop.
- Bone marrow infiltration exceeds 30% lymphocytes.
- **The lymphocytes are mature with less than 55% atypical or blast forms.**
- CLL is incurable; chemotherapy can be started for late symptomatic disease.

## 3. ACUTE LYMPHOCYTIC LEUKEMIA (ALL)
- It is a malignant clonal disorder of the bone marrow lymphopoietic precursor cells. In ALL, progressive medullary and extramedullary accumulations of lymphoblasts are present that lack the potential for differentiation and maturation.
- **The Philadelphia chromosome** (balanced translocation between chromosomes 9 and 22) is present in 5% of children and 25% of adults with ALL.
- The clinical presentation is dominated by progressive weakness and fatigue secondary to anaemia, infection secondary to leukopenia, and bleeding secondary to thrombocytopenia.
- When 50% of the bone marrow is replaced, then peripheral blood cytopenias are observed.
- Homogeneous infiltrate of lymphoblasts replaces the normal bone marrow elements.
- *Lymphoblasts stain negative for Sudan Black and peroxidase but positive with Periodic Acid-Schiff (PAS).*
- *Initial Rx to induce remission is chemotherapy with Prednisolone and Vincristine. Intrathecal Methotrexate is also used.*
- *Cure rate approximately 80%.*
- **Poor Prognosis Factors**:
  - ✓ **M**ale gender.
  - ✓ **W**hite cell count > 50 x 10$^9$/l at diagnosis
  - ✓ **A**ge < 1 or > 10 yrs.
  - ✓ **C**NS involvement
  - ✓ **A**ssociated Chromosome /Genetic disorder.

## 4. ACUTE MYELOGENOUS LEUKEMIA (AML)
- Is the most common acute leukaemia affecting adults
- It is a group of neoplastic disorders of the hematopoietic precursor cells of the bone marrow.
- AML is subdivided by the French-American-British (FAB) system into 6 categories depending on the morphology.
- The bone marrow is gradually replaced by blast cells.
- The most important complications are *progressive anaemia, leukopenia, and thrombocytopenia.* 30% of the nucleated cells in the aspirate must be blast cells of myeloid origin.
- *The presence of Auer rods is virtually diagnostic of AML, because these condensed lysosomal cytoplasmic azurophilic rod-shaped structures do not appear in ALL.*

- o *Myeloblasts stain Positive for Sudan Black and peroxidase but Negative with Periodic Acid-Schiff (PAS).*
- o Rx: Chemotherapy and Bone marrow transplantation in children (Methotrexate rarely required).
- o Generally poor prognosis.

## 2. EPIDEMIOLOGY

- ALL is the most common type of leukaemia in children **(2-5years)**.
- 4/5 of all leukaemia diagnosed in children is this type.
- Although leukaemia is the most common cancer of childhood, more than 9 in 10 cases are diagnosed in adults.
- Almost 4 in 10 cases (40%) of leukaemia are diagnosed in people aged 75 or older, and around half (50%) are in people aged 70 or older.
- **Mortality/ Morbidity**
  - o When all leukemias are lumped together, the global 5-year survival is 20%.
  - o In the UK in 2012, around 4,800 people died from leukaemia, that's 13 people every day.
  - o More than half (56%) of deaths from leukaemia are in people aged 75 and over.
- **Races** : Whites> blacks
- **Sex** : Males> females
- **Age** : Most childhood leukemias are acute.

- o **ALL** is the most common malignancy in children, especially affecting those aged 2-10 years. **ALL** is seen in only **20%** of adult acute leukemias and behaves more aggressively than the childhood type.
- o **AML** constitutes **15-20%** of acute leukemias in children.
- o Incidence of **AML** increases with age; in persons younger than 65 years, the incidence is 1.3, and in persons older than 65 years, the incidence is 12.2.
- o **CML** constitutes less than **5%** of childhood leukemias.
- o The incidence of CML increases slowly with age until the middle 40s, when the incidence starts to rise rapidly.
- o Incidence of **CLL** is over 10 per 100,000 for persons older than 70 years but is less than 1 per 100,000 for those younger than 50 years.
- o Mean age at diagnosis of CLL is 60 years.

## 3. LABORATORY STUDIES

➢ **FBC and Differential**
- **To diagnose CLL:**
  - Lymphocytosis > 5000/mm³.
  - Neutrophil count normal
  - RBC counts and Platelet counts are mildly decreased.
  - In addition, **the peripheral smear or bone marrow should show normal mature small lymphocytes with less than 55% atypical or blast forms.**
- **To diagnose CML:**
  - Leukocytosis > 100,000/mm³.
  - The differential count shows that neutrophil precursors are present.
  - This is accompanied by basophilia and eosinophilia.
  - 90% of cases have the **Philadelphia chromosome.**
  - Unlike those in AML, these cells are mature and functional.
➢ **Bone Marrow Aspiration**

# III. MULTIPLE MYELOMA

- Also known as **plasma cell myeloma**, **myelomatosis**, or **Kahler's disease,** is a cancer of plasma cells. In multiple myeloma, collections of abnormal plasma cells accumulate in the bone marrow, where they interfere with the production of normal blood cells.
- *Most cases of multiple myeloma also feature the production of a paraprotein (IgG), an abnormal antibody which can cause kidney problems.*
- *Bone lesions and hypercalcemia are often encountered.*
- *Decreased albumin level and increased protein level as a result of high IgG.*

**DIAGNOSIS:**
- o   Serum protein electrophoresis.
- o   Serum free kappa/lambda light chain assay.
- o   Bone marrow examination.
- o   Urine protein electrophoresis (Bence jones proteins).
- o   X-rays of commonly involved bones.
- Multiple myeloma is considered to be incurable but treatable.
- Remissions may be induced with **steroids**, **chemotherapy**, **Proteasome Inhibitors**, **Immunomodulatory Drugs** such as **Thalidomide or Lenalidomide**, and **stem cell transplants.**
- Radiation therapy is sometimes used to reduce pain from bone lesions.

**EPIDEMIOLOGY:**
- o   More common in men.
- o   With conventional treatment, median survival is 3–4 years, which may be extended to 5–7 years or longer with advanced treatments.
- o   The five-year survival rate is 45%.

**CLINICAL PRESENTATIONS:**
- o   **Bone pain:** 70% of patients (most common symptom).
- o   **Anaemia:**  Normocytic and Normochromic.
- o   **Kidney failure:**
  - ▪   Due to proteins secreted by the malignant cells.
  - ▪   Other causes include hyperuricemia, recurrent infections (pyelonephritis), and local infiltration of tumor cells.
- o   **Infections:** Pneumonias and Pyelonephritis.
- o   **Neurological:**
  - ▪   Weakness, confusion and fatigue may be due to anaemia or hypercalcemia.
  - ▪   Headache, visual changes and retinopathy may be the result of hyperviscosity of the blood.

# IV. LYMPHOMA

### 1. DEFINITION
- Lymphoma is cancer of the lymph system (or lymphatic system), which is part of our immunity.
- It is characterized by the formation of solid tumors in the immune system.
- Lymphoma is currently the fifth most common cancer diagnosed by clinicians in the UK (after breast, lung, colon and prostate cancers).
- It is the most common blood cancer.
- Lymphoma can occur at any age; it is the most common cancer affecting those under the age of 30 and around 1 in 10 cancers diagnosed in children are lymphomas.
- About 90% of lymphomas are the non-Hodgkin's type while about 10% are Hodgkin's

### 2. CLASSIFICATION
- Lymphatic cancers are classified by the type of immune cells affected.

## A. NON-HODGKIN'S LYMPHOMA
- o   It is more common in people aged over 55.
- o   Can be classified by the type of lymphocyte they develop from.
- o   Lymphocytes are either B cells or T cells, so non-Hodgkin lymphomas can be divided into either B-cell lymphoma (the majority) or T-cell lymphomas.
- o   Some types grow slowly (low-grade lymphomas) and others grow at a faster rate (high-grade lymphomas).
- o   Sometimes, a lymphoma changes ('transforms') from a slow-growing type to a faster-growing type. This is known as *transformation*.
- o   The lymphoma then has to be treated as a high-grade lymphoma.

## 1. HIGH-GRADE NON-HODGKIN LYMPHOMA

- Also called "aggressive" lymphomas.
- Cells appear to be dividing quite quickly.
- Some types will grow faster than others.
- More common in people aged over 50, but they can occur at any age, including in children.
- Generally, respond very well to treatment.
- The high-grade non-Hodgkin lymphomas include:
  - **B-cell non-Hodgkin lymphomas**
    - ✓ Diffuse large B-cell lymphoma – this is the most common type of high-grade lymphoma
    - ✓ Burkitt lymphoma
    - ✓ Mantle cell lymphoma
    - ✓ Primary mediastinal B-cell lymphoma
    - ✓ Primary central nervous system lymphoma.
  - **T-cell non-Hodgkin lymphomas**
    - ✓ Peripheral T-cell lymphoma
    - ✓ Anaplastic large cell lymphoma
    - ✓ Angioimmunoblastic T-cell lymphoma (AITL)
    - ✓ Enteropathy-associated T-cell lymphoma
    - ✓ Adult T-cell leukaemia/lymphoma
    - ✓ Nasal-type NK/T-cell lymphoma.

## 2. LOW-GRADE NON-HODGKIN LYMPHOMA

- Also called 'indolent' non-Hodgkin lymphomas.
- Cells appear to be dividing slowly.
- This means that low-grade non-Hodgkin lymphoma can take a long time to develop.
- The low-grade non-Hodgkin lymphomas include:
  - ✓ Follicular lymphoma – the most common type of low-grade non-Hodgkin lymphoma.
  - ✓ Chronic lymphocytic leukaemia/small lymphocytic lymphoma
  - ✓ Lymphoplasmacytic lymphoma (Waldenström's macroglobulinaemia)
  - ✓ Gastric MALT lymphoma
  - ✓ Non-gastric MALT lymphoma
  - ✓ Splenic marginal zone lymphoma
  - ✓ Nodal marginal zone lymphoma.
- Most people have advanced-stage low-grade non-Hodgkin lymphoma by the time they are diagnosed. Advanced-stage low-grade non-Hodgkin lymphomas (stage III or IV) are more difficult to cure completely.
- Low-grade non-Hodgkin lymphomas are more common in older people and are very rare in children and young adults.

## B. HODGKIN'S LYMPHOMA:

- The cancer cells are usually an abnormal type of B lymphocyte, named ***Reed-Sternberg cells***.
- Affects more men than women.
- There are a number of different types of Hodgkin lymphoma:
  - Nodular sclerosis
  - Mixed cellularity
  - Lymphocyte-rich (Predominant): Good Prognosis
  - Lymphocyte-depleted: worst prognosis
- The majority of people with Hodgkin lymphoma will be completely cured.
- The **Ann Arbour** clinical staging is as follows:
  - **Stage I:** one involved lymph node group.
  - **Stage II:** two involved lymph node groups on one side of the diaphragm.
  - **Stage III:** lymph node groups involved on both sides of the diaphragm.
  - **Stage IV:** Involvement of extra-nodal tissues, such as the liver or bone marrow.
- **Risk factors for Hodgkin's lymphoma:**
  - Male gender
  - Age 15-40 and age >55
  - Positive family history
  - Epstein - Barr virus infection
  - Immunosuppression including HIV
- **Good Prognostic indicators in Hodgkin's lymphoma:**
  - Young age at presentation
  - Histology: lymphocyte predominant (best prognosis) > nodular sclerosing > mixed cellularity > lymphocyte depleted (worst prognosis)
  - Lower Ann Arbour staging

## 3. SIGNS AND SYMPTOMS OF LYMPHOMA

- The most common sign of lymphoma is a painless lump or swelling, often in the neck, armpit or groin.
- Some lymphomas can develop without any obvious lump.
- Instead, the first thing noticed may be symptoms which can include: **FEW**
  - **F**evers
  - **E**xcessive sweating, especially at night
  - **W**eight loss (unexplained)
    (The above three are known as 'B symptoms')
  - unusual tiredness and persistent itching

o    coughing or breathlessness
o    Abdominal pain or diarrhoea.

## 4. INVESTIGATIONS
- The first test is an examination of any lump noticed.
- a lymph node biopsy
- Blood tests.
- CT scan (computed tomography)
- PET/CT scan
- MRI scan (magnetic resonance imaging) and Ultrasound scan.

## 5. TREATMENT
## A. TREATMENT OF HODGKIN LYMPHOMA
- Many people who have Hodgkin lymphoma will be cured.
- **Early-stage:**
  o    Short course of chemotherapy and radiotherapy to the enlarged lymph nodes.
- **Advanced-stage:**
  o    Longer course of chemotherapy.
  o    Some people will have radiotherapy.
- The chemotherapy is usually made up of several different chemotherapy drugs and is known as '**combination chemotherapy**'.
- Combination chemotherapies are often named after the initials of the drugs used.
- One of the most commonly used regimens is called **ABVD** because it consists of **A**driamycin, **B**leomycin, **V**inblastine and **D**acarbazine.

## B. TREATMENT OF HIGH-GRADE NON-HODGKIN LYMPHOMA
- Many people who have high-grade non-Hodgkin lymphoma will be cured.
- High-grade non-Hodgkin lymphoma is almost always treated with intravenous combination chemotherapy.
- The type of chemotherapy most commonly used for high-grade non-Hodgkin lymphoma is called **CHOP**, so called because it is made up of the four drugs:
  ✓    **C**yclophosphamide
  ✓    **H**ydroxydaunorubicin
  ✓    **O**ncovin® (also called vincristine)
  ✓    **P**rednisolone.
- Most people with a B-cell lymphoma will be given their **CHOP** with the addition of the drug **R**ituximab, so the treatment is known as '**R-CHOP**'.
- Rituximab is an antibody that helps the immune system to kill the lymphoma cells.
- Rituximab is not suitable for T-cell lymphomas so CHOP chemotherapy alone or a different combination regimen will be used for these lymphomas.
- Some people with high-grade non-Hodgkin lymphoma will have treatment with high doses of chemotherapy or radiotherapy and a stem cell transplant.

## C. TREATMENT OF LOW-GRADE NON-HODGKIN LYMPHOMA
- '**Watch and wait**': this is known as active monitoring of patients with low-grade non-Hodgkin lymphoma when they feel well.
- The active treatments in use are:
- *Combination chemotherapy plus rituximab*:
  o    **R-CVP**
      ✓    **R**ituximab
      ✓    **C**yclophosphamide,
      ✓    **V**incristine
      ✓    **P**rednisolone
  o    **R-CHOP**
  o    **CVP**: Combination chemotherapy on its own
- *Tablet chemotherapy.*
- *Rituximab maintenance therapy*: given once every 2–3 months for a maximum of 2 years.
- *Radiotherapy* may be offered to people whose low-grade non-Hodgkin lymphoma is confined to one area. This is uncommon.
- Sometimes rituximab is used on its own for people who have disease that does not respond to chemotherapy.
- Some people with low-grade non-Hodgkin lymphoma may be offered treatments such as a *stem cell transplant.*

# V. BLEEDING AND BLOOD CLOTTING

## 1. SIGNIFICANCE OF HEMOSTASIS

- When vessels are damaged, there are three mechanisms that promote haemostasis:
- **Vasoconstriction**: there is an immediate reflex, following damage that promotes reducing blood loss.
- **Platelet adhesion**: Collagen exposed from the damaged site will promote adhesion of platelets.
  - When platelets adhere to the damaged vessel, they undergo degranulation and release cytoplasmic granules, which contain serotonin, ADP and Thromboxane $A_2$.
    - Serotonin: vasoconstrictor
    - ADP: attracts more platelets to the area
    - Thromboxane $A_2$: promotes platelet aggregation, degranulation, and vasoconstriction.
- Thus, ADP and thromboxane A2 promote more platelet adhesion and therefore more ADP and thromboxane.
- **Formation of platelet plug**: by the *positive feedback mechanism*. The process of coagulation can now start:
  - *Damaged tissue releases factor III (tissue factor or tissue thromboplastin), which with the aid of $Ca^{++}$ will activate factor VII, thus initiating the Extrinsic Mechanism.*
  - *Factor XII from active platelets will activate factor XI, thus initiating the Intrinsic Mechanism.*
  - Both active factor VII and active factor XI will promote cascade reactions, eventually activating factor X.
  - Active factor X, along with factor III, factor V, $Ca^{++}$, and platelet thromboplastic factor ($PF_3$), will activate prothrombin activator.
  - Prothrombin activator converts prothrombin to thrombin.
  - Thrombin converts fibrinogen to fibrin.
  - Fibrin initially forms a loose mesh, but then factor XIII causes the formation of covalent cross links, which convert fibrin to a dense aggregation of fibers.
  - Platelets and red blood cells become caught in this mesh of fiber, thus the formation of a blood clot.

## 2. COAGULATION CASCADE

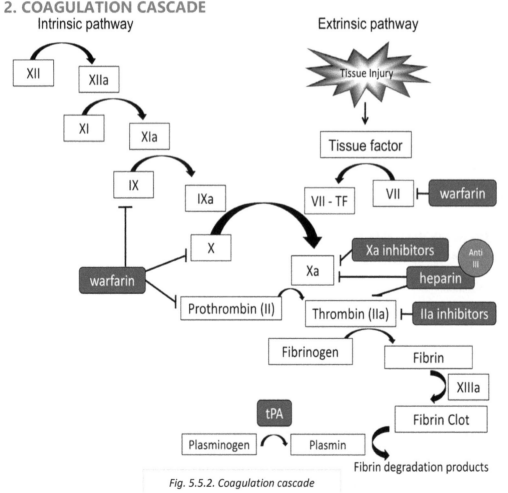

*Fig. 5.5.2. Coagulation cascade*

- **Factor I:** Fibrinogen
- **Factor II:** Prothrombin
- **Factor III:** Thromboplastin/ Tissue factor
- **Factor IV:** Calcium ion
- **Factor V:** Proaccelerin / Labile factor / Ac-globulin (Ac-G)
- **Factor VII:** Cothromboplastin, Proconvertin, stable factor
- **Factor VIII:** Anti-haemolytic factor / Antihemophilic factor (AHF) or globulin (AHG) / antihemophilic factor A
- **Factor IX:** Christmas factor / Plasma thromboplastin component (PTC) / Antihemophilic factor B
- **Factor X:** Stuart Prower factor / Stuart factor
- **Factor XI:** Plasma thromboplastin antecedent (PTA)/antihemophilic factor C
- **Factor XII:** Hageman factor
- **Factor XIII:** Fibrin stabilizing factor

# 3. INHIBITION OF CLOTTING

- After the activation of the blood-clotting system, the active enzymes must be turned off and the clotting process contained locally to the area of tissue injury.
- The details of the regulation of blood coagulation remain obscure, but it is clear that a series of blood proteins play a specialized role in disengaging the activated blood-clotting system.

## A. ANTITHROMBIN III
- o  A plasma protein that combines with thrombin as well as most of the other activated blood-clotting proteins (e.g. factors Xa and IXa) to form inert complexes.
- o  This action is greatly enhanced by the presence of heparin, a substance formed by mast cells of the connective tissue.
- o  The hereditary deficiency of antithrombin III is associated with an excessive tendency toward clot formation, and manifestations of this defect are recurrent thrombophlebitis and pulmonary embolism.

## B. HEPARIN COFACTOR II
- o  Another plasma protease inhibitor that specifically forms a complex with thrombin, thus inactivating this enzyme.
- o  Heparin is an Antithrombin agent.

## C. PROTEIN C AND S
- o  Vitamin K-dependent proteins.
- o  A zymogen that requires vitamin K for its activation by thrombin complexed to thrombomodulin, a protein on the endothelial cell membrane. Activated protein C is capable of inactivating the active cofactor forms of factors VIII and V.
- o  Its action is enhanced when bound to protein S, a vitamin K-dependent protein that is attached to cell membranes (platelet or possibly endothelial cells).
- o  A deficiency in the level of protein C or protein S is associated with an excessive tendency to form clots.

## D. PLASMIN
- o  An enzyme that catalyses the removal of old fibrin at injury sites and any which may be deposited in normal vessels.
- o  Plasmin is derived from plasminogen, an inert protein precursor that can be activated by tissue plasminogen activator.
- o  Streptokinase, urokinase, and tissue plasminogen activator are drugs that activate plasminogen and lead to the dissolution of clots.

# 4. SYNTHESIS OF BLOOD-CLOTTING PROTEINS

- Most of the blood coagulation proteins are synthesized in the liver (**Except III & IV (34))**.
- In addition, factor VIII is synthesized in a large number of other tissues.
- Six proteins involved in blood coagulation require vitamin K for their complete synthesis: factor IX, factor X, prothrombin (II), factor VII, protein C, and protein S. (**910-27CS**).
- In a region of the liver cell called the rough endoplasmic reticulum, specific glutamic acid residues form a modified glutamic acid known as *γ-carboxyglutamic acid.* This enzyme reaction, known as γ-carboxylation, requires vitamin K as a cofactor.
- *γ-Carboxyglutamic acid is a unique amino acid that binds to calcium*.
- In the protein, γ-carboxyglutamic acids form the calcium-binding sites that characterize this form of calcium-binding protein, the vitamin K-dependent proteins.
- Calcium stabilizes certain structural forms of the vitamin K-dependent proteins, enabling these proteins to bind to cell membranes.
- In the absence of vitamin K or in the presence of vitamin K antagonists such as warfarin, γ-carboxylation is inhibited and proteins are synthesized that are deficient in γ-carboxyglutamic acid.

# 5. ERYTHROPOIETIN

- Erythropoietin is produced by the **liver** during fetal life.
- After birth, the **kidneys** constitute the major source of production.
- Erythropoietin as an antiapoptotic, a member of **class 1 cytokines**.
- Erythropoietin is secreted by **fibroblasts in the renal cortex**.
- These cells possess specific regulatory mechanisms, called **hypoxia-inducible factors (HIFs)**, which, under hypoxic conditions, stimulate the production of erythropoietin, which stimulates the production of erythrocytes.
- **INDICATIONS/APPLICATIONS:**
  - o  Erythropoietin testing, in combination with other tests, can be used to differentiate polycythaemia vera from secondary polycythemia.
  - o  It can also help differentiate between appropriate and inappropriate secondary polycythemia.
  - o  In some conditions, erythropoietin testing can be used in the assessment and differentiation of anemia, especially in patients receiving erythropoietin replacement therapy with an inadequate response.
  - o  Erythropoietin has been used as a doping agent, since it can improve performance by improving tissue oxygenation.

# VI. COAGULATION DISORDERS

## 1. DEFINITION
- Coagulation disorders deal with disruption of the body's ability to control blood clotting. The most commonly known coagulation disorder is hemophilia, a condition in which patients bleed for long periods of time before clotting.

## 2. DESCRIPTION
- Coagulation, or clotting, occurs as a complex process involving several components of the blood.
- Plasma, the fluid component of the blood, carries a number of proteins and coagulation factors that regulate bleeding.
- Platelets, small colorless fragments in the blood, initiate contraction of damaged blood vessels so that less blood is lost.
- They also help plug damaged blood vessels and work with plasma to accelerate blood clotting.
- A disorder affecting platelet production or one of the many steps in the entire process can disrupt clotting.
- Coagulation disorders arise from different causes and produce different complications.
- Some common coagulation disorders are:

## A. HAEMOPHILIA
- Haemophilia A affects 1 in 5000 males (1/10 000 males).
- Haemophilia B affects 1 in 50,000 males. Haemophilia C is a mild form of haemophilia that occurs in both sexes. It predominantly affects Ashkenazi Jews.
- Haemophilia A is an **X-linked recessive disorder**.
- Mild and severe haemophilia A are inherited through a complex genetic system that passes a recessive gene on the female chromosome.
- **Women usually do not show signs of haemophilia but are carriers of the disease.** Each male child of the carrier has a 50% chance of having haemophilia, and each female child has a 50% chance of passing the gene on.
- Factor IX has a longer half-life than factor VIII, therefore patients with haemophilia B require treatment less frequently than those with Haemophilia A. Because of its hereditary nature, haemophilia A may be suspected before symptoms occur.
- Some signs of haemophilia A are numerous large, deep bruises and pain and swelling of joints caused by internal bleeding.
  - *In both haemophilia, A and B, there is spontaneous bleeding and:*
    - *Normal bleeding time (BT)*
    - *Normal prothrombin time (PT)*
    - *Normal thrombin time (TT)*
    - *Prolonged partial thromboplastin time (PTT)*
- A person with mild haemophilia may first discover the disorder with prolonged bleeding following a surgical procedure.

## B. CHRISTMAS DISEASE
- Christmas disease, or haemophilia B, is also hereditary but less common than haemophilia A.
- The severity of Christmas disease varies from mild to severe, although mild cases are more common.
- The severity depends on the degree of deficiency of the Factor IX (clotting factor).
- Haemophilia B symptoms are similar to those of haemophilia A, including numerous, large and deep bruises and prolonged bleeding.
- The more dangerous symptoms are those that represent possible internal bleeding, such as swelling of joints, or bleeding into internal organs upon trauma.
- Haemophilia most often occurs in families with a known history of the disease, but occasionally, new cases will occur in families with no apparent history.

## C. THROMBOCYTOPENIA
- Thrombocytopenia may be acquired or congenital.
- Heparin, quinine and sulphonamides are commonly implicated drugs in thrombocytopenia.
- It represents a defective or decreased production of platelets.
- Symptoms include sudden onset of small spots of hemorrhage on the skin, or bleeding into mucous membranes.
- Some patients show none of these symptoms, but complain of fatigue and general weakness.
- There are several causes of thrombocytopenia, which is more commonly acquired as a result of another disorder.
- Common underlying disorders include leukaemia, drug toxicity, or aplastic anaemia, all of which lead to decreased or defective production of platelets in the bone marrow.
- Other diseases may destroy platelets outside the marrow.
- These include severe infection, disseminated intravascular coagulation, and cirrhosis of the liver.

## IDIOPATHIC THROMBOCYTOPENIC PURPURA (ITP)

- **Acute ITP** is more common in children and has an equal sex distribution.
- **Chronic ITP** is more common in young to middle aged women.
- Idiopathic (Immune) thrombocytopenic purpura (ITP) is a clinical syndrome in which a decreased number of circulating platelets **(thrombocytopenia)** manifests as a **bleeding tendency, easy bruising (purpura)**, or **extravasation of blood** from capillaries into skin and mucous membranes **(petechiae)**.
- In many cases ITP's cause **is autoimmune** not idiopathic, with antibodies against platelets being detected in approximately 60% patients. A preceding illness is the usual likely trigger. Idiopathic thrombocytopenic purpura (ITP) is a condition of an abnormally low platelet count with no known cause, although in approximately 60% of cases antibodies against platelets are detected.
- **Clinical features include:**
  - *Purpuric rash.*
  - *Mucous membrane bleeding*
  - *Conjunctival haemorrhage*
  - *Occasionally gastrointestinal bleeding*
- *Children may be suspected of suffering from non-accidental injury due to the ease of bruising and bleeding*
- ***Note—the presence of lymphadenopathy, hepatomegaly or splenomegaly suggests an alternative diagnosis e.g. leukaemia.***
- The most important investigation is a **full blood count.**
- Platelets will be **< 30×10$^9$/L.**
- Children should be referred on for paediatric review.
- Treatment is usually expectant because most cases resolve spontaneously over 3 months. Occasionally life-threatening haemorrhage occurs and patients should be managed in the usual ABCDE manner and resuscitated accordingly.

## D. VON WILLEBRAND'S DISEASE

- Is caused by a defect in the Von Willebrand clotting factor, often accompanied by a deficiency of Factor VIII as well.
- It is a hereditary disorder that affects both males and females.
- In rare cases, it may be acquired. Symptoms include easy bruising, bleeding in small cuts that stops and starts, abnormal bleeding after surgery, and abnormally heavy menstrual bleeding.
- Nosebleeds and blood in the stool with a black, tarlike appearance are also signs of Von Willebrand's disease.

## E. HYPOPROTHROMBINEMIA

- This disorder is a deficiency in prothrombin, or Factor II, a glycoprotein formed and stored in the liver.
- Prothrombin, under the right conditions, is converted to thrombin, which activates fibrin and begins the process of coagulation.
- Some patients may show no symptoms, and others will suffer severe haemorrhaging. Patients may experience easy bruising, profuse nosebleeds, postpartum hemorrhage, excessively prolonged or heavy menstrual bleeding, and postsurgical hemorrhage.
- Hypoprothrombinaemia may also be acquired rather than inherited, and usually results from a Vitamin K deficiency caused by liver diseases, newborn haemorrhagic disease, or a number of other factors.

### 3. DIAGNOSIS

- **Hemophilia A** will be diagnosed with laboratory tests detecting presence or absence of clotting factor VIII, factor IX, and others, as well as the presence or absence of clotting factor inhibitors.
- **Christmas disease** will be checked against normal bleeding and clotting time, as well as for abnormal serum reagents in factor IX deficiency. Other tests of prothrombin time and thromboplastic generation may also be ordered.
- **Thrombocytopenia** tests include coagulation tests revealing a decreased platelet count, prolonged bleeding time, and other measurements.
- If these tests indicate that platelet destruction is causing the disorder, bone marrow examination may be ordered.
- **Von Willebrand's disease** will be diagnosed with the assistance of laboratory tests which show prolonged bleeding time, absent or reduced levels of factor VIII, normal platelet count, and others.
- **Hypothrombinemia** is diagnosed with history information and the use of tests that measure vitamin K deficiency, deficiency of prothrombin, and clotting factors V, VII, IX, and X.
- **Factor XI deficiency** is diagnosed most often after injury-related bleeding. Blood tests can help pinpoint factor VII deficiency.

### 4. TREATMENT

- **Hemophilia A** in mild episodes may require infusion of a drug called **Desmopressin or DDAVP**.
- Severe bleeding episodes will require transfusions of human blood clotting factors.
- **Christmas disease** patients are treated similarly to hemophilia A patients. Superficial wounds can be cleaned and bandaged. Parents of hemophiliac children receiving immunizations should inform the vaccination provider in advance to decrease the possibility of bleeding problems. These children should probably not receive injections which go into the muscle.
- **Secondary acquired thrombocytopenia** is best alleviated by treating the underlying cause or disorder.
- The specific treatment may depend on the underlying cause. Sometimes, corticosteroids or immune globulin may be given to improve platelet production.

- **Von Willebrand's** disease is treated by several methods to reduce bleeding time and to replace factor VIII, which consequently will replace the Von Willebrand factor.
- This may include infusion of cryoprecipitate or fresh frozen plasma. Desmopressin may also help raise levels of the Von Willebrand factor.
- **Hypoprothrombinemia** may be treated with concentrates of prothrombin.
- Vitamin K may also be produced, and in bleeding episodes, the patient may receive fresh plasma products.
- **Factor XI** (hemophilia C) is most often treated with plasma, since there are no commercially available concentrates of factor XI.
- **Factor VII** patients may be treated with prothrombin complex concentrates.

### Causes of a prolonged bleeding time include:
- ✓ Thrombocytopenia,
- ✓ DIC
- ✓ Vitamin C deficiency
- ✓ Von Willebrand disease
- ✓ Glanzmann's thrombasthenia
- ✓ Bernard-Soulier syndrome
- ✓ Aspirin and NSAIDS

### BLOOD TESTS
- ✓ **INR:** testing extrinsic system
- ✓ **APTT:** testing intrinsic system
- ✓ **PT:** Extrinsic and common pathways

### Investigation of bleeding disorders: if:
- ✓ **Low Platelet:** do FBC, Film, Bone Marrow biopsy
- ✓ **High INR:** look for liver disease, use of anticoagulant
- ✓ **High APTT:** consider factor VIII/IX deficiency or heparin
- ✓ **Elevated Bleeding Time:** consider vWD or Platelet Disorder

### TESTS OF COAGULATION

| Screening test | Coagulation abnormality | Normal time | Disorder |
|---|---|---|---|
| **Thrombin time (TT)** | Defisciency or abnormality of fibrinogen or inhibition of thrombin by fibrin | 14-16sec | **DIC** **Heparin** |
| **Prothrombin time (PT)** **Extrinsic and common pathways** | Defisciency or inhibition of factors VII, X, V, II | 10-14sec | **DIC** **Liver** **Warfarin** |
| **Activated partial Thromboplastin time (aPTT)** **Intrinsic Pathway** | Defisciency or inhibition of factors XII, IX (Xmas disease), VIII (haemophilia), X, V, II, fibrinogen | 30-40sec | **Haemophilia** **Christmas Disease and as above** |

### CAUSES OF PROLONGED PROTHROMBIN TIME (PT) AND ACTIVATED PARTIAL THROMBOPLASTIN TIME (APTT)

| Prolonged PT | Prolonged aPTT | Prolonged PT and aPTT |
|---|---|---|
| **Inherited** | | |
| Factor VII deficiency | vWF, factor VIII, IX, XI, or XII deficiency | Prothrombin, fibrinogen, factor V, X or combined factor deficiency |
| (7) | (v89-11/12) | (21-510) |
| **Acquired** | | |
| Vitamin K deficiency | Heparin use | Liver disease |
| Liver disease | Inhibitor of vWF, factors VIII, IX, XI or XII | DIC |
| Warfarin use | Antiphospholipid antibodies | Supratherapeutic heparin or warfarin |
| Factor VII inhibitor | | Combined heparin or warfarin use |
| | | Inhibitor of prothrombin fibrinogen, factor V or X |
| | | Direct thrombin inhibitor |

# VII. THROMBOSIS

**CAUSES:**
- Factor V Leiden (5% population)
- Protein C or S deficiency (these inhibit factors V and VIII)
- Antithrombin deficiency
- Antiphospholipid syndrome

## A. PROTEIN C DEFICIENCY

- It is a congenital or acquired condition that leads to increased risk for thrombosis. Congenital protein C deficiency is one of several inherited thrombophilias, which are a heterogeneous group of genetic disorders associated with an elevated risk of venous thromboembolism.

### 1. GENETICS OF PROTEIN C DEFICIENCY

- Heterozygous protein C deficiency is **inherited in an autosomal dominant fashion.** The mutations are divided into 2 types (type I and type II) on the basis of whether they cause a quantitative (type I) or functional (type II) deficiency of protein C.

### A. TYPE I DEFICIENCY

- Type I protein C deficiency refers to a quantitative deficiency in the plasma protein C concentration.

### B. TYPE II DEFICIENCY

- Type II protein C deficiency is less common than type I disease, and is associated with decreased functional activity and normal immunologic levels of protein C.

### 2. MORTALITY/MORBIDITY

- Clinical manifestations of heterozygous protein C deficiency include **VTE** (venous thromboembolism) and warfarin-induced skin necrosis (**WISN**). *Heterozygous protein C deficiency does not appear to be associated with an elevated risk of arterial thrombosis*
- Whether the risk of pregnancy loss is increased in this disorder is controversial.
- Homozygous and compound heterozygous protein C deficiency are classically associated with neonatal purpura fulminans (**NPF**).
- Occasionally, patients present with VTE in childhood or adolescence.

## B. PROTEIN S DEFICIENCY

- Protein S, a vitamin K-dependent protein, is made by the liver and acts as the principal cofactor to protein C.
- Hereditary protein S is an **autosomal dominant trait.** Protein S exists as two forms in the blood circulation: **Free form** and **bound form.**
- Approximately 60% to 65% of total protein S in the circulation exists in the bound form and ~35% to 40% in the free form.
- Free protein S is the form involved in the activated protein C (APC) blood thinning activity.
- There are three subtypes of protein S deficiency.
  - **Type I deficiency:** The decrease in the activity of protein S is proportional to the decrease in the level of protein S.
  - **Type II deficiency:** The levels of the free and bound forms of the protein are normal, but they do not function properly because of a gene alteration.
  - **Type III deficiency:** There is a normal level of total protein S, but the level of free protein S is abnormally low.
- Protein S deficiency can also be acquired due to vitamin K deficiency or treatment with warfarin, systemic sex hormone therapy and pregnancy, liver disease, and certain chronic infections (example HIV).
- Vitamin K deficiency or treatment with warfarin generally also impairs the coagulation system itself (factors II, VII, IX and X), and therefore predisposes to bleeding rather than thrombosis. Protein S deficiency is the underlying cause of a small proportion of cases of disseminated intravascular coagulation (DIC), deep venous thrombosis (DVT) and pulmonary embolism (PE).

## C. ANTIPHOSPHOLIPID SYNDROME (APS)

- The antiphospholipid syndrome is a disorder of the immune system that is characterized by excessive clotting of blood and/or certain complications of pregnancy (premature miscarriages, unexplained fetal death, or premature birth) and the presence of antiphospholipid antibodies in the blood.
- Clotting disorders associated with antiphospholipid syndrome include deep venous thrombosis (DVT) and pulmonary embolism (PE).
- Patients with antiphospholipid syndrome have both blood clots and antiphospholipid antibodies that are detectable with blood testing.
- It is a disorder that manifests clinically as recurrent venous or arterial thrombosis and/or fetal loss.
- Characteristic laboratory abnormalities in APS include:
  - Persistently elevated levels of antibodies directed against membrane anionic phospholipids (ie, anticardiolipin [aCL] antibody, antiphosphatidylserine) or their associated plasma proteins,
  - Predominantly beta-2 glycoprotein I (apolipoprotein H).
  - Evidence of a circulating anticoagulant.

- APS is more common in young to middle-aged adults; however, it also manifests in children and elderly people.
- *APL syndrome is the cause of 14% of all strokes, 11% of myocardial infarctions, 10% of deep vein thromboses, 6% of pregnancy morbidity, and 9% of pregnancy losses.*
- Up to 5% of healthy individuals are known to have APL antibodies.
- Life-long treatment with **warfarin** is standard for recurrent thrombotic events.
- For obstetric patients with antiphospholipid syndrome (APS), the standard therapy is **subcutaneous LMWH and low-dose aspirin**.
- Patients who require heparin administration throughout pregnancy should receive calcium and vitamin D supplementation to help avoid heparin-induced osteoporosis. When monitoring heparin therapy, note that the **aPTT may be unreliable** in the presence of circulating LA with a baseline elevated aPTT.
- In this case, factor Xa may be helpful. The antithrombotic properties of **hydroxychloroquine** have long been recognized and may be considered in the prophylactic treatment of a patient with SLE and a positive aPL antibody test result.

## FACTOR V LEIDEN
- *A rare autosomal dominant condition resulting in thrombophilia.*
- *Most patients are heterozygous for the condition and present with venous thromboembolism.*
- *The risk is increased even further for those on Oestrogen-containing contraceptives and HRT, but still remain low and general screening is not indicated.*

# Past Asked Questions

| In patients with sickle cell disease | |
|---|---|
| It is an autosomal dominant disease | F |
| The primary defect is in the heme moieties of haemoglobin molecules | F |
| HbS undergoes polymerization when deoxygenated | T |
| During a crisis, microvascular occlusion depends upon the number of sickle cells | F |
| **A Patient with Hemolytic Anaemia may also have:** | |
| Helmet cells seen on the blood film | T |
| Jaundice | T |
| A positive direct Coombs test | T |
| Sternotomy Scar | T |
| **Appropriate function of the coagulation cascade requires:** | |
| Factor VIII binding to exposed collagen of damaged blood vessels | F |
| Carboxylation of factors II, VII, IX and X by vitamin K dependant enzymes | T |
| Conversion of fibrinogen to fibrin by plasmin | F |
| Activation of protein C and Protein S | T |
| **Regarding Heparin and its role in anticoagulation** | |
| Causes thrombocytopaenia | T |
| aPTT is a measure of extrinsic clotting pathway | F |
| Exerts its anticoagulant effect through binding and activating thrombin and factor Xa | F |
| In high dose, can be used to lyse established thrombus | F |
| **Erythropoeitin:** | |
| Is a cytokine? | T |
| Is released from the peritubular fibroblasts of the bone marrow? | F |
| Stimulates maturation of normoblasts into reticulocytes? | T |
| Is upregulated by persistent hypercabia? | F |
| **Investigation of a tiredness in an otherwise well 60yr old patient reveals the following FBC results: Hb 7.1, WCC 6.4, Platelets 256, MCV 114:** | |
| The anaemia results from a failure of DNA synthesis | T |
| A deficiency of intrinsic factor is the most likely cause of the abnormal results | T |
| This patient should be treated with blood transfusion | F |
| **The following statements are true of the blood grouping:** | |
| A personal with blood group O can donate blood to individuals of any ABO blood group (universal donor) but receive blood only from a group O individual | T |
| Donors with blood group B will carry antibodies to the A antigen in their serum | T |
| Maternal anti_RhD antibodies can pass across the placenta | T |
| Donor platelets must be screened for ABO compatibility but not Rh compatibility | F |

# Part Six: Evidence Based Medicine

Compiled and Edited by:
**Dr Moussa Issa**
MBChB MRCEM
Senior ED Registrar

# SECTION 1. BASIC OF EVIDENCE BASED MEDICINE

## I. DEFINITIONS

- Evidence-based medicine (EBM) is the process of systematically reviewing, appraising and using clinical research findings to aid the delivery of optimum clinical care to patients.

## 2. THE EVIDENCE HIERARCHY: WHAT IS THE "BEST EVIDENCE"?

- What is "the best available evidence"? The hierarchy of evidence is a core principal of Evidence-Based Practice (EBP) and attempts to address this question. The evidence hierarchy allows you to take a top-down approach to locating the best evidence whereby you first search for a recent well-conducted systematic review and if that is not available, then move down to the next level of evidence to answer your question.

- EBP hierarchies rank study types based on the rigour (strength and precision) of their research methods. Different hierarchies exist for different question types, and even experts may disagree on the exact rank of information in the evidence hierarchies. The following image represents the hierarchy of evidence provided by the National Health and Medical Research Council.

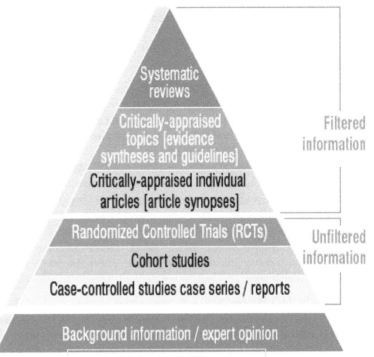

Fig. 6.1.1. Evidence Hierarchy

- Most experts agree that the higher up the hierarchy the study design is positioned, the more rigorous the methodology and hence the more likely it is that the study design can minimise the effect of bias on the results of the study.

- In most evidence hierachies current, well designed systematic reviews and meta-analyses are at the top of the pyramid, and expert opinion and anecdotal experience are at the bottom.

## 1. CASE SERIES AND CASE REPORTS

- These consist either of collections of reports on the treatment of individual patients with the same condition, or of reports on a single patient.

- Case series/reports are used to illustrate an aspect of a condition, the treatment or the adverse reaction to treatment.

- **Example:** You have a patient that has a condition that you are unfamiliar with. You would search for case reports that could help you decide on a direction of treatment or to assist on a diagnosis

- **Disadvantages:** Case series/reports have no control group (one to compare outcomes), so they have no statistical validity.

- **Advantages:** The benefits of case series/reports are that they are easy to understand and can be written up in a very short period of time.

## 2. CASE CONTROL STUDIES

- Patients who already have a certain condition are compared with people who do not.

- Case control studies are generally designed to estimate the odds (using an odds ratio) of developing the studied condition/disease.

- They can determine if there is an associational relationship between condition and risk factor.

- **Example:** A study in which colon cancer patients are asked what kinds of food they have eaten in the past and the answers are compared with a selected control group.

- Case control studies are less reliable than either randomized controlled trials or cohort studies.

- **Disadvantage** to case control studies is that one cannot directly obtain absolute risk (i.e. incidence) of a bad outcome.

- **The advantages** of case control studies are they can be done quickly and are very efficient for conditions/diseases with rare outcomes.

## 3. COHORT STUDIES

- Also called longitudinal studies, involve a case-defined population who presently have a certain exposure and/or receive a particular treatment that are followed over time and compared with another group who are not affected by the exposure under investigation.

- Cohort studies may be either prospective (i.e., exposure factors are identified at the beginning of a study and a defined population is followed into the future), or historical/retrospective (i.e., past medical records for the defined population are used to identify exposure factors).
- Cohort studies are used to establish causation of a disease or to evaluate the outcome/impact of treatment, when randomized controlled clinical trials are not possible.
- **Example:** One of the more well-known examples of a cohort study is the **Framingham Heart Study**, which followed generations of residents of Framingham, Massachusetts.
- Cohort studies are not as reliable as randomized controlled studies, since the two groups may differ in ways other than the variable under study.
- Other problems with cohort studies are that they require a large sample size, are inefficient for rare outcomes, and can take long periods of time.

## 4. RANDOMIZED CONTROLLED STUDIES

- This is a study in which:
- ➢ There are two groups, one treatment group and one control group. The treatment group receives the treatment under investigation, and the control group receives either no treatment (placebo) or standard treatment.
- ➢ Patients are randomly assigned to all groups.
- They lend themselves best to answering questions about the effectiveness of different therapies or interventions.
- Randomization helps avoid the bias in choice of patients-to-treatment that a physician might be subject to.
- It also increases the probability that differences between the groups can be attributed to the treatment(s) under study.
- Having a control group allows for a comparison of treatments – e.g., treatment A produced favorable results 56% of the time versus treatment B in which only 25% of patients had favorable results.
- There are certain types of questions on which randomized controlled studies cannot be done for ethical reasons, for instance, if patients were asked to undertake harmful experiences (like smoking) or denied any treatment beyond a placebo when there are known effective treatments.

## 5. DOUBLE-BLIND METHOD

- This is a type of randomized controlled clinical trial/study in which neither medical staff/physician/researcher nor the patient knows which of several possible treatments/therapies the patient is receiving.
- **Example:** Studies of treatments that consist essentially of taking pills are very easy to do double blind – the patient takes one of two pills of identical size, shape, and color, and neither the patient nor the physician needs to know which is which.

*Randomized controlled trials are considered the "gold standard" in medical research. Randomization helps avoid the bias in choice of patients-to-treatment that a physician might be subject to.*

*A double-blind study is the most rigorous clinical research design because, in addition to the randomization of subjects, which reduces the risk of bias, it can eliminate or minimize the placebo effect which is a further challenge to the validity of a study.*

## 6. SYSTEMATIC REVIEWS

- A systematic review is a comprehensive survey of a topic that takes great care to find all relevant studies of the highest level of evidence, **published and unpublished**, assess each study, synthesize the findings from individual studies in an unbiased, explicit and reproducible way and present a balanced and impartial summary of the findings with due consideration of any flaws in the evidence.
- In this way it can be used for the evaluation of either existing or new technologies or practices.
- A systematic review is more rigorous than a traditional literature review and attempts to reduce the influence of bias.
- In order to do this, a systematic review follows a formal process:
  - o Clearly formulated research question; Published & unpublished (conferences, company reports, "file drawer reports", etc.) literature is carefully searched for relevant research;
  - o Identified research is assessed according to an explicit methodology; Results of the critical assessment of the individual studies are combined; Final results are placed in context, addressing such issues are quality of the included studies, impact of bias and the applicability of the findings.

## 7. META-ANALYSES

- Meta-analysis is a systematic, objective way to combine data from many studies, usually from randomized controlled clinical trials, and arrive at a pooled estimate of treatment effectiveness and statistical significance.
- Meta-analysis can also combine data from case/control and cohort studies.
- The advantage to merging these data is that it increases sample size and allows for analyses that would not otherwise be possible.
- They should not be confused with reviews of the literature or systematic reviews.
- Two problems with meta-analysis are publication bias (studies showing no effect or little effect are often not published and just "filed" away) and the quality of the design of the studies from which data is pulled.
- This can lead to misleading results when all the data on the subject from "published" literature are summarized.

*The difference between a systematic review and a meta-analysis is that a systematic review looks at the whole picture (qualitative view), while a meta-analysis looks for the specific statistical picture (quantitative view).*

## 8. SENSITIVITY AND SPECIFICITY

- **Sensitivity** is the probability of a positive test amongst patients with the disease. A very sensitive test will have few false negatives and be good at picking up disease.
- **Specificity** is the probability of a negative test among patients without the disease. A very specific test will have few false positives and be good at ruling a disease out.
- **SnNOUT** means if a test is very sensitive (Sn) a Negative test rules the diagnosis out.
- **SpPIN** means if a test is highly specific (Sp) a Positive result rules the diagnosis in.

### IMPORTANT FORMULAS

|  | Test result | |
|---|---|---|
|  | **Present** | **Absent** |
| **Positive** | a | b |
| **Negative** | c | d |

$$Sn = \frac{a}{a+c} \qquad Sp = \frac{d}{d+b} \qquad PPV = \frac{a}{a+b} \qquad NPV = \frac{d}{c+d}$$

$$OR = \frac{ad}{bc} \qquad RR = \frac{EER}{CER} \qquad NNT = \frac{1}{ARR} \qquad ARR = CER - EER$$

- **The sensitivity** of the test **is** a/a+c;
- **The specificity** of the test **is** d/b+d.
- **The positive predictive value (PPV)** of the test **is** a/a+b;
- **The negative predictive value (NPV)** of the test **is** d/c+d
  - E.g. The PPV is the percentage of patients who test positive for HIV who really do have HIV.
  - The NPV is the percentage who test negative for HIV who really do not have it.
- **Experimental Event Rate (EER)** = Event rate in treated group
- **Control Event Rate (CER)** = Event rate in control group
- **Odds Ratio =** (ad) / (bc)

*PPV and NPV are depending on the background prevalence of the disorder in the population.*
*When prevalence is low, there are few true positives in the population, and false positives can be large compared to the number of true positives. Hence the positive predictive value falls.*
*If a disease is rare, the PPV will be lower (but sensitivity and specificity remain constant).*

## 9. INCIDENCE AND PREVALENCE

### A. INCIDENCE
- Incidence is the rate of new (or newly diagnosed) cases of the disease.
- It is generally reported as the number of new cases occurring within a period of time (e.g., per month, per year).
- E.g. a study that found an incidence of HIV amongst UK Doctors was 4% per annum, means that 4% of UK Doctors contracted HIV during the year.

### B. PREVALENCE
- Prevalence is the probability of a disease in a population at any one point in time.
- It is the actual number of cases alive, with the disease either during a period of time (period prevalence) or at a particular date in time (point prevalence).
- Example, the prevalence of HIV in the population is 5% simply means that 5% of the population *at the time of the study* have HIV.

## 10. ABSOLUTE RISK (AR) AND ABSOLUTE RISK REDUCTION (ARR)

- **The absolute risk** is the actual, arithmetic risk of an event happening.
- **The ARR** (sometimes also called the Risk Difference) is the difference between 2 event rates.
  E.g. AR of a MI with placebo over 5 years is 5% and with drug A is 3%, the ARR is simply 2%.
- This is the difference between the CER (control event rate) and the EER (experimental event rate).
- Knowing the absolute risk is essential when deciding how clinically relevant a study is.
- **Absolute risk increase** (ARI) similarly calculates an absolute difference in bad events happening in a trial:
  E.g. when the experimental treatment harms more patients than the control.
  E.g. Drug B reduces the chance of a stroke from 20% (CER) to 17% (EER). What is the ARR? Answer 3%.

## 11. NUMBER NEEDED TO TREAT OR HARM (NNT AND NNH)

- A clinically useful measure of the absolute benefit or harm of an intervention expressed in terms of the number of patients who have to be treated for one of them to benefit or be harmed.
- *NNT is the inverse of the absolute risk reduction.*
- The ideal NNT is 1, where everyone improves with treatment and no-one improves with control. NNT = 1/ARR      ARR = CER– EER
- NNTs are always rounded up to the nearest whole number.

- *The higher the NNT, the less effective is the treatment.*
- *The lower the NNT, the better.*
- *The Higher the NNH, the better.*
- Example: the ARR of a stroke with warfarin is 2% (=2/100 = 0.02), the NNT is 1/0.02 = 50.
- E.g. Drug A reduces risk of a MI from 10% to 5%, what is the NNT? **The ARR is 5% (0.05), so the NNT is 1/0.05 = 20.**

## 12. RELATIVE RISK, RELATIVE RISK REDUCTION (RRR) & RISK RATIO (RR)

- ***The relative risk, or risk ratio***, is the ratio of the risk of an event in experimental group compared to the control group i.e. RR = EER/CER.
- ***The RRR*** is the proportional reduction seen in an event rate between the experimental and control groups.
- For example if a drug reduces your risk of an MI from 6% to 3%, it halves your risk of a MI i.e. the RRR is 50%.
- But note that the ARR is only 3%.
- Relative risks and odds ratios are used in meta-analyses as they are more stable across trials of different duration and in individuals with different baseline risks. They remain constant across a range of absolute risks.
- Crucially, if not understood, they can create an illusion of a much more dramatic effect.
- Saying that this drug reduces your risk of a MI by 50% sounds great; but if your absolute risk was only 6%, this is the same as reducing it 3%.
- So, saying this drug reduces your risk by 50% or 3% are both true statements but sound very different, so guess which one that drug companies tend to prefer! However relative risks are still useful to know as you can then apply them yourself to an individual's absolute risk.
- So, if you know an intervention reduces the relative risk by a third, you can easily calculate and inform your two patients with a 30% and a 9% risk of heart disease that the intervention will reduce their individual risk by about a third i.e. to 20% and 6% respectively.

## 13. EXPERIMENTAL EVENT RATE

- The rate at which events occur in the experimental group
  E.g. in the CER example above, an EER of 9% (or 0.09) means that 9% of the aspirin group had MI.

## 14. CONTROL EVENT RATE

- The rate at which events occur in the control group
  E.g. in a RCT of aspirin v placebo to prevent MI, a CER of 10% means that 10% of the placebo group had MI.
- It is sometimes represented as a proportion (10%= 10/100= 0.1).

## 15. ODDS RATIOS (AD/BC)

- It is another way of expressing a relative risk and it is simply the odds of an event (either beneficial or harmful) happening versus it not happening.
- For statistical reasons they are favoured in meta-analysis and case-control studies.
- They are calculated from the CER and EER OR=RR= EER/CER
  E.g. consider a trial of a new drug: 10 out of 200 patients died in the control arm; 5 out of 200 died in the treatment arm.
- What are the odds of death in the treatment arm? The EER is 5/200 i.e. 2.5% which is 0.025
- What are the odds of death with control? The CER is 10/200 i.e. 5% which is 0.05
- What is the OR of the study? This is the ratio of the odds, i.e. 0.025/0.05 = 0.5 i.e. the treatment halves the risk of death compared to control

## 16. ALLOCATION CONCEALMENT

- This is considered by many to be the most important thing to check when appraising a RCT.
- To minimize bias in a blinded RCT it is essential that patients are allocated completely at random between the two groups.
- Researchers must conceal which group the patients will be allocated to from their clinicians, otherwise the clinicians will inevitably distort the randomization process and it is no longer truly 'blind'.
- For example: if patients in hospital were being entered into a RCT of antibiotic vs. placebo for acute cough, and one could tell (by means fair or foul) which group our patient was going to be allocated to we would naturally want our sicker patients to go into the antibiotic group and the not-so-sick ones into the placebo group.
- So, researchers have to conceal allocation from the clinicians to avoid bias.

## 17. P VALUE

- A measure that an event happened by chance alone.
  E.g. **p = 0.05** *means that there is a 5% chance that the result occurred by chance.*
- *For entirely arbitrary reasons p< 0.05 means statistically significant and p<0.01 means highly significant.*
- *The p-value is the estimated probability of rejecting the null hypothesis and therefore reflects type I error.*
- *The p value is misleadingly low with a type I error and misleadingly high with a type II error.*

- *The lower the value, the more likely the effect is real.*

## 18. TYPE 1 AND 2 ERRORS
- *A Type 1 error* (False Positive)
  - ○ Occurs if a result is statistically significant, but this is a chance finding and in fact there is no real difference.
  - ○ Type 1 error is more serious than Type 2 error because it results in the Null Hypothesis being rejected when it is, in fact, true.
- *A Type 2 error* (False Negative)
  - ○ Occurs if the study finds no-significant difference when in fact there is a real treatment difference.
  - ○ It occurs where there is a failure to reject the Null Hypothesis when it is false and no conclusion is drawn from the result.
  - ○ *Small studies with wide CI are prone to these errors.*
  - ○ *Increasing the sample size will reduce both type 1 and 2 errors.*

*Null hypothesis: denoted by $H_0$, is usually the hypothesis that sample observations result purely from chance, there is no relationship between two measured phenomena, or no difference among groups.*
*The null hypothesis is generally assumed to be true until evidence indicates otherwise.*

## 19. CLUSTER RANDOMIZATION
- It means a natural group, or cluster, which is randomized to the same intervention and then compared to a control group.
- A cluster may be a family, a school, an area or (commonly) a group of Doctors or practices which are then compared to another group.

## 20. CONFIDENCE INTERVALS (CI)
- A CI is a range of numbers within which there is a 95% chance that the true result lies.
- if the result is a NNT 30 (95% CI 12-56) it tells us that the result of this trial is a NNT of 30 but the true result could lie anywhere between 12 and 56.
  i.e. if we repeated this trial 100 times, 95 times the result would lie between 12 and 56.
- **95% CI =+/- 1.96 times the standard error of the mean.**
- CI can easily tell if statistical significance has been reached, without doing any maths! If the CI includes the value that reflects 'no-effect' the result is statistically non-significant.
- This value of no-effect is obviously 1 for results that are expressed as ratios (e.g. Relative Risk, Odds Ratio) and 0 for measurements (e.g. NNT, percentages or ARR).
- So, CI give two very useful bits of information: firstly, they tell if a result has reached statistical significance, like a p value does, but they also give an idea of the precision of the result.
- *A wide CI means a less precise result and a narrow CI a more precise result.*
- *Generally speaking the larger the numbers in the study, the smaller the CI and the more sure you are that the result is true.*
- This is why meta-analyses are considered at the top of the evidence hierarchy because they have tighter CI.

## 21. LIKELIHOOD RATIO (LR)
- A measure used in studies looking at diagnosis. It tells us how useful a test, symptom or sign is for establishing a diagnosis and is considered the most useful overall measure of its efficacy.
- LR is the ratio of the probability of a positive result amongst patients who really do have the disease to the probability of a positive result in patients who do not have the disease.
- They are a clinical application of **Bayes' Theorem**.
- LR can be applied to a pre-test probability to estimate the post-test probability.
- LR tell us how much we should shift our suspicion for a particular test result.
- Because tests can be positive or negative, there are at least two likelihood ratios for each test.
- **The "positive likelihood ratio" (LR+)** tells us how much to increase the probability of disease if the test is positive.
- **The "negative likelihood ratio" (LR-)** tells us how much to decrease it if the test is negative.
- The formula for calculating the likelihood ratio is:
  *LR= probability of an individual with the condition having the test result over probability of an individual without the condition having the test result.*
- Thus, the positive likelihood ratio is:
  - ○ **LR+** = probability of an individual **with** the condition having a **positive** test **over** probability of an individual **without** the condition having a **positive** test.
- Similarly, the negative likelihood ratio is:
  - ○ **LR-** = probability of an individual **with** the condition having a **negative** test **over** probability of an individual **without** the condition having a **negative** test.
- You can also define the LR+ and LR- in terms of sensitivity and specificity:
- Positive Likelihood ratio **(LR+) =sensitivity/(1-specificity)**

$$LR+ = \frac{sensitivity}{1 - specificity}$$

- Negative Likelihood ratio (**LR-**)= (1-sensitivity)/specificity

$$LR- = \frac{1 - sensitivity}{specificity}$$

- ○ **LR > 1:** test associated with the disease
- ○ **LR < 1:** test associated with the absence of the disease
- ○ **LR =1:** test is of no clinical utility. However, it is not until **LR+ is > 5** and **LR- is < 0.2** that they become most useful.

## 22. CONFOUNDING VARIABLE

- Important to consider when appraising a study, confounding variables are factors that you are not actually interested in but will affect the result.
- They should be spread equally amongst the control and experimental groups but are very difficult to control for, especially in case-control studies.

## 23. CROSS SECTIONAL STUDY OR SURVEY

- An observational study that observes a defined population at a single point in time or time interval and measures the prevalence of risk factors.
- Cheap and simple but subject to bias.

## 24. DESCRIPTIVE STUDIES

- What they say on the tin. These include case reports, case series, qualitative studies and surveys.
- At the bottom of the evidence hierarchy, but can produce useful learning points and can help answer some of the questions that RCTs or systematic reviews cannot.

## 25. DIAGNOSTIC VALIDATION STUDY

- Answers questions about the efficacy of a diagnostic test, symptom or sign.
- Expresses results using *Likelihood ratio* (LR), **sensitivity and specificity**.

## 26. DIAGNOSTIC ODDS-RATIO (DOR)

- Used when evaluating diagnostic tests.
- *The DOR is the odds of a positive test in patients with the disease, compared to the odds of a positive test in those without the disease*
- E.g. if the DOR is 6, the odds of having a positive test are 6 times higher in someone with the disease than in someone without.

## 27. END-POINT

- **The primary end-point** of a study is the main point of interest of the study in question.
- **A surrogate end point** is a measurement that may correlate with a clinical end-point but is not guaranteed to do so.
- **Composite end-points** combine a number of different measurements into a single composite end-point.
- **Validity** is a means of measuring the end-points chosen by a study. It is the extent to which a conclusion, or measurement, is well founded and corresponds accurately to the real world. Validity can be internal or external.

## 28. EXCLUSION CRITERIA

- Essential information when appraising a RCT for relevance to your patient. This is very pertinent in primary care where often we see patients with co-morbidity, and these tend to be excluded from RCTs.
- For example, an early statin study showed an increase in breast cancer cases (CARE study), and since then all patients with a previous history of cancer have been excluded from statin trials.

## 29. FOLLOW-UP

- Very important when appraising a RCT, is looking for drop-out rates.
- If the drop-out rates are high, how confident can you be in the final results? What if all the drop-outs had a bad outcome?
- **If less than 80% are followed up it is generally recommended that the result is ignored.**

## 30. FOREST PLOT

- The pictorial representation, also known as a blobbogram, of the results of a meta-analysis. Forest plots are easy and very useful to interpret.
- Each individual study should be annotated, and it has a square, or 'blob', with a horizontal line representing the 95% CI.
- The blob in the middle is the reported result of the study, and the relative size of it represents the weighting that this individual study has in the overall analysis.
- The vertical line down the middle is the' line of no effect', which for a ratio is 1.
- **Studies are statistically significant if the CI line does not cross the value of no-effect i.e. the vertical line.**
- If the horizontal line of the study crosses the vertical 'line of no effect' it is non-significant.
- The overall result pooled by meta-analysis is represented by a diamond, the length of which represents the CI.
- If the diamond does not cross the line of no effect, this is a positive result. If it does, it means the overall result is non-significant.

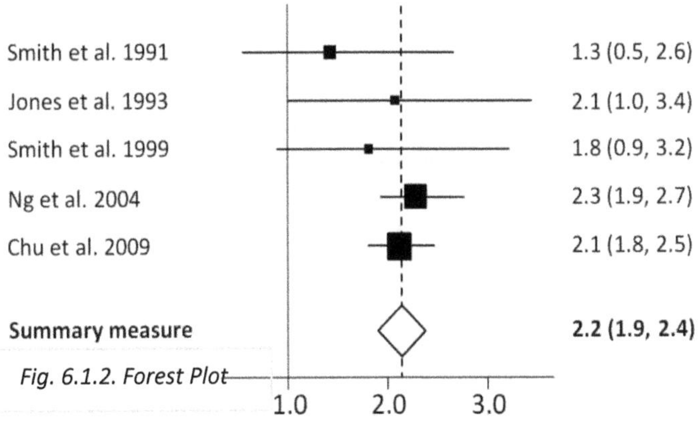

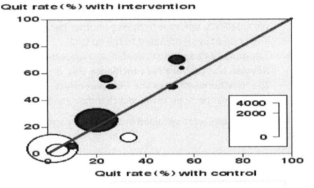

Smith et al. 1991     1.3 (0.5, 2.6)
Jones et al. 1993     2.1 (1.0, 3.4)
Smith et al. 1999     1.8 (0.9, 3.2)
Ng et al. 2004     2.3 (1.9, 2.7)
Chu et al. 2009     2.1 (1.8, 2.5)

Summary measure     **2.2 (1.9, 2.4)**

*Fig. 6.1.2. Forest Plot*

1.0    2.0    3.0

## 31. BOX AND WHISKERS PLOTS

- Box and whiskers plots are used to display quantitative variables that have a skewed distribution.
- The Box is divided by the median and represents 50% of the data.
- 75% of the values lie below the upper quartile and 25% lie below the lower quartile.

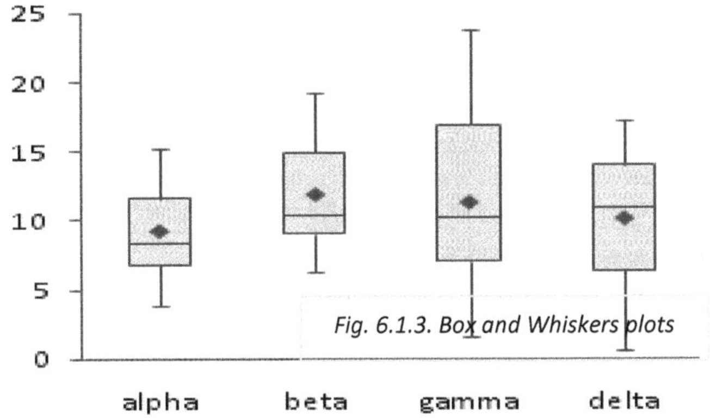

*Fig. 6.1.3. Box and Whiskers plots*

alpha    beta    gamma    delta

## 32. L'ABBE PLOTS

- Commonly used to display data visually in a meta-analysis of clinical trials that compare treatments against control intervention or placebos.
- They are essentially scatter-plots of results of individual studies with the treatment group results on the vertical axis and the control group results on the horizontal axis.
- Trials in which control or placebo are better than the experimental treatment are displayed on the lower right of the plot.
- The size of the trial is reflected by the size of the circle used.

Quit rate(%) with intervention

Quit rate(%) with control

*Fig. 6.1.4. L'Abbe plots*

## 33. FUNNEL PLOTS

- A method of graphing results in a meta-analysis to see if the results have been affected by publication bias.
- A funnel plot is a simple scatter plot of the intervention effect estimates from individual studies against some measure of each study's size or precision.
- In common with forest plots, it is most common to plot the effect estimates on the horizontal scale, and thus the measure of study size on the vertical axis.
- This is the opposite of conventional graphical displays for scatter plots, in which the outcome (e.g. intervention effect) is plotted on the vertical axis and the covariate (e.g. study size) is plotted on the horizontal axis.

## 34. HAZARD RATIO

- A way of expressing the relative risk of an adverse event i.e. if an adverse event was twice as likely to happen with a particular intervention, it would have a HR of 2.

## 35. HETEROGENICITY

- This is important when appraising systematic reviews.
- Consider how heterogeneous the results are both clinically and statistically.
- Clinically you have to use your judgment to see how heterogeneous the studies are to warrant combining them (e.g. is a systematic review of sinusitis that includes groups of patients with just facial pain and those with a CT scan confirmed diagnosis valid?).
- Statistically consider if the individual results contradict each other. This can be assessed by 'eye balling' the Forest plot.
- Anoraks use formal statistical tests such as the Cochran Q (chi-squared) test to do this.

## 36. INTENTION TO TREAT

- This is a method of analyzing results of a RCT which is intended to minimize bias. It is very counter-intuitive.
- If a patient is allocated drug B at the start of the trial, at the end he must be included in the drug B group for the final analysis EVEN IF he never ended up taking drug B or even switched to drug A or C.
- It happens quite often that patients have to drop-out or swap drugs during a trial but they have to be analyzed according to how they were intended to be treated at the beginning. Otherwise researchers could pick and choose who makes it or not to the final analysis which would bias results. Intention to treat ensures that the original randomized groups remain comparable.
- The alternative ('per protocol analysis'), is known to cause bias.

## 37. NESTED CASE-CONTROL STUDY

- This is a case control study which is 'nested' within a defined cohort.
- Cases of a disease which occur within this cohort are identified, and compared to matched controls within the same cohort which do not develop the disease. Although a less robust level of evidence than a cohort study, they are cheaper and easier to do than a full cohort study and can help answer useful questions about factors which contribute to the development of a condition.

## 38. 'NON-INFERIORITY TRIALS' AND 'EQUIVALENCE' TRIALS

- These are trials specifically designed to see if the new drug is 'no worse than' or at least 'as good as' the standard treatment.
- Non-inferiority trials require smaller sample sizes, are cheaper and quicker to do and less likely to produce disappointing results for new drugs so are increasingly used in Pharma sponsored research! The hope is that by demonstrating non-inferiority the new drug will then become a 'me too' option, a second-line therapy or stimulate further research.

## 39. PUBLICATION BIAS

- An important source of bias. Negative trials are just as valid as positive ones, but are less likely to be published.
- Also, occurs in a SR if the search for studies is incomplete.
  - **Instrument bias** occurs when the measuring instrument is not properly calibrated.
  - **Performance bias** occurs when systematic differences exist between the care provided to the different intervention groups in the study.
  - **Berkson bias** or **Admission bias**: It is a form of selection bias that causes hospital cases and controls in a case control study to be systematically different from one another because the combination of exposure to risk and occurrence of disease increases the likelihood of being admitted to the hospital.
  - This produces a systematically higher exposure rate among hospital patients, so it distorts the odds ratio.
  - **Neyman bias** or **Prevalence-Incidence bias**, occurs when the prevalence of a condition does not reflect its incidence.
  - **The Hawthorne effect** or **the Observer effect** refers to a phenomenon by which people alter or modify their behavior, usually in a positive manner, due to the fact that they are being observed.

The following results were obtained in a trial of treatment A vs placebo where treatment A is a new drug for myocardial infarction (MI).

|            | Alive | Dead |
|------------|-------|------|
| A          | 90    | 10   |
| PLACEBO    | 80    | 20   |

a. The absolute risk reduction is 0.2          F
b. The NNT is 10          T
c. The relative risk reduction is 0.5          T
d. All MI patients should be placed on treatment A          F

#### Explanation

- Risk is the number of times an event occurs divided by the total number of events. Absolute risk reduction (ARR) is the actual difference in risk between two groups.
- Thus, in this case, Risk of death post MI in the control group given the placebo is 20/(80+20) = 0.2. This is the control event rate, CER.
- Risk of death post MI in the group who receive drug A is 10/(90+10) = 0.1.
- This is the experimental event rate, EER.
- Therefore, the absolute risk reduction (AAR) is the control event rate (CER) – experimental event rate (EER).
- In this case, CER - EER = 0.2 – 0.1 = 0.1
- The AAR is useful as it allows us to calculate the number needed to treat (NNT)
- The number needed to treat is the number of people who need to be treated to achieve one positive outcome. It is calculated as 1/the absolute risk reduction (AAR). In this case the NNT = 1/AAR = 1/0.1 = 10. Thus, we would need to treat 10 patients post MI with drug A to save one life.
- The relative risk reduction (RR) is the ratio of the risks in both the control and experimental groups: in this case RR is EER/CER = 0.1/0.2 = 0.5
- Although this trial demonstrates a very favourable NNT for drug A in reducing death post MI, there are many other factors - such as its safety and side effects - that must be considered before it is licensed as a treatment.

# SECTION 2. NORMAL/GAUSSIAN & SKEWED DISTRIBUTIONS

## I. GAUSSIAN DISTRIBUTION

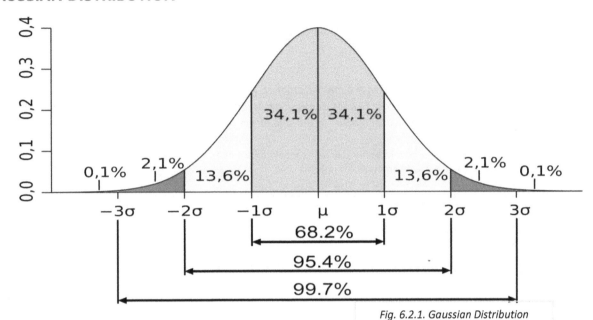

*Fig. 6.2.1. Gaussian Distribution*

- Normal distributions are symmetrical with a single central peak at the mean (average) of the data.
- The shape of the curve is described as bell-shaped with the graph falling off **evenly** on either side of the mean.
- 50% of the distribution lies to the left of the mean and 50% lies to the right of the mean.
- The spread of a normal distribution is controlled by the standard deviation, $\sigma$.
- A random variable with a Gaussian distribution is said to be normally distributed and is called a **normal deviate**.
- *The smaller the standard deviation the more concentrated the data.*
- **Important points**:
  - The area under the normal curve is equal to 1.0.
  - Normal distributions are denser in the center and less dense in the tails.
  - Normal distributions are defined by two parameters, the mean ($\mu$) and the standard deviation ($\sigma$).
  - About 68% of values drawn from a normal distribution are within 1 standard deviation $\sigma$ away from the mean.
  - About 95% of the values lie within 2 standard deviations.
  - About 99.7% are within 3 standard deviations.
  - **This fact is known as the 68-95-99.7 (empirical) rule, or the *3-sigma rule*.**
    *Normal distributions are symmetric around their mean.*
    *The mean, median, and mode of a normal distribution are equal.*

## II. SKEWED DISTRIBUTION

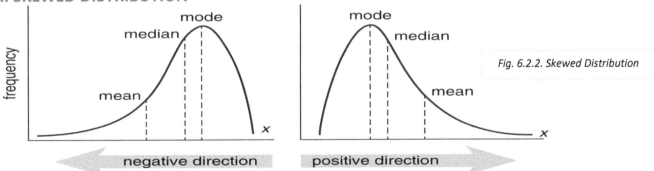

*Fig. 6.2.2. Skewed Distribution*

- Now the picture is not symmetric around the mean anymore.

- For a **Right skewed (Positive Skew)** distribution, the mean is typically greater than the median.
- Also notice that the tail of the distribution on the right hand (positive) side is longer than on the left-hand side.
- A distribution that is **skewed left (Negative Skew)** has exactly the opposite characteristics of one that is skewed right:
  - the mean is typically less than the median;
  - the tail of the distribution is longer on the left-hand side than on the right-hand side; and
  - The median is closer to the third quartile than to the first quartile.

## 1. THE "MEAN"

- It is the "average" used to, where you add up all the numbers and then divide by the number of numbers.

## 2. THE "MEDIAN"

- It is the "middle" value in the list of numbers.
- To find the median, your numbers have to be listed in numerical order, so you may have to rewrite your list first.
- When the totals of the list are odd, the median is the middle entry in the list after sorting the list into increasing order.
- When the totals of the list are even, the median is equal to the sum of the two middle (after sorting the list into increasing order) numbers divided by two.
- Thus, remember to line up your values, the middle number is the median! Be sure to remember the odd and even rule.
  - Find the Median of: 8, 5, 34, 7, 13 (Odd amount of numbers)
  - Line up your numbers: 5, 7,8, 13, 34 (smallest to largest)
  - 5+1=6/2=3$^{rd}$ number, The Median is: 8 (The number in the middle)
  - Find the Median of: 8, 5, 34, 7, 14, 12, 17, 24 (Even amount of numbers)
  - Line up your numbers: 5, 7,8,12, 14, 17, 24, 34
  - Add the 2 middles numbers and divide by 2:
  - 12+14 = 26 ÷ 2 = 13, The Median is 13.

## 3. THE "MODE"

- It is the value that occurs most often. If no number is repeated, then there is no mode for the list.
- It is important to note that there can be more than one mode and if no number occurs more than once in the set, then there is no mode for that set of numbers.

## 4. THE "RANGE"

- It is just the difference between the largest and smallest values.

## 5. VARIANCE

- It is the average of the squared differences from the Mean.
- The variance is a measure of the spread of the observations around the mean value (Variance measures how far a set of numbers are spread out from their mean). It only applies to normally distributed data.

## 6. STANDARD DEVIATION

- Square root of the variance, measures amount of variation of values around the mean.

## 7. STANDARD ERROR

- Measure of variability of sample means around a population mean.
- The standard error decreases with increasing sample size and can be used to construct confidence intervals.
- **The standard error is the standard deviation divided by the square root of the sample size:**
  Standard error  =  Standard deviation / √n

## 8. COEFFICIENT OF VARIATION

- Used to compare variability among different variables that vary in magnitude of the values (elephant weight versus mouse weight)

## 9. SPREAD OF DATA

- Variances and standard deviations can be used to determine the spread of the data.
- If the variance or standard deviation is large, the data are more dispersed.
- The information is useful in comparing two or more data sets to determine which is more variable.

## 10. EFFICACY

- It is the capacity for beneficial change (or therapeutic effect) of a given intervention, most commonly used in the practice of medicine and pharmacology. It is not the same as effectiveness.
- A treatment is effective if it works in real life in non-ideal circumstances.

## 12. EFFECTIVENESS

- Can be defined as 'the extent to which a drug achieves its intended effect in the usual clinical settings.
- It can be evaluated through observational studies of real practice.
- This allows practice to be assessed in qualitative as well as quantitative terms.
  *Effectiveness refers to how well an intervention would work in the 'real world'.*
  *Efficacy studies are concerned with how well an intervention works under ideal circumstances and not in a 'real world' setting.*

## 13. EFFICIENCY

- Depends on whether a drug is worth its cost to individuals or society.
- The most efficacious treatment, based on the best evidence, may not be the most cost-effective option.

## 14. CORRELATION COEFFICIENT, "r"

- The quantity *r*, called the ***linear correlation coefficient***, measures the strength and     the direction of a linear relationship between two variables.
- The linear correlation coefficient is sometimes referred to as the ***Pearson product moment correlation coefficient*** in honor of its developer Karl Pearson.
  - **If the r is close to 1**: it would indicate that the variables are positively linearly related.
  - **If r= -1**, it indicates that the variables are negatively linearly related.
  - **If r= 0**, it would indicate a weak linear relationship between the variables (no correlation between variables*).*

## 15. PARAMETRIC AND NON-PARAMETRIC TESTS

- Parametric statistical test is one that makes assumptions about the parameters (defining properties) of the population distribution(s) from which one's data are drawn, while a non-parametric test is one that makes no such assumptions.
- In this strict sense, "non-parametric" is essentially a null category, since virtually all statistical tests assume one thing or another about the properties of the source population(s).
- For practical purposes, you can think of "parametric" as referring to tests, such as **t-tests** and **the analysis of variance**, that assume the underlying source population(s) to be normally distributed; they generally also assume that one's measures derive from an equal-interval scale.
- And you can think of "non-parametric" as referring to tests that do not make on these particular assumptions.
- **Examples of non-parametric tests include**:
  - *The various forms of chi-square tests*
  - *The Fisher Exact Probability test*
  - *The Mann-Whitney Test*
  - *The Wilcoxon Signed-Rank Test*
  - *The Kruskal-Wallis Test*
  - *The Friedman Test*
- **Examples of parametric tests include**:
  - *Two-sample t-test*
  - *Paired t-test*
  - *Analysis of variance (ANOVA)*
  - *Pearson coefficient of correlation*

| Regarding the number needed to treat (NNT) | |
|---|---|
| The higher the value the more effective the treatment | F |
| The NNT is calculated from the absolute risk reduction | T |
| The NNT can be evaluated for studies of prophylactic treatments | T |
| The number needed to harm (NNH) is the inverse of the NNT | F |
| **The following definition of statistical terms are correct** | |
| Incidence is the number of people with the disease at a given point in time divided by the population size | F |
| The mode is the middle number of a data set that has been ranked in numerical order | F |
| Variance measures how far a set of numbers are spread out from their mean | T |
| A skewed data set is one where the values in a data set are not symmetrically distributed about the middle | T |

# Section 3. Phases of Clinical (Drug) Trials

## PHASE I: SAFETY AND EFFECTS (METABOLISM) OF DRUG
○ Studies assess the safety of a drug or device.
○ Can take several months to complete.
○ Includes a small number of healthy volunteers (20 to 100), who are generally paid for participating in the study.
○ The study is designed to determine the effects of the drug (or device) on humans including how it is absorbed, metabolized, and excreted.
○ This phase also investigates the side effects that occur as dosage levels are increased. About **70% pass** this phase of testing.

## PHASE II: EFFICACY OF THE DRUG
○ Studies test the efficacy of a drug or device.
○ Can last from several months to two years.
○ Involves up to several hundred patients.
○ Most phase II studies are randomized trials.
○ Provide information about the relative safety and effectiveness of the new drug.
○ About **33%** successfully complete both Phase I and Phase II studies.

## PHASE III: EFFECTIVENESS, BENEFITS AND SIDE EFFECTS OF THE DRUG
○ Studies involve randomized and blind testing in several hundred to several thousand patients.
○ Can last several years.
○ Provides with a more thorough understanding of the effectiveness of the drug or device, the benefits and the range of possible adverse reactions.
○ **70% to 90%** of drugs that enter Phase III studies successfully complete this phase of testing.
○ Once Phase III is complete, a pharmaceutical company can request approval for marketing the drug.

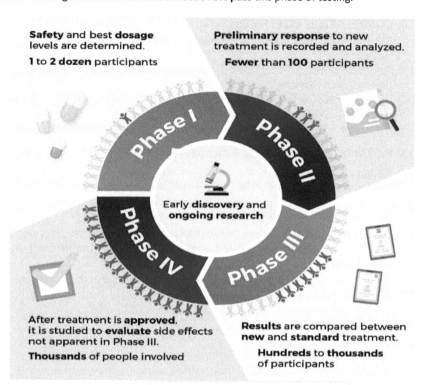

**Safety** and best **dosage** levels are determined.
**1** to **2 dozen** participants

**Preliminary response** to new treatment is recorded and analyzed.
**Fewer** than **100** participants

Early **discovery** and **ongoing research**

After treatment is **approved**, it is studied to **evaluate** side effects not apparent in Phase III.
**Thousands** of people involved

**Results** are compared between **new** and **standard** treatment.
**Hundreds** to **thousands** of participants

*Fig. 6.3.1. Phases of Clinical trial*

## PHASE IV: POST MARKETING SURVEILLANCE TRIALS.
○ Conducted after a drug or device has been approved for consumer sale.
○ Have **70-90%** success rate.
○ Objectives at this stage:
   ✓ To compare a drug with other drugs already in the market.
   ✓ To monitor a drug's long-term effectiveness and impact on a patient's quality of life.
   ✓ To determine the cost-effectiveness of a drug therapy relative to other traditional and new therapies.
○ Phase IV studies can result in a drug or device being taken off the market or restrictions of use could be placed on the product depending on the findings in the study.

# FRCEM PRIMARY PAST PAPERS

## MRCEM PART A DEC 2015

1. Pathogens causing Reiter's syndrome: yersinia? Salmonella? Campylobacter? Shigella?
2. Malaria: can G6PD provide immunity to falciparum? P. vivax malaria? Blackwater fever?
3. Tuberculosis: is the M. tuberculosis a non-spore forming pathogen? Can it get denatured while exposed on room air? All patients present with hemoptysis?
4. Adenosine: is it a purine nucleotide? Is it contraindicated with beta blocker usage? Dose must be reduced by half with dipyridamole?
5. Drug passing first metabolism: poorly absorbed by gut? Fully excreted by kidneys?
6. Drugs causing dyskinesia: procyclidine? Metoclopramide? Fluoxetine?
7. Platelets: aspirin inhibits TX A2? Platelets activated by thrombin? Clopidogrel inhibits GP IIb/IIIa? Serotonin is a vasoconstrictor?
8. Middle cerebral artery syndrome: bitemporal hemianopsia? Hemiplegia of the lower half of the contralateral face? Sensory loss of the contralateral face, arm and leg? Vertebral artery dissection gives ipsilateral facial dysesthesia?
9. Kidney reabsorption at different levels of nephrons: water at the ascending loop of henle?
10. Biochemistry manifestations of hypoadrenalism: hypernatraemia? Hypokalaemia? Hypercalcaemia? Hyperglycaemia?
11. Coronary vessels: RCA origin from the Aorta? Supply of SA Node, AVN, inferior MI.
12. ECG wave forms
13. Nerve at upper limbs injuries: ulna nerve injury at wrist with loss of dorsal sensation? (know level of injury of the 3 nerves as per this book)
14. Inguinal canal borders and spermatic cord
15. Ureters relations.
16. Spinal/ vertebral levels:
17. Dermatomes: thumb, nipple, xiphisternum and lateral knee
18. Fluid compartment: intracellular, plasma, total body fluid
19. Lung volumes: what is Vital Capacity? What is Minute volume? TLV can be measured with spirometer?
20. Frank starling mechanism and curve: is cardiac output decreases with End-Systolic volume?
21. Oxygen dissociation curve: know all left and right shifts
22. Larynx and vocal cord anatomy
23. Anatomy of big vessels for IV line: is saphenous 1-2cm anterior to medial malleolus? Is femoral vein lateral to femoral nerve? Is jugular medial to common carotid?
24. Ankle sprains: know all ligaments involved and their attachments
25. Foot innervation: deep peroneal nerve at 1st web space? Is sural nerve at medial aspect of foot? Calcaneal nerve branch of saphenous nerve? Is plantar nerve branch of tibial nerve?
26. Ligaments knee: quadriceps attachments to the knee?
27. Tetanus: non-spore forming? Exotoxin? Incubation period? Is the wound causing local inflammation?
28. Action potential: effect of lignocaine? Influence of length of neurone? Influence of myelinated vs unmyelinated?
29. Physiological changes in pregnancy: decreased cardiac output? Increased insulin resistance? Increased GFR?
30. Flexor retinaculum wrist
31. Carpal tunnel borders and contents
32. Anatomical snuff box: contains the scaphoid and the trapezium? Flexor carpi ulnaris? Flexor carpi radialis? Ulnar nerve?
33. Anaphylaxis: activated by IgE? One needs first to be sensitized?
34. Innervation face and tongue
35. Scoline: non-depolarizing? Needs reversal for prolonged action? Propofol: has an analgesic property? Is contraindicated with cow milk allergy?
36. Vertebral level of: left kidney on inspiration? The pancreas? The liver?
37. Lactic acidosis: causes?
38. Evidence based Medicine: specificity, PPV, Likelihood ratio?
39. Evidence based Medicine: P value and Null hypothesis
40. Evidence based Medicine: Gaussian distribution, standard deviation: Mean-Median and mode are all equal?
41. Fluid composition: normal saline contains 110mmol of Na? lignocaine1% contains 10mg lignocaine? Dextrose 5% contains 50mg Dextrose in 1liter? Adrenaline 1:10000 contains 100 mcg of adrenaline?
42. Oxygen distribution from the wall: face mask, nasal cannula, venturi mask (questions about flow rate and O2 percentage delivered)
43. Haemorrhage and hypovolemic shock: Heart rate stays unchanged until you lose 40% of your blood? Know all stages of hemorrhagic shock
44. Exit foramen skull: Trigeminal nerve exit (V2) at the foramen ovale?
45. Action potential: effect of lignocaine? Myelinated vs unmyelinated effects?
46. ECG basics: normal axis +30 to -60?
47. Anterior triangle of neck
48. Alveolar pressure

## MRCEM PART A JUNE 2016

1. Ankle ligaments injuries
2. Insertions Foot and leg tendons
3. ECG changes in hyperkalaemia: prolonged QT, Prolonged QRS, prolonged PR, T inversion
4. Fluid concentration: Nacl with 130mmol of Na, D/W 5% 1l= 5g dextrose, adrenaline 1/10000=100mcg adrenaline, bicarbonate 8.4% 1l=1000meq
5. Anaesthesia drugs: propofol has analgesic property, propofol contraindicated with cowmilk allergy, scoline is a non-depolarising, scoline needs reversal for prolonged action
6. Oxygen dissociation curve (always asked topic)
7. Tetanus: opisthotonus gives eye gaze, it is a gram positive, secretes neurotoxin, needs ABX to prevent further complication
8. Shoulder muscles and movemts: rotator cuff, movement from 0-15 degrees, movement beyond 120 degrees
9. Carpal bones anatomy and relations to each other
10. Brain strokes: MCA, ACA, PCA, Posterior inferior cerebellar artery
11. Ureter relations to transverse process on xray, is the ureter moves medial at the pelvis, VUJ is one the constricted part.
12. Vocal cord anatomy during intubation
13. Respiratory differences between children and adult
14. Action potential: ranvier axons prevent spontaneous depolarisation, lignocaine blocks calcium channel, depolarisation initiated by influx of K, myelinated is faster than unmyelinated
15. Inguinal canal: femoral hernia position, femoral artery lateral to nerve, direct hernia sac through the canal, direct hernia sac is lateral to inferior epigastric artery
16. Knee anatomy: patella dislocation always medial, collateral ligament taught in flexion, suprapatellar bursa connects to the knee joint, ACL prevent anterior dislocation tibia
17. Glandular fever: incubation period, jaundice very rare
18. Physiological changes in Pregnancy
19. Emergency thoracotomy: subcostal nerve more likely to be damage, Rt ventricle forms the right border of heart, left phrenic nerves is lateral to pericardium
20. Lobar pneumonia: klebsiella gives lung abscess; maroxella more sensitive to penicillin, in young is caused by staph. aureus
21. Trauma with Extradural hematoma: ICP rises with bleeding, autoregulation will be maintained, CBF decreases if PCo2 increases, CPP formula
22. Blood gas: causes of metabolic alkalosis

23. Hemorrhagic shock: pulse pressure earliest sign to be decreased, aldosterone will be stimulated, renin secreted by juxtaglomerular apparatus
24. Insertions of Hand muscles: extensor digitorum profondus, central slip, extensor indecis
25. ACS: ticagrelor contraindicated in diabetic, nitroglycerine is a vasodilator, aspirin and prasugrel increases bleeding risk
26. Upper limbs nerves injury: axillary injury at axilla with waste of deltoid, radial nerve with thenar eminence, median nerve at elbow with adduction of wrist
27. Frank starling
28. JVP pressure
29. Malaria: transmitted by male anopheles, hypnozoite is the dormant phase
30. Anticoagulant: platelets activated by thrombin. Aspirin inhibits COX1, prasugrel inhibits GP IIa/IIb, serotonin is vasoconstrictor
31. Statistic
32. Inflammation
33. Brown sequard injury signs
34. Alveolar pressure
35. Wound healing phases characteristics
36. Route of contamination: N. Meningitides via droplets, salmonella via droplets, leptospirosis via intact skin, legionella via fecooral route
37. Antidote of diazepam, cyanide, paracetamol and betablockers
38. Antipsychotics side effects: what is bradykinaesia, metoclopramide is the drug of choice, benzodiazepines for dystonia, dyskinaesia is more in young than adults
39. Lung volumes: FEV1/FVC is used to differentiate restrictive to obstructive lung disorders, VC=IRV+VT+ERV, RV is measured by spirometry
40. Increased Respiratory rate is caused by: peripheral chemoreceptors in hypoxia, in hypercarbia, J receptors
41. Gonorrhoea septic knee arthritis: more in males than females, hematogenous spread, treated with single dose of ciprofloxacine, purpuric rash is characteristic
42. Upper limb blood supply
43. Drug passing first metabolism
44. Vertebra anatomy: pedicles, C7 vertebra, ligamentum flavum

## MCEM PART A JUNE 2009

**1. Anterior Cruciate Ligament:**
- Has rich bood supply.
- Commonly tear
- Attach to anterior Intercondylar ridge of the tibia and to the postero-medial aspect of lateral condyle of the femur
- Taught in extension

**2. Regarding the GE by Rotavirus:**
- abdominal Pain is a predominant feature
- Can spread from respiratory tract
- Norwalk virus can cause epidemic in the institution
- Infection transmission simply prevented by hand wash by soap

**3. Regarding the hepatitis B virus:**
- 10% will become carriers
- Spreads through feco-oral route
- HbeAg indicate high infectivity
- Chronic cases can be treated by B interferone

**4. Regarding the platelets:**
- Clopidogrel blocks GP IIb/IIIa receptors on platelets.
- Aspirin inhibits platelets cyclo-oxigenase irreversibly
- Platelets are activated by thrombin
- Platelets release serotonin which causes vasoconstriction.

**5. G6PD:**
- G6PD can cause methaemoglobineamia
- Porphyrias cause defect in functional heme molecule.
- G6PD causes spherocytosis.
- G6PD causes destruction of the cell wall

**6. Aorta branches:**
- splenic artery
- Inferior mesenteric artery
- Testicular artery
- Renal artery

**7. Level of C6:**
- cricoid cartilage
- Origin of vertebral artery
- Bifurcation of carotid
- Stellate ganglion

**8. Trigeminal nerve:**
- supply the corneal sensation
- Supply sensation to the posterior 1/3 of the tongue
- Ophthalmic Division has motor fibers.
- Maxillary division coming out through foramen ovale

**9. Structures under the extensor Retinaculum of the ankle:**
- Peroneus tertius
- Tibialis poserior.
- Extensor Hallus longus
- Deep peroneal nerve.

**10. Structure under carpal tunnel:**
- Median nerve
- Flexor carbi ulnaris
- Flexor policies longus
- Ulnar nerve.

**11. Nerve supply:**
- Deltoid by axillary nerve
- Anterior Interoseius nerve supply flexor policis longus
- Adduction of the thumb needs the ulnar nerve
- Lumbricals supplied by the median nerve.

**12. Rotator cuff:**
- supraspinatus, infraspinatus, teres major and subscapularis muscles
- Named like this because it is rotating the humerus
- Injuried by forced abduction
- Shoulder is common site for degenerative tendonitis.

**13. Heart physiology:**
- Thermodiluton method needs pulmonary artery catheterization
- Ficks method can be used to measure cardiac output
- CO affected by heart rate only

**14. Respiratory volumes:**
- Vital capacity is the sum of ERV & IRV.
- Respiratory Minute volume is RR X TV
- Residual volume can be measured by spirometry
- Lung volumes is independent on sex and height

**15. Pt with ph 7.19 pco2 60  po2 60  Hco3 24  BE -8 on 35% o2:**
- Is picture of compensated acidosis
- Can represent DKA
- In alkalosis, BE is positive
- This patient is ventilated proper way.

**16. Pt found confused with T° of 41.6:**
- Rapid descent of 2 degree indicate viral cause rather than bacterial one.
- All cases of high fever must receive IV AB because of possibility of sepsis
- Ecstasy can cause hyperthermia
- Chronic use of antipsychotic can cause hyperpyrexia

**17. Clostridium causes:**
- botulinum
- Q fever
- Anthrax
- Pseudomembranous colitis

**18. Tetanus:**
- Is notifiable disease
- Tetanus Toxoid and Immunoglobulin must be given in pt with wound prone and poor immunization schedule
- Act by releasing endotoxin

**19. Malaria:**
- Cerebral malaria mainly caused by falciparum
- Malaria vivax can relapse after becoming dorminat in the liver
- Spherozoite is the infection to human after bite
- One test of thin and thick film can exclude malaria

**20. Herpes simplex virus:**
- Type II commonly causes genital herpes
- Reactivation of dormant virus in nerve route causes shingles
- If affecting the cornea so topical cortisone is the drug of choice.
- CT is the modality of choice to viral encephalitis.

**21. Nappy area:**
- Involvement of the flexor side indicate candidal cause
- Presence of satellite lesions indicate candidal cause
- Extensive form of napkin dermatitis indicates systemic antibiotic
- Presence of golden crusts indicate staph infection

**22. Renal failure:**
- urine osmolarity of 350 indicate pre-renal cause
- Urine Na of 56 indicate renal cause
- Obstruction is the most common cause

**23. Magnesium:**
- Mg is predominant in the serum
- Hypomagnesaemia worsen digitalis toxicity
- The most common cause of hypomagnesaemia is renal loss
- Can cause tetany and carpopedal spasm

**24. Warfarin is affected by:**
- Ampicillin
- NSAID
- Aspirin
- Morphine

**25. Erythromycin:**
- combination with amiodarone must be avoided
- Active against haemophilus influenza
- 1st drug of choice for whooping cough
- Most common side effect is hypersensetivity

**26. Anatomical Snuffbox**
- Extensor indicis share in its boundaries
- Trapezium sharing in part of the floor
- Site of radial artery to pass to the dorsum of the hand
- Best viewed in adduction and extension of the wrist.

**27. Blood**
- Vit K dependant factors are II, VII, IX, XII
- Heparin work on anti-thrombin III to produce its anticoagulant effect
- Streptokinase activate plasminogen to produce its anti-coagulant effect
- Extrinsic pathway activated by tissue thromboplastin.

**28. Lobar pneumonia:**
- Macrophage appears after 72 hours
- Strep. Pneumonia is the most common cause
- Most common in alcoholics
- Most common complicated by lung abscess

**29. Osteomyelitis:**
- Haematogenous spread most common in the elderly
- Reactive phase of healing producing involucrum
- Periosteum changes will appear in x-ray after 2 days
- Hypertrophic non-union has poor prognosis

**30. Acromegaly feature:**
- Prognathism
- Glucose intolerance
- Homonymous haemianopia
- Myopathy

**31. Iron:**
- Reabsorbed mainly in the terminal ileum
- Low plasma iron making iron easily separated from ferritin
- Intrinsic factor produced in the terminal ileum
- Vitamin C deficiency affects bone healing

**32. Patient with IDDM not on treatment:**
- Hypertriglyceridaemia
- Increase lipolysis
- Total body potassium is high but serum level is normal
- Will cause deep slow respiration

**33. Blood transfusin complication:**
- Metabolic Acidosis
- Hyperkaleamia
- Hypercalcaemia
- using of warmer device with mesh increase the possibility of clots

**34. Patient with bleeding from redial artery BP 122/82 Pulse 102 capillary refill 3sec**
- It represents type I heamorrhage
- MAP is 102
- Best managed by blood
- Pulse rate is most reliable for restoring blood volume

**35. Cerebral perfusion:**
- increase ICP will increase cerebral perfusion
- Increase MAP will increase cerebral perfusion
- Head down decrease perfusion
- Pco2 increase perfusion

**36. Inotropics**
- Noradrenaline is more beta than alpha
- Dobutamine is selective alpha agonist
- Sympathomimetics cause constriction in the veins and venules of the intestine

**37. Adenosine**
- Temporary blocks AV node
- Contraindicated with b-blockers
- Dispyramole reduce its half life
- Best given slowly IV

**38. Statistics**
- A- P value    b- p value    c- confidence interval

**39. TCA features:**
- seizures
- Constricted pupil
- Arrhythmia
- Hyperthermia

**40. Fractures:**
- Monteggia fracture is fracture of proximal ulna with dislocation of radial head
- Extensor central slip tear giving swan neck appearance

- Pt with fracture humerus shaft is unable to extend the wrist.
- Musculcutenous nerve injury pt will loose elbow flexion

**41. Conduction through nerve:**

- conduction increases with diameter
- C fibers localize the pain
- 45 degree making pain with touch
- Myeline sheath will prevent movement of the current to the adjacent tissue

**42. Neuritis**

- Increase scotoma in retrobulbar neuritis
- Pain with eye movement

**43. ADH:**

- ADH increase the permeability of distal convoluted tubule to water

- Angiotensin II activate ADH release from post pituitary
- (Hypotension) hypovolaemia increase the secretion of ADH
- Decrease in Rt atrial pressure will stimulate ADH release

**44. Pediatric traumatic elbow joint**

- Presence of swelling with normal x-ray in the elbow most commonly due to haemophilia
- Sensation of the medial side of the forearm is supplied by C7

**45. Regarding shock:**

- All types of shock have low cardiac output
- Blood will be pooled to the brain and the heart on the expense of the liver & kidney.
- There is coronary and cerebral vasodilatation.
- Carotid body and acidosis

## FRCEM PRIMARY DEC 2016

1. Contra-indications of vaccination in AIDS patients
2. Ulnar nerve anatomy
3. Median nerve anatomy
4. Fibular nerve anatomy
5. Sciatic nerve anatomy
6. Facial nerve and chorda tympani and tongue innervations
7. Tetanus and Rabies immunisation
8. Mechanism of action of Furosemide
9. Tuberculosis: most sensitive and specific test
10. Coronary arteries of the heart Anatomy
11. Wound healing
12. Attachements of peroneus Longus tendon

13. Lidocaine pharmacokinetics
14. Rotator cuff muscles anatomy
15. First line treatment, contraindications and interactions of NSAIDS in acute Gout.
16. Visual field loss and corresponding blood supply
17. Optic chiasm lesions: Parietal and temporal infarct
18. Clinical signs associated with MCA, ACA and PCA strokes
19. Frank Starling mechanism is best explained by?
20. Causes of Pneumonia in Elderly
21. Iron deficiency anaemia
22. Diastolic murmurs

## FRCEM PRIMARY JUNE 2017

1. Musuculocutaneous nerve – stab wound to axilla, causing weakness of elbow flexion and supination
2. Platysma – stab wound to anterior triangle of neck – which muscle would be injured (choices were sternocleidomastoid, scalenous anterior, trapezius, platysma and one other)
3. Ankle movement loss –? Location of lesion
4. Lower lip numbness, nerve involved? Inferior alveolar
5. Scenario of impetigo in child, what factor causes its spread? Faecal- oral, droplet, intact skin, broken skin?
6. Achilles tendon rupture – ciprofloxacin
7. Boy with hemophilia scenario, what deficiency?
8. Digoxin toxicity, worsens – hypokalemia
9. Swollen painful knee joint youngish male (35 or so?) No other history, what would you find on gram stain? Gram positive pairs of cocci in clusters, or gram-positive cocci in chains, or gram-negative rods or gram-positive rods or gram negative intracellular organisms arranged like kidney beans (correct answer – gonococcal arthritis)
10. Succinylcholine mechanism of action – depolarizing neuromuscular blockage
11. Anaphylaxis, adrenaline dose? 1:1000
12. Optic tract lesion, right or left – scenario depicting right homonymous hemianopia Small wound on ankle, swollen acutely inflamed next day – what is the most abundant cell type present? Neutrophils
13. Neck of fibula fracture – common peronial nerve injury
14. Valgus deformity of knee joint following football injury. What ligament damaged – medial collateral
15. Hyperextension of knee joint – horse-riding incident, unable to weight bear swollen painful knee etc, injury to? – anterior cruciate
16. Orbital blowout fracture – inferior orbital fissure fracture, which will be damaged?
17. Starling's law
18. Scenario of pancytopenia? Causative drug? – choices included celecoxib and mefenamic acid
19. Lip/peri-oral swelling not improving with adrenaline, which drug implicated mainly as cause?
20. Orbital blowout fracture, diplopia on upward gaze. Which is entrapped? Superior oblique, inferior oblique, inferior rectus, superior rectus, medial rectus
21. Oculomotor nerve – consensual light reflex scenario where light shined in right eye, reflex present, light moved to left eye but right pupil dilates, lesion?
22. Precipitant of gout in a patient's drug regimen? – hydrochlorthiazide
23. Gout treatment, scenario given elderly, heart failure, diabetes, acute gout treatment? – colchicine, allopurinol, diclofenac, etc
24. Scenario or warafrinized patient with head injury? Reversal with?
25. Head injury with fractured internal acoustic meatus, which two nerves would be affected – facial and glossopharyngeal
26. Female with mass on anterior 2/3rd of tongue, where is lymph drainage?
27. Headache, increased intracranial pressure symptoms, bitemporal hemianopia? Lesion site – optic chiasm
28. Mass in optic chiasm, symptomatic, hyperglycemia, likely hormone excess? Growth hormone
29. Hemorrhage, life threatening, what will be the effect on kidneys? – decrease urine production
30. Scenario of heart failure, furosemide given, site of action? – loop of henle
31. Someone in type 2 respiratory failure, how will body realise it needs to increase breathing rate? – chemoreceptors
32. Digoxin toxocity, when to give digibind? – prolonged seizures, severe bradyarhythmia
33. Hyperkalemia, ECG changes just before cardiac arrest?
34. ECG shown, which vessel involved based on ECG changes?
35. Angiography of chest pain patient, occlusion of left circumflex branch, which cardiac area affected
36. 3-month-old, diagnosed pertussis, most horrible complication? – apneic spells
37. Alcoholic male, cough, bloody sputum, fevers, consolidation on xray, microorganism? – klebsiella
38. Alcoholic, male, ascites, cause? – portal hypertension
39. Mechanism of action Propofol?